THE NEUROFIBROMATOSES

THE NEUROFIBROMATOSES

A pathogenetic and clinical overview

Edited by
S. M. Huson
and
R. A. C. Hughes

CHAPMAN & HALL MEDICAL
London · Glasgow · New York · Tokyo · Melbourne · Madras

Published by Chapman & Hall, 2–6 Boundary Row, London SE1 8HN, UK

Chapman & Hall, 2–6 Boundary Row, London SE1 8HN, UK

Blackie Academic & Professional, Wester Cleddens Road, Bishopbriggs, Glasgow G64 2NZ, UK

Chapman & Hall Inc., One Penn Plaza, 41st Floor, New York, NY10119, USA

Chapman & Hall Japan, Thomson Publishing Japan, Hirakawacho Nemoto Building, 6F, 1–7–11 Hirakawa-cho, Chiyoda-ku, Tokyo 102, Japan

Chapman & Hall Australia, Thomas Nelson Australia, 102 Dodds Street, South Melbourne, Victoria 3205, Australia

Chapman & Hall India, R. Seshadri, 32 Second Main Road, CIT East, Madras 600 035, India

First edition 1994

Typeset in 10/12 Palatino by Type Study, Scarborough
Printed in Great Britain at the University Press, Cambridge

ISBN 0 412 38920 7

A catalogue record for this book is available from the British Library

Library of Congress Cataloging-in-Publication data

The Neurofibromatoses : a pathogenetic and clinical overview / edited by S.M. Huson and R.A.C. Hughes.
p. cm.
Includes bibliographical references and index.
ISBN 0–412–38920–7
1. Neurofibromatosis – Genetic aspects. 2. Neurofibromatosis.
I. Huson, S. M. II. Hughes, R. A. C. (Richard Anthony Cranmer)
RC280.N4N4865 1993
616.99′383 – dc20 93–6465
CIP

Printed on acid-free text paper, manufactured in accordance with ANSI/NISO Z39.48–1992 (Permanence of Paper).

To our neurofibromatosis patients and their families

Contents

Colour plates appear between pages 240 and 241.

Contributors

M.F. Angel
Division of Plastic, Reconstructive and Maxillo Facial Surgery
Johns Hopkins Medical School
Baltimore
Maryland 21287, USA

J.C. Carey
Division of Medical Genetics
Department of Pediatrics
University of Utah
Salt Lake City
Utah 84132, USA

R.D. Clark
Children's Hospital Los Angeles
Division of Medical Genetics
Box 90
P.O. Box 54700
Los Angeles
California 90054–0700, USA

F.S. Collins
Director of the National Center for Genome Research
National Institutes of Health
Building 38A
Room 605
Bethesda
Maryland 20892, USA

D.W. Dunn
c/o Psychiatry Department
Indiana University Medical Center
Indianapolis
Indiana 46223, USA

M.T. Edgerton
Division of Craniofacial Surgery
University of Virginia
Health Sciences Center
Charlottesville
Virginia 22908, USA

J. Fairbank
Nuffield Orthopaedic Centre
Windmill Road
Headington
Oxford OX3 7LD, UK

R.E. Ferner
United Medical Dental School
Department of Neurology
Guy's Hospital
St Thomas' Street
London SE1 9RT, UK

R.A.C. Hughes
Department of Neurology
Guy's Hospital
St Thomas' Street
London SE1 9RT, UK

S.M. Huson
Department of Medical Genetics
Churchill Hospital
Oxford OX3 7LJ, UK

K.R. Jessen
Department of Anatomy and Developmental Biology
University College London
Gower Street
London WC1E 6BT, UK

D.A. Marchuk
Department of Genetics
Duke University Medical Center
Box 3175
Room 265
CARL Building
Durham NC 27710, USA

R.L. Martuza
Department of Neurosurgery
Georgetown University
Medical Center
3800 Reservoir Road NW
Washington, DC 20007, USA

R. Mirsky
Department of Anatomy and Developmental Biology
University College London
Gower Street
London WC1E 6BT, UK

J.J. Mulvihill
Department of Human Genetics
University of Pittsburgh
Pittsburgh
Pennsylvania 15261, USA

J.A. Persing
Division of Plastic Surgery
School of Medicine
Yale University
New Haven
Connecticut 06510–8062, USA

V.A. Purvin
Midwest Eye Institute
Indiana University
1800 North Capitol Avenue
PO Box 1367
Indianapolis
Indiana 46206–1367, USA

H. Radner
Institut für Neuropathologie
Universitatskliniken Bonn
Sigmond-Freud-Strasse 25
D-5300
Bonn 1, Germany

G.A. Rouleau
Centre for Research in Neuroscience
McGill University
1650 Cedar Ave
Montreal
Quebec H3G 1A4 Canada

G.R. Seward
Department of Oral and Maxillo-Facial Surgery
The London Hospital Medical College
Turner Street
London E1 2AD, UK

P.M. Short
Molecular Neurogenetics Laboratory
Massachusetts General Hospital East
Building 149
13th Street Charlestown
Massachusetts 02129, USA

J. Smith
Centre de Biologie du Développement
Université Paul Sabatier
Bât. 4R3
118 route de Narbonne
31062 Toulouse Cedex
France

M. Upadhyaya
Institute of Medical Genetics
University of Wales
College of Medicine
Heath Park
Cardiff CF4 4XN, UK

D. Viskochil
Division of Medical Genetics
Department of Pediatrics
University of Utah
Salt Lake City
Utah 84132, USA

O.D. Wiestler
Institut für Neuropathologie
Universitätskliniken Bonn
Sigmond-Freud-Strasse 25
D-5300
Bonn 1, Germany

Preface

For the past 100 years neurofibromatosis has attracted reports in the specialist journals of every medical discipline. Van der Hoeve declared in 1932 that neurofibromatosis and other similar conditions characterized by multiple birth marks, such as tuberous sclerosis, 'are worthy of the attention of neurologists, psychiatrists, neurosurgeons, surgeons, internists, paediatrists, pathologists, embryologists, teratologists, dermatologists, and otologists – that means the attention of the whole medical profession'. He called these conditions 'phakomatoses' derived from *phakos*, the Greek word for a birth mark. Unfortunately, neurofibromatosis remained merely a medical curiosity, of interest to nearly every specialty but the special responsibility of none. Until recently, neurofibromatosis attracted little clinical and laboratory research compared with other genetic conditions such as cystic fibrosis or Duchenne muscular dystrophy.

Fortunately this has changed over the last two decades. The study of this disorder of birth marks promises to increase our understanding of neural crest development and control of cell proliferation. Much of the credit must go to neurofibromatosis patient groups, the National Neurofibromatosis Foundation founded in the USA in 1978 and its British cousin founded in 1981. These groups have increased public and medical awareness of neurofibromatosis, stimulated research and led to the development of specialist neurofibromatosis centres throughout the world.

We have invited an international panel so as to cover authoritatively as many aspects of neurofibromatosis as possible. In the introduction, one of us (S.M.H.) explains how neurofibromatosis has been differentiated into the common neurofibromatosis 1 (NF1), which causes café au lait patches, dermal neurofibromas and many other manifestations; the uncommon neurofibromatosis 2 (NF2), which causes bilateral vestibular Schwannomas (acoustic neuromas); and other rare forms of neurofibromatosis. In Chapter 2 Marchuk and Collins describe the experimental work, in which they were centrally involved, which identified the *NF1* gene on chromosome 17, and showed that it coded for a protein, neurofibromin, which controls cell proliferation. In Chapter 3, Rouleau describes how the *NF2* gene has been localized to the long arm of chromosome 22 and functions as a tumour suppressor gene. In subsequent chapters, Smith explains the development of the neural crest from which the cells at fault in NF1 are derived, Mirsky and Jessen discuss the biology of Schwann cells, which form the basis of neurofibromas, and Wiestler and Radner describe and illustrate the pathology of neurofibromatosis. These chapters provide a basis for understanding the pathogenesis of the clinical manifestations of neurofibromatosis.

The multiple clinical manifestations of NF1 are reviewed in Chapter 7. In Chapters 8 to 13 appropriate specialists describe the presentation and management of its neurological, intellectual, ophthalmological, orthopaedic and internal medical complications. Mulvihill puts in epidemiological context the often exaggerated association between NF1 and malignant disease. Angel, Persing and Edgerton describe the opportunities and limitations of reconstructive surgery. Optimal care of patients with neurofibromatosis requires close cooperation between many different medical specialties. The problems are so variable that effective care of patients requires much good will and cooperation. We conclude this section by returning to the whole patient as an individual with an overview of the overall management and counselling of patients with NF1.

The attribution of the diagnosis of neurofibromatosis 1 to Joseph Merrick, an incorrect diagnosis in our view, drew largely unwelcome attention to the disease. Joseph Merrick was a man whose gross deformities earned him the nickname of the Elephant Man, the derision of the crowds at the Victorian fairstall and finally the sympathy of Sir Frederick Treves and contemporary society figures. In Chapter 16, Seward describes his case, which has become inextricably mixed with the history of neurofibromatosis. One of the most frequent questions from the concerned parents of a newly diagnosed child is, 'Will my child grow to be like the Elephant Man?' In Chapter 17, Clark describes an alternative diagnosis for the Elephant Man, the Proteus syndrome, a developmental abnormality named after the Greek god who could adopt many forms. Whatever the truth about the Elephant Man's diagnosis, neither of us has seen a patient with NF1 who bore a close resemblance to Joseph Merrick, nor are we aware of anyone else who has done so.

NF2 has now been clearly differentiated from NF1 on genetic grounds. It is very much less common and most of this book is devoted to NF1. However, the two conditions were not distinguished until the last decade and disentangling some early accounts of the clinical features of neurofibromatosis is sometimes difficult or even impossible. Chapter 18 concentrates on the clinical features and management of NF2. Its major defining feature is bilateral vestibular Schwannomas, which cause progressive deafness and present a formidable neurosurgical problem. In the last chapter, Viskochil and Carey describe the problems of diagnosing and classifying uncommon variants of neurofibromatosis, especially segmental neurofibromatosis, and conditions that resemble neurofibromatosis.

The pace of research has been such that important new information has appeared even while we have been editing the manuscripts submitted. The gestation of this book has been longer than we would have liked. We thank our contributors for their pains and patience in helping to cover as much of the very extensive field represented by these fascinating diseases as was possible in a reasonably sized volume.

The impact of molecular biology on neurofibromatosis, as on many other genetic diseases, has resulted in greater steps towards our eventual understanding of its pathogenesis than anything since the original disease descriptions. The *NF1* gene and its gene product have been discovered. The *NF2* gene and gene product were identified while this book was in preparation and we are grateful to Dr Rouleau for updating his chapter at proof stage. We anticipate that in the next decade the biological basis of both major forms of neurofibromatosis will be elucidated, which will eventually lead to useful disease treatment. We hope this book will provide a useful overview of current clinical and scientific knowledge about the different forms of neurofibromatosis, and be a reference source both for clinicians in every discipline caring for patients and for researchers entering the field.

S.M. Huson
R.A.C. Hughes

Acknowledgements

The editors are grateful to the contributors for their patience with the long gestation of this book. We would like to thank the staff of Chapman & Hall, particularly Annalisa Page and the sub-editorial and production departments, for their helpful and efficient role in its publication. Dr Huson is grateful to Dr D.C. Thrush and Professors D.A.S. Compston and P.S. Harper for encouraging her initial research on neurofibromatosis. Both editors are involved in ongoing neurofibromatosis research and would like to thank their colleagues for productive collaboration and helpful discussions about the book; Dr Huson collaborates with Dr M. Upadhyaya, Dr J. Sampson, Dr I. Cordeiro and Ms J. Castle, Professor Hughes with Dr R. Ferner and Dr T. Cox. Lorna Fisher, Barbara Jenkins and Margaret Shade (Oxford) and Sheila Button (London) have given excellent secretarial assistance to the project. Finally, we would like to thank our families for their support during the preparation of the book.

Neurofibromatosis lay organizations

The editors are aware of neurofibromatosis lay organizations in the following countries: Australia, Belgium, Canada, Croatia, the Czech Republic and Slovakia, Denmark, Egypt, Eire, Finland, France, Germany, Holland, Indonesia, Israel, Italy, New Zealand, Norway, Poland, Spain, Sweden, Switzerland, the United Kingdom and the United States of America. Because of the difficulty of maintaining updated address lists, we suggest that for further information readers contact one of the organizations below which have established offices with permanent staff.

Colonel John Blackwell, CBE
Director
The Neurofibromatosis Association *
120 London Road
Kingston upon Thames
Surrey KT2 6QJ
UK
Telephone and facsimile (0)81 547 1636

Mr Peter Bellermann
President
National Neurofibromatosis Foundation
141 Fifth Avenue, Suite 7–9
New York, NY 10010
USA
Telephone 212 460 8980
Facsimile 212 529 6094

* The UK Neurofibromatosis Association was formerly called LINK (Let's Increase Neurofibromatosis Knowledge). Some chapters still refer to LINK as this change in name happened in 1993.

1

Neurofibromatosis: historical perspective, classification and diagnostic criteria

S.M. Hudson

1.1 INTRODUCTION

> As a medical curiosity, the disease has excited a voluminous literature, in which there are reflected wide differences of opinion. The present contribution makes no attempt at a comprehensive review of the literature, a sizeable proportion of which serves, in the authors' opinion, more to confuse than enlighten.
>
> *Crowe, Schull and Neel (1956)*

In preparing this book it was tempting to devote more space to molecular biology and possible future developments and to gloss over historical detail. However, a review of the past literature highlights the problem of disease classification and our lack of knowledge about the natural history of this group of disorders. Both areas are important to the clinical understanding of patients with neurofibromatosis, which forms the basis of modern molecular biological research. Throughout this book we have adopted the nomenclature for the different forms of neurofibromatosis recommended by the National Institutes of Health (NIH) Consensus Conference on Neurofibromatosis (1988). The most common form of the disease, as described by von Recklinghausen (1882), is neurofibromatosis 1 (NF1). Neurofibromatosis 2 (NF2) is the form in which bilateral vestibular Schwannomas (acoustic neuromas) are the major feature. Some of the names that have been suggested for each form at various times are shown in Table 1.1. In the early literature little attempt was made to distinguish the different forms and they were usually reported under the umbrella term 'von Recklinghausen's disease'. Prior to the NIH

Table 1.1 Names used for NF1 and NF2 in the past

NF1
'von Recklinghausen's disease'[a]
The Elephant Man disease
Elephantiasis neuromatosis
Multiple neurofibromatosis
Peripheral neurofibromatosis
von Recklinghausen neurofibromatosis
NF2
Bilateral acoustic neurofibromatosis
Central neurofibromatosis
Hereditary bilateral vestibular Schwannoma syndrome[b]
Wishart–Gardner–Eldridge syndrome[b]

[a] Until relatively recently, both NF1 and NF2 were referred to under this title.
[b] Names suggested by Mulvihill (1988), the first to reflect the true pathology and the second to accord appropriate eponymous credit.

Conference, NF1 was most commonly called von Recklinghausen's, multiple or peripheral neurofibromatosis, and NF2 bilateral acoustic or central neurofibromatosis. The old terms all had problems (Mulvihill, 1988). The eponyms told us nothing about the nature of the underlying disease; the concept of peripheral and central disease seemed superficially sound but created confusion in those cases of NF1 with central nervous system (CNS) involvement. Bilateral acoustic neurofibromatosis now seems unsatisfactory since the 'neuromas' are actually Schwann cell tumours or Schwannomas, and arise from the vestibular not the acoustic part of the eighth cranial nerve. Throughout this book we have chosen to refer to acoustic neuromas as vestibular Schwannomas.

1.2 HISTORICAL PERSPECTIVE

1.2.1 Neurofibromatosis 1

As in many diseases, exactly which was the first case report and who truly deserved the eponymous credit has been a matter of debate (Zanca and Zanca, 1980; Mulvihill, 1988; Hecht, 1989). Zanca and Zanca (1980) recorded possible illustrations of NF1 sufferers with plexiform neurofibromas dating back as far as the second century. They claimed that the earliest clinical description of a case was by Ulisse Aldrovandi, an Italian physician and naturalist, in the sixteenth century (published posthumously, 1642). Aldrovandi described a man of short stature with tumours growing from the left side of his head and upper trunk (Figure 1.1;

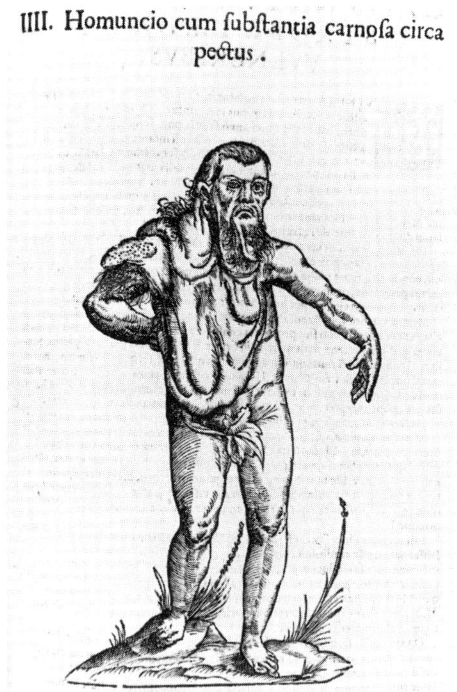

Figure 1.1 Illustration accompanying Aldrovandi's case report (1642, published courtesy of P. Madigan). The original Latin caption is translated as 'A dwarf with flesh substance around the chest'. (Reprinted with permission of S. Karger AG, Basel from Madigan and Masello, 1989.)

Madigan and Masello, 1989). Zanca and Zanca (1980) postulated that this was a plexiform neurofibroma, although Hecht (1989) questioned this diagnosis in the absence of other features. Hecht drew attention to the drawings (dated 1749) in *Buffon's Histoire Naturelle* of a child with both skin tumours and pigment anomalies as being more typical of NF1 (Figure 1.2) and I would agree. The first clinical reports of patients with multiple small dermal tumours date from the eighteenth century literature (Akenside, 1768; Ludwig and Tilesius, 1793). Both descriptions identified important aspects of the disease. Akenside's patient had inherited the condition and had developed a method of treatment:

> He was generally healthy, and apparently of a good habit of body; but had been accustomed, during the greater part of his life, to a constant succession of wens, that shot out in several places; on his head, trunk, arms, and legs; which indisposition he inherited from his father. As often as these wens became inconvenient from their size, his method was, to cut them off with a razor; at which times, he

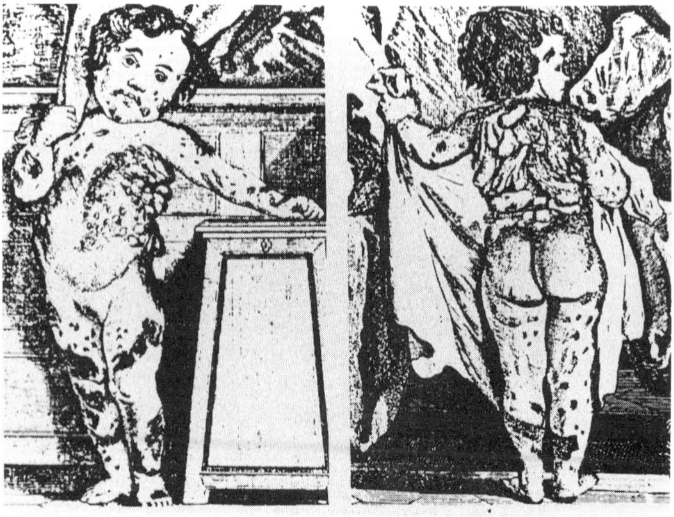

Figure 1.2 Illustration of a girl with neurofibromatosis from *Buffon's Histoire Naturelle* (1749). (Reprinted with permission of S. Karger AG, Basel from Hecht, 1989.)

> constantly found that they grew upon the part by five or six suckers, as he called them.
>
> *Akenside (1768)*

The observation that neurofibromas regrow in increased numbers at the site where one has been removed is something we are still unclear about. Several patients have reported this to me, but I have not personally observed the phenomenon. In the other eighteenth century description, Ludwig and Tilesius (1793) drew attention both to the unpleasant physical stigmata of NF1 and the difficulty with nosology, which we are still wrestling with today! Their patient, Johann Gottfried Rheinhard, was referred to by Ludwig as his wart man and reported under the title 'Case history of extraordinarily unsightly skin'. The preface discussed classification as follows:

> Although nosologists for centuries have repeatedly strived seriously to bring these . . . chronic diseases of the skin into an appropriate system, they still have not been able to provide an entirely complete overview of the diseases . . . To specify the disease of Rheinhard, . . . I cannot select an entirely suitable name.
>
> *Ludwig and Tilesius (1793)*

In the nineteenth century, illustrations of pathological studies of NF1 began to appear. In his *Anatomie Pathologique du Corps Human*, Jean Cruveilhier (1791–1874) clearly described and illustrated NF1 (Figure 1.3).

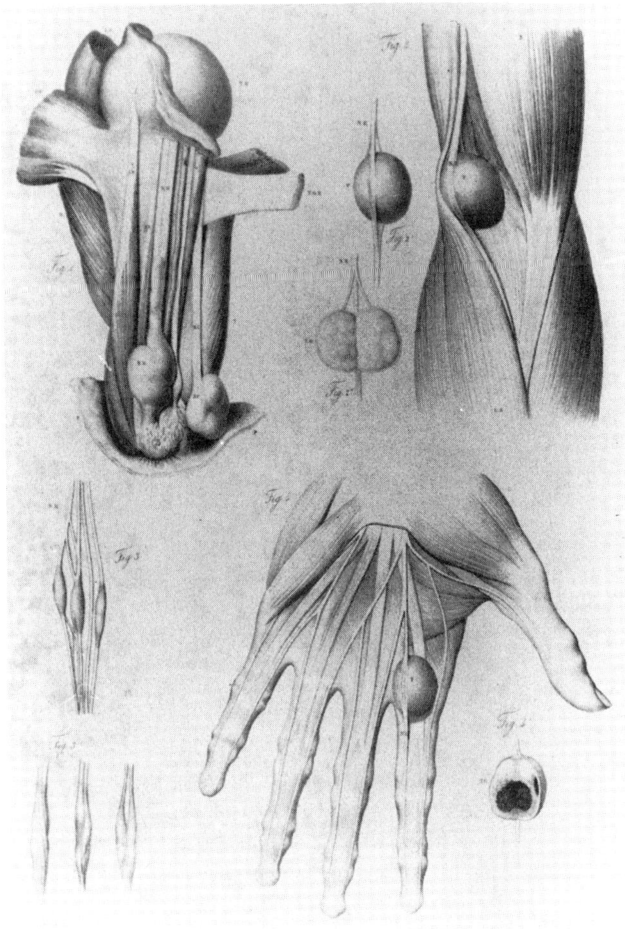

Figure 1.3 Illustration of multiple peripheral nerve tumours from Cruveilhier's atlas.

By 1849, Smith was able to cite 75 references in a review of the literature; he presented two further cases (Figure 1.4) and postulated, but was unable to prove, that the tumours arose from the fibrous connective tissue of small nerves. Thirty-three years later, von Recklinghausen (1882) confirmed their origin and named the tumours neurofibromas. Von Recklinghausen also emphasized that one of his two cases had an affected sibling. Following this important work, the disease became known as von Recklinghausen's disease.

Von Recklinghausen (1882) also described 'innumerable brown pigmentation spots' in one of his cases, but did not appreciate their

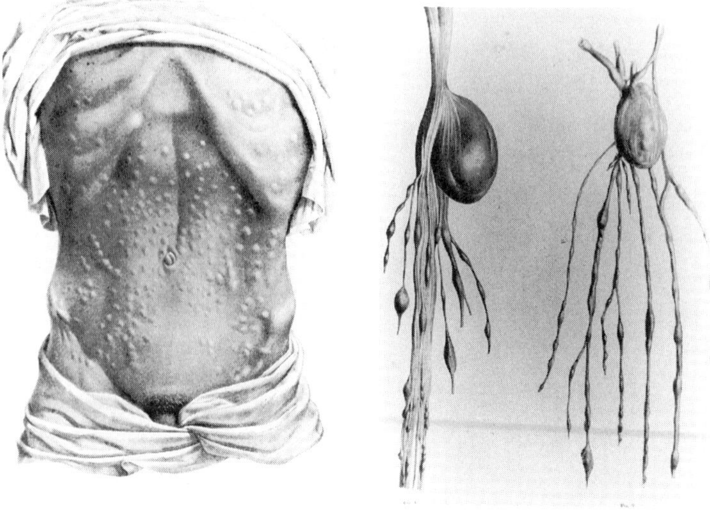

Figure 1.4 Illustrations from Smith (1849). These copies were taken from the republished edition of 1898 (New Sydenham Society, London). (A) The appearance of the abdomen of one of his cases showing multiple cutaneous tumours. (B) Multiple tumours in the right sciatic nerve, reflecting a form of plexiform neurofibroma.

significance. The credit for this falls to Marie and Bernard (1896) and Chauffard (1896). However, it was not until the studies of Crowe, Schull and Neel (Crowe and Schull, 1953; Crowe, Schull and Neel, 1956) that it was accepted that café au lait spots were the first manifestations of the disease to appear. Parkes Weber (1909) had described young patients with only café au lait spots as having a *forme fruste* of the disease. Much later, Crowe (1964) reported that axillary freckling was a clinical feature unique to NF1. The other major features of NF1, Lisch nodules, were probably first reported in 1918 by Waardenburg, who described small wart-like lesions of the iris. In 1937 Lisch reported three cases of NF1, all of which had nodular lesions of the iris that had a distinct appearance. He concluded that they were pathognomonic of the disease and that if the irides of more NF1 patients were examined, they would be a frequent finding. His hypothesis, although not tested until 1981, was found to be correct (Lewis and Riccardi, 1981).

The first reports of NF1 occurring in more than one family member are those of Akenside (1768) and Virchow (1847). Thomson undertook a systematic genetic survey in 1900, demonstrating that the disease was familial in 30 of the 77 reported cases. Preiser and Davenport (1918) studied the frequency of NF1 in children of affected individuals in the literature. Because 50 out of 115 individuals (44%) were affected, with no difference in the sex distribution and many instances of male to male transmission, they concluded that inheritance was autosomal dominant. Subsequent authors accepted that inheritance was autosomal dominant in some families, but were confused by the high reported incidence of sporadic cases and failed to appreciate the significance of multiple café au lait spots in relatives of affected individuals (Siemens, 1926; Peyron, Kobozieff and Zimmer, 1937). The question of mode of inheritance was resolved by the studies of Borberg (1951) and Crowe, Schull and Neel (1956). Both concluded that inheritance was autosomal dominant with high penetrance, and that sporadic cases represented new gene mutations.

After the recognition of NF1 as a distinct entity, reports of complications affecting most of the body systems began to appear in the medical literature, but it was only with the first large clinical studies of Borberg (1951) and Crowe, Schull and Neel (1956) that the spectrum and prevalence of complications became more clear. However, even then, the studies were confounded by bias as a result of the method of patient ascertainment and failure to distinguish the different forms of neurofibromatosis. The late 1970s saw an escalation of activity specific to neurofibromatosis both in clinical and laboratory research and the formation of lay organizations for disease sufferers (e.g. the National Neurofibromatosis Foundation in the USA, formed in 1978; Neurofibromatosis Association in the UK, formed in 1981). The proceedings of the first ever multidisciplinary workshop on neurofibromatosis (Riccardi and Mulvihill, 1981) bore witness to the developing interest at this time. The developments since then are described throughout this book.

1.2.2 Neurofibromatosis 2

The earliest clinical descriptions of NF2 (Wishart, 1822; Knoblauch, 1843) predate the publications of both Smith (1849) and von Recklinghausen (1882) on NF1. However, the condition was only described in detail by Henneberg and Koch in 1903. Authors reviewing cases of bilateral acoustic neuromas (which we now prefer to call vestibular Schwannomas) recognized that the cutaneous features were similar to those in von Recklinghausen's disease, which was becoming increasingly recognized. Reviewing the literature in 1915, Henschen reported a series of 245 cases with unilateral acoustic neuromas and 24 with bilateral lesions. Five of the former compared with 19 of the latter were said to have signs of von Recklinghausen's disease. Cushing, in his 1917 review of acoustic neuromas, concluded that bilateral acoustic neuromas represented a form of neurofibromatosis.

Following reports of the familial occurrence of NF2 (Feiling and Ward, 1920; Gardiner and Frazier, 1930) showing autosomal dominant inheritance, acoustic neuromas became accepted as one of the complications of von Recklinghausen's disease. Gardiner and Frazier did point out that the uniform expression of acoustic neuromas in their family and limited cutaneous involvement was unusual. Despite this, cases with multiple nervous system tumours, regardless of their association with cutaneous or other system involvement, were usually subsequently labelled as having 'von Recklinghausen's disease'. When Young, Eldridge and Gardner (1970) reported a follow-up of the Gardiner and Frazier family, NF2 at last became established as a distinct entity. This report and a later study from the same group (Kanter *et al.*, 1980) emphasized that the major feature of NF2 is bilateral acoustic neuromas and that the cutaneous features, present in some patients, are much less prominent than in NF1. Other NF1 complications were notably absent.

When reviewing older reports of neurofibromatosis one must always reassess the cases according to modern diagnostic criteria. For example, Crowe, Schull and Neel (1956) reported that 5% of patients with 'multiple neurofibromatosis' have acoustic neuromas. However, on critical review the deafness was caused by an acoustic neuroma in only four out of 10 cases, none of whom would satisfy current criteria for the diagnosis of NF1. 'Splitting off' the various forms of neurofibromatosis from the all-embracing umbrella of von Recklinghausen's disease may seem at first an academic exercise (and one geneticists are fond of!). Its clinical importance will become obvious on reading the relevant chapters on management and genetic counselling, which are quite different in the two diseases.

1.3 CLASSIFICATION OF THE DIFFERENT TYPES OF NEUROFIBROMATOSIS

The term neurofibromatosis covers a number of different conditions that are clinically related because of overlapping manifestations. However, at the genetic level the two best defined conditions, NF1 and NF2, have already been shown to be distinct (Chapters 2 and 3). This section reviews the classifications that have been proposed for the different forms of neurofibromatosis.

1.3.1 Riccardi's classification

Riccardi was one of the first clinical investigators to realize the importance of coordinating care for neurofibromatosis sufferers and the need for long-term follow-up. As (Riccardi 1981a) assessed more cases, he realized that not all patients fell into the NF1 and NF2 categories. In 1982, he proposed a classification that included seven different types of neurofibromatosis and an eighth category for cases 'not otherwise specified'; this classification has been updated in each edition of his book (Riccardi, 1992). The definition of the different forms depended on variations in the occurrence, number and distribution of the major defining features and associated complications, particularly tumours of the nervous system. Riccardi's classification is summarized in Table 19.1. It has not come into widespread use, partly because the type III 'mixed', type VI 'variant' and type VII 'late onset' forms are not defined sufficiently to permit their general use. In his recent book on neurofibromatosis, Riccardi (1992) also mentioned three other conditions under the heading 'Other NF types': gastrointestinal neurofibromatosis, multiple Schwannomatosis and familial brain tumours. Riccardi's classification and these related disorders are discussed further in Chapter 19.

1.3.2 The National Institutes of Health Consensus Development Conference classification and diagnostic criteria

The NIH Consensus Conference on Neurofibromatosis (1988) addressed the questions 'What are the various clinical types of neurofibromatosis, and what are their frequencies and diagnostic criteria?' The panel concluded that at that time only NF1 and NF2 could be precisely classified though other forms did exist. They recommended a numerical rather than descriptive or eponymous nomenclature. One of the advantages was that as other forms become more clearly defined they could be added. The consensus statement included diagnostic criteria for NF1 and NF2 (Table 1.2). The NF2 criteria have since been slightly modified as discussed in Chapter 18. NF1 is by far the most common of the neurofibromatoses with an estimated birth incidence of 1 in 2500 to 1 in 3300 (Crowe, Schull and Neel, 1956; Huson *et al.*, 1989). Population-based studies have found the prevalence of NF1 to be between 1 in 4000 and 1 in 5000 (Samuelsson and Axelsson, 1981; Huson *et al.*, 1989). NF2 has a prevalence of between 4.7 and 8.6 per million of population and an estimated birth incidence of 1 in 33–40000 (Evans *et al.*, 1992). The medical literature suggests that the other forms of neurofibromatosis are all rarer than both NF1 and NF2, although no formal prevalence studies have been undertaken. My impression is that with increasing awareness of variant forms, segmental NF is at least as prevalent as NF2; this observation is based on almost equal numbers of referrals for each condition to the Oxford Regional Genetics Service in the last 3 years.

1.4 PATHOGENESIS OF NF1: AN INTRODUCTORY OVERVIEW

For such a common genetic disease, the number of scientific papers published about NF prior to the last decade was surprisingly small. This

Table 1.2 NIH Consensus Statement (1988): diagnostic criteria for NF1 and NF2

NF1

The diagnostic criteria for NF1 are met in an individual if two or more of the following are found:

Six or more café au lait macules of over 5 mm in greatest diameter in prepubertal individuals and over 15 mm in greatest diameter in postpubertal individuals
Two or more neurofibromas of any type or one plexiform neurofibroma
Freckling in the axillary or inguinal regions
Optic glioma
Two or more Lisch nodules (iris hamartomas)
A distinctive osseous lesion such as sphenoid dysplasia or thinning of the long bone cortex with or without pseudoarthrosis
A first-degree relative (parent, sibling or offspring) with NF1 by the above criteria

NF2

The diagnostic criteria for NF2 are met by an individual who has:

1 Bilateral eighth nerve masses seen with appropriate imaging techniques (e.g. CT or MRI) **or**
2 A first-degree relative with NF2 and either:
   (a) unilateral eighth nerve mass **or**
   (b) two of the following:
      - neurofibroma
      - meningioma
      - glioma
      - Schwannoma
      - juvenile posterior subcapsular lenticular opacity

was probably for the same reason that clinical care was previously poorly coordinated. NF patients present to so many different specialties that no one group realized the overall disease burden and was thus stimulated to develop a research interest. Fortunately, with the application of molecular genetic techniques to the localization and characterization of the *NF1* and *NF2* genes this situation has changed dramatically. This section is written to provide a brief overview of work that may be relevant to our eventual understanding of the pathogenesis of NF. Now that it is appreciated that the clinical features of NF1 and NF2 are usually distinct and the genes on different chromosomes (NIH Consensus Conference Statement, 1988), one major question of interest is the nature of any overlapping pathogenetic mechanisms. From a clinician's viewpoint, there are enough common features to expect some overlap (Table 1.3). Although the tumours in NF1 and NF2 are histologically distinct (Chapter 6), the tumours that are the major features of each disorder (dermal

Table 1.3 Major clinical features of NF1 and NF2 and embryonic origin of tissue

Disease feature	*Embryonic origin of involved tissue*
NF1	
Major disease features	
Café au lait spots	
Neurofibromas	Neural crest
Lisch nodules	
Minor disease features	
Macrocephaly	Primary tissue
Short stature	involved uncertain
Major complications	
Intellectual handicap	Neural tube
Plexiform neurofibromas	Neural crest
Orthopaedic problems (scoliosis, pseudoarthrosis)	Mesoderm
Disease associated tumours	
Optic glioma	Neural tube
Peripheral nerve malignancy	Neural crest
Rhabdomyosarcoma	Mesoderm
Phaeochromocytoma	Neural crest
Duodenal carcinoid	Endoderm
NF2	
Major disease features	
Bilateral vestibular Schwannomas (acoustic neuromas)	Neural crest
Minor disease features	
Café au lait spots	Neural crest
Peripheral nerve Schwannomas	Neural crest
Cataracts/disease-specific lens opacities	Mesoderm
Complications	
Meningiomas	Neural crest (for prosencephalic + part of mesencephalic derived tissue) Neural tube (other meninges)
Spinal nerve root Schwannomas	Neural crest
Glial cell tumours	Neural tube

neurofibromas in NF1, vestibular Schwannomas in NF2) both have Schwann cells as a major component.

1.4.1 Clinical observations as clues to pathogenesis

The clinician's contribution to elucidating pathogenesis has been the careful description of different types of neurofibromatosis and their natural histories. If NF1 had not been distinguished clinically from other forms before genetic linkage studies were used to localize the gene, confusing results suggesting locus heterogeneity would have resulted. As a result of uniform and relatively rigid diagnostic criteria, pooling of data from a number of centres was possible, which gave a very precise linkage map and confidently excluded locus heterogeneity (Goldgar *et al.*, 1989).

The rate of progression of different lesions in NF1 and NF2 may offer clues to pathogenesis. Why do café au lait spots appear during childhood, but then remain static or even disappear in adults? Why do neurofibromas not appear until around the time of puberty? What hormonal influences cause neurofibromas to grow in pregnancy? The work of Riccardi in this field is to be applauded. In a series of papers over the last two decades, his clinical observations stimulated thought-provoking questions about pathogenesis (Riccardi and Kleiner, 1977; Riccardi, 1979; Riccardi, Kleiner and Lubs, 1979; Riccardi, 1980, 1981b, 1982, 1990). Riccardi's stimulus and encouragement to other investigators (including myself), particularly in the early stages of their own studies, has been a major contribution to the increasing interest in neurofibromatosis worldwide.

1.4.2 Neurofibromatosis as a neurocristopathy

Bolande (1974, 1981) proposed that various dysgenetic hamartomatous and neoplastic conditions had a common origin in abnormal neural crest development. The disease manifestations resulted from abnormal migration, growth or cytodifferentiation of primitive neural crest cells at various stages of human development. Bolande described this group of conditions as neurocristopathies, and distinguished them into two groups:

- Simple neurocristopathies – characterized by a single pathological process, e.g. Hirschsprung's disease (dysgenetic) and phaeochromocytoma (neoplastic).
- Complex neurocristopathies – syndromes of multiple and variegated simple neurocristopathies, e.g. neurofibromatosis, the multiple endocrine neoplasia syndromes and neurocutaneous melanosis.

The major clinical features of NF1 and NF2 are listed in Table 1.3 with their tissues of origin; most features arise in tissue of neural crest origin. Considering NF1 as a neurocristopathy, it is difficult to explain those complications arising in tissues of other origins. In Chapter 4, Dr Smith discusses how a primary neural crest abnormality causing secondary changes in other tissues would explain this. Schwann cells are of neural crest origin and are the principal cells in the tumours of NF1 and NF2. In

Chapter 5, Drs Jessen and Mirsky review Schwann cell biology and its application to the pathogenesis of neurofibromatosis.

1.4.3 Nerve growth factor

Nerve growth factor (NGF) is a polypeptide necessary for the growth and maintenance of sympathetic and certain sensory neurons. Abnormalities of NGF were proposed as important in the pathogenesis of neurofibromatosis. Early studies in small numbers of patients (reviewed by Eldridge, 1981) suggested that NGF activity was increased in the serum of patients with NF1 and NF2. The increased NGF activity was detected by a different assay in NF1 from that in NF2, and Fabricant, Todaro and Eldridge (1979) proposed that the two diseases may result from different abnormalities of NGF. This suggestion has now been disproved. Riopelle *et al.* (1984), using an improved assay system in a much larger number of NF1 patients, found that NGF activity was normal. Darby *et al.* (1985) found that there were multiple crossovers between the *NGF* and *NF1* genes in a linkage study with the β-NGF DNA probe, and so excluded *NGF* as a candidate gene for NF1. The studies of Seizinger, Martuza and Gusella (1986) and Rouleau *et al.* (1987) localized the *NF2* gene to chromosome 22, and excluded *NGF* (on chromosome 1) as a candidate gene. However, NGF could still have a modifying effect on *NF1* or *NF2* gene expression.

1.4.4 Mechanisms of tumorigenesis

In both NF1 and NF2, one of the major features is tumour formation at various sites. In NF2 the tumours are the sole cause of significant morbidity and mortality. In NF1, although other complications such as intellectual handicap and skeletal problems occur, the development of multiple dermal tumours is one of the major defining features. In addition, NF1 patients are at an increased risk of developing other tumours such as optic gliomas, astrocytomas, neurofibrosarcomas, phaeochromocytomas and carcinoid tumours. The understanding of the mechanism of tumour formation in both diseases is critical to the development of disease treatments. As the tumours in NF1 and NF2 are not usually present at birth, it is attractive to postulate some form of presymptomatic treatment to block the pathways involved in tumorigenesis.

To date, three main mechanisms of tumorigenesis have been studied, with most work being on NF1. Despite this, we are uncertain as to the primary trigger to neurofibroma formation and in which cell type the abnormality develops. Neurofibromas are comprised of 60–85% Schwann cells, 10–20% fibroblasts and lesser numbers of pericytes, perineurial cells, mast cells, endothelial cells and smooth muscle cells. These are enveloped by an extensive extracellular matrix (Peltonen *et al.*, 1988). Several observations suggest that Schwann cells may be the primary target of factors stimulating neurofibroma formation (Ratner *et al.*, 1990). In normal adult nerve, Schwann cells are usually closely associated with axons (Webster and Favilla, 1984); in neurofibromas they are associated with bundles of axons or free in the extracellular matrix (Stefansson, Wollmann and Jerkovic, 1982; Waggener, 1966). Schwann cells are the major cell type amplified in neurofibromas and the malignant nerve sheath tumours that occur in NF1 (Ducatman *et al.*, 1984). Both neurofibromas from NF1 patients (Ratner *et al.*, 1990) and vestibular Schwannomas from NF2 patients (Brockes, Breakefield and Martuza, 1986) contain Schwann cell mitogens.

(a) The 'double hit' hypothesis of Knudson

In both NF1 and NF2 the feature that causes morbidity and mortality is the development of multiple tumours. The neurofibromatoses are often considered to share pathogenetic similarities with other inherited cancer syndromes such as von Hippel-Lindau disease and the multiple endocrine neoplasia syndromes. At the cellular level, the cause of any tumour is genetic. A change in gene expression must occur to permit abnormal growth. The development of tumours may be associated with mutation or inappropriate expression of specific normal cellular genes, which are referred to as oncogenes. Oncogene activation results in malignant transformation of the cells containing them, and the genetic changes causing them have recently been elucidated (Friend, Dryja and Weinberg, 1988). An example is seen in chronic myeloid leukaemia, where one of the translocation breakpoints that gives rise to the Philadelphia chromosome falls within an oncogene (Kurzrock, Gutterman and Talpaz, 1988). As oncogenes are dominant at a cellular level, phenotypic expression requires only one mutant copy; an abnormal oncogene would therefore not be a likely candidate as the cause of the inherited susceptibility to tumour formation in neurofibromatosis. Recessive mutations causing a functional loss of genes that control cell growth and differentiation seem more likely.

De Mars (1970) first proposed this mechanism for certain familial cancers. He suggested that gene carriers might be heterozygous for a recessive mutation and that cancer developed because a subsequent somatic mutation caused an individual cell to become homozygous for the gene. In 1971, Knudson studied the age-specific incidence of familial and sporadic forms of retinoblastoma. He noted that in familial cases the tumours developed at a younger age and were often multiple and that in sporadic cases tumours were single. This led him to suggest that the development of these cancers requires two events (or 'hits'). Those with the hereditary form have a germline mutation at the locus and cancer develops when a second somatic mutation occurs. However, for a sporadic tumour, two sporadic mutations are necessary, which is why they usually develop at a later age and are rarely multiple. The inherited cancers appear dominant within a family, because it is highly likely that each gene carrier will develop a second 'hit' in at least one tissue and therefore express the gene. This type of gene is now called a tumour suppressor gene.

From a clinical viewpoint, NF2 fits this model very well. In the general population unilateral vestibular Schwannomas develop in middle or old age. In NF2, vestibular Schwannomas occur bilaterally and are often associated with other neoplasms, all of which develop at a relatively young age. Applied to NF1, the 'two hit' model would suggest that each café au lait spot and dermal neurofibroma represents a second somatic mutation. This would explain why the lesions are discrete. However, NF1 has a number of features (short stature, intellectual handicap, learning difficulties) that are difficult to explain using the two hit model and that suggest a single abnormal copy of the *NF1* gene has some phenotypic effect.

Cytogenetic analysis and DNA markers have shown Knudson's hypothesis to be correct for a number of inherited cancers including retinoblastoma (Cavanee *et al.*, 1983, 1986; Ponder, 1988). Molecular studies have shown that the *NF2* gene acts as a tumour suppressor gene (reviewed by Dr Rouleau in Chapter 3). Despite the more complicated phenotype, Drs Marchuk and Collins conclude in Chapter 2 that the *NF1* gene is a tumour suppressor gene.

(b) The role of mast cells in neurofibroma formation

Mast cells are a major component of neurofibromas (Lascano, 1958; Cawley and Hoch-Ligitti, 1961). Riccardi (1981b) postulated that mast cells may contribute to the origin and growth of neurofibromas. He has also suggested (1990) that trauma may have a role in the origin and/or progression of neurofibromas. His proposal is that trauma disrupts the normal relationship between Schwann cells and neurons, which causes inappropriate initiation of wound healing. Normally the result would be formation of a discrete scar. However, the NF1 mutation interferes with the signal that the wound healing phase is complete so that growth continues and a neurofibroma forms. Local somatic mutation would explain why isolated neurofibromas arise in the general population. Riccardi (1992) reviews the scientific work on mast cells that contributes to the understanding of their role in NF1.

(c) Angiogenesis in neurofibroma formation

The growth of any solid tumour is dependent on stimulation of angiogenesis (Folkman, 1974; Folkman and Klagsbrun, 1987; Folkman *et al.*, 1989). Solid tumours do not make their own blood vessels but induce them from their host; antiangiogenic factors have therefore been explored in the treatment of various human tumours. Neurofibroma Schwann cells from NF1 patients, unlike normal Schwann cells, promote angiogenesis and invade basement membranes in the chick chorioallantoic membrane model system (Sheela, Riccardi and Ratner, 1990). Animal models have been developed for growing Schwann cell tumours (Lee *et al.*, 1990a) and meningiomas (Medhkour *et al.*, 1989) from both neurofibromatosis patients and the general population in the subrenal capsule of nude mice. The technique allows direct observation of tumour size and neovascularity. Lee *et al.* (1990b) have used this model to study the effect of heparin and hydrocortisone on an implanted neurofibrosarcoma from an NF1 patient. Heparin treatment alone stimulated angiogenesis and resulted in tumour growth greater than in the control group. Hydrocortisone alone caused a minimal reduction in tumour growth and had a minimal effect on angiogenesis. However, heparin and hydrocortisone administered together inhibited both angiogenesis and tumour growth, suggesting that angiogenesis modulators are worthy of study as a means of tumour control in neurofibromatosis.

1.4.5 Animal models

(a) Naturally occurring models

The occurrence of single or multiple neurofibromas has been reported in birds (Bossart, 1983) and mammals, including cows, horses and dogs (Luginbuhl *et al.*, 1968; Goedegeburre, 1975; Canfield, 1978). Of particular interest is the occurrence of multiple neurofibromas in Holstein cows. Slanina and co-workers (1978) identified a herd with a relatively large number of animals with multiple congenital cutaneous neurofibromas. All affected individuals had been sired by a single bull. Doran *et al.* (1993) have reported a further herd of Holstein cows with multiple cutaneous neurofibromas. Lesions on one of the cows have undergone early malignant degeneration similar to a low-grade neurofibrosarcoma. Molecular studies are in progress to determine whether these neurofibromas are genetically determined and develop because of mutations in the bovine *NF1* gene.

The only animal known to have abnormalities of pigmentation and to develop neurofibromas is the bicolour damsel fish (Schmale, Udey and Hensley, 1986). As these fish reach maturity they develop areas of thickened hyperpigmented epithelium, which is followed by the development of nerve cell tumours (neurofibromas, Schwannomas and neurofibrosarcomas). Epidemiological studies of these fish suggest an infectious rather than a genetic aetiology. Schmale and Hensley (1988) demonstrated transmissibility of the condition by inoculating homogenized tumour into healthy bicolour damsel fish. Similar tumours developed at the injection site of approximately 84% of inoculated fish. The tumours appeared within an average of 5 months of inoculation in juvenile fish and 14 months in adult fish. The tumours arose by the neoplastic transformation of host nerve cells rather than by transplantation and proliferation of tumour cells from the donor fish. An infectious transmissible agent such as a virus may be the cause of neurofibromas and other Schwann cell tumours in the bicolour damsel fish when it occurs naturally. These studies do not suggest a pure genetic mechanism for the fish disease. However, the fish may have a genetic susceptibility to nerve sheath tumour development that results from introduction of a viral oncogene or alteration in expression of a cellular gene.

(b) Mutagen-induced and transgenic models

Alternative animal models have been constructed in the laboratory, either by intrauterine or postnatal exposure to mutagens or the creation of transgenic mice. Mice and rats provide attractive models because of the ease of breeding, large litters and short generation span. However phenotypic expression of the NF1 mutation may be limited in these species: pigmentary changes are not seen in the scalp in humans and may not be expected in the skin of hairy animals.

Ethylnitrosurea (ENU) induces Schwannomas in a high percentage of rats following late fetal or early postnatal exposure (Vinores, 1986). Riccardi (1988, 1992) tried to develop an inheritable Mendelian mutation following ENU exposure. The rats developed both Schwannomas and neurofibrosarcomas in two generations. The first generation had been exposed to ENU *in utero*. In the second generation one of 80 live-born offspring had developed neurofibrosarcoma at the time of reporting, suggesting the possibility of an inherited germline mutation predisposing to sarcoma formation, the germline mutation having arisen secondary to ENU exposure.

Even prior to the cloning of the *NF1* gene, a transgenic mouse experiment had accidentally produced an animal with an NF1-like phenotype. The *tat* gene of human T-lymphotropic virus type 1 (HTLV-1) under the control of its own long terminal repeat induces two phenotypes in transgenic mice in the absence of other viral genes (Nerenberg *et al.*, 1987). One of these transgenics developed fibromas frequently associated with peripheral nerve sheaths (Hinrichs *et al.*, 1987). The tumours tended to occur at sites of trauma and sometimes underwent malignant degeneration. These observations led Nerenberg and colleagues to suggest that, at least in some cases, NF1 may be associated with HTLV-1 infection. They subsequently analysed neurofibromas from Japanese (where HTLV-1 is endemic) and North American NF1 patients (Nerenberg *et al.*, 1991). The virus was not seen in the tumour tissue in either group, making an association unlikely. Further analysis of the mouse also showed differences with NF1. Firstly, HTLV-1 integrates at random into the mouse genome, not to one specific locus. No other complications, other than the tumours, have developed and on further histological analysis the tumours appear less like neurofibromas (Nerenberg *et al.*, 1991).

With the cloning of the *NF1* gene and demonstration that the mouse *NF1* locus is homologous to the human one, the creation of animals with the *NF1* locus 'knocked-out' by homologous recombination became possible. The outcome of these experiments to date is reviewed by Drs Marchuk and Collins in Chapter 2.

1.4.6 Conclusions

This introduction has provided a brief overview of theories of pathogenesis and experimental approaches that may provide insights into our understanding of neurofibromatosis. Little progress was made until molecular genetic techniques were applied to the localization and cloning of the *NF1* and *NF2* genes. These developments are reviewed in detail in the subsequent two chapters, which are followed by overviews of the biology of the neural crest and of Schwann cells. Over the next decade it is anticipated that these 'pieces' will fall into place to complete the jigsaw that represents our understanding of NF pathogenesis.

> . . . The reverse genetics trail that is currently being blazed for NF1 shows a greater promise of providing an understanding of the true basis of this major genetic disease than has any previous endeavour in more than a century since the original description of the disease.
>
> *Collins* et al. *(1989)*

ACKNOWLEDGEMENTS

The author wishes to thank Patricia Madigan for providing Figure 1.1 and Alastair Compston for Figures 1.3 and 1.4.

REFERENCES

Akenside, M. (1768) Observations on cancers. *Med. Trans. Coll. Phys. Lond.*, **1**, 64–92.

Aldrovandi, U. (1642) *Monstrorum Historia cum Paralipomenis Historiae Omnium Animalium*, Typis Nicolai Tibaldini, Bononiae.

Bolande, R.P. (1974) The neurocristopathies. A unifying concept of disease arising in neural crest maldevelopment. *Hum. Pathol.*, **5**, 409–29.

Bolande, R.P. (1981) Neurofibromatosis – the quintessential neurocristopathy: pathogenetic concepts and relationships. *Adv. Neurol.*, **29**, 67–75.

Borberg, A. (1951) Clinical and genetic investigations into tuberous sclerosis and Recklinghausen's neurofibromatosis. *Acta Psychiat. Neurol. [Suppl.]*, **71**, 1–239.

Bossart, G.D. (1983) Neurofibromatosis in a macaw (*Arachloroptera*): morphologic and immunocytochemical diagnosis. *Vet. Pathol.*, 20, 773–6.

Brockes, J.P., Breakefield, X.O. and Martuza, R.L. (1986) Glial growth factor-like activity in Schwann cell tumors. *Ann. Neurol.*, **20**, 317–22.

Canfield, P. (1978) A light microscopic study of bovine peripheral nerve sheath tumours. *Vet. Pathol.*, **15**, 283–91.

Cavenee, W.K., Dryja, T.P., Phillips, R.A. *et al.* (1983) Expression of recessive alleles by chromosomal mechanisms in retinoblastoma. *Nature*, **305**, 779–84.

Cavenee, W.K., Muphree, A.L., Skull, M.M. *et al.* (1986) Prediction of familial predisposition in retinoblastoma. *N. Engl. J. Med.*, **314**, 1201–7.

Cawley, E.P. and Hoch-Ligitti, C. (1961) Association of tissue mast cells and skin tumours. *Arch. Dermatol.*, **83**, 92–6.

Chauffard, M.A. (1896) Dermato-fibromatose pigmentaire (ou neurofibromatose generalisée.) *Soc. Med. Hop. Paris*, **13**, 200.

Collins, F.S., Ponder, B.A.J., Seizinger, B.R. and Epstein, C.J. (1989) Editorial: The von Recklinghausen neurofibromatosis region on chromosome 17. Genetic and physical maps come into focus. *Am. J. Hum. Genet.*, **44**, 1–5.

Crowe, F.W. (1964) Axillary freckling as a diagnostic aid in neurofibromatosis. *Ann. Intern. Med.*, **61**, 1142–3.

Crowe, F.W. and Schull, W.J. (1953) Diagnostic importance of the café au lait spot in neurofibromatosis. *Arch. Intern. Med.*, **91**, 758–66.

Crowe, F.W., Schull, W.J. and Neel, J.V. (1956) *A Clinical, Pathological and Genetic Study of Multiple Neurofibromatosis*, Charles C. Thomas, Springfield, Illinois.

Cruveilhier, J. (1829–42) *Anatomie Pathologique du Corps Humain*, Baillière, Paris.

Cushing, H. (1917) *Tumors of the Nervus Acusticus and the Syndrome of the Cerebellopontine Angle*, W.B. Saunders, Philadelphia.

Darby, J.K., Feder, J., Selby, M. *et al.* (1985) A discordant sibship analysis between bega-NGF and neurofibromatosis. *Am. J. Hum. Genet.*, 37, 52–9.

De Mars, R. (1970) In *23rd Annual Symposium on Fundamental Cancer Research*, Williams and Wilkins, Baltimore, pp. 105–6.

Doran, S., Sartin, E., Gregory, P., Liu, P. and Collins, F. (1993) Of fish and cows: the search for mutations in the NF1 gene. Poster presentation, NNFF international consortium on gene cloning and gene function for NF1 and NF2 meeting, Ann Arbor, April 1993.

Ducatman, B.S., Scheithauer, B.W., Piepgras, D.G. and Reiman, H.M. (1984) Malignant peripheral nerve sheath tumours in childhood. *J. Neurooncol.*, **2**, 241–8.

Eldridge, R. (1981) Central neurofibromatosis. *Adv. Neurol.*, **29**, 57–65.

Evans, D.G.R., Huson, S.M., Donnai, D. *et al.* (1992) A genetic study of type 2 neurofibromatosis in the United Kingdom: prevalence, mutation rate, fitness and confirmation of maternal transmission effect on severity. *J. Med. Genet.*, **29**, 841–6.

Fabricant, R.N., Todaro, G.T. and Eldridge, R.E. (1979) Increased levels of a nerve growth factor cross-reacting protein in central neurofibromatosis. *Lancet*, **i**, 4–7.

Feiling, A. and Ward, E. (1920) A familial form of acoustic tumour. *Br. Med. J.*, **1**, 496–7.

Folkman, J. (1974) Tumour angiogenesis. *Adv. Cancer Res.*, **19**, 331–58.

Folkman, J. and Klagsbrun, M. (1987) Angiogenic factors. *Science*, **235**, 442–7.

Folkman, J., Watson, K., Ingber, D. and Hanahan, D. (1989) Induction of angiogenesis during the transition from hyperplasia to neoplasia. *Nature*, **339**, 58–61.

Friend, S.H., Dryja, T.P. and Weinberg, R.A. (1988) Oncogenes and tumor-suppressor genes. *N. Engl. J. Med.*, **318**, 618–22.

Gardiner, W.T. and Frazier, C.H. (1930) Bilateral acoustic neurofibromas: a clinical study and field survey of a family of five generations with bilateral deafness in 38 members. *Arch. Neurol. Psych.*, **23**, 266–300.

Goedegeburre, S.A. (1975) A case of neurofibromatosis in the dog. *J. Small Anim. Pract.*, **16**, 329–35.

Goldgar, D.E., Green, P., Parry, D. and Mulvihill, J.J. (1989) Multipoint linkage analysis in neurofibromatosis type 1: an international collaboration. *Am. J. Hum. Genet.*, **44**, 6–12.

Hecht, F. (1989) Recognition of neurofibromatosis before von Recklinghausen. *Neurofibromatosis*, **2**, 180–4.

Henneberg, R. and Koch, M. (1903) Ueber 'centrale' neurofibromatose und die Geschwülste des Kleinhirnbrückenwinkels (Acusticusneurome). *Arch. F. Psychiatr.*, **36**, 251.

Henschen, F. (1915) Zur histologie und pathogenese der Kleinhirnbruckenwinkel tumoren. *Arch. F. Psychiatr.*, **56**, 21.

Hinrichs, S.H., Nerenberg, M., Reynolds, R.K. *et al.* (1987) A transgenic mouse model for human neurofibromatosis. *Science*, **237**, 1330–43.

Huson, S.M., Clark, P., Compston, D.A.S. and Harper, P.S. (1989) A genetic study of von Recklinghausen neurofibromatosis in South East Wales. I: Prevalence, fitness, mutation rate and effect of parental transmission on severity. *J. Med. Genet.*, **26**, 704–11.

Kanter, W.R., Eldridge, R., Fabricant, R. *et al.* (1980) Central neurofibromatosis with bilateral acoustic neuroma: genetic, clinical and biochemical distinctions from peripheral neurofibromatosis. *Neurology*, **30**, 851–9.

Knoblauch, J. (1843) De neuromate et gangliis accessories. Frankfurt. Dissertation.

Knudson, A.G. Jr (1971) Mutation and cancer: statistical study of retinoblastoma. *Proc. Natl. Acad. Sci. USA*, **68**, 829–33.

Kurzrock, R. Gutterman, J.U. and Talpaz, M. (1988) The molecular genetics of Philadelphia chromosome-positive leukemias. *N. Engl. J. Med.*, **319**, 990–8.

Lascano, E.F. (1958) Mast cells in human tumors. *Cancer*, **6**, 1110–13.

Lee, J.K., Kim, T.S., Chiocca, E.A. *et al.* (1990a) Growth of human Schwannomas in the sub-renal capsule of the nude mouse. *Neurosurgery*, **26**, 598–605.

Lee, J.K., Choi, B., Sobel, R.A. *et al.* (1990b) Inhibition of growth and angiogenesis of human neurofibrosarcoma by heparin and hydrocortisone. *J. Neurosurg.*, **73**, 429–35.

Lewis, R.A. and Riccardi, V.M. (1981) Von Recklinghausen neurofibromatosis: incidence of iris hamartomata. *Ophthalmology*, **88**, 348–54.

Lisch, K. (1937) Ueber Beteiligung der Augen, insbesondere das vorkommen von Irisknotchen bei der neurofibromatose (Recklinghausen). *Z. Augenheilkde*, **93**, 137–43.

Ludwig, C.F. and Tilesius, W.G. (1793) *Historia Pathologica Singularis Cutis Turpitudinis*, Siegried Lebrecht Crusius, Leipzig.

Luginbuhl, H., Frankhauser, R. and McGrath, J.T. (1968) Spontaneous neoplasms of the nervous system in animals. *Prog. Neurol. Surg.*, **2**, 85–164.

Madigan, P. and Masello, M.J. (1989) Report of a neurofibromatosis-like case: Monstrorum Historia, 1642. *Neurofibromatosis*, **2**, 53–6.

Marie, P. and Bernard, A. (1896) Neurofibromatose generalisée. *Soc. Med. Hop. Paris*, **13**, 777.

Medhkour, A., Van Roey, M., Sobel, R.A. *et al.* (1989) Implantation of human meningiomas into the subrenal capsule of the nude mouse. A model for studies of tumour growth. *J. Neurosurg*, **71**, 545–50.

Mulvihill, J.J. (1988) Neurofibromatosis: history, nomenclature, and natural history. *Neurofibromatosis*, **1**, 124–31.

Nerenberg, M., Hinrichs, S.H., Reynolds, R.K. *et al.* (1987) The *tat* gene of human T-lymphotropic virus type 1 induces mesenchymal tumors in transgenic mice. *Science*, **237**, 1324–9.

Nerenberg, M.I., Minor, T., Nagashima, K. *et al.* (1991) Absence of association of HTLV-1 infection with type 1 neurofibromatosis in the United States or Japan. *Neurology*, **41**, 1687–9.

NIH Consensus Development Conference Statement (1988) Neurofibromatosis. *Arch. Neurol.*, **45**, 575–8.

Parkes Weber, F. (1909) Cutaneous pigmentation as an incomplete form of Recklinghausen's disease, with remarks on the classification of incomplete forms of Recklinghausen's disease. *Br. J. Dermatol.*, **21**, 49–51.

Peltonen, J., Jaakkola, S., Lebwohl, M. *et al.* (1988) Cellular differentiation and expression of matrix genes in type 1 neurofibromatosis. *Lab. Invest.*, **59**, 760–71.

Peyron, A., Kobozieff, N. and Zimmer, L. (1937) Sur l'hérédité de la neurofibromatose. *Bull. de l'Assoc. franc. p. l'étude du cancer*, **26**, 168.

Ponder, B.A.J. (1988) Gene loss in human tumours. *Nature*, **335**, 400–2.

Preiser, S.A. and Davenport, C.B. (1918) Multiple neurofibromatosis (von Recklinghausen disease) and its inheritance. *Am. J. Med. Sci.*, **156**, 507–41.

Ratner, N., Lieberman, M.A., Riccardi, V.M. and Hong, D. (1990) Mitogen accumulation in von Recklinghausen neurofibromatosis. *Ann. Neurol.*, **27**, 496–501.

Riccardi, V.M. (1979) Cell–cell interaction as an epigenetic determinant in the expression of mutant neural crest cells. *Birth Defects*, **15**(8), 89–98.

Riccardi, V.M. (1980) The pathophysiology of neurofibromatosis: IV. Dermatologic insights into heterogeneity and pathogenesis, *J. Am. Acad. Dermatol.*, **3**, 157–66.

Riccardi, V.M. (1981a) Von Recklinghausen neurofibromatosis. *N. Engl. J. Med.*, **305**, 1617–27.

Riccardi, V.M. (1981b) Cutaneous manifestations of neurofibromatosis: cellular interaction, pigmentation, and mast cells. *Birth Defects*, **17**(2), 129–45.

Riccardi, V.M. (1982) Neurofibromatosis: clinical heterogeneity. *Curr. Prob. Cancer*, **VII**(2), 1–34.

Riccardi, V.M. (1988) A germline mutation rodent model for neurofibromatosis. Neurofibrosarcoma in the untreated offspring of rats exposed *in utero* to ethylnitrosurea. *Am. J. Hum. Genet.*, **42**, A32.

Riccardi, V.M. (1990) The potential role of trauma and mast cells in the pathogenesis of neurofibromas, in *Tuberous Sclerosis and Neurofibromatosis: Epidemiology, Pathophysiology, Biology and Management* (eds Y. Ishibashi and Y. Horis), Elsevier, Amsterdam, pp. 167–90.

Riccardi, V.M. (1992) *Neurofibromatosis: Phenotype, Natural History and Pathogenesis*, 2nd edn (1st edn 1986), The Johns Hopkins University Press, Baltimore.

Riccardi, V.M. and Kleiner, B. (1977) Neurofibromatosis: a neoplastic birth defect with two age peaks of severity. *Birth Defects*, **13**(3C), 131–8.

Riccardi, V.M. and Mulvhill, J.J. (eds) (1981) Neurofibromatosis (von Recklinghausen's disease). *Adv. Neurol.*, **29**.

Riccardi, V.M., Kleiner, B. and Lubs, M.L. (1979) Neurofibromatosis: variable expression is not intrinsic to the mutant gene. *Birth Defects*, **15**, 283–9.

Riopelle, R.J., Riccardi, V.M., Faulkner, S. and Martin, M.C. (1984) Serum neuronal growth factor levels in von Recklinghausen's neurofibromatosis. *Ann. Neurol.*, **16**, 54–9.

Rouleau, G.A., Wertelecki, W., Haines, J. L. *et al.* (1987) Genetic linkage analysis of bilateral acoustic neurofibromatosis to a DNA marker on chromosome 22. *Nature*, **329**, 246–8.

Samuelsson, B. and Axelsson, R. (1981) Neurofibromatosis. A clinical and genetic study of 96 cases in Gothenburg, Sweden. *Acta Derm. (Stockh.) [Suppl.]*, **95**, 67–71.

Schmale, M.C. and Hensley, G.T. (1988) Transmissibility of a neurofibromatosis-like disease in bicolor damselfish. *Cancer Res.*, **48**, 3828–33.

Schmale, M.C., Udey, L.R. and Hensley, G.T. (1986) Neurofibromatosis in the bicolor damselfish (*Pomacentrus partitus*) as a model for von Recklinghausen's neurofibromatosis. *Ann. N. Y. Acad. Sci.*, **486**, 386–402.

Seizinger, B.R., Martuza, R.L. and Gusella, J.F. (1986) Loss of genes on chromosome 22 in tumorigenesis of human acoustic neuroma. *Nature*, **322**, 644–7.

Sheela, S., Riccardi, V.M. and Ratner, N. (1990) Angiogenic and invasive properties of neurofibroma Schwann cells. *J. Cell. Biol.*, **111**, 645–53.

Siemens, H.W. (1926) Klinisch-dermatologische Studien ueber die Recklinghausensche Krankheit. *Archiv Derm. u. Syph.*, **150**, 80–103.

Slanina, L., Konrad, V., Vajda, V. *et al.* (1978) Congenital neurofibromatosis of the skin in calves. *Dtsch. Tierartzl. Wochenschr.*, **85**, 41–5.

Smith, R.W. (1849) *A Treatise on the Pathology, Diagnosis and Treatment of Neurofibroma*, Hodges and Smith, Dublin.

Stefansson, K., Wollmann, R. and Jerkovic, M. (1982) S-100 protein in soft tissue tumours derived from Schwann cells and melanocytes. *Am. J. Pathol.*, **106**, 261–8.

Thomson, A. (1900) *On Neuroma and Neurofibromatosis*, Turnbull and Spears, Edinburgh.

Vinores, S.A. (1986) Nerve growth factor modification of the ethylnitrosurea model for multiple Schwannomas. *Ann. N.Y. Acad. Sci.*, **486**, 124–31.

Virchow, R. (1847) Ueber die reform der patholigischen und therapeutische Anschauungen durch die mikroskopischen Untersuchungen. *Virchows Arch. Pathol. Anat. Phys.*, **1**, 207–55.

von Recklinghausen, F.D. (1882) *Ueber die multiplen Fibrome der Haut und ihre Beziehung zu den multiplen Neuromen*, Hirschwald, Berlin.

Waardenburg, P.J. (1918) Heterochramie en melanosis. *Ned. Tijdschr. Geneeskd.*, **2**, 1453–5.

Waggener, J.D. (1966) Ultrastructure of benign peripheral nerve sheath tumours. *Cancer*, **19**, 699–709.

Webster, H.F. De and Favilla, T.J. (1984) Development of peripheral nerve fibers, in *Peripheral Neuropathy* (eds P.J. Dyck, P.K. Thomas, E.H. Lambert and R.P. Bunge), W.B. Saunders, Philadelphia, pp. 329–59.

Wishart, J. (1822) Cases of tumors in the skull, dura mater and brain. *Edinb. Med. Surg. J.*, **18**, 393–7.

Young, D.F., Eldridge, R. and Gardner, W.J. (1970) Bilateral acoustic neuromas in a large kindred. *JAMA*, **214**, 347–53.

Zanca, A. and Zanca, A. (1980) Antique illustrations of neurofibromatosis. *Int. J. Dermatol.*, **19**, 55–8.

2

Molecular genetics of neurofibromatosis 1

D.A. Marchuk and F.S. Collins

2.1 GENETICS

Neurofibromatosis 1 (NF1) is one of the most common inherited disorders in humans, with an incidence of about 1 in 2500 to 3300, and affecting all ethnic groups (Crowe *et al.*, 1956; Riccardi, 1981; Riccardi and Eichner, 1986). The spontaneous mutation rate is very high, and 30–50% of cases are new mutations (Crowe *et al.*, 1956; Riccardi and Eichner, 1986). This leads to a calculated mutation rate of 1/10 000 alleles per generation (Crowe *et al.*, 1956), which is about 100-fold higher than the usual mutation rate for a single locus. Linkage analysis and the subsequent cloning of the gene (see below) have not demonstrated any other loci responsible for NF1, so that the high mutation rate cannot be due to multiple loci (Goldgar *et al.*, 1989; Weiming *et al.*, 1991).

Although the hereditary nature of NF1 was not recognized in initial descriptions, its autosomal dominant mode of inheritance has been established (Borberg, 1951; Crowe *et al.*, 1956). What has not been established is whether NF1 is a true dominant disorder, i.e. whether heterozygotes and homozygotes display the same phenotype. This requires careful molecular genetic analysis of the offspring of rare matings of two NF1 individuals. It is possible, however, that the *NF1* gene product is absolutely required at some point during early development, and homozygosity for NF1 may therefore be lethal. In support of this, transgenic mice homozygous for an *NF1* knockout mutation die in early embryogenesis (section 2.8).

There have been rare reports of families where the disorder has skipped a generation, but these may be due to misdiagnosis of mildly affected family members, or to independent mutation. Rigorous diagnostic criteria for NF1 have been established (Stumpf *et al.*, 1987) and with careful examination it is extremely rare to identify an obligate carrier who does not meet these criteria (Riccardi and Lewis, 1988). The disorder is thus considered fully penetrant (Sergeyev, 1975; Riccardi and Eichner, 1986).

The clinical features of the disorder can be quite variable, even among affected family members, indicating that factors other than the specific mutation inherited must play a role in the disease phenotype. If the gene has a tumour suppressor mode of action, the tissue type receiving the second (somatic) mutation and the time during development that the mutation occurs may determine the actual phenotype displayed. These factors would be quite variable among different individuals and even within the same individual in different tissues. One report indicates that severity may be more similar in monozygotic than dizygotic twins (Cartwright, 1982), indicating that genetic factors other than the specific NF1 mutation may also determine the severity of phenotype, at least in part. The severity of the features progresses with age, and seems to be affected by hormonal changes such as puberty or pregnancy. Some individuals may not present with the disorder until adulthood (Riccardi and Eichner, 1986).

There has been a suggestion of a maternal effect in NF1, where the severity of the phenotype is more pronounced if inherited from the mother (Miller and Hall, 1978; Hall, 1981), although this has been disputed (Riccardi and Wald, 1987). The majority of new mutations are paternal in origin (Jadayel *et al.*, 1990; Stephens *et al.*, 1992), but it has been difficult to determine whether this is the effect of advanced paternal age on mutation frequency (Riccardi and Eichner, 1986).

2.2 POSITIONAL CLONING

The lack of reasonable candidate genes for the disorder made the NF1 gene a good prospect for positional cloning. In this scheme the gene location is determined by linkage analysis to polymorphic chromosomal markers using families segregating the disorder. The region can be further narrowed to a small interval on a given chromosome by more refined linkage. When further linkage becomes futile owing to the lack of recombinant individuals between markers, a physical (restriction) map of the region is constructed and the DNA in the region is cloned. Physical mapping is aided by somatic cell hybrids containing reduced portions of the chromosome in question. These provide landmarks for mapping during initial phases of the map when large distances are being surveyed. Any gross chromosome abnormality that is co-segregating with the disorder in a family, such as a cytogenetically visible deletion or translocation, can act as a signpost to the location of the gene and provide a shortcut to mapping efforts. This was indeed the case for NF1.

Eventually the gene is found by searching for transcripts within the region. Evolutionarily conserved regions often point to coding regions of the genome. These regions can be used as probes against Northern (RNA) blots to see if they represent expressed sequences. Probes that are conserved and expressed are used to isolate cDNAs from libraries synthesized from messenger RNA from appropriate tissues. Candidate genes must pass the mutation test, i.e. patients with the disorder must harbour mutations within the candidate gene that are never found in the normal population. In this regard the high percentage of new-mutation NF1 patients provided a convenient way to distinguish causative mutations from co-segregating polymorphisms within the gene. Any deviation from the normal sequence in a new mutation patient that is not seen in the individual's parents is quite likely to be the causative mutation.

2.3 LINKAGE ANALYSIS

Linkage analysis for NF1 was aided by two important contributions from the neurofibromatosis research and medical community. One was the establishment of diagnostic criteria for the disorder (Stumpf *et al.*, 1987). Accurate diagnosis was critical for linkage studies so that normal and affected individuals in a pedigree could be identified with certainty. The second was the establishment of national and international organizations involved in NF1 research, such as the National Neurofibromatosis Foundation in the USA, LINK (Let's Increase Neurofibromatosis Knowledge; now called the Neurofibromatosis Association) in the UK and the International Consortium for Neurofibromatosis Linkage Analysis. These organizations provided funds for research and conferences, and encouraged pooling of crucial resources such as families and probes for linkage studies.

Initial linkage analysis using restriction fragment length polymorphisms (RFLPs), although not demonstrating the chromosomal location of the NF1 gene, excluded candidate genes such as the nerve growth factor beta gene at 1p (Darby *et al.*, 1985; Spence *et al.*, 1986) and the *sis* gene on chromosome 22 (Seizinger *et al.*, 1986). Chromosome 19 was examined as a result of reports of potential co-segregation of NF1 with myotonic dystrophy (Ichikawa *et al.*, 1981; Rivas and DiLiberti, 1984), but linkage proved negative here as well (Dietz *et al.*, 1986; Huson *et al.*, 1986). A LINK sponsored conference in February 1987 resulted in the establishment of a linkage consortium for NF1 (Harper, 1987; Huson, 1987). RFLPs associated with various genes (including many oncogenes and growth factors that were considered possible candidate genes) as well as random probes were used in nine independent linkage studies (Barker *et al.*, 1987a; Diehl *et al.*, 1987a; Ferrell *et al.*, 1987; Kittur *et al.*, 1987; Mathew

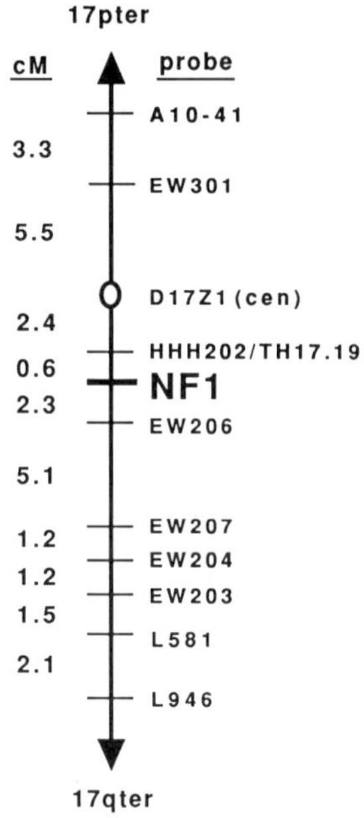

Figure 2.1 A multipoint linkage map of the *NF1* region of chromosome 17. The alpha satellite marker D17Z1 marks the position of the centromere. The order of markers shown is favoured by at least 100:1 odds over alternatives that involve exchanging a pair of markers. The genetic distances are shown in centimorgans and are sex-averaged. (Source: Goldgar *et al.*, 1989.)

et al., 1987; Pericak-Vance *et al.*, 1987a; Seizinger *et al.*, 1987a; Spence *et al.*, 1987; Upadhyaya *et al.*, 1987a). By pooling the data of the members of the consortium and previously published data, an exclusion map was generated. The chromosomes most likely to contain the NF1 locus included 5, 10, 17 or 18, with 17 being the best candidate (Sarfarazi, Huson and Edwards, 1987).

Linkage to the pericentromeric region of chromosome 17 was very soon established. Barker *et al.* (1987b) reported linkage to the centromeric alpha-satellite probe *D17Z1* as well as a second marker near the centromere. Seizinger *et al.* (1987b) found linkage to the nerve growth factor receptor (NGFR) on the long arm of chromosome 17. However, crossovers were observed between NF1 and NGFR, excluding this locus as a candidate gene. A large number of additional RFLPs were rapidly generated in the region to provide probes for more refined linkage analysis. The results of these analyses were published concurrently in December 1987 (Diehl *et al.*, 1987b; Fain *et al.*, 1987; Pericak-Vance *et al.*, 1987b; Seizinger *et al.*, 1987c; Stephens *et al.*, 1987; Upadhyaya *et al.*, 1987b; White *et al.*, 1987) along with a summary of the compiled data

(Skolnick, Ponder and Seizinger, 1987). Although flanking markers were identified for NF1, they were thought to be located on either side of the centromere. Thus it could not be established whether NF1 mapped to the long or short arm of chromosome 17. The most closely linked probe, pHHH202 (White *et al.*, 1987), showed no recombinants with NF1. Also significant was the complete lack of locus heterogeneity.

At a third meeting of the International Consortium for Neurofibromatosis Type 1 Linkage Analysis in June 1988, an exhaustive linkage map of the pericentromeric region of chromosome 17 was compiled. These results were published together early in 1989 (Diehl *et al.*, 1989; Fain *et al.*, 1989a; Kittur *et al.*, 1989; Mathew *et al.*, 1989; Seizinger *et al.*, 1989; Stephens *et al.*, 1989; Vance *et al.*, 1989; Upadhyaya *et al.*, 1989). A multipoint analysis of all the linkage data was performed involving 142 families with over 700 affected individuals using 31 pericentromeric probes and analysing a total of 13838 genotypes (Goldgar *et al.*, 1989). At this point the NF1 gene was mapped to within a 3cM interval on 17q. Flanking markers were pHHH202 on the centromeric side with one recombinant chromosome, and EW206 distally with three recombinants (Figure 2.1). It was now possible, given informative markers in the parents, to provide prenatal or presymptomatic diagnosis for individuals at risk within NF1 families.

2.4 PHYSICAL MAPPING

Concurrent with the refined linkage analysis, several groups embarked on constructing a physical map of this region of 17q. Somatic cell hybrids containing portions of human 17 were established, each with unique breakpoints along the chromosome. Establishment of hybrids containing portions of 17q was aided by the selectable thymidine kinase gene, which mapped distal to the NF1 region. One set of hybrids was established from individuals with chromosome 17 translocations not associated with NF1 (van Tuinen *et al.*, 1987). A second set of hybrids was constructed from microcell fusion of chromosome 17, tagged with a selectable neomycin resistance gene (Lugo, Leach and Fournier, 1986; Leach *et al.*, 1989). These hybrids effectively delineated the NF1 region into smaller subregions. Each breakpoint provided a position for ordering probes. In this case any probe could be mapped even if it was not polymorphic.

The panel of these reduced hybrids was useful in ordering closely linked probes in the region (Fain *et al.*, 1989b; Fountain *et al.*, 1989a; O'Connell *et al.*, 1989a). Comparison of the genetic and physical maps of probes was remarkably similar, further strengthening the assignment of position for the probes. The non-polymorphic *erb*B2 oncogene, which maps to 17q, was also excluded as a candidate gene by the mapping data.

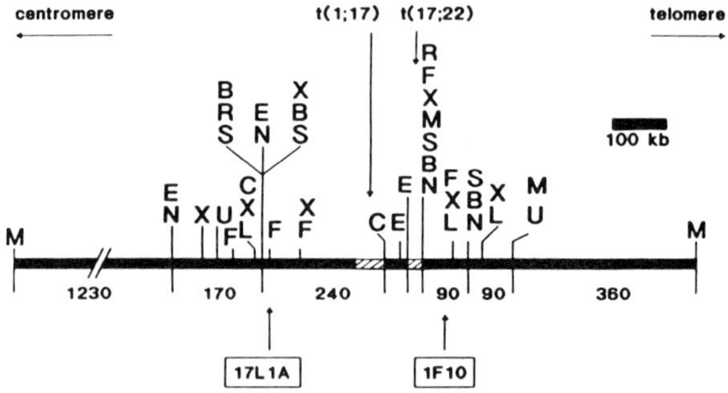

Figure 2.2 A physical map of the region around the two NF1 translocation breakpoints. 17L1A is the distal half of the NotI linking clone 17L1 (Fountain *et al.*, 1989b) and c11-1F10 is a cosmid mapping to the region (O'Connell *et al.*, 1989b). Both probes detect the translocation breakpoints, which lie within the cross-hatched region. Sizes are shown in kilobases. The key for restriction sites is: B = BssHII; C = C1aI; E = EagI; F = SfiI; L = Sa1I; M = M1uI; N = NotI; U = NruI; R = NarI; S = SacII; X = XhoI. (Modified from Fountain *et al.*, 1989b.)

The key breakthrough in the mapping and cloning of the NF1 gene was the discovery of two NF1 patients with balanced chromosome translocations involving 17q. One patient carried a balanced translocation involving 1p34.3 and 17q11.2 (Schmidt, Michels and Dewald, 1987). A second patient was subsequently discovered carrying a balanced translocation involving 17q11.2 and 22q11.2 (Ledbetter *et al.*, 1989). The fact that both patients contained breakpoints within 17q11.2, the region identified by linkage and physical mapping, suggested that the breakpoints were within the NF1 gene, and would provide a physical target for molecular cloning of the gene. Somatic cell hybrids were constructed from both patients that contained only the translocation chromosomes. The hybrid DCR-1, derived from the t(1;17), contained 17q11.2-qter as its only complement of chromosome 17 (Menon *et al.*, 1989). A similar hybrid, NF13, was constructed from the t(17;22), containing only the material distal to the breakpoint on chromosome 17 (Ledbetter *et al.*, 1989). These hybrids became useful tools in the delineation of the NF1 region and eventual cloning of the gene. Importantly, probes previously mapped centromeric to NF1 by genetic methods were proximal to the DCR-1 and NF13 breakpoints, and probes mapped telomeric to these were distal.

In order to identify precisely the translocation breakpoints on the physical map, more probes were generated in the region. A NotI linking library was constructed from flow-sorted chromosome 17 DNA with the hope of using the clones to construct a NotI restriction map of this region of the chromosome (Wallace *et al.*, 1989). One of these NotI linking clones, 17L1, was subsequently shown to lie within 300 kb to the centromeric side of the t(1;17) translocation breakpoint by detecting abnormal fragments using pulsed-field gel electrophoresis (Fountain *et al.*, 1989b). A large number of cosmid clones generated from microcell hybrids were also mapped to the region to generate probes for the NF1 gene (O'Connell *et al.*, 1989a). One of these, c11-1F10, was also shown to detect both the t(1;17) and t(17;22) breakpoints from the telomeric side using pulsed-field gel electrophoresis (O'Connell *et al.*, 1989b). Since both probes were mapped to a 600 kb NruI genomic fragment, the region containing the NF1 gene was narrowed considerably. Furthermore, the distance between the two translocation breakpoints was estimated to be about 60 kb (Figure 2.2).

2.5 CANDIDATE GENES

With the NF1 region narrowed, a systematic search was initiated for transcripts arising from this rather small genomic region. The assumption was made that the NF1 gene was interrupted by both breakpoints and therefore must be a relatively large gene. Since it was unclear how far the gene might extend in either direction, the safest course to follow was to concentrate on the region between the breakpoints.

The first candidate gene isolated from the positional cloning strategy was the result of a serendipitous discovery. The human homologue of the mouse *Evi-2A* gene (Buchberg *et al.*, 1988), associated with esotropic viral insertions and implicated in retrovirus-induced murine myeloid tumours, was mapped to the region between the t(1;17) and t(17;22) breakpoints (O'Connell *et al.*, 1990). The human *EV12A* gene was shown to be expressed in brain, blood and bone marrow, although its function remains unknown (Cawthon *et al.*, 1990b). The gene did not cross either of the breakpoints, so that, if it was the NF1 gene, the breakpoints were causing a position effect on its expression. However, no mutations were found in this gene in other NF1 patients, ruling it out as the gene responsible for NF1.

A second gene, *EVI2B*, was subsequently found by walking between the NF1 breakpoints (Cawthon *et al.*, 1990b, 1991). This locus also has a mouse homologue, which may be associated with esotropic retroviral insertions. This gene of unknown function is similar to *EVI2A* in its size, general structure and expression, although it is not found expressed in brain. However, this gene also failed to show mutations in NF1 patients.

A third gene was subsequently cloned in the region and found to lie within the breakpoint regions. The oligodendrocyte-myelin glycoprotein (*OMGP*) gene had previously been described (Mikol *et al.*, 1990), but was later independently isolated as a candidate gene within the NF1 region (Viskochil *et al.*, 1991). The OMGP has been postulated to be a cell adhesion molecule in myelin of the nerve sheath, and is expressed only in oligodendrocytes and Schwann cells. Although this biological function strengthened its promise as a candidate gene, again no mutations in this gene were found in NF1 patients.

Subsequent analysis showed that these three genes are embedded within one large intron (greater than 40 kb) of the true NF1 gene and transcribed from the opposite strand (Xu *et al.*, 1990a). It is possible that transcription of *NF1* and the embedded genes may be mutually exclusive in any given cell. This may be due to steric hindrance of RNA polymerase as proposed by Wallace *et al.* (1990b). A second possibility is that transcription could be affected by an imprinting effect, where the *NF1* gene and the embedded genes are transcribed from opposite chromosome homologues. The parental origin of the transcribed homologue may vary during development and from tissue to tissue, and may contribute to the variable phenotypes seen in the disorder. It is also possible that the embedded genes play some role in the pathogenesis of NF1. Loss of *NF1* transcription may promote abnormal expression or overexpression of the embedded genes by the loss of antisense nuclear RNA. It is intriguing that the mouse homologues to *EVI2A* and *EVI2B* are implicated in myeloid tumours in mice, though the mechanism remains to be clarified. This may have some bearing on the slightly elevated risk of juvenile myeloid leukaemia in NF1 patients (Clark and Hutter, 1982).

2.6 THE NF1 GENE

The fourth candidate gene cloned was the authentic NF1 gene (Cawthon *et al.*, 1990a; Viskochil *et al.*, 1990; Wallace *et al.*, 1990a) (Figures 2.2 and 2.3). Probes used in the isolation of the gene came from three different sources. An evolutionarily conserved genomic fragment mapping distal to the t(17;22) breakpoint was isolated from a cosmid contig extending through the breakpoint region (Cawthon *et al.*, 1990a; Viskochil *et al.*, 1990). A second probe came from a conserved fragment subcloned from the end of a chromosome jump clone that began within the breakpoint region and ended distal to the t(17;22) breakpoint (Wallace *et al.*, 1990a,b). An entire yeast artificial chromosome (YAC) encompassing the region between the translocation breakpoints and extending over 100 kb toward the telomere was also used as a probe (Wallace *et al.*, 1990a; Marchuk *et al.*, 1992). Each of these probes identified cDNAs that were part of a large gene interrupted by the two translocation breakpoints.

Initial reports on mutations within the gene have described large deletions (Upadhyaya *et al.*, 1990; Viskochil *et al.*, 1990; Kayes *et al.*, 1992), point mutations, including nonsense mutations (Cawthon *et al.*, 1990a; Estivill *et al.*, 1991; Upadhyaya *et al.*, 1992), and a *de novo* insertion in a new mutation patient (Wallace *et al.*, 1990a). This insertion has subsequently been shown to be an *Alu* repetitive element lying within an intron that causes an exon to be skipped during splicing. The resulting aberrantly

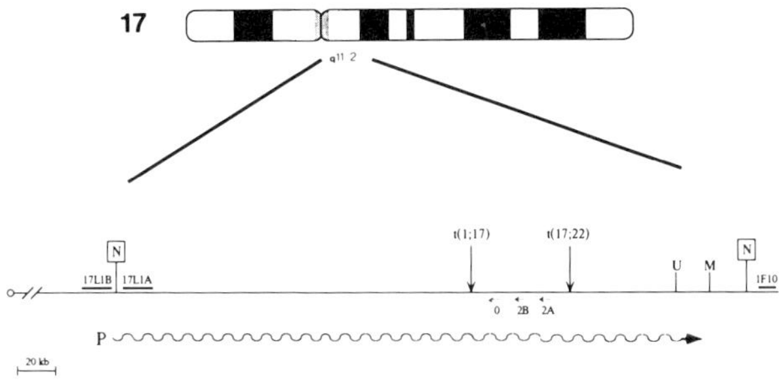

Figure 2.3 Extent of the *NF1* transcript on the genomic map of chromosome 17. Shown above is a schematic diagram of chromosome 17. Below is an enlargement of the region of 17q11.2 containing the NF1 gene. The code for restriction sites is N for NotI, U for NruI and M for MluI. The boxed sites represent the positions of undermethylated CpG islands in genomic DNA. The 5′ end of the transcript begins in the centromeric half of the NotI linking clone 17L1B (Fountain *et al.*, 1989a,b; Wallace *et al.*, 1989). It extends through the position of a t(1; 17) NF1 translocation breakpoint (Fountain *et al.*, 1989b; O'Connell *et al.*, 1989) and beyond the position of a t(17; 22) NF1 translocation breakpoint (O'Connell *et al.*, 1989). The transcript ends within the region bordered by the NruI and MluI sites. The gene therefore extends between 270 and 310 kb. Three other transcripts are embedded within a single intron and are transcribed off the complementary strand (Xu *et al.*, 1990). The three genes are *EVI2A* (Cawthon *et al.*, 1990b; O'Connell *et al.*, 1990), *EVI2B* (Cawthon *et al.*, 1991) and *OMGP* (Mikol *et al.*, 1990; Viskochil *et al.*, 1991).

spliced transcript causes a frameshift resulting in a premature termination codon (Wallace *et al.*, 1991). These mutation results confirm that the *NF1* gene has been cloned and suggest a loss of function of the gene product as the causative mutation. Further evidence for the inactivation hypothesis came from expression studies of the *NF1* transcript in somatic cell hybrids. The gene was shown to be expressed from a normal human chromosome 17 in a rodent–human hybrid cell line, but not in somatic cell hybrids containing the t(1;17) and t(17;22) translocation chromosomes. These observations are consistent with *NF1* acting as a tumour suppressor gene (Knudson, 1971, 1985), suggesting that the mechanism of action is actually recessive at the cellular level.

The *NF1* transcript is estimated to be 11–13 kb by its migration on a Northern blot (Wallace *et al.*, 1990a). Over 9 kb of this message has been cloned and sequenced, which includes the entire coding region (Marchuk *et al.*, 1991). Primer extension results (Marchuk *et al.*, 1991) indicate that most of the uncloned sequence from this transcript must arise from a long (approximately 4 kb) 3′ untranslated region. Alternatively, estimates of transcript size may be incorrect, as size estimates in this range of Northern blotting are difficult. The *NF1* gene was found to be expressed in all tissues examined by RNA-polymerase chain reaction (RNA-PCR) and is therefore judged to be ubiquitously expressed (Wallace *et al.*, 1990).

The size of the *NF1* gene has been determined by mapping cDNA clones back to a YAC contig that spans over 600 kb surrounding the gene (Marchuk *et al.*, 1992). The gene is almost entirely contained within the approximately 300 kb genomic NotI fragment identified by the 17L1A half-linking clone. The 5′ end is just centromeric to the NotI site, within the first 500 bp of half-linking clone 17L1B. More refined mapping of the cDNA against the YAC contig shows that the gene extends toward the telomere a minimum of 270 kb, with a maximum gene size of 310 kb. These estimates are based on rare cutting restriction sites that cut in the unmethylated YAC clones but not in native genomic DNA. The gene contains approximately 50 exons (R. White, personal communication).

The large *NF1* transcript and 300 kb gene size represent a large target for mutations. Since the NF1 phenotype results from loss of function mutations, causative mutations may be dispersed throughout the coding and regulatory region. In the patients surveyed thus far, this seems to be the case (Cawthon *et al.*, 1990a; Wallace *et al.*, 1990a; R. Cawthon, personal communication; Wallace *et al.*, unpublished observations). The size of the gene alone, however, cannot fully account for the high mutation rate, since its transcript is only of the order of 10 times larger than that of an average gene. Therefore other factors must be involved. There are presently not enough mutation data to determine whether there are highly mutable or unstable regions within the gene. Some of the mutations may be due to gene conversion events from non-processed pseudogenes mapping to other chromosomes. NF1 pseudogenes have been located on chromosomes 2, 20 and 21 (Cummings and Marchuk, unpublished observations), 15 (Legius *et al.*, 1992) as well as 14 and 22 (Marchuk *et al.*, 1992). The pseudogenes may potentially act as a reservoir of mutation that can be crossed into the *NF1* locus, thereby increasing the mutation rate, but this has yet to be demonstrated.

2.7 THE *NF1* GENE PRODUCT

Initial partial sequences of the 3′ end of the *NF1* gene (Cawthon *et al.*, 1990s; Wallace *et al.*, 1990a) revealed very little in the way of sequence homologies that could provide a clue to the function of the gene product. Further cloning and sequence analysis (Buchberg *et al.*, 1990; Xu *et al.*, 1990a) revealed a region of approximately 30% homology with the mammalian GTPase activating protein (GAP) (Trahey and McCormick, 1987; Trahey *et al.*, 1988; Vogel *et al.*, 1988) and yeast *IRA1* and *IRA2* (inhibitory regulators of the *RAS*-cAMP pathway) gene products (Tanaka *et al.*, 1989, 1990, 1991). These proteins accelerate the rate at which the p21 *ras* protein hydrolyses GTP to become inactive *ras*-GDP (Figure 2.4). This

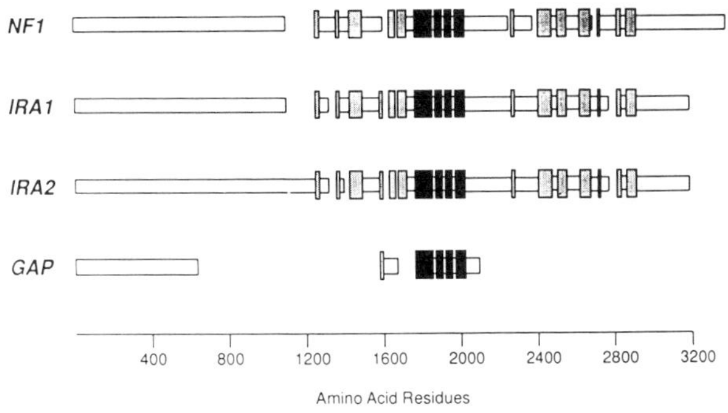

Figure 2.4 Sequence domains and motifs among *NF1*-related proteins. Unfilled rectangles indicate regions with little or no sequence conservation. Blank spaces between rectangles signify gaps introduced to align the sequences. The stippled boxes represent regions homologous in only three of the proteins. The black boxes show the regions conserved in all four members and taken together represent the GTPase activating (GAP-related) domain. (Source: Ballester *et al.*, 1990.)

provided the first glimpse of the function of *NF1*; like GAP, it may be an upstream regulatory protein for *ras* (or a *ras*-related protein) and its normal function may be to down-regulate one or more members of the *ras* family involved in mitogenic signal transduction. Loss of *NF1* function might therefore keep *ras* continually in an active (GTP-bound) state, resulting in unrestrained mitogenic signalling (Figure 2.5).

This model received further support when it was shown that the proposed GAP-related-domain of *NF1* (*NF1*-GRD) was functionally related to both mammalian GAP and the yeast *IRA* gene products *in vivo* and *in vitro*. The *NF1*-GRD expressed in yeast has been shown to promote hydrolysis of GTP by *ras* expressed in yeast (Ballester *et al.*, 1990; Xu *et al.*, 1990b). Interestingly, this domain was unable to down-regulate the yeast *RAS2*$^{\text{val-19}}$ mutant, which is analogous to the human oncogenic H-*ras*$^{\text{val-12}}$ (Ballester *et al.*, 1990). The *NF1*-GRD has been expressed in a baculovirus–insect cell expression system, and was shown to interact with *ras* to promote hydrolysis of GTP to GDP *in vitro* (Martin *et al.*, 1990). Finally, it has been demonstrated that the *NF1*-GRD expressed in yeast can complement the phenotype due to *ira1* and *ira2* mutations (Ballester *et al.*, 1990; Martin *et al.*, 1990; Xu *et al.*, 1990).

GTPase stimulation of *ras* by the *NF1*-GRD has been shown to be inhibited by certain lipids produced in response to mitogenic stimulation (Bollag and McCormick, 1991; Golubić *et al.*, 1992; Han *et al.*, 1991). Phosphatidate, arachidonate and phosphatidylinositol 4,5 bisphosphate were shown to inhibit GTPase activity of *ras* coincubated with the *NF1*-GRD in an *in vitro* assay, whereas phosphatidylcholine, arachidate and diacylglycerol had no effect. Inhibition by the detergent n-dodecyl

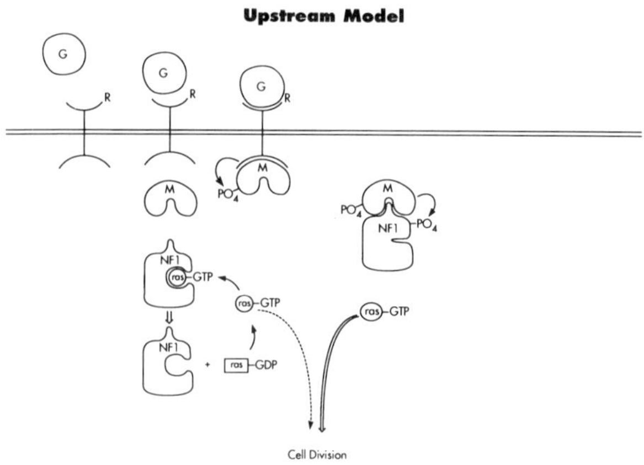

Figure 2.5 An upstream model of *NF1* function. In this model the *NF1* protein exerts its effect primarily on *ras* to accelerate GTP hydrolysis and thus inactivate *ras*. A growth factor (G) (possibly nerve growth factor) binds to its receptor (R) on the cell surface to promote an intracellular phosphorylation of an intermediate protein (M, possibly a member of the *ERK* family). This intermediate in turn will phosphorylate the *NF1* protein at threonine and serine residues to inactivate the GTPase-promoting function of *NF1*. Therefore *ras* will remain in the active (GTP-bound) state and cell division will occur. When *NF1* is not phosphorylated, it promotes hydrolysis of GTP by *ras* and cell division is blocked.

beta-D maltoside can be used to discriminate between the contributions of GAP and *NF1* upon *ras* GTP hydrolysis, and this assay has been used to estimate the relative contributions of *NF1* to total GAP activity in a variety of tissues (Bollag and McCormick, 1991). Significantly, the rat phaeochromocytoma cell line PC12 shows predominantly *NF1* GAP activity. This cell line has been shown to differentiate in response to activated *ras* (see below).

An alternative model of *ras–NF1* interaction postulates that *NF1* may instead (or in addition) be a downstream effector (target) for *ras* (Figure 2.6). A downstream model has also been proposed for the related GAP, with support from the following observations. Mutations in the putative *ras* effector domain (the region of *ras* thought to interact with its target during signal transduction) inactivate the transformation ability of *ras* and block GTPase activation by GAP, yet retain guanine nucleotide binding capacity (Adari *et al.*, 1988; Cales *et al.*, 1988). Second, GAP binds to oncogenic *ras* mutants but does not activate GTP hydrolysis (Vogel *et al.*, 1988). Third, GAP is required for *ras* to inhibit G-protein activation of atrial potassium channels (Yatani *et al.*, 1990). These results taken together suggest that proper signal transduction requires that GAP bind to the effector domain of *ras* (irrespective of GTP hydrolysis) and therefore GAP may be a target of activated *ras*. *NF1*-GRD interactions with effector and oncogenic mutants of *ras* have shown results similar to GAP, suggesting that the *NF1* protein may also interact with p21 *ras* through its effector domain and be a target of activated *ras*. The *NF1*-GRD binds very poorly to an effector domain mutant of H-*ras* in a competitive inhibition binding assay (Martin *et al.*, 1990). It binds very tightly to oncogenic and effector mutants of *ras*, yet has no effect on GTPase activity (Xu *et al.*, 1990b; Bollag and McCormick, 1991). It should be cautioned, however, that these studies were not undertaken with the full-length *NF1* protein.

None the less, the downstream effector model is attractive for its ability to account for the role of *ras* in certain cells of neuroectodermal origin. In the rat phaeochromocytoma cell line PC12, activated *ras* induces differentiation and blocks proliferation (Bar-Sagi and Feramisco, 1985; Noda *et al.*, 1985). Inhibition of *ras* in these cells blocks neural differentiation normally induced by nerve growth factor (Hagag *et al.*, 1986; Szeberenyi *et al.*, 1990). Activated *ras* has also been shown to induce cell cycle arrest when introduced into rat Schwann cells (Ridley *et al.*, 1988). This is significant because Schwann cells may be the original cells that recruit other cell types in the formation of neurofibromas and neurofibrosarcomas (Ratner *et al.*, 1990; Sheela *et al.*, 1990). Therefore, if *NF1* is the target (effector) of *ras*, then loss of *NF1* function could lead to a block of normal differentiation resulting in unrestrained proliferation of Schwann cells.

At first glance it may seem contradictory for *NF1* to be both a downstream effector and negative regulator of *ras*. The interaction of the two, however, may be analogous to the interaction with a growth factor and its receptor: after the signal is sent downstream, the receptor is desensitized. This may be due to a GDP/GTP exchange reaction, limiting signal transduction to a single interaction between *ras*-GTP and *NF1*. Here, *NF1* would simultaneously send a downstream signal and downregulate the input signal. A similar model has been proposed for GAP-*ras* interactions (McCormick, 1989).

Either of these two models, with *NF1* as the upstream negative regulator or downstream effector, are consistent with *NF1* being a tumour suppressor gene, where the phenotype results from the loss of both alleles of the gene (Knudson, 1971, 1985). Early studies of NF1 tumours did not show a consistent loss of heterozygosity for *NF1* in 17q11.2 (Skuse *et al.*, 1989; Menon *et al.*, 1990; Glover *et al.*, 1991), but these interpretations were made difficult by frequent losses on 17p, apparently reflecting the major role that loss of the p53 gene plays in tumour progression in this disorder (Nigro *et al.*, 1989; Menon *et al.*, 1990). More recent analyses have indicated that loss of heterozygosity involving only 17q can be demonstrated at least for some tumours. Skuse *et al.* (1990) observed a loss of heterozygosity for 13 out of 17 NF1 tumours analysed,

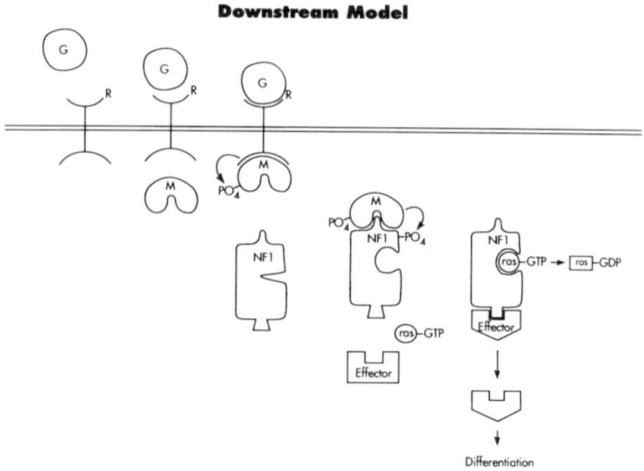

Figure 2.6 A downstream model of *NF1* function. In this model the *NF1* protein acts both to promote hydrolysis of GTP by *ras* and to receive the signal from activated *ras* to promote differentiation. Here a growth factor (G) (again possibly nerve growth factor) binds to its receptor (R) on the cell surface to promote phosphorylation of an intermediate protein (M). This intermediate in turn phosphorylates the *NF1* protein to convert it into an active conformation. The *ras*–GTP–*NF1* complex then interacts with an effector to continue the signal transduction pathway leading to differentiation. When *NF1* is not phosphorylated it remains unable to deactivate *ras* and cell division occurs.

with no complicating loss on the short arm of chromosome 17. In addition, Xu *et al.* (1992) have demonstrated loss of heterozygosity for markers surrounding the *NF1* locus in 7 NF1-associated phaeochromocytomas. In the three for which phase could be determined, the loss involved the wild-type chromosome. In those tumours not showing loss of heterozygosity, the mutation in the second allele may be an independently acquired mutation. Since the germline mutation rate for NF1 is so high, the somatic rate may also be elevated, so that for this particular locus mechanisms leading to the loss of heterozygosity (loss and reduplication, mitotic crossing over) are less common than independent second mutations. In addition, one neurofibrosarcoma has been analysed showing homozygous deletions of portions of the NF1 gene (Legius *et al.*, 1993). These results taken together provide molecular evidence for the tumour suppressor model of *NF1* action.

The evidence that the *NF1* gene is a tumour suppressor gene is strengthened by an unusual chromosomal aberration found in a sporadic case of NF1 (Andersen *et al.*, 1990). A karyotype from this mildly affected patient showed the formation of a minichromosome by excision of the proximal region of 17q, which was lost in about 6% of somatic cells grown in culture. With one allele lost in a fraction of the somatic cells, this patient effectively became hemizygous in those cells for the *NF1* gene. Subsequent somatic mutations could account for the second mutation and development of neurofibromas.

It is also possible that the second hit mutation may not be within the *NF1* gene. Mutations within other genes involved in the pathway toward development of benign neurofibromas may be in other as yet undefined loci. This model requires that a gene dosage of one-half is sufficient to create an abnormal phenotype. In order to determine whether this is the case it is important to establish whether neurofibromas are clonal. Studies on the fibroblasts from neurofibromas from females heterozygous for an X-chromosome-encoded biochemical marker indicated that the cells were non-clonal (Fialkow *et al.*, 1971). However, this study was potentially flawed by assaying a mixture of cell types from the benign tumour rather than the Schwann cells. The other cell types, including fibroblasts, may be recruited by the abnormal Schwann cells (Sheela *et al.*, 1990). A more recent study using a DNA probe that is subject to X-chromosome inactivation showed that neurofibromas may indeed be clonal (Skuse *et al.*, 1991). Neurofibromas from eight females that were heterozygous for an RFLP detected by a phosphoglycerokinase (PGK) probe showed methylation of only one allele, suggesting that the neurofibroma arose via clonal expansion of a single cell. However, the malignant neurofibrosarcomas may still require both *NF1* alleles to be inactivated. A primary neurofibrosarcoma and metastases from the same female NF1 patient showed a probable clonal origin of the tumour in a clonality assay using an X-chromosome-encoded biochemical marker (Friedman *et al.*, 1982).

The identification of the *NF1* gene product (DeClue *et al.*, 1991; Gutmann *et al.*, 1991), now named neurofibromin, has enabled further dissection of the role of the gene product in the development of malignancy. Antibodies raised against the GAP-related domain as well as peptides throughout the protein have revealed a high-molecular-weight, predominantly cytoplasmic protein with an apparent molecular mass (Mr) of 235–280 kDa. The highest level of expression of neurofibromin is seen in tissues of the nervous system. Antibodies to neurofibromin label neurons, oligodendrocytes and non-myelinating Schwann cells but not astrocytes or myelinating Schwann cells (Daston *et al.*, 1992). Neurofibromin was undetectable or detected at only low levels in spleen, skeletal muscle, thymus, kidney, liver, heart and skin (Daston *et al.*, 1992; Hattori *et al.*, 1992). It is unclear how this highly restricted distribution of neurofibromin relates to the nearly ubiquitous expression of its message (Buchberg *et al.*, 1990; Wallace *et al.*, 1990). One possibility is that the presence of *NF1* transcript detected by RNA-PCR reflects low-level contamination of nerve or other tissue within the samples. However, cell lines purified by multiple passages of growth *in vitro* still show expression of the transcript. This might be explained by up-regulation of the message during growth *in vitro*.

Neurofibrosarcomas and cell lines derived from tumours of NF1 patients have shown greatly reduced to undetectable levels of neurofibromin on Western blots and by immunoprecipitation (Basu *et al.*, 1992; DeClue *et al.*, 1992). The level of total GAP activity in these cells is also greatly reduced, resulting in elevated levels of *ras*-bound GTP. These results lend further support for the tumour suppressor model of *NF1* action.

The increased rate of malignancy of a number of tissues in NF1 patients raises the question of the role of the *NF1* gene in sporadic cancers. Li *et al.* (1992) have discovered mis-sense mutations in the *NF1* gene in three sporadic tumour types: colon adenocarcinoma, myelodysplastic syndrome and anaplastic astrocytoma. These mutations affect codon number 1423, which is an invariant lysine residue within the GAP-related domain of the GAP family (Wang *et al.*, 1991). A mutation at the same codon has also been described as the germline mutation in an NF1 patient (Li *et al.*, 1992). *In vitro* assays of the amino acid substitutions inserted within the GAP-related domain showed a 200–400 fold decrease in GAP activity, although binding affinity was unaffected. Independent analysis of mutations at this residue indicate that the mutant protein may be unstable (Wiesmuller and Wittinghofer, 1992). Recent investigation of melanoma cell lines (Andersen *et al.*, 1993a) has uncovered frequent abnormalities of *NF1* expression including one case of homozygous deletion of part of the gene. Low or undetectable neurofibromin levels were demonstrated in four of 10 neuroblastoma cell lines, and two of these lines showed evidence of partial deletion of the *NF1* locus (The *et al.*, 1993). Thus NF1 joins the retinoblastoma gene (Weichselbaum, Beckett and Diamond, 1988), the p53 gene (Nigro *et al.*, 1989), which is associated with the heritable Li-Fraumeni syndrome (Malkin *et al.*, 1990), and the APC gene (Nishisho *et al.*, 1991; Powell *et al.*, 1992) responsible for familial adenomatous polyposis, as genes that play a role in the development of both heritable and sporadic cancer. Given the ubiquitous expression of the *NF1* gene and its potential role in a signal transduction pathway involving *ras*, this is not surprising. In addition, there is evidence that NF1 patients show a higher risk than the general population for certain leukaemias and neuronal tumours (Bader, 1986; Sorensen *et al.*, 1986; Georg *et al.*, 1989; Lefkowitz, Obringer and Meadows, 1990) (see also Chapter 12). The contribution of *NF1* mutations to these and other sporadic tumours remains to be determined.

The complete amino acid sequence of the primary *NF1* gene product has been determined (Marchuk *et al.*, 1991). The protein consists of 2818 amino acids with a calculated molecular weight of 327 kDa. Estimates of the size of the protein on Western blots are in the range of 250 kDa

(Gutmann *et al.*, 1991). This discrepancy may be due to processing of the protein or may be an artefact due to protein folding or the difficulty of making an accurate molecular weight estimate in this size range. Within the GAP-related domain are four blocks of homology highly conserved between the GAP family of proteins (Figure 2.4; Wang *et al.*, 1991). Invariant amino acid residues within these blocks may provide important information on the structure–function relationship of the protein sequence. Mutations within some of these residues have been shown to inhibit GAP activity of the *NF1*-GRD in a yeast *ira1* complementation assay (Gutmann *et al.*, 1993). The sequence shows no significant homology to the *Bcr*-related GAP family, which includes n-chimaerin, and GAP^{rho} (Diekmann *et al.*, 1991) and possibly the p85 of bovine brain phosphatidylinositol 3-kinase (Otsu *et al.*, 1991). There is also no homology to *rap*1GAP (Rubinfeld *et al.*, 1991).

The complete sequence of the *NF1* protein product has provided few additional clues to its function. The protein shows no apparent membrane spanning region, and is predicted to be cytosolic by discriminant analysis (Marchuk *et al.*, 1991). Fluorescent *in situ* hybridization using antibodies to the *NF1* protein shows staining predominantly in the cytoplasm, which in some cases seem to resemble the pattern of microtubule staining (Gregory *et al.*, 1993). Other studies indicate that the pattern of neurofibromin staining suggests an association with elements of the endoplasmic reticulum (Golubić *et al.*, 1992). There are no SH2 or SH3 domains (*src* homology domains), which are present in GAP (Koch *et al.*, 1991). These domains are homologous to non-catalytic regions of the oncogene *src* and may direct interactions with phosphotyrosine proteins involved in signal transduction (Koch *et al.*, 1991). Their absence in *NF1* implies that *NF1* and GAP are not interchangeable in the cell, and that *NF1* is probably not directly modulated through tyrosine phosphorylation by activated growth factor receptors. Immunoprecipitated *NF1* shows no evidence of tyrosine phosphorylation, but is phosphorylated on serine and threonine residues. Phosphorylation increases in response to treatment with various mitogens including activators of protein kinase C (Basu *et al.*, 1992; Boyer *et al.*, 1993). Phosphorylation at these sites may mean that an intermediate between the activated tyrosine kinase receptor and *NF1* modulates *NF1* activity. A potential candidate for this intermediate could be one of the microtubule-associated ERK family, which are activated by tyrosine phosphorylation by nerve growth factor and are themselves serine/threonine protein kinases (Boulton *et al.*, 1991).

Certainly, the large size of the *NF1* product in relation to the small portion conferring GAP activity indicates that other domains may be involved in modulating the *ras*-GTPase activity of this protein, or carrying out entirely different functions. The sequence homology with yeast *IRA1* and especially *IRA2* extends beyond the GAP catalytic domain toward both termini, with strong homology in the carboxy terminus. There may therefore be more extensive functional homology with these members of the GAP family than with GAP itself. It may be useful to think of the *NF1* product as consisting of three domains: an amino-terminus of unknown function, a GAP-related middle domain and a carboxy-terminus related to the *IRA1* and *IRA2* gene products. Unfortunately, the functions of these domains of the *IRA* gene products are not known even in this simple eukaryote. For *NF1*, these undefined regions may be responsible for interaction with other factors in the pathway leading to differentiation, such as the low-affinity NGFR and the *trk* oncogene product, or factors such as ERK that may mediate between these and *NF1*. Interactions at these other domains may also ultimately provide a clue as to the reasons why a mutation in a ubiquitously expressed gene reveals its character predominantly in cells derived from the embryonic neural crest.

Two alternatively processed forms of this primary transcript have been discovered. One is a 54bp insertion coding for an additional 18 amino acids near the 3′ end of the transcript (Xu *et al.*, 1990a). A 63bp insertion coding for an additional 21 amino acids within one of the most conserved regions of the GAP-related domain has also been discovered (Nisha *et al.*, 1991; Andersen *et al.*, 1993a). The insertion of these mostly basic amino acids completely abolished the homology of the subdomain, but the *NF1*-GRD containing this insertion still retains GTPase activity (Andersen *et al.*, 1993a). It is presently unknown how the alternatively spliced transcripts are regulated, and there has not yet been an exhaustive search of the tissues where each of these transcripts can be found. At least in some tissues their expression is not mutually exclusive (Andersen *et al.*, 1993a). These alternative forms may also play a role in the diverse clinical manifestations of the disorder. Germline mutations in some of the alternatively spliced exons may produce some of the more unusual NF1 phenotypes. In support of this, 13 of 16 primary brain tumours expressed the 63bp insert whereas normal brain did not (Suzuki *et al.*, 1991).

2.8 ANIMAL MODELS OF NF1

The development of an animal model for NF1 has a high priority, since such a model would allow clear understanding of the pathogenesis of the disease and an ideal system with which to test new treatments. With the cloning of the NF1 gene, the demonstration that most germline mutations involve inactivation of the gene and that the mouse NF1 locus is homologous to the human, the possibility of creating a mouse model by homologous recombination in embryonic stem cells was immediately raised. Using this approach, Tyler Jacks, Robert Weinberg and colleagues were able successfully to target the mouse NF1 locus, using a construct that inserted into the mouse homolog of human exon 31. Chimeric animals were produced and bred, and germline incorporation was demonstrated. Heterozygotes (*nf*/–) have demonstrated no apparent abnormal phenotype up to 1 year of age, which is somewhat disappointing. Careful examination, including a search for Lisch nodules, skin spotting or any evidence of tumour formation, has not yielded any compatible features. Researchers are now exposing these animals to mutagens on the chance that an increased rate of somatic mutation may bring out the phenotype in these *nf*/– animals.

Heterozygotes were bred together to investigate the phenotype of a homozygous knockout. Genotyping live born mice indicated a complete deficiency of –/– mice, suggesting that this genotype caused death at the embryonic stage. More careful investigation has demonstrated that the –/– animals developed essentially normally until about day 12 of embryogenesis, when they became oedematous and pale, and died by day 13.5. Pathologic examination of these animals indicates normal formation of the central and peripheral nervous systems, which is rather surprising in the complete absence of neurofibromin. However, there appears to be a defect of the heart and major vessels, leading to massive pericardial effusion, cardiac failure and death.

It will be of interest to breed the heterozygous mutation into a variety of other mouse strains to see whether a phenotype will emerge. There is a precedent for such a situation, namely the *min* mouse, which develops multiple intestinal neoplasms and has a mutation in the gene homologous to the human familial polyposis (APC) locus (Luongo *et al.*, 1993). The number of tumours developed in a given mouse depends on the strain background, being few or even absent in some strains. Recently, this information has been used to map a major locus responsible for modifying severity. Were this to be possible using the *nf*/– mouse system, much could be potentially learned about other loci that modify severity.

2.9 PROSPECTS FOR DIAGNOSIS AND THERAPY

The cloning of the NF1 gene brought hope that routine prenatal and presymptomatic diagnosis would soon be possible. Before this, diagnosis was limited to families with NF1 where parents were informative for linked markers (Ward *et al.*, 1990; Hoffman and Boehm, 1992). If one or a few mutations were responsible for the majority of NF1 mutations, it would be possible to screen for mutations regardless of family history, even in potential new mutation patients. However, the large size of the gene and transcript, coupled with the seeming wide variety of possible mutations, makes this prospect less likely. A number of polymorphisms within the NF1 gene have been discovered (Andersen *et al.*, 1991; Watkins *et al.*, 1991; Xu *et al.*, 1991). Undoubtedly more will be discovered, including simple sequence repeats that can be analysed by PCR (Andersen *et al.*, 1993b). These will potentially be useful for more accurate diagnosis using linkage analysis in families showing a history of NF1. However, given the high mutation rate and frequency of new mutation patients, this approach will not be useful in most cases. Direct DNA mutation detection will eventually be feasible for clinical purposes, but probably not for a few years given the large size of the gene.

One potential use of presymptomatic diagnosis might be the prediction of the severity of the disorder. However, the phenotype is so variable within a nuclear family, it is unclear whether the outcome of a given mutation can be predicted in most situations, which will greatly hamper genetic counselling. As more mutations are discovered and catalogued, this question can be addressed.

Although DNA diagnosis for clinical application may be slow in coming, other avenues are available that may be more fruitful. It may be possible to develop a protein assay based on Western (protein) blot analysis, to determine whether an abnormal protein product is made. This would potentially identify gross rearrangements of the gene as well as nonsense mutations that produce a truncated protein product. It is likely, however, that many of the altered neurofibromin products would be unstable in the cell and not appear as an abnormally sized band on a Western blot.

Perhaps a more promising avenue is the prospect for developing a biochemical assay for neurofibromin. These assays can often be more easily quantitated and may be capable of detecting reduced dosages of functional gene product in the heterozygous state. One biochemical assay already exists for neurofibromin, namely, the acceleration of GTP hydrolysis by *ras* in an *in vitro* system. It remains to be determined whether this assay will identify the majority of NF1 mutations. It is likely that as more information concerning neurofibromin accumulates, other assays can be developed that will be widely useful.

It is too early to predict the outcome of cloning the NF1 gene on therapy. Prospects for gene therapy for a heritable disorder affecting such a broad range of tissues may be very dim for the foreseeable future, as an effective therapy would require close to 100% efficiency of gene delivery. However, more conventional therapies may be worth pursuing. The discovery of the link between *NF1* and *ras* has brought NF1 research into a very active field of study. New chemotherapeutic agents are under development that interfere with *ras* C-terminal processing (Gibbs, 1991). These may someday prove useful for NF1 patients. As more is learned about the role of neurofibromin in the cell, other approaches may be discovered for therapy and an eventual cure for the disorder.

ACKNOWLEDGEMENTS

We gratefully acknowledge the many contributions of Drs Margaret Wallace, Lone Andersen, David Gutmann, Susan Wilson-Gunn and Paula Gregory, as well as other members of the NF1 research team of the Collins laboratory. We are grateful to our colleagues who have shared information with us prior to publication. Support for our research has been provided by the Howard Hughes Medical Institute, and the National Institutes of Health grant numbers NS23410 (FSC) and HG00018 (DAM).

REFERENCES

Adari, H. *et al.* (1988) Guanosine triphosphate activating protein (GAP) interacts with the p21 *ras* effector binding domain. *Science*, **240**, 518–21.

Andersen, L.B. *et al.* (1990) Formation of a minichromosome by excision of the proximal region of 17q in a patient with von Recklinghausen neurofibromatosis. *Cytogenet. Cell Genet.*, **53**, 206–10.

Andersen, L.B. *et al.* (1991) A highly polymorphic cDNA probe in the *NF1* gene. *Nucleic Acids Res.*, **19**, 197.

Andersen, L.B. *et al.* (1993a) A conserved alternative splice in the von Recklinghausen neurofibromatosis (*NF1*) gene produces two neurofibromin isoforms, both with GAP activity. *Mol. Cell Biol.*, **13**, 487–95.

Andersen, L.B. *et al.* (1993b) A compound nucleotide repeat in the neurofibromatosis (*NF1*) gene. *Hum. Mol. Genet.*, **2**, 1083.

Bader, J.L. (1986) Neurofibromatosis and cancer, *Ann. N.Y. Acad. Sci.*, **486**, 57–65.

Ballester, R. *et al.* (1990) The *NF1* locus encodes a protein functionally related to mammalian GAP and yeast *IRA* proteins. *Cell*, **63**, 851–9.

Barker, D. *et al.* (1987a) A genomic search for linkage of neurofibromatosis to RFLPs. *J. Med. Genet.*, **24**, 536–8.

Barker, D. *et al.* (1987b) Gene for von Recklinghausen neurofibromatosis is in the pericentromeric region of chromosome 17. *Science*, **236**, 1100–2.

Bar-Sagi, D. and Feramisco, J. (1985) Microinjection of the *ras* oncogene protein into PC12 cells induces morphological differentiation. *Cell*, **42**, 841–8.

Basu, T.N. *et al.* (1992) Aberrant regulation of *ras* proteins in malignant tumor cells from type 1 neurofibromatosis patients. *Nature*, **356**, 713–15.

Bollag, G. and McCormick, F. (1991) Differential regulation of *ras*-GAP and neurofibromatosis gene product activities. *Nature*, **351**, 576–9.

Borberg, A. (1951) Clinical and genetic investigations into tuberous sclerosis and Recklinghausen's neurofibromatosis. *Acta. Psychiatr. Neurol.* (suppl.), **71**, 1–239.

Boulton, T.G. *et al.* (1991) *ERK*s: a family of protein-serine/threonine kinases that are activated and tyrosine phosphorylated in response to insulin and NGF. *Cell*, **65**, 663–75.

Boyer, M. *et al.* (1993) Differential modulation of neurofibromin and p120-GAP by immunoglobulin receptor in B-lymphocytes. *Oncogene*, submitted.

Buchberg, A.M. *et al.* (1988) Localization of *evi-2* to chromosome 11: linkage to other proto-oncogene and growth factor loci using interspecific backcross mice. *Oncogene Res.*, **2**, 149–65.

Buchberg, A. *et al.* (1990) Sequence homology shared by neurofibromatosis type-1 gene and *IRA*-1 and *IRA*-2 negative regulators of the *RAS* cyclic AMP pathway. *Nature*, **347**, 291–4.

Cales, C. *et al.* (1988) The cytoplasmic protein GAP is implicated as the target for regulation by the *ras* gene product. *Nature*, **332**, 548–51.

Cartwright, S.C. (1982) Concordant optic glioma in a pair of monozygotic twins with neurofibromatosis. *Clin. Pediatr.*, **21**, 236–8.

Cawthon, R. *et al.* (1990a) A major segment of the neurofibromatosis type 1 gene: cDNA sequence, genomic structure and point mutations. *Cell*, **62**, 193–201.

Cawthon, R. *et al.* (1990b) Identification and characterization of transcripts from the neurofibromatosis 1 region: the sequence and genomic structure of *EV12* and mapping of other transcripts. *Genomics*, **7**, 555–65.

Cawthon, R.M. *et al.* (1991) cDNA sequence and genomic structure of *EV12B*, a gene lying within an intron of the neurofibromatosis type 1 gene. *Genomics*, **9**, 446–60.

Clark, R.D. and Hutter, J.J. (1982) Familial neurofibromatosis and juvenile chronic myelogenous leukemia. *Hum. Genet.*, **60**, 230–2.

Crowe, F. *et al.* (1956) *A Clinical, Pathological and Genetic Study of Multiple Neurofibromatosis*, C.C. Thomas, Springfield, IL.

Darby, J.K. *et al.* (1985) A discordant sibship analysis between beta-NGF and neurofibromatosis. *Am. J. Hum. Genet.*, **37**, 52–9.

Daston, M.M. *et al.* (1992) The protein product of the neurofibromatosis type 1 gene is expressed at highest abundance in neurons, Schwann cells and olgidendrocytes. *Neuron*, **8**, 415–28.

DeClue, J.E. *et al.* (1991) Identification and characterization of the neurofibromatosis type 1 protein product. *Proc. Natl. Acad. Sci. USA*, **88**, 9914–18.

DeClue, J.E. *et al.* (1992) Abnormal regulation of mammalian $p21^{ras}$ contributes to malignant tumor growth in von Recklinghausen (type 1) neurofibromatosis. *Cell*, **69**, 265–73.

Diehl, S.R. *et al.* (1987a) Linkage analysis of peripheral neurofibromatosis to DNA markers on chromosome 8. *J. Med. Genet.*, **24**, 532–4.

Diehl, S.R. *et al.* (1987b) Linkage analysis of von Recklinghausen neurofibromatosis to DNA markers on chromosome 17. *Genomics*, **1**, 361–3.

Diehl, S.R. *et al.* (1989) A refined genetic map of the region of chromosome 17 surrounding the von Recklinghausen neurofibromatosis (*NF1*) gene. *Am. J. Hum. Genet.*, **44**, 33–7.

Diekmann, D. *et al.* (1991) *Bcr* encodes a GTPase-activating protein for p21 *ras*. *Nature*, **351**, 400–2.

Dietz, J.N. *et al.* (1986) Linkage analysis of von Recklinghausen neurofibromatosis: chromosomes 4 and 19. *Genet. Epidemiol.*, **3**, 313–21.

Estivill, X. *et al.* (1991) Recurrence of a nonsense mutation in the *NF1* gene causing classical neurofibromatosis type 1. *Hum. Genet.*, **88**, 185–8.

Fain, P.R. *et al.* (1987) Genetic analysis of NF1: identification of close flanking markers on chromosome 17. *Genomics*, **1**, 340–5.

Fain, P.R. *et al.* (1989a) The order of loci in the pericentric region of chromosome 17, based on evidence from physical and genetic breakpoints. *Am. J. Hum. Genet.*, **44**, 68–72.

Fain, P.R. *et al.* (1989b) Refined physical and genetic mapping of the *NF1* region on chromosome 17. *Am. J. Hum. Genet.*, **45**, 721–8.

Ferrell, R.E. *et al.* (1987) Von Recklinghausen neurofibromatosis: a linkage study of candidate and random marker genes. *J. Med. Genet.*, **24**, 522–4.

Fialkow, P.J. *et al.* (1971) Multiple cell origin of hereditary neurofibromatosis. *N. Engl. J. Med.*, **284**, 298–300.

Fountain, J.W. *et al.* (1989a) Physical mapping of the von Recklinghausen neurofibromatosis region on chromosome 17. *Amer. J. Hum. Genet.*, **44**, 58–67.

Fountain, J.W. *et al.* (1989b) Physical mapping of a translocation breakpoint in neurofibromatosis. *Science*, **244**, 1085–7.

Friedman, J.M. *et al.* (1982) Probable clonal origin of neurofibrosarcoma in a patient with hereditary neurofibromatosis. *J. Natl. Cancer Inst. USA*, **69**, 1289–91.

Gibbs, J.B. (1991) *Ras* C-terminal processing enzymes – new drug targets? *Cell*, **65**, 1–4.

Glover, T.W. *et al.* (1991) Molecular and cytogenetic analysis of tumors in von Recklinghausen neurofibromatosis. *Genes, Chrom. Cancer*, **3**, 62–70.

Goerg, C. *et al.* (1989) Neurofibromatosis and acute monocytic leukemia in adults. *Cancer*, **64**, 1717–19.

Goldgar, D.E. *et al.* (1989) Multipoint linkage analysis in neurofibromatosis type 1: an international collaboration. *Am. J. Hum. Genet.*, **44**, 6–12.

Golubić, M. *et al.* (1992) Catalytic properties, tissue and intracellular distribution of neurofibromin. *Oncogene*, **7**, 2151–9.

Gregory, P.E. *et al.* (1993) The neurofibromatosis type 1 gene product 'Neurofibromin' associates with microtubules. *Somatic Cell Mol. Genet.*, **19**, 265–74.

Gutmann, D.H. *et al.* (1991) Identification of the neurofibromatosis type 1 gene product. *Proc. Natl. Acad. Sci. USA*, **88**, 9658–62.

Gutmann, D.H. *et al.* (1993) Analysis of the neurofibromatosis type 1 (*NF1*) GAP-related domain by site-directed mutagenesis. *Oncogene*.

Hagag, N. *et al.* (1986) Inhibition of growth factor induced differentiation of PC12 cells by microinjection of antibody to *ras* p21. *Nature*, **319**, 680–2.

Hall, J.G. (1981) Possible maternal and hormonal factors in neurofibromatosis. *Adv. Neurol.*, **29**, 125–31.

Han, J.-W. *et al.* (1991) Regulation of *Ras*-GAP and the neurofibromatosis gene product by eicosanoids. *Science*, **252**, 576–9.

Harper, P.S. (1987) Gene mapping and neurogenetics. *J. Med. Genet.*, **24**, 513–14.

Hattori, S. *et al.* (1992) Identification of neurofibromatosis type 1 gene product as an insoluble GTPase-activating protein toward *ras* p21. *Oncogene*, **7**, 481–5.

Hoffman, K.J. and Boehm, C.D. (1992) Familial neurofibromatosis type 1: clinical experience with DNA testing. *J. Pediatr.*, **120**, 394–8.

Huson, S.M. (1987) The first European symposium on neurofibromatosis. *J. Med. Genet.*, **24**, 572–3.

Huson, S.M. *et al.* (1986) Evidence against linkage of von Recklinghausen neurofibromatosis and chromosome 19 markers. *Ann. N.Y. Acad. Sci.*, **486**, 349–53.

Ichikawa, K. *et al.* (1981) Coincidence of neurofibromatosis and myotonic dystrophy in a kindred. *J. Med. Genet.*, **18**, 134–8.

Jadayel, D. *et al.* (1990) Paternal origin of new mutations in von Recklinghausen neurofibromatosis. *Nature*, **343**, 558–9.

Kayes, L.M. *et al.* (1992) Large *de novo* DNA deletion in a patient with sporadic neurofibromatosis 1, mental retardation and dysmorphism. *J. Med. Genet.*, **29**, 686–90.

Kittur, S. *et al.* (1987) Linkage analysis of neurofibromatosis. *J. Med. Genet.*, **24**, 526–7.

Kittur, S.D. *et al.* (1989) Linkage analysis of neurofibromatosis type 1, using chromosome 17 DNA markers. *Am. J. Hum. Genet.*, **44**, 48–50.

Knudson, A.G. (1971) Mutation and cancer: statistical study of retinoblastoma. *Proc. Natl. Acad. Sci. USA*, **68**, 820–3.

Knudson, A.G. (1985) Hereditary cancer, oncogenes and antioncogenes. *Cancer Res.*, **45**, 1437–43.

Koch, C.A. *et al.* (1991) SH2 and SH3 domains: elements that control interactions of cytoplasmic signaling proteins. *Science*, **252**, 668–74.

Leach, R.J. *et al.* (1989) Physical mapping of human chromosome 17 using fragment-containing microcell hybrids. *Genomics*, **5**, 167–76.

Ledbetter, D.H. *et al.* (1989) Precise localization of *NF1* to 17q11.2 by balanced translocation. *Am. J. Hum. Genet.*, **44**, 20–4.

Lefkowitz, I.B., Obringer, A.C. and Meadows, A.T. (1990) Neurofibromatosis and cancer: incidence and management, in *Neurofibromatosis: A Handbook for Patients, Families, and Health-care Professionals* (eds A.E. Rubenstein and B.R. Korf), Thieme Medical, New York, pp. 99–111.

Legius, E. *et al.* (1992) *NF1*-related locus on chromosome 15. *Genomics*, **13**, 1316–18.

Legius, E. *et al.* (1993) Somatic deletion of neurofibromatosis type 1 gene in a neurofibrosarcoma supports a tumor suppressor gene hypothesis. *Nature Genetics*, **3**, 122–5.

Li, Y. *et al.* (1992) Somatic mutations in the neurofibromatosis 1 gene in human tumors. *Cell*, **69**, 275–81.

Lugo, T.G., Leach, R.J. and Fournier, R.E.K. (1986) Parasexual approaches to the study of human genetic disease. *Ann. N.Y. Acad. Sci.*, **486**, 293–303.

Luongo, C. *et al.* (1993) Mapping of multiple intestinal neoplasms (MIN) to proximal chromosome 18 of mouse. *Genomics*, **15**, 3–8.

Malkin, D. *et al.* (1990) Germ line p53 mutations in a familial syndrome of breast cancer, sarcomas, and other neoplasms. *Science*, **250**, 1233–8.

Marchuk, D.A. *et al.* (1991) cDNA cloning of the type 1 neurofibromatosis gene: complete sequence of the *NF1* gene product. *Genomics*, **11**, 931–40.

Marchuk, D.A. *et al.* (1992) A yeast artificial chromosome contig encompassing the type 1 neurofibromatosis gene. *Genomics*, **13**, 672–80.

Martin, G.A. *et al.* (1990) The GAP-related domain of the neurofibromatosis type 1 gene product interacts with *ras* p21. *Cell*, **63**, 843–9.

Mathew, C.G.P. *et al.* (1987) Linkage analysis of British and Indian families with von Recklinghausen neurofibromatosis. *J. Med. Genet.*, **24**, 524–6.

Mathew, C.G.P. *et al.* (1989) Linkage analysis of chromosome 17 markers in British and South African families with neurofibromatosis type 1. *Am. J. Hum. Genet.*, **44**, 38–40.

McCormick, F. (1989) *ras* GTPase activating protein: signal transmitter and signal terminator. *Cell*, **56**, 5–8.

Menon, A. *et al.* (1989) Characterisation of a translocation within the von Recklinghausen neurofibromatosis region of chromosome 17. *Genomics*, **5**, 245–9.

Menon, A.G. *et al.* (1990) Chromosome 17p deletions and *p53* gene mutations associated with the formation of malignant neurofibromas in von Recklinghausen neurofibromatosis. *Proc. Natl. Acad. Sci. USA*, **87**, 5435–9.

Mikol, D.D. *et al.* (1990) The oligodendrocyte-myelin glycoprotein belongs to a distinct family of proteins and contains the HNK-1 carbohydrate. *J. Cell Biol.*, **110**, 471–9.

Miller, M. and Hall, J.G. (1978) Possible maternal effect on severity of neurofibromatosis, *Lancet*, **ii**, 1071–4.

Nigro, J.M. *et al.* (1989) Mutations in the *p53* gene occur in diverse human tumor types. *Nature*, **342**, 705–8.

Nisha, T. *et al.* (1991) Differential expression of two types of the neurofibromatosis type 1 (*NF1*) gene transcripts related to neuronal differentiation. *Oncogene*, **6**, 1555–9.

Nishisho, I. *et al.* (1991) Mutations of chromosome 5q21 genes in FAP and colorectal cancer patients. *Science*, **253**, 665–9.

Noda, M. *et al.* (1985) Sarcoma viruses carrying *ras* oncogenes induce differentiation-associated properties in a neuronal cell line. *Nature*, **318**, 73–5.

O'Connell, P. *et al.* (1989a) Two von Recklinghausen neurofibromatosis translocations map within a 600-kb segment of 17q11.2. *Science*, **244**, 1087–8.

O'Connell, P. *et al.* (1989b) Fine structure DNA mapping studies of the chromosomal region harboring the genetic defect in neurofibromatosis type 1, *Am. J. Hum. Genet.*, **41**, 51–7.

O'Connell, P. *et al.* (1990) The human homolog of murine *Evi-2* lies between two von Recklinghausen neurofibromatosis translocations. *Genomics*, **7**, 547–54.

Otsu, M. *et al.* (1991) Characterization of two 85 kd proteins that associate with receptor tyrosine kinases, middle-T/pp60 c-*src* complexes, and PI3 kinase. *Cell*, **65**, 91–104.

Pericak-Vance, M.A. *et al.* (1987a) Linkage studies in peripheral neurofibromatosis. *J. Med. Genet.*, **24**, 530–2.

Pericak-Vance, M.A. *et al.* (1987b) Genetic linkage studies of chromosome 17 RFLPs in von Recklinghausen neurofibromatosis (NF1). *Genomics*, **1**, 349–52.

Powell, S.M. *et al.* (1992) *APC* mutations occur early during colorectal tumorigenesis. *Nature*, **359**, 235–7.

Ratner, N. *et al.* (1990) Mitogen accumulation in von Recklinghausen neurofibromatosis. *Ann. Neurol.*, **27**, 496–501.

Riccardi, V.M. (1981) Von Recklinghausen neurofibromatosis. *New Engl. J. Med.*, **305**, 1617–27.

Riccardi, V.M. and Eichner, J.E. (1986) *Neurofibromatosis: Phenotype, Natural History, and Pathogenesis*, Johns Hopkins University Press, Baltimore, MD.

Riccardi, V.M. and Lewis, R.A. (1988) Penetrance of von Recklinghausen neurofibromatosis: a distinction between predecessors and descendants. *Amer. J. Hum. Genet.*, **42**, 284–9.

Riccardi, V.M. and Wald, J.S. (1987) Discounting an adverse maternal effect on severity of neurofibromatosis. *Pediatrics*, **79**, 386–93.

Ridley, A.J. *et al.* (1988) *ras*-mediated cell cycle arrest is altered by nuclear oncogenes to induce Schwann cell transformation. *EMBO J.*, **7**, 1635–45.

Rivas, M.L. and DiLiberti, J.H. (1984) Genetic linkage between myotonic dystrophy and neurofibromatosis. *Cytogenet. Cell Genet.*, **37**, 570–1.

Rubinfeld, B. *et al.* (1991) Molecular cloning of a GTPase activating protein specific for the *Krev*-1 protein $p21^{rap1}$. *Cell*, **65**, 1033–42.

Sarfarazi, M., Huson, S.M. and Edwards, J.H. (1987) An exclusion map for von Recklinghausen neurofibromatosis, *J. Med. Genet.*, **24**, 515–20.

Schmidt, M.A., Michels, V.V. and Dewald, G.W. (1987) Cases of neurofibromatosis with rearrangements of chromosome 17 involving band 17q11.2. *Am. J. Med. Genet.*, **28**, 771–7.

Seizinger, B.R. *et al.* (1986) Genetic linkage analysis of neurofibromatosis with DNA markers. *Ann. N.Y. Acad. Sci.*, **486**, 304–10.

Seizinger, B.R. *et al.* (1987a) DNA linkage analysis in von Recklinghausen neurofibromatosis. *J. Med. Genet.*, **24**, 529–530.

Seizinger, B.R. *et al.* (1987b) Genetic linkage of von Recklinghausen neurofibromatosis to the nerve growth factor receptor gene. *Cell*, **49**, 589–94.

Seizinger, B.R. *et al.* (1987c) Linkage analysis in von Recklinghausen's neurofibromatosis (NF1) with DNA markers for chromosome 17. *Genomics*, **1**(4), 346–8.

Seizinger, B.R. *et al.* (1989) Flanking markers for the gene causing von Recklinghausen neurofibromatosis (NF1). *Am. J. Hum. Genet.*, **44**, 30–2.

Sergeyev, A.S. (1975) On the mutation rate of neurofibromatosis. *Hum. Genet.*, **28**, 129–38.

Sheela, S. *et al.* (1990) Angiogenic and invasive properties of neurofibroma Schwann cells. *J. Cell Biol.*, **111**, 645–53.

Skolnick, M.H., Ponder, B. and Seizinger, B. (1987) Linkage of NF1 to 12 chromosome 17 markers: a summary of eight concurrent reports. *Genomics*, **1**, 382–3.

Skuse, G.R. (1990) Type 1 neurofibromatosis gene: correction. *Science*, **250**, 1749.

Skuse, G.R. *et al.* (1989) Molecular genetic analysis of tumors in von Recklinghausen neurofibromatosis: loss of heterozygosity for chromosome 17. *Genes, Chrom. Cancer*, **1**, 36–41.

Skuse, G.R. *et al.* (1991) The neurofibroma in von Recklinghausen neurofibromatosis has a unicellular origin. *Am. J. Hum. Genet.*, **49**, 600–7.

Sorensen, S.A., Mulvihill, J.J. and Neilsen, A. (1986) Long-term follow-up of von Recklinghausen neurofibromatosis. *N. Engl. J. Med.*, **314**, 1010–15.

Spence, *et al.* (1986) Genetic linkage analysis of neurofibromatosis. *Ann. N.Y. Acad. Sci.*, **486**, 287–92.

Spence, *et al.* (1987) Linkage analysis of neurofibromatosis (von Recklinghausen disease). *J. Med. Genet.*, **20**, 334–7.

Stephens, K. *et al.* (1987) Linkage studies with chromosome 17 DNA markers in 45 neurofibromatosis 1 families. *Genomics*, **1**, 353–7.

Stephens, K. *et al.* (1989) Genetic analysis of eight loci tightly linked to neurofibromatosis 1. *Am. J. Hum. Genet.*, **44**, 13–19.

Stephens, K. *et al.* (1992) Preferential mutation of the neurofibromatosis type 1 gene in paternally derived chromosomes. *Hum. Genet.*, **88**, 279–82.

Stumpf, D.A. *et al.* (1987) NIH Consensus Development Conference Statement. *Neurofibromatosis*, **6**(12).

Suzuki, Y. *et al.* (1991) Brain tumors predominantly express the neurofibromatosis type 1 gene transcripts containing the 63 base insert in the region coding for GTPase activating protein-related domain. *Biochem. Biophys. Res. Commun.*, **181**, 955–61.

Szeberenyi, J. *et al.* (1990) Effect of a dominant inhibitory Ha-*ras* mutation on neuronal differentiation of PC12 cells. *Mol. Cell. Biol.*, **10**, 5324–32.

Tanaka, K. *et al.* (1989) *IRA1*, an inhibitory regulator of the *RAS*/cyclic AMP pathway in *Saccharomyces cerevisiae*. *Mol. Cell Biol.*, **9**, 757–68.

Tanaka, K. *et al.* (1990) *IRA2*, a second gene of *Saccharomyces cerevisiae* that encodes a protein with a domain homologous to mammalian *ras*-GTPase activating protein. *Mol. Cell. Biol.*, **10**, 4303–13.

Tanaka, K. *et al.* (1991) *IRA2*, an upstream negative regulator of RAS in yeast, is a *RAS* GTPase-activating protein. *Proc. Natl. Acad. Sci. USA*, **88**, 468–72.

The, I. *et al.* (1993) Neurofibromatosis type 1 gene mutations in neuroblastoma. *Nature Genetics*, **3**, 62–6.

Trahey, M. and McCormick, F. (1987) A cytoplasmic protein stimulates normal N-*ras* p21 GTPase, but does not affect oncogenic mutants. *Science*, **238**, 542–5.

Trahey, M. *et al.* (1988) Molecular cloning of two types of GAP from complementary DNA from human placenta. *Science*, **242**, 1697–700.

Upadhyaya, M. *et al.* (1987a) Further exclusion data for the von Recklinghausen neurofibromatosis gene: a genetic linkage study of 19 polymorphic markers. *J. Med. Genet.*, **24**, 534–6.

Upadhyaya, M. *et al.* (1987b) Chromosome 17 markers and von Recklinghausen neurofibromatosis: a genetic linkage study in a British population. *Genomics*, **1**, 358–60.

Upadhyaya, M. *et al.* (1989) Close flanking markers for neurofibromatosis type 1 (NF1). *Am. J. Hum. Genet.*, **44**, 41–7.

Upadhyaya, M. *et al.* (1990) A 90 kb DNA deletion associated with neurofibromatosis type 1. *J. Med. Genet.*, **27**, 738–41.

Upadhyaya, M. *et al.* (1992) Analysis of mutations at the neurofibromatosis (NF1) locus. *Hum. Mol. Gen.*, **1**, 735–40.

van Tuinen, P. *et al.* (1987) Regional mapping panel for human chromosome 17, application to neurofibromatosis type 1. *Genomics*, **1**, 371–81.

Vance, J.M. *et al.* (1989) Genetic linkage mapping of chromosome 17 markers and neurofibromatosis type 1. *Am. J. Hum. Genet.*, **44**, 25–9.

Viskochil, D. *et al.* (1990) Deletions and a translocation interrupt a cloned gene at the neurofibromatosis type 1 locus. *Cell*, **62**, 187–92.

Viskochil, D. *et al.* (1991) The oligodendrocyte-myelin glycoprotein is embedded within the neurofibromatosis type 1 gene. *Mol. Cell Biol.*, **11**, 906–12.

Vogel, U. *et al.* (1988) Cloning of bovine GAP and its interaction with oncogenic *ras* p21. *Nature*, **335**, 90–3.

Wallace, M.R. *et al.* (1989) Direct construction of a chromosome-specific *Not*I linking library from flow-sorted chromosomes. *Nucleic Acids Res.*, **17**, 1665–77.

Wallace, M.R. *et al.* (1990a) Type 1 neurofibromatosis gene: identification of a large transcript disrupted in three NF1 patients. *Science*, **249**, 181–6.

Wallace, M.R. *et al.* (1990b) A chromosome jump crosses a translocation breakpoint in the von Recklinghausen neurofibromatosis region. *Genes, Chrom. Cancer*, **2**, 271–7.

Wallace, M.R. *et al.* (1991) A *de novo* Alu insertion results in neurofibromatosis type 1. *Nature*, **353**, 865–6.

Wang, Y. *et al.* (1991) *SAR1*, a gene from *Schizosaccharomyces pombe* encoding a GAP-like protein that regulates *RAS*1. *Cell Regulation*, **2**, 453–65.

Ward, *et al.* (1990) Diagnosis of neurofibromatosis 1 by using tightly linked flanking DNA markers. *Am. J. Hum. Genet.*, **46**, 943–9.

Watkins, W.S. *et al.* (1991) A BgIII RFLP near the human neurofibromatosis type 1 (*NF1*) gene. *Nucleic Acids Res.*, **19**, 6662.

Weichselbaum, R.R., Beckett, M. and Diamond, A. (1988) Some retinoblastoma, osteosarcomas and soft tissue sarcomas may share a common etiology. *Proc. Natl. Acad. Sci. USA*, **85**, 2106–9.

Weiming, X. *et al.* (1991) The gene for von Recklinghausen neurofibromatosis (NF1) maps to the pericentromeric region of chromosome 17 in Chinese families. *Genomics*, **10**, 1090–2.

White, R. *et al.* (1987) Tightly linked markers for the neurofibromatosis type 1 gene. *Genomics*, **1**, 364–7.

Wiesmuller, L. and Wittinghofer, A. (1992) Expression of the GTPase activating domain of the neurofibromatosis type 1 (*NF1*) gene in *Escherichia coli* and role of the conserved lysine residue. *J. Biol. Chem.*, **267**, 10207–10.

Xu, G. *et al.* (1990a) The neurofibromatosis type 1 gene encodes a protein related to GAP. *Cell*, **62**, 599–608.

Xu, G. *et al.* (1990b) The catalytic domain of the neurofibromatosis type 1 gene product stimulates *ras* GTPase and complements *ira* mutants of *S. cerevisiae*. *Cell*, **63**, 835–41.

Xu, G. *et al.* (1991) An Alu polymorphism intragenic to the neurofibromatosis type 1 gene (*NF1*). *Nucleic Acids Res.*, **19**, 3764.

Xu, G. *et al.* (1992) Loss of *NF1* alleles in phaeochromocytomas from patients with type 1 neurofibromatosis. *Genes Chromo. Cancer*, **4**, 337–42.

Yatani, A. *et al.* (1990) *ras* p21 and GAP inhibit coupling of muscarinic receptors to atrial K^+ channels. *Cell*, **61**, 769–76.

3

Molecular genetic studies of neurofibromatosis 2

G.A. Rouleau

3.1 INTRODUCTION

Neurofibromatosis 2 (NF2) is an autosomal dominant disease characterized by an inherited predisposition to develop tumours of the nervous system. Although NF2 was described over a century ago, molecular studies have only recently begun to elucidate its pathogenesis.

In this chapter I will begin by reviewing the current state of understanding of the genesis of meningiomas and vestibular Schwannomas, common sporadic tumours also seen in NF2. I will then describe molecular studies of tumours removed from NF2 patients as well as genetic linkage studies in a very large family. These results, which mapped the *NF2* gene to chromosome 22, were consistent with the hypothesis that the *NF2* gene is a tumour suppressor gene, analogous to the retinoblastoma gene. Subsequent fine mapping assigned the *NF2* gene to a small region of chromosome 22, thereby allowing the gene to be approached using positional cloning. Certain unresolved issues, such as the existence of a separate meningioma susceptibility locus and genetic heterogeneity, will be discussed.

3.2 SPORADIC TUMOURS ASSOCIATED WITH NF2

The most important feature of NF2 is the frequent occurrence of meningioma and vestibular Schwannoma (formerly called acoustic neuroma). These tumours, when seen in NF2 patients, typically occur in the third decade, in contrast to the sporadic tumours, which appear in the fourth or fifth decade. Although NF2 is an uncommon disease, sporadic meningioma and vestibular Schwannoma are common, representing approximately 30% of primary adult brain tumours, making them an important cause of morbidity and mortality in man (Butler, Brooks and Netsky, 1982). I will briefly review the pathological, clinical and molecular aspects of these tumours.

3.2.1 Sporadic meningioma

Meningiomas are histologically benign tumours derived from the arachnoidal cells of the meninges. They are common, representing 25% of spinal tumours and 15% of cranial tumours. They occur more frequently in females, with a female: male ratio of 2:1. Meningiomas typically occur in middle age with a peak incidence at approximately 45 years of age (Russell and Rubenstein, 1972; Quest, 1978).

Monosomy for chromosome 22 in meningioma was first reported by Zang and Singer (1967), who found loss of one copy of this chromosome by cytogenetic analysis of short-term cultures of fresh tumours. Subsequent studies by many authors have confirmed the association of monosomy 22 and meningioma (for a review see Zang, 1982; Casalone *et al.*, 1987). Partial loss of distal portions of the long arm of chromosome 22 is described in 10–30% of the tumours studied cytogenetically, suggesting that the critical region of this chromosome, which when lost allows tumour formation, is located on the distal long arm.

Molecular studies confirming the loss of genes on chromosome 22 in meningiomas have been described in four papers. All these studies were based on the same methodology. Briefly, Southern blot analysis was performed on DNA from normal tissue, usually blood, and DNA from tumour tissue. These blood/tumour pairs were then probed with polymorphic DNA markers, and the allelic pattern of the blood and tumour DNA compared. A polymorphic DNA marker is informative when the individual is heterozygous (has two different alleles, one for each chromosome) in the normal tissue; thus analysis of the tumour tissue DNA discloses if there has been loss of one of the alleles at this locus in the tumour. One important advantage of this technique over cytological analysis is that by analysing DNA obtained directly from fresh tumours, the problem of differential growth rates of different cells (clonal selection) inherent to the analysis of cultured tumours is avoided.

Seizinger *et al.* (1987b) reported loss of alleles on chromosome 22 in 17 of 40 meningiomas. No partial loss of the chromosome was observed in this study. Dumanski *et al.* (1987) reported loss of alleles on chromosome 22 in 19 of 35 meningiomas. In a subsequent paper, Dumanski *et al.* (1990) expanded this study to 81 meningiomas using 25 separate loci on chromosome 22. In this large study the authors found that 30 tumours (37%) retained all loci on chromosome 22, 42 tumours (52%) lost one

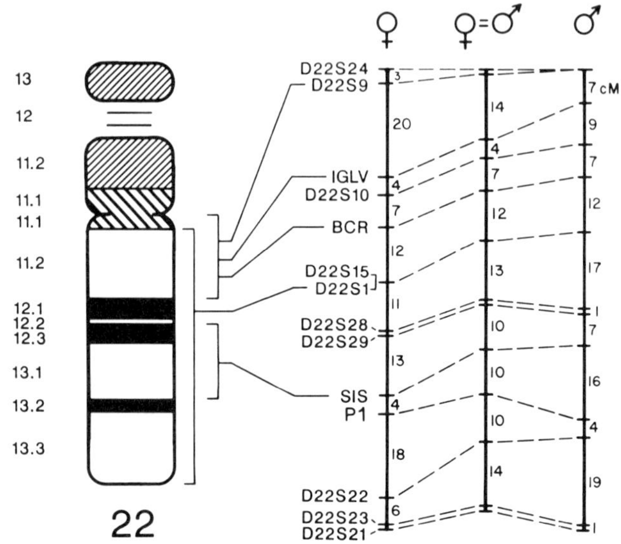

Figure 3.1 Human chromosome 22 genetic map. The sex-averaged genetic map (male = female recombination) is shown, flanked by maps constructed on the basis of only male or female meioses, respectively. The map distances are shown in centimorgans. The bracketed regions indicate the physical regions to which particular loci have been assigned. The polymorphic loci shown are either anonymous fragments (the 'D' numbers, D22S . . .) or genes, designated by their official locus symbol (a series of letters). IGLV represents the immunoglobulin light chain variable region gene, BCR represents the breakpoint cluster region gene, SIS represents the platelet-derived growth factor β chain gene (formerly known as the SIS oncogene) and P1 represents a polymorphic blood marker.

allele for all informative loci (monosomy for chromosome 22) and nine tumours (11%) lost only part of chromosome 22. These nine tumours, which retained constitutional heterozygosity at one or more chromosome 22 loci with loss of heterozygosity for at least one other locus, can be used for mapping by assuming that the meningioma locus must be within the minimum common deleted region. In these tumours the lost alleles were always located distal to the conserved alleles, consistent with variable terminal deletion of one copy of chromosome 22 in tumour tissue DNA. The only segment of chromosome 22 consistently lost in the tumour tissue DNA is distal to the locus D22S28, placing the meningioma locus telomeric to this marker (Figure 3.1). In a fourth paper, Okazaki *et al.* (1988) studied 14 meningiomas with four polymorphic markers. Three tumours were uninformative, eight tumours showed no loss of alleles (seven of these were informative at only one locus) and three tumours showed loss of alleles. In contrast to the results of Seizinger *et al.* (1987b) and Dumanski *et al.* (1990), all three tumours (100%) showed partial loss of the chromosome. Remarkably, the pattern of loss in all three tumours would indicate a deletion involving the region distal to PDGFB and proximal to IGLV, with retention of a central section of the long arm (Figure 3.1). This unexpected result needs to be confirmed. Such complex chromosomal rearrangements were not found in any other studies. In summary, loss of chromosome 22 is frequently seen in meningioma; partial loss is occasionally seen with consistent loss of telomeric loci; and deletion mapping is most consistent with the meningioma locus mapping distal to D22S28.

Recently, Lekanne Deprez *et al.* (1991) reported the mapping of a translocation breakpoint in a meningioma cell line that had lost one entire copy of chromosome 22 and had a t(4;22) involving the second chromosome 22. They constructed somatic cell hybrids which segregated the 4p+ and 22q− chromosomes, thereby allowing them to map the breakpoint to the interval bracketed by D22S1 and D22S15, a region proximal to D22S28. They postulate that a tumour suppressor gene, presumably *NF2*, has been inactivated by this translocation. If this assumption is correct, this tumour suppressor gene maps between D22S1 and D22S15 (Figure 3.1).

3.2.2 Sporadic vestibular Schwannoma

Vestibular Schwannomas, also called acoustic neuromas, are histologically benign tumours derived from Schwann cells of the vestibular branch of the eighth cranial nerve (Martuza *et al.*, 1985). Rarely, Schwannomas may occur on spinal roots, usually dorsal roots, or on other cranial nerves such as the fifth, ninth or tenth. They are common, representing 10% of primary central nervous system (CNS) tumours and occurring in middle age with a peak incidence at approximately 45 years of age (Martuza *et al.*, 1985; Tator, 1985).

In 1986, Seizinger, Martuza and Gusella reported loss of genes on chromosome 22 in vestibular Schwannoma. Using polymorphic DNA markers they showed loss of alleles on chromosome 22 in seven of 16 (44%) sporadic vestibular Schwannomas. No loss of heterozygosity was seen for 11 other chromosomes tested, suggesting that loss of chromosome 22 is a very specific event in this tumour. These results were confirmed by Couturier *et al.* (1990), who found loss of chromosome 22 in four of 14 vestibular Schwannomas tested using polymorphic DNA markers and/or cytogenetically. Further support for loss of chromosome 22 in vestibular Schwannomas was provided by Fontaine *et al.* (1991a), who reported allelic losses in 28 of 72 (39%) vestibular Schwannomas tested. Couturier *et al.* (1990) also tested sporadic Schwannomas removed from locations other than the eighth cranial nerve for loss of heterozygosity. Three of nine tumours tested using DNA markers lost chromosome 22.

Fontaine *et al.* (1991b) also found monosomy for chromosome 22 in three of three sporadic non-vestibular Schwannomas, confirming a common mechanism for tumorigenesis in all Schwannomas, regardless of their location.

3.3 MOLECULAR ANALYSIS OF NF2 TUMOURS

Molecular analysis of sporadic meningioma and vestibular Schwannoma, both NF2-associated tumours, implicated chromosome 22 as a likely site for the *NF2* gene. However, the studies described above involved sporadic tumours, not tumours of NF2 patients. Therefore, analysis of tumours obtained from NF2 patients was needed in order to confirm the link between loss of chromosome 22 and NF2. Seizinger *et al.* (1987a) reported analysis for loss of heterozygosity of six tumours from patients with NF2: two vestibular Schwannomas, one meningioma and three Schwannomas. Loss of alleles on chromosome 22 was identified in five out of the six tumours, indicating that specific loss of genes on this chromosome is a frequent event not only in sporadic cases of vestibular Schwannoma and meningioma, but also in the heritable form of these tumours. This observation suggests that both sporadic and familial vestibular Schwannomas result from similar mechanisms involving the same gene locus. In addition, this specific chromosomal alteration implies a common pathogenetic mechanism for different histological tumour types in NF2.

3.4 FAMILY STUDIES

The association of loss of alleles on chromosome 22 and tumour formation suggests, but does not establish, that this chromosomal mechanism represents the primary cause, and not simply the secondary consequence, of tumorigenesis. Significant overlap of symptoms exists between NF1 (localized to chromosome 17) and NF2, with some patients fulfilling the diagnostic criteria for both diseases (Kanter *et al.*, 1980; Deutsch, 1984; Martuza and Eldridge, 1988; Garretto *et al.*, 1989; Michels *et al.*, 1989). Both disorders share certain genetic features, such as autosomal dominant inheritance, high penetrance, variable clinical expressivity, a high rate of new mutation and a predisposition to multiple tumours of neural crest origin. These similarities raise the possibility that NF1 and NF2 may result from different mutations involving the same gene (allelic genetic heterogeneity). Finally, a recent report by Cawthon *et al.* (1990) describing a mutation in the *NF1* gene in a patient with NF2, suggests that the inherited disease may be caused by specific mutations on chromosome 17.

To resolve these critical issues, genetic linkage analysis was performed using DNA markers to determine whether the primary inherited defect in NF2 is located on chromosome 17 or 22. Details of this study are described in Rouleau *et al.* (1987). Significant linkage was found (Lod score = 3.42) with D22S1, an anonymous DNA marker on chromosome 22, which definitely establishes NF1 and NF2 as different disorders (non-allelic genetic heterogeneity) and suggests that loss of the *NF2* gene is in fact the primary cause of vestibular Schwannoma and perhaps meningioma.

3.5 FLANKING MARKERS

In order to define further the limits of the *NF2* locus, additional polymorphic markers for chromosome 22 were generated and a genetic map was constructed for this autosome (Rouleau *et al.*, 1989; Figure 3.1). With these additional resources we were able to expand the number of tumours that are informative by deletion analysis, and a tumour with an interstitial deletion was identified that included sequences telomeric to the marker D22S1, including D22S28 (Rouleau *et al.*, 1990; Figure 3.1). This deletion strongly suggests that the *NF2* locus is distal to D22S1, and so establishes this locus as a centromeric flanking marker. In addition, the genetic map of chromosome 22 has allowed us to optimize the informativeness of a large NF2 pedigree using multipoint linkage analysis (Rouleau *et al.*, 1990). Using this method we have established that D22S28 is the telomeric flanking marker by odds of 30 000 : 1. Recently, we have identified a recombination between D22S1 and NF2 in this same kindred. Reconstruction of the NF2 chromosome haplotype segregating in this family has confirmed that the disease locus is indeed telomeric to D22S1 (unpublished results). Therefore, genetic studies place the *NF2* locus between the markers D22S1 and D22S28 (Figure 3.1).

Recently, Wolff *et al.* (1992) tested NF2-associated tumours from 39 patients with polymorphic DNA markers. These include mostly vestibular Schwannomas, plus a few meningiomas, Schwannomas and ependymomas. They found two tumours with terminal deletions where most of the NF2 region is lost. One of these tumours, a vestibular Schwannoma from an NF2 patient, had a breakpoint between D22S41/D22S46 and D22S56. Though the precise location of these markers is not known, they have been mapped using irradiation-reduced hybrids to the D22S1–D22S28 interval (Wolff *et al.*, 1992). Therefore, this study helps to sublocalize the *NF2* locus to the interval flanked by D22S41/D22S46 and D22S28.

3.6 MENINGIOMA AND NF2: ONE OR TWO LOCI?

Meningioma, the first tumour associated with loss of genes on chromosome 22, is seen with a high frequency in NF2. However, in NF2, vestibular Schwannomas are seen much more frequently than meningiomas. In addition, there are instances where patients develop multiple meningiomas in the absence of vestibular Schwannomas, such as one patient with a ring chromosome 22 and multiple precocious meningiomas (Arinami *et al.*, 1986), and a few families who have an inherited predisposition for multiple meningiomas (Gaist and Piazza, 1959; Joynt and Perret, 1961, 1965; Sedzimir, Frazer and Roberts, 1973; Memon, 1980; Bolger *et al.*, 1985; McDowell, 1990). These two sets of observations would suggest that between the loci responsible for NF2 and multiple meningioma there may be: (1) allelic heterogeneity (one gene with different mutations) or (2) non-allelic heterogeneity (different genes altogether). Data presented by Dumanski *et al.* (1990) place the meningioma locus distal to D22S28, outside the NF2 region, favouring the hypothesis of non-allelic heterogeneity. However, the results of Lekanne Deprez *et al.* (1991), where a translocation breakpoint in a meningioma maps to the NF2 region, favour the hypothesis of allelic heterogeneity (one gene) based on the assumption that the translocation interrupts a tumour suppressor gene, presumably the *NF2* gene itself. Ultimately, cloning of the responsible gene(s) will definitively resolve this issue.

3.7 GENETIC HETEROGENEITY

The question of non-allelic heterogeneity in NF2 needs to be addressed. It is theoretically possible that several genes could, when mutated, lead to the clinical syndrome we define as NF2. In fact, many instances of genetic non-allelic heterogeneity have been described, one of the most striking being hereditary motor and sensory neuropathy type 1 (Charcot–Marie–Tooth disease) where mutations at loci on chromosome 1, 17 and elsewhere all lead to similar syndromes (Bird, Ott and Giblett, 1982; Guiloff *et al.*, 1982; Vance *et al.*, 1989). A patient with NF2 has been found to have a mutation in the *NF1* gene on chromosome 17 (Cawthon *et al.*, 1990) suggesting that certain mutations in the *NF1* gene may lead to the clinical phenotype NF2. However, the biological significance of the reported *NF1* mutation is unknown, and segregation analysis was not performed to demonstrate that the chromosome 17 mutation is linked to the NF2 phenotype (see section 18.3 for further discussion).

The selective and frequent involvement of chromosome 22 seen in the deletion studies of meningiomas and vestibular Schwannomas strongly argues against involvement of another gene, not on chromosome 22, in NF2. Confirmation of the absence of non-allelic genetic heterogeneity required analysis of 13 NF2 families using markers on both chromosomes 22 and 17. We confirmed the assignment of the *NF2* locus to the long arm of chromosome 22 and, using the admixture test (HOMOG computer program), we rejected the hypothesis of genetic heterogeneity (Narod *et al.*, 1992). Indeed, we believe that chromosome 22 markers can now be used for presymptomatic diagnosis in selected families.

3.8 NF2 IS A TUMOUR SUPPRESSOR GENE

Deletion studies of meningiomas and vestibular Schwannomas suggested that loss of a locus, or several loci, on chromosome 22 is a frequent event in their tumorigenesis. Establishing that the inherited defect in NF2 maps to the same region of chromosome 22 strongly supports the hypothesis that the primary defect leading to the formation of these tumours is on chromosome 22. Therefore, by analogy to the pathogenetic mechanism proposed for the well-studied retinoblastoma tumour suppressor gene, tumorigenesis in NF2 involves: (1) a somatic mutation inactivating the wild-type *NF2* gene, at a critical time in specific cell types, unmasking the mutant allele; and (2) clonal expansion of this cell because the absence of a functional *NF2* gene product leads to a growth advantage (Cavenee *et al.*, 1983; Friend *et al.*, 1986). Sporadic meningiomas and vestibular Schwannomas would develop when two somatic mutations, such as non-disjunction, mitotic recombination, deletion or inactivating point mutation, inactivate both copies of the *NF2* gene in a single cell of the appropriate type at the appropriate time, thereby leading to clonal expansion and a tumour. We would expect that one somatic event inactivating one NF2 allele would be much more frequent than two mutations, explaining why individuals inheriting a mutant *NF2* gene (therefore requiring only one somatic mutation) have multiple tumours, in contrast to normal individuals who rarely develop one of these neoplasms, and never two or more tumours.

This proposed mechanism explains why NF2 mutations are recessive at the cellular level, but lead to a dominantly inherited disease. The key to this seeming paradox is that somatic mutations, which normally do not lead to a phenotype, result in clonal expansion and tumour formation in NF2 patients. Additional evidence that *NF2* is a tumour suppressor gene comes from the analysis of five tumours (one vestibular Schwannoma and four independent neurofibromas) from a single NF2 patient. The observed loss of the same allele of the D22S28 locus in all five tumours demonstrates that the somatic event in each tumour involved loss of the chromosome 22 containing this allele. The 2 allele of this locus, which is non-randomly retained, therefore marks the chromosome carrying the defective NF2 allele (Rouleau *et al.*, 1990).

3.9 PREDICTIVE TESTING

NF2 is a serious disease that is often not detected until tumours develop and symptoms appear. A predictive test would significantly modify patient management, prognosis and family planning. 'At-risk' individuals found to carry the gene could be monitored for the earliest signs of tumour formation, potentially permitting surgical intervention before the development of hearing loss or other permanent neurological dysfunction (Martuza *et al.*, 1985).

Testing 'at-risk' individuals is now possible for any family where the co-segregating chromosome can be identified (Narod *et al.*, 1992; unpublished results). Eventually, the cloning of the gene and characterization of the *NF2* gene mutations will most likely open new avenues for diagnosis, particularly for sporadic cases.

3.10 CONCLUSION

Mapping the *NF2* locus to chromosome 22 and identifying flanking markers were the essential first steps towards the cloning and characterization of the gene defect. The *NF2* gene has now been localized to a sufficiently small region of chromosome 22 to allow application of many new techniques, such as pulsed-field gel electrophoresis (Schwartz and Cantor, 1984) and yeast artificial chromosome cloning (Burke, Carle and Olsen, 1987) for positional cloning of the defect. The availability of an abundance of tumours and the isolation of many new DNA sequences on chromosome 22 make the identification of the *NF2* gene likely within 1 or 2 years. The cloning and sequencing of the *NF2* gene will allow detailed analysis of the function of this recessive oncogene, and hopefully will lead to new treatments.

NOTE

During preparation of this book two important papers have been published which describe the cloning of the *NF2* gene. Rouleau *et al.* (1993) and Trofatter *et al.* (1993) identified a number of germ-line deletions in NF2 patients, leading to the isolation of a candidate cDNA which was interrupted by these rearrangements. This gene was tested for the presence of subtle germ-line mutations in NF2 individuals. Rouleau *et al.* identified 16 such mutations, establishing with certainty that the candidate cDNA encodes for the *NF2* gene. All of these mutations, except one, lead to a truncated protein, strongly supporting the model that *NF2* is a tumour suppressor gene. The candidate gene encodes for a protein which has very high homology to the protein 4.1 family including moesin and radixin. Based on these homologies we predict that the NF2 protein acts at the membrane cytoskeleton interface linking components of the membrane with components of the actin skeleton. These findings suggest that NF2 is a structural membrane associated protein, the loss of which may represent a new mechanism for tumour development. The identification of the *NF2* gene will lead to further characterization of the role of this protein in the development of NF2 and associated tumours.

ACKNOWLEDGEMENTS

G.A.R. is supported in part by the Fonds de Recherche en Santé de Québec, by the Medical Research Council of Canada and by the National Neurofibromatosis Foundation. The author wishes to thank Albert Aguayo, Jean-Pierre Julien and Denise Figlewicz for useful discussion and comments.

REFERENCES

Arinami, T., Kondo, I., Hamaguchi, H. and Nakajima, S. (1986) Multifocal meningiomas in a patient with a constitutional ring chromosome 22. *J. Med. Genet*, **23**, 178–80.

Bird, T.D., Ott, J. and Giblett, E.R. (1982) Evidence for linkage of Charcot–Marie–Tooth neuropathy to the Duffy locus on chromosome 1. *Am. J. Hum. Genet.*, **34**, 388–94.

Bolger, G.B., Stamberg, J., Hollis, G.F. *et al.* (1985) Chromosome translocation t(14;22) and oncogene (c-*sis*) variant in a pedigree with familial meningioma. *N. Engl. J. Med.*, **312**, 564–7.

Burke, D.T., Carle, G.T. and Olsen, M.V. (1987) Cloning of large segments of exogenous DNA into yeast by means of artificial chromosome vectors. *Science*, **236**, 806–12.

Butler, J., Brooks, R. and Netsky, D. (1982) Classification and biology of brain tumours. In *Neurological Surgery* (ed. J.R. Youmans), W.B. Saunders, Philadelphia.

Casalone, R., Granata, P., Simi, P. *et al.* (1987) Recessive cancer genes in meningiomas – an analysis of 31 cases. *Cancer Genet. Cytogenet.*, **27**, 145–59.

Cavenee, W.K., Dryja, T.P., Phillips, R.A. *et al.* (1983) Expression of recessive alleles by chromosomal mechanisms in retinoblastoma. *Nature*, **305**, 779–84.

Cawthon, R.M., Weiss, R., Xu, G. *et al.* (1990) A major segment of the neurofibromatosis type 1 gene: cDNA sequence, genomic structure, and point mutations. *Cell*, **62**, 193–201.

Couturier, J., Delattre, O., Kujas, M. *et al.* (1990) Assessment of chromosome 22 anomalies in neurinomas by combined karyotype and RFLP analyses. *Cancer Genet. Cytogenet.*, **45**, 55–62.

Deutsch, E.C. (1984) Von Recklinghausen's neurofibromatosis with multiple intracranial tumours. *Ear Nose Throat J.*, **63**, 141–8.

Dumanski, J.P., Carlbom, E., Collins, V.P. and Nordenskjöld, M. (1987) Deletion mapping of a locus on human chromosome 22 involved in the oncogenesis of meningioma. *Proc. Natl. Acad. Sci. USA*, **84**, 9275–9.

Dumanski, J.P., Rouleau, G.A., Nordenskjöld, M. and Collins, V.P. (1990) Molecular genetic analysis of chromosome 22 in meningioma. *Cancer Res.*, **50**, 5863–7.

Friend, S.H., Bernards, R., Rogelj, S. *et al.* (1986) A human DNA segment with properties of the gene that predisposes to retinoblastoma and osteosarcoma. *Nature*, **323**, 643–6.

Fontaine, B., Sanson, M., Delattre, O. *et al.* (1991a) Parental origin of chromosome 22 loss in sporadic and NF2 neuromas. *Genomics*, **10**, 280–3.
Fontaine, B., Hanson, M.P., VonSattel, J.P. *et al.* (1991b) Loss of chromosome 22 alleles in human sporadic spinal schwannomas. *Ann. Neurol.*, **29**, 183–6.
Gaist, G. and Piazza, G. (1959) Meningiomas in two members of the same family (with no evidence of neurofibromatosis). *J. Neurosurg.*, **16**, 110–13.
Garretto, N.S., Ameriso, S., Molina, H.A. *et al.* (1989) Type 2 neurofibromatosis with Lisch nodules. *Neurofibromatosis*, **2**, 315–21.
Guiloff, R.J., Thomas, P.K., Contreras, M. *et al.* (1982) Linkage of autosomal dominant type 1 hereditary motor and sensory neuropathy to the Duffy locus on chromosome 1. *J. Neurol. Neurosurg. Psychiatr.*, **45**, 669–74.
Joynt, R.J. and Perret, J.E. (1961) Meningiomas in a mother and daughter: cases without evidence of neurofibromatosis. *Neurology*, **11**, 164–5.
Joynt, R.J. and Perret, J.E. (1965) Familial meningiomas, *J. Neurol. Neurosurg. Psychiatr.*, **28**, 163–4.
Kanter, W.R., Eldridge, R., Fabricant, R. *et al.* (1980) Central neurofibromatosis with bilateral acoustic neuroma: genetic, clinical and biochemical distinctions from peripheral neurofibromatosis. *Neurology*, **30**, 851–9.
Lekanne Deprez, R.H., Groen, N.A., van Biezen, N.A. *et al.* (1991) A t(4;22) in a meningioma points to the localization of a putative tumour-suppressor gene. *Am. J. Hum. Genet.*, **48**, 783–90.
Martuza, R.L. and Eldridge, R. (1988) Neurofibromatosis 2 (bilateral acoustic neurofibromatosis). *N. Engl. J. Med.*, **318**, 684–8.
Martuza, R.L., Parker, S.W., Nadol, J.B. *et al.* (1985) Diagnosis of cerebellopontine angle tumours. *Clin. Neurosurg.*, **32**, 177–213.
McDowell, J.R. (1990) Familial meningioma. *Neurology*, **40**, 312–14.
Memon, M.Y. (1980) Multiple and familial meningiomas without evidence of neurofibromatosis. *Neurosurgery*, **7**, 262–4.
Michels, V.V., Whisnant, J.P., Garrity, J.A. *et al.* (1989) Neurofibromatosis type 1 with bilateral acoustic neuromas. *Neurofibromatosis*, **2**, 213–17.
Narod, S.A., Parry, D.M., Parboosingh, J. *et al.* (1992) Neurofibromatosis type 2 appears to be a genetically homogeneous disease. *Am. J. Hum. Genet.*, **51**, 486–96.
Okazaki, M., Nishisho, I., Tateishi, H. *et al.* (1988) Loss of genes on the long arm of chromosome 22 in human meningiomas. *Mol. Biol. Med.*, **5**, 15–22.
Quest, D.O. (1978) Meningiomas: an update. *Neurosurgery*, **3**, 219–25.
Rouleau, G.A., Wertelecki, W., Haines, J.L. *et al.* (1987) Genetic linkage of bilateral acoustic neurofibromatosis to a DNA marker on chromosome 22. *Nature*, **329**, 246–8.
Rouleau, G.A., Haines, J.L., Bazanowski, A. *et al.* (1989) A genetic linkage map of the long arm of human chromosome 22. *Genomics*, **4**, 1–4.
Rouleau, G.A., Seizinger, B.R., Wertelecki, W. *et al.* (1990) Flanking markers bracket the neurofibromatosis type 2 (NF2) gene on chromosome 22. *Am. J. Hum. Genet.*, **46**, 323–8.
Rouleau, G.A., Merel, P., Lutchman, M. *et al.* (1993) Alteration in a new gene encoding a putative membrane organizing protein causes neurofibromatosis type 2. *Nature*, **363**, 515–21.
Russell, D.S. and Rubenstein, L.J. (1972) *Pathology of Tumours of the Nervous System*, 3rd edn, Williams & Wilkins, Baltimore, pp. 48–73.
Schwartz, D.C. and Cantor, C.R. (1984) Separation of yeast chromosome-sized DNAs by pulsed field gel electrophoresis. *Cell*, **37**, 67–75.
Sedzimir, C.B., Frazer, A.K. and Roberts, J.P. (1973) Cranial and spinal meningiomas in a pair of identical twin boys. *J. Neurol. Neurosurg. Psychiatr.*, **36**, 368–76.

Seizinger, B.R., Martuza, R.L. and Gusella, J.F. (1986) Loss of genes on chromosome 22 in tumorigenesis of human acoustic neuroma. *Nature*, **332**, 644–7.

Seizinger, B.R., Rouleau, G.A., Ozelius, L.J. *et al.* (1987a) Common pathogenetic mechanism for three tumour types in bilateral acoustic neurofibromatosis. *Science*, **236**, 317–19.

Seizinger, B.R., de la Monte, S., Atkins, L. *et al.* (1987b) Molecular genetic approach to human meningioma: loss of genes on chromosome 22. *Proc. Natl. Acad. Sci. USA*, **84**, 5419–23.

Tator, C.H. (1985) Acoustic neuromas: management of 204 cases. *Can. J. Neurol. Sci.*, **12**, 353–7.

Trofatter, J.A., MacCollin, M.M., Rutter, J.L. *et al.* (1993) A novel moesin-, ezrin-, radixin-like gene is a candidate for the neurofibromatosis 2 tumour suppressor. *Cell*, **72**, 791–800.

Vance, J.M., Nicholson, G.A., Yamaoka, L.H. *et al.* (1989) Linkage of Charcot–Marie–Tooth neuropathy type 1a to chromosome 17. *Exp. Neurol.*, **104**, 186–9.

Wertelecki, W., Rouleau, G.A., Superneau, D.W. *et al.* (1988) Neurofibromatosis 2: clinical and DNA linkage studies. *N. Engl. J. Med.*, **319**, 278–83.

Wolff, R.K., Frazer, K.A., Jackler, R.K. *et al.* (1992) Analysis of chromosome 22 deletions in neurofibromatosis type 2-related tumors. *Am. J. Hum. Genet.*, **51**, 478–85.

Zang, K.D. (1982) Cytological and cytogenetical studies on human meningioma. *Cancer Genet. Cytogenet.*, **6**, 249–75.

Zang, K.D. and Singer, H. (1967) Chromosomal constitution of meningiomas. *Nature*, **216**, 84–5.

4

The neural crest: migration and differentiation*

J. Smith

4.1 INTRODUCTION

Neurofibromatosis 1 (NF1) is characterized by the remarkable diversity of its clinical manifestations. Abnormal maculation of the skin (pigmented café au lait spots) is variably associated with superficial or deep neurofibromas, astrocytomas, phaeochromocytomas (benign or, less often, malignant tumours), vascular and skeletal abnormalities, and learning disorders. Neurofibromatosis 2 (NF2) causes Schwannomas, especially vestibular Schwannomas, meningiomas and astrocytomas. More than 15 years ago, Bolande (1974) suggested that a common denominator between these different manifestations and between neurofibromatosis and certain other afflictions (grouped together under the heading of phakomatoses) was to be found in the neural crest. Consequently, the term 'neurocristopathy' was coined to include the more or less complex syndromes involving pathological development of neural crest derivatives. However, although there is no doubt that the cell types predominantly concerned by neurofibromatosis (melanocytes and peripheral glial cells, in particular) do indeed arise from the neural crest, the site and nature of the postulated developmental defect(s) are not known. In which cells is the abnormality seated? Is it in the neurectoderm in general, in the neural crest in particular or, more specifically, in certain lineages derived from it? Alternatively, is it localized, not in the neural crest itself, but in some of the cells that constitute the environment that is essential for the normal migration and differentiation of the neural crest? Which biological process is deranged in neurofibromatosis: migration, multiplication or differentiation? Answers to these questions can come only from a concerted effort on the part of molecular geneticists, cell biologists and embryologists. The recent cloning of the neurofibromatosis

* This chapter was submitted in November 1990.

gene (Cawthon *et al.*, 1990; Viskochil *et al.*, 1990; Wallace *et al.*, 1990) represents an important breakthrough in the molecular analysis of the disorder. It is therefore all the more important to return to the embryo in an attempt to fill in some of the gaps in our perception of the normal development of the neural crest. Fortunately, this is an area of research that has, over the last 10 years or so, been the object of a resurgence of interest, accompanied by the emergence of innovative technology. As a consequence, significant advances have been made in our understanding of when and where crest cells migrate and what they differentiate into, as well as in the identification of factors that can influence these processes. Some of the most recent studies have focused on deciphering the events involved in the segregation of the various lineages that arise during embryogenesis. This review will touch upon each of these points, with particular emphasis on the steps where the effects of ontogenetic dysregulation could be most important.

4.2 THE FORMATION AND FATE OF THE NEURAL CREST

The neural crest is a rudiment phylogenetically restricted to vertebrates. It forms very early in embryogenesis, but only after the creation and segregation of three germ layers (ectoderm, mesoderm and endoderm) and the neuralization by the chordamesoderm of the dorsal ectoderm. Neuralization consists of the formation of the neural plate and the hollowing of the latter to form a tube. The neural crest materializes in an anteroposterior fashion at the dorsal summit of the neural tube, which corresponds to the lateral margins of the neural plate. The crest is short-lived and rapidly loses its initial epithelial organization as its component cells embark on migrations that sometimes take them far from their point of departure. At certain specific sites, migration ceases and the progeny of the crest cells differentiate into several characteristic cell types.

Much of the early experimental work on neural crest development (see Hörstadius (1950) and Le Douarin (1982) for references) was carried out on amphibians. Early fate maps were constructed by ablating a particular region of the neural crest and studying the resulting anatomical deficiency. However, the ability of vertebrate embryos to replace missing portions by cells from neighbouring regions meant that the results of these studies only gave a coarse (although essentially correct) view of the precursor–product relationships between the neural crest and various differentiated tissues. In fact, the rapid dissemination of crest cells throughout the developing embryo can only be followed and analysed if the cells have been previously labelled in such a way that they can be identified during embryogenesis. Several more or less satisfactory marking methods have been used (Le Douarin, 1982). However, the introduction (Le Douarin, 1969, 1973) of a technique based on permanent, histologically recognizable structural differences between interphase nuclei of quail and chick was undoubtedly instrumental in refining the analysis of the developmental fate of the neurectoderm in general and the neural crest in particular. A characteristic of the quail nucleus is the presence of a small number of nucleolus-associated clumps of heterochromatin. In the chick, as in most other avian species examined, the nucleolar chromatin is dispersed throughout the nucleoplasm. This peculiarity of the quail nucleus can be revealed by classical histochemical staining methods and with the electron microscope (Figure 4.1). Chimaeric embryos are constructed by replacing a portion of neural tube from a chick embryo (before the neural crest has begun to migrate) with the equivalent stretch of a quail neural tube (isotopic and isochronic transplantation). The migration and development of cells originating in the neural crest are then studied in progressively older embryos. This work was carried out intensively in the laboratory of N. Le Douarin and elsewhere (Narayanan and Narayanan, 1978a,b, 1980; Noden, 1978; Richardson *et al.*, 1989). Investigations of this sort can be extended beyond the period of embryonic life; quail-chick 'neural tube chimaeras'

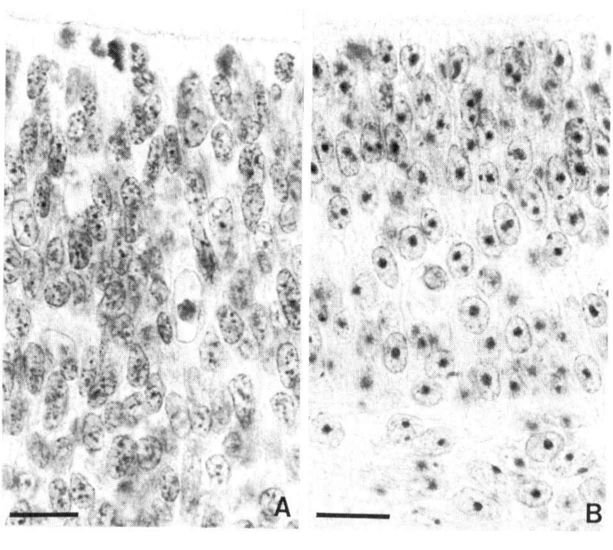

Figure 4.1 Cells of two closely related species of birds can be distinguished by a simple histochemical reaction. Chick nuclear heterochromatin is dispersed throughout the nucleus (A), whereas in the quail (B) it is condensed into one or two spots that are readily revealed by the Feulgen-Rossenbeck method for staining DNA. This striking cytological difference between chick and quail cells allows unambiguous identification of the species of origin of individual cells in chimaeric tissue. The sections shown here are of spinal cord from 7-day embryos. Scale bar 25 μm. (Photo by courtesy of Dr M.-A. Teillet.)

can hatch and behave apparently normally for some time after birth (Kinutani and Le Douarin, 1985, Balaban, Teillet and Le Douarin, 1988).

Recently, a new technology whereby cells are injected *in vivo* with a fluorescent dye has been applied to the mapping of neural crest derivatives (Bronner-Fraser, 1988, 1989). Although this method suffers from the primary drawback of other artificial marking systems, i.e. the rapid dilution of the label with successive cell divisions, it has the more than compensatory advantage of enabling the fate(s) of single cells (when only one cell was injected in the first instance) to be followed *in embryo*.

Derivatives of the neural crest include neurons and non-neuronal cells of the entire (i.e. sensory, autonomic and enteric) peripheral nervous system, one nucleus of the central nervous system (CNS), pigment cells, adrenal medulla, certain other types of endocrine cells and part of the skeletal, muscular and connective tissue of the head and neck (the so-called mesectodermal derivatives) (Table 4.1). This list has been compiled from data obtained from experiments on birds and lower vertebrates. There is reason to believe that it also applies to other species, including humans with the possible exception of certain craniofacial derivatives, e.g. certain skeletal elements of the middle ear, the origin of which may be crucially dependent on the precise location of the crest–mesoderm interface (Noden, 1987).

An important result of studies involving stably labelled neural transplants has been the accurate pinpointing of the sites of origin along the embryonic axis of numerous derivatives of the neural crest (Le Douarin and Teillet, 1973, 1974). For example, the ganglia and plexuses of the sympathetic nervous system derive from the neural crest caudad to the level of the fifth pair of somites. The adrenal medulla arises from crest cells migrating exclusively from the levels of somites 18–24. The enteric ganglia originate from crest cells located, for the most part, at the 'vagal' level of the neuraxis (i.e. encompassing somites 1–7), with a minor contribution, limited to the postumbilical gut, of crest cells from the 'sacral' level (i.e. beyond the 28th pair of somites). The cranial ganglia derive, at least in part, from the cephalic neural crest. The spinal (dorsal root) ganglia are formed (one pair per pair of somites) from the level of the 6th somite caudad.

It is useful to end this section by mentioning what the neural crest does *not* give rise to, particularly in view of some misconceptions that may persist. The neural crest does not give rise to the entire APUD cell series. These polypeptide hormone-secreting cells, designated by an acronym defining two of their common properties, i.e. amine precursor uptake and decarboxylation (Pearse, 1968, 1976), are widespread throughout the body; some are found in the endocrine glands, and others are localized in non-endocrine tissue. It was suggested that these cells, by virtue of their metabolic similarities, share a common embryological origin (Pearse, 1968, 1976). However, careful scrutiny of quail-chick chimaeras showed

Table 4.1 Non-exhaustive list of derivatives of the neural crest

Central nervous system	Neurons of the mesencephalic nucleus of the trigeminal nerve
Peripheral nervous system	Neurons of sensory ganglia (spinal ganglia and ganglia of trigeminal, glossopharyngeal and vagal nerves)
	Neurons of all sympathetic, parasympathetic and enteric ganglia
	Satellite cells in all sensory, sympathetic, parasympathetic and enteric ganglia
	Schwann cells
Mesectodermal derivatives	Nasal and orbital skeleton, palate, maxillary and visceral skeleton, parts of the cranial vault and otic capsule, mandibular and hyoid bones and cartilage
	Sclera and choroid, ciliary muscles, corneal endothelium and stromal fibroblasts
	Dermis, smooth muscle and adipose tissue in the face and ventrolateral side of the neck
	Small contribution to the striated muscle of the face and neck
	Connective tissue of walls of the large vessels derived from the aortic arches
	Meninges in the prosencephalon and part of the mesencephalon
	Odontoblasts
	Connective tissue of the pituitary, thymus, thyroid, parathyroid, lacrymal and salivary glands
Endocrine system	Carotid body type I cells, calcitonin-producing cells and adrenal medulla
Pigment cells	Melanocytes of the epidermis, dermis and internal organs
	Chromatophores of the iris

conclusively that, of this numerous family (which includes pancreatic α_2 and β cells, intestinal argyrophil and enterochromaffin cells, and pituitary adrenocorticotrophic hormone (ACTH)- and melanocyte-stimulating hormone (MSH)-secreting cells), only the adrenal medulla, the calcitonin-secretory cells of the thyroid and carotid body type I cells originate from the neural crest (Andrew, 1974; Fontaine and Le Douarin, 1977a; Fontaine, Le Lièvre and Le Douarin, 1977) or, for that matter, from the neurectoderm as a whole (Fontaine and Le Douarin, 1977b; Le Douarin, 1988).

Again, the neural crest is not the source of all the neurons of the cranial peripheral sensory ganglia. Early investigators showed that the ectodermal placodes (which are localized epithelial thickenings that appear laterally in the cephalic ectoderm of the young embryo) contribute significantly to these ganglia (Le Douarin and Smith, 1988), although only construction of quail-chick chimaeras enabled the respective contributions of neural crest and placodes to be determined for each (Noden, 1978; Narayanan and Narayanan, 1980; Ayer-Le Lièvre and Le Douarin, 1982; D'Amico-Martel and Noden, 1983). It is now known that all the glial cells of all the cranial sensory ganglia are neural crest-derived, whereas their neurons originate, according to the ganglion considered, in the crest, the placodes or in both structures. Neurons are entirely placode-derived in the nodose, petrosal and geniculate ganglia, are exclusively crest-derived in the jugular/superior complex and are of mixed origin in the trigeminal and vestibuloacoustic ganglia. (Mosaicism of the latter is due, in fact, to the coalescence of the rudimentary proximal ganglion of nerve VII, all the neurons of which originate in the neural crest, with the vestibular ganglion of nerve VIII, in which all the neurons derive from the ectodermal placodes.)

Finally, it has been demonstrated recently, by means of a retroviral cell-marking technique (Bunge *et al.*, 1989), that the perineurial cells of peripheral ganglia do not arise from the neural crest, but from a fibroblastic (i.e. mesodermal) origin. If this conclusion, reached by the use of an *in vitro* cell culture system, can be shown to apply equally to *in vivo* development, it may be pertinent to the aetiology of neurofibromatosis inasmuch as it has been claimed that some neurofibromas may be composed of perineurial rather than Schwann cells (Harkin, 1986).

4.3 THE DEVELOPMENTAL FATE OF THE ANTERIOR NEURAL PRIMORDIUM

The recent mapping of the anterior neurectoderm in avian chimaeras (Couly and Le Douarin, 1985, 1987) has provided results relevant to disorders such as neurofibromatosis that affect diverse derivatives in both central and peripheral areas. Cephalic structures form as a result of extensive, complex morphogenetic processes that can completely mask close positional relationships in the early primordium before the large-scale movements have begun. Examination of chimaeras, constructed at 0- to 3-somite stages by the transfer of defined areas of the antero-lateral neural ridge and adjacent neural plate, revealed a previously unsuspected early contiguity of the primordium of the hypothalamus with the adenohypophyseal placode. Similarly, the olfactory placode (source of the olfactory sensory epithelium) was shown to lie juxtaposed to the floor of the telencephalon, from which the olfactory bulb subsequently develops. The precise developmental significance of this initial apposition of plate and ridge territories that will subsequently form parts of integrated functional units, i.e. the hypothalamo–hypophyseal complex and the central and peripheral olfactory structures, remains to be determined. As speculated by Couly and Le Douarin (1985), all the cells composing these structures may arise from a few progenitors (perhaps only one) which rapidly become restricted in their developmental capacities to several related cell types.

The rostral limits of the neural crest are at the caudal prosencephalic level (Couly and Le Douarin, 1987). Anterior to this zone, the neural folds do not yield mesectodermal derivatives (bones and dermis), but provide (somewhat unexpectedly) the superficial ectoderm of the roof of the mouth, olfactory cavities and face. Neural crest from the caudal prosencephalic/rostral mesencephalic level was found to give rise to nasofrontal mesectoderm, sclera and choroid membrane of the eye, and forebrain meninges. However, the meninges of the hindbrain and spinal cord are of mesodermal origin (Le Douarin, 1982).

From these studies, a rationale was proposed for the genesis of certain pathological disorders in man, uniting malformations of the face with those of the brain and/or adenohypophyseal deficiencies (Couly and Le Douarin, 1987). The origin of the choroid from neural crest is relevant to the occurrence of choroidal hamartomas and Lisch nodules in NF1 (Chapter X).

4.4 MIGRATION OF NEURAL CREST CELLS AND THE ORGANIZATION OF PERIPHERAL STRUCTURES

A striking characteristic that sets neural crest cells apart from their immediate neighbours in the superficial ectoderm or the neural tube is their ability to migrate extensively. Although some cells, e.g. those that give rise to the meninges or the dorsal root ganglia (DRG), do not move very far before settling and differentiating, others, such as the precursors of Schwann cells ensheathing peripheral nerves, of enteric nervous system ganglion cells and of melanocytes throughout the body, migrate considerable distances from their point of departure.

4.4.1 Mapping of the pathways followed by migrating neural crest cells

Various methods are available for following neural crest cell migration *in situ*. The construction of chimaeric embryos, already described, has provided much valuable information, but other techniques involving no surgical manipulations are also commonly used. The most widespread is based on the expression by migrating avian neural crest cells of surface glycoproteins that are recognized by several independently obtained monoclonal antibodies, NC1 (Vincent, Duband and Thiery, 1983), HNK-1 (Abo and Balch, 1981) and GlN2 (Barbu *et al.*, 1986), all of which apparently recognize similar or identical epitopes. Although these antibodies do not possess an absolute specificity for neural crest cells and their derivatives, do not stain the entire crest cell population (Vincent and Thiery, 1984; Teillet, Kalcheim and Le Douarin, 1987; Newgreen, Powell and Moser, 1990) and do not react in all vertebrate species (Tucker *et al.*, 1988), they have been used profitably to define migration pathways in avian (Bronner-Fraser, 1986; Loring and Erickson, 1987; Teillet, Kalcheim and Le Douarin, 1987), rodent (Erickson, Loring and Lester, 1989) and teleostean (Sadaghiani and Vielkind, 1990) embryos. Preliminary observations have also been made in humans (Tucker *et al.*, 1988). A recent report suggests that the cytoskeleton-associated molecule vinculin may be an efficient and perhaps universal tracer for following crest cell migration and peripheral ganglion formation (Duband and Thiery, 1990). Another recently introduced technique involves the injection of a fluorescent carbocyanine dye into the lumen of the neural tube (Serbedzija, Bronner-Fraser and Fraser, 1989), thus labelling all cells, including premigratory crest cells, whose endfeet contact the lumen. Although all these methods have their advantages and drawbacks, they provide a remarkably concordant picture of neural crest cell migration.

At the onset of migration in the trunk of the avian embryo, which proceeds with a craniocaudal chronology, crest cells cover the dorsal half of the neural tube before reaching the segmented somite region, where they follow distinct pathways (Weston, 1963; Tosney, 1978; Teillet, Kalcheim and Le Douarin, 1987). One stream of cells consisting of presumptive melanocytes passes laterally beneath the ectoderm and above the somites; it displays no apparent segmental organization (Serbedzija, Bronner-Fraser and Fraser, 1989). The dorsoventral pathways, in contrast, are strongly conditioned by the metamerization of the somitic mesoderm. One route leads cells through the space located between two adjacent somites (Thiery, Duband and Delouvée, 1982a; Vincent and Thiery, 1984; Teillet, Kalcheim and Le Douarin, 1987; Newgreen, Powell and Moser, 1990), taking them ventrally to sites dorsolateral to the aorta, where they aggregate to form the sympathetic ganglia (one pair per pair of somites). The major pathway followed by crest cells moving ventrad passes through the rostral half of the somite and, more precisely, the sclerotomal (ventral) as opposed to the dermomyotomal (dorsal) moiety of the somite (Keynes and Stern, 1984; Rickmann, Fawcett and Keynes, 1985; Bronner-Fraser, 1986; Loring and Erickson, 1987; Teillet, Kalcheim and Le Douarin, 1987; Newgreen, Scheel and Kastner, 1986; Newgreen, Powell and Moser, 1990). The cells following this route form the DRG and the Schwann cells in the dorsal and ventral roots. They also contribute to the sympathetic ganglion

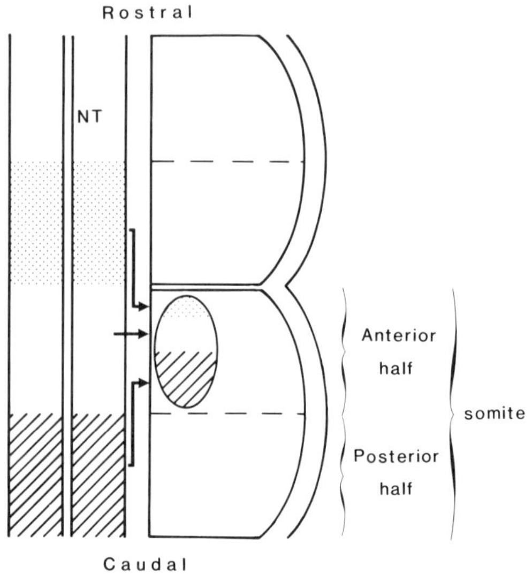

Figure 4.2 Schematic frontal section through the trunk region of a young avian embryo showing the pathways (arrows) taken by migrating neural crest cells before condensing to form a dorsal root ganglion (DRG). The ganglion arises from crest cells that migrate through the anterior half of the somite. These cells come initially from a length of neural tube (NT) that extends continuously from the posterior half of the somite that lies rostral to the future DRG down to the caudal region of the somite at the same segmental level as the ganglion. As indicated in the figure, their localization in the ganglion corresponds approximately to their original position along the rostrocaudal axis. (Reproduced from Teillet, Kalcheim and Le Douarin, 1987, with permission.)

chains (Teillet, Kalcheim and Le Douarin, 1987; Newgreen, Powell and Moser, 1990). Virtually identical observations have been made in the mouse (Serbedzija, Fraser and Bronner-Fraser, 1990).

Teillet, Kalcheim and Le Douarin (1987) refined the analysis of neural crest migration to the sites of DRG formation by grafting into chick hosts short lengths of quail neural primordium ending at mid-somitic or intersomitic levels. Using the quail nuclear marker in conjunction with HNK-1 staining, these authors demonstrated clearly that DRG do not form opposite the middle of a somite, but rather facing its rostral half. Furthermore, they showed that any given DRG is composed of neural crest cells originating not only from the rostral level of the corresponding somite (found mainly in the rostral part of the ganglion), but also of cells that leave the neural primordium opposite the caudal half of the same somite and the caudal half of the preceding one (Figure 4.2). In other words, prior to gangliogenesis, while DRG precursor cells arising opposite rostral half-somites migrate essentially laterally, those originating opposite caudal half-somites move longitudinally in both anterior and posterior directions. The migration pattern of Schwann cell precursors lining the segmental dorsal and ventral root fibres was seen to be virtually identical to that described for DRG, whereas the precursors of the sympathetic ganglia and melanocytes were more widely disseminated, ending up as many as three somites rostrad or caudad of their point of departure.

4.4.2 Cell-surface and matrix molecules involved in neural crest cell migration

The recent realization that neural crest cells migrate preferentially at the level of and into the anterior region of the sclerotomal mesenchyme has initiated a series of studies aimed at identifying molecular differences between anterior and posterior somite halves that could explain this. Components of the extracellular matrix, molecules at the surface of crest cells and/or of cells lining the pathways along which they migrate must, via modulation of cell–substrate or cell–cell adhesion, be important contributory factors in the patterned dispersal of crest-derived cells. Our understanding of this is far from complete and additional molecules involved in adhesion and motility doubtless await characterization. Nevertheless extracellular and surface components have been identified that potentially play important roles in the interactions of neural crest cells with their environment. The experimental approaches to this problem combine histochemical or immunocytochemical analysis *in vivo*, exposure *in vitro* of isolated neural crest cells to potentially relevant molecules and the targeted perturbation of migration *in situ*.

Early work showed that neural crest cells migrate into cell-free spaces rich in the glycosaminoglycans chondroitin sulphate and hyaluronate (Derby, 1978; Pintar, 1978). Hyaluronate, in particular, appears to be important in maintaining hydrated cell-free spaces into which crest cells can move (Pratt, Larsen and Johnston, 1975); furthermore, according to its concentration, it may either prevent or facilitate the release of the cells from the neural tube (Luckenbill-Edds and Carrington, 1988). Other experiments demonstrated that pathways of migration contain high concentrations of fibronectin, that crest cells migrate preferentially on fibronectin lanes *in vitro* (Newgreen and Thiery, 1980; Rovasio *et al.*, 1983) and that injection into embryos of antibodies or peptides capable of blocking interactions of neural crest cells with fibronectin inhibits migration (Boucaut *et al.*, 1984; Bronner-Fraser, 1985). Crest cells themselves initially possess the adhesion molecules N-cadherin and N-CAM, lose both as they leave the neural tube and re-express them as they aggregate at the end-points of their migration (Thiery *et al.*, 1982b; Lallier and Bronner-Fraser, 1988).

The distribution of fibronectin within the somite is too homogeneous to explain the selective channelling of crest cells in the anterior portion

(Newgreen and Thiery, 1980; Thiery, Duband and Delouvée, 1982a; Rickmann, Fawcett and Keynes, 1985; Mackie *et al.*, 1988). Likewise, laminin and N-CAM are uniformly present within the sclerotomal mesenchyme (Rickmann, Fawcett and Keynes, 1985; Duband *et al.*, 1987). On the other hand, the specific localization of a number of other macromolecules to rostral or caudal half-somites has been reported. Thus butyrylcholinesterase activity is concentrated rostrally (Layer, Alber and Rathjen, 1988), as are cytotactin and tenascin (basement membrane-associated glycoproteins that are probably identifical to each other and that are believed to be involved in neuron-glia adhesion), whereas a cytotactin-binding proteoglycan is restricted to caudal half-somites (Tan *et al.*, 1987; Mackie *et al.*, 1988). However, the conclusion that cytotactin/tenascin is a major factor in patterning crest cell migration has been dismissed by Stern *et al.* (1989), who found no temporal or spatial correlations between the expression of the glycoprotein and the migration of crest cells. They suggest instead that tenascin-related molecules (which seem to have an inhibitory effect on migration) may play a role at later stages of ontogeny, e.g. during gangliogenesis. A molecule (probably a glycolipid) bearing an epitope recognized by HNK-1 has also been demonstrated to appear transiently at the surface of rostral somite cells concomitantly with the immigration of crest cells (Newgreen, Powell and Moser, 1990); in view of the apparent role in cell adhesion of some other molecules recognized by this monoclonal antibody (Riopelle, McGarry and Roder, 1986; Bronner-Fraser, 1987), it has been proposed that the somite glycolipid may interact heterotypically with neural crest cells and so be one of the agents responsible for their patterned repartitioning (Newgreen, Powell and Moser, 1990). Co-operative interactions between crest and somite cells, resulting in the production of a high-molecular-weight form of tenascin, have also been invoked as a possible means of regulating neural crest migration in the sclerotomal mesenchyme (Stern *et al.*, 1989).

Molecules at the cell surface and in extracellular spaces are not the only factors involved in cell motility. A recent report has underlined the potential importance of cytoskeletal components as regulators of adhesive behaviour (Duband and Thiery, 1990). Clearly, the problem is complex and much further analysis will be required before all the subtleties underlying the control of crest cell migration can be grasped.

4.4.3 Experimentally provoked anomalies of peripheral ganglion patterning

As predicted from the existence of obligate pathways of migration, disorganization of the environment through which crest cells migrate radically disturbs gangliogenesis. Gross deletion of several successive somites caused motor axons and neural crest cells to migrate with a non-segmental pattern (Lewis *et al.*, 1981; Tosney, 1988). In a technically more demanding approach, less drastic modifications of the milieu at the trunk level were produced unilaterally by the surgical construction of compound somites, consisting of multiple rostral or caudal halves (Stern and Keynes, 1987; Kalcheim and Teillet, 1989). The initial phases of neural crest migration were seen to be similar irrespective of the rostral or caudal nature of the somitic mesenchyme; the cells appeared as a continuous unsegmented strip along the dorsal aspects of the neural tube. However, whereas crest cells penetrated multiple rostral sclerotomes massively in an unsegmented manner, they hardly migrated at all into compound caudal sclerotomes. These phenomena were reflected in strikingly atypical formation of the spinal ganglia. The DRG that formed in the context of multiple caudal sclerotomes were much reduced in size, abnormally segmented and situated in an unusually dorsal position. In contrast, embryos grafted with multiple rostral half-somites developed a single giant DRG spanning the entire implant (Kalcheim and Teillet, 1989) (Figure 4.3). These findings provide a forceful illustration of the importance of differential interactions between crest cells and the two halves of a somite in the correct patterning of the spinal ganglia.

4.5 DEVELOPMENTAL POTENTIALITIES OF NEURAL CREST CELLS AND THEIR PROGENY

The establishment of fate maps has revealed that the neural crest is organized axially into regions which will develop into different derivatives. In contrast, the total number of cell types that each region is capable of giving rise to under appropriate environmental conditions is less restricted. This can be shown by transposing regions of the neuraxis *in vivo* (heterotopic and heterochronic grafts; Le Douarin and Teillet, 1974) or by culturing them *in vitro* (see later). With the exception of its mesectodermal capabilities, which are confined to the cephalic region, the neural crest can be considered as a fairly uniformly pluripotential structure. The fact that the entire range of developmental possibilities is not normally implemented at each level of the neuraxis implies that the differentiation of neural crest-derived cells is in great part conditioned by their environment during and after their migration. These findings pose fundamental embryological questions relating to the state of determination, or commitment to a particular developmental fate, of individual crest cells at the time they set out from the neural primordium. Does the overall pluripotentiality of the neural crest population mean that each cell is pluripotential? Or is the neural crest a mosaic structure, made up of subsets of cells each of which is determined to differentiate in a particular manner? Learning the answers to these questions should reveal how environmental factors act. In the first case, environmental factors would impose a particular developmental option on toti- or multipotent

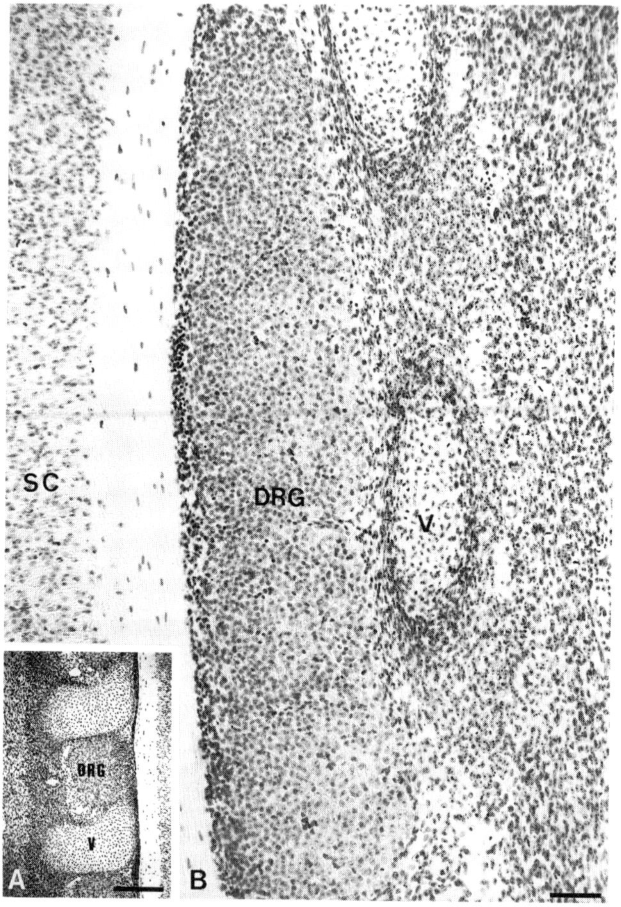

Figure 4.3 A 'polyganglion' resulting from the manipulation of the environment in which neural crest cells migrate and differentiate. Frontal section through an 8-day chick embryo from which four somites had been removed unilaterally 6 days earlier and replaced by an equivalent length of rostral half-somites from a 2-day quail embryo. (A) Control side. Normal DRG alternate with vertebrae (V). Scale bar 150 μm. (B) Operated side at the same level, showing a giant unsegmented dorsal root ganglion (DRG) in contact with the spinal cord (SC) throughout its length. Scale bar 40 μm. (Reproduced from Kalcheim and Teillet, 1989, with permission.)

progenitors. In the second case environmental factors selectively promote the survival and multiplication of specific subpopulations of cells whose subsequent differentiation would unfold according to a genetically determined plan. The answers will also enable us to predict the consequences of biological disorders affecting only part of the neural crest cell population (e.g. resulting from somatic mutation or teratogenic insults). Lesions of pluripotential cells will affect a wider spectrum of derivatives than those afflicting cells with restricted developmental potentialities.

4.5.1 Evidence for heterogeneity in the neural crest cell population

During recent years, much effort has been spent in trying to determine exactly when different neural crest-derived cell lineages become segregated and, in particular, whether or not this phenomenon has already begun in the premigratory or migrating crest. It is becoming increasingly clear that the neural crest is far from homogeneous in the potentialities of its individual constituent cells.

(a) Indirect evidence from observations in vivo *and* in vitro

With few exceptions (Smith *et al.*, 1979; Cochard and Coltey, 1983; Payette, Bennet and Gershon, 1984), no phenotypic features characteristic of any of its terminally differentiated derivatives are expressed by cells of the neural crest while they are still in the process of migrating. However, certain monoclonal antibodies raised against determinants expressed by peripheral ganglion cells also react with neural crest, and in some cases they have revealed individual differences at the molecular level between cells in the migrating population *in situ* (Barbu *et al.*, 1986) or after a very short period of culture *in vitro* (Ciment and Weston, 1982; Barald, 1988).

Although the non-mesectodermal developmental capacities of the crest cell population are qualitatively equivalent throughout the neuraxis, certain quantitative differences have been noted. Thus, trunk crest is a less abundant potential source of enteric ganglia than is cranial crest (Le Douarin and Teillet, 1974; Smith, Cochard and Le Douarin, 1977; Newgreen *et al.*, 1980). Conversely, trunk crest differentiates into adrenergic cells and melanocytes with greater facility than the cranial crest (Newgreen *et al.*, 1980; our unpublished results).

Cultures of neural crest have been used in a number of laboratories as model systems (for a review, see Le Douarin and Smith, 1988). It is possible, by manipulating the medium in which the cells are grown, to obtain the differentiation of most, if not all, neural crest derivatives. However, neural crest cells do not react identically to a given set of culture conditions. For instance, only a small proportion ever expresses neuronal properties and the neurons that do develop are of neurochemically diverse types (Maxwell, Sietz and Rafford, 1982; Maxwell, Sietz and Jean, 1984; Garcia-Arraras *et al.*, 1986, 1987; Ziller *et al.*, 1987; Fauquet and Ziller, 1989). This heterogeneity does not necessarily imply the existence of an equivalent number of precommitted precursors, because, as will be shown in the next section, similarly varied derivatives can be obtained when single crest cells are grown under clonal conditions. The phenotypes in mass cultures of neural crest cannot therefore provide much information relating to the state of determination of the cells when they are removed from the embryo. On the other hand, results of experiments involving the sequential culturing of neural crest in different media strongly support the hypothesis of an early segregation of two neuronal lineages whose precursor cells have demonstrably different requirements for differentiation (Ziller *et al.*, 1983, 1987).

(b) *Direct evidence from clonal cultures*

An ideal way of examining directly the potentialities of single cells is to isolate them and test individually their capacities for differentiation under controlled, permissive conditions in culture. Clonal cultures of neural crest were first carried out, using the limiting dilution technique, by Sieber-Blum and Cohen (1980), who described three qualitatively different kinds of clone in the colonies they obtained. Recently, Baroffio, Dupin and Le Douarin (1988) and Dupin *et al.* (1990) published the results of a comprehensive investigation in which they used a technology guaranteeing that only one cell is seeded. Their protocol involves the dissociation of mesencephalic neural crest (dissected out of quail embryos while it is migrating laterally under the surface ectoderm) to single cells, which are then cultured individually on a feeder layer of growth-inhibited 3T3 cells (a line derived from mouse fibroblasts), in a medium including serum, chick embryo extract and growth factors. These conditions were found to be permissive, not only for survival and multiplication, but also for the expression of phenotypes representative of the principal lineages arising from the neural crest.

Analysis by several phenotypic markers of clones derived from single neural crest cells provided interesting conclusions. First, neural crest cells taken at the migrating stage have strikingly differing abilities to multiply: after 10 days in culture, some clones contained fewer than 10 cells while others comprised 20000 or more. Second, a great many individual neural crest cells are multipotential, since the vast majority of clones that they gave rise to contained more than one identifiable derivative (up to six were found, in variable proportions). Third, cells in the migrating neural crest are heterogeneous in their developmental potentialities. Most are apparently pluripotential, but not identically so; 20 or so classes of clone were characterized according to the phenotype, or combination of phenotypes, that they expressed. Furthermore, although clones displaying multiple phenotypes predominated, some (approximately 20% of the total) were composed of only a single cell type, implying derivation from fully determined precursors. Rare colonies containing less than 10 cells were entirely neuronal; others, larger and more common, were exclusively made up of glial cells. However, in contrast to the results obtained earlier with clonal cultures of trunk neural crest (Sieber-Blum and Cohen, 1980), no evidence was obtained for the existence of a fully determined precursor of melanocytes.

Several additional interesting points were brought to light in the course of this investigation. For instance, neurons, found in somewhat less than half of the clones, were almost always associated with non-neuronal cells, some of which were identified as Schwann cells on the basis of their immunoreactivity with a monoclonal antibody recognizing a surface glycoprotein (Schwann cell myelin protein, SMP) present on all Schwann cells but not on ganglionic satellite cells or neurons (Dulac *et al.*, 1988). This result clearly implies that common precursors for non-neuronal cells and neurons occur frequently in the migrating neural crest. Interestingly, a number of clones contained only Schwann cells, indicating that determined progenitors of this cell type also exist at the same stage of development. In a subsequent series of experiments (Baroffio and Blot, 1992), it was found that neural (neurons and Schwann or satellite cells) and mesectodermal cells coexisted in approximately 3% of the cultures examined. This result demonstrates that mesectodermal and neural lineages are not completely segregated by the time crest cell migration is under way, as had been proposed previously (Le Lièvre and Le Douarin, 1975).

Finally, a single clone (0.3% of the total number examined) was found to contain the complete range of phenotypes that could be identified with the available markers, i.e. cartilage, neuronal, Schwann, satellite and pigment cells. The founder cell of such a clone may be representative of a small totipotent population akin to the stem cells from which lymphoid and haemopoietic cells arise during ontogeny of the blood system (Anderson, 1989; Baroffio and Blot, 1992).

4.5.5 Evidence for the accumulation of heterogeneous populations of developmentally restricted precursors at peripheral sites *in vivo*

The preceding section demonstrates how individual cells in the migrating neural crest population differ in their abilities to proliferate and differentiate under conditions that provide factors necessary for mitosis and signals required for the development of most of their derivatives. This suggests a model in which subpopulations of migrating and dividing neural crest cells become rapidly, but asynchronously, committed to different and progressively more restricted developmental fates. The relationships between the different types of precursor, i.e. their respective hierarchies on a lineage tree, have not yet been clarified. The absence of any clear pattern in the combinations of potentialities intermediate between those of the totipotent progenitor and the monopotent, determined precursors suggests that restriction does not proceed in a stereotyped sequence, but that potentialities are segregated in a stochastic manner.

Since there is no evidence to suggest that differently committed precursors follow distinct routes of migration in the embryo, one of the probable consequences of the early developmental heterogeneity of the neural crest population would be the arrival, at the sites in which differentiation occurs, of a mixed population of precursors corresponding to different lineages, only some of which have potentialities that are normally expressed in a given location. Consequently, the regional differences in phenotypic expression that characterize neural crest derivatives would be due to site-specific selection (in response to relevant permissive environmental factors) of only those progenitors whose potentialities 'correspond' to a particular location; 'inappropriate' precursors would remain latent or ultimately disappear, according to their requirements for survival.

No clonal analysis similar to that performed with migrating neural crest cells has been carried out with crest derivatives and so little or no information is available about the persistence of pluripotentiality in cells that have migrated to peripheral sites. The method that has been most often used to search for normally unexpressed programmes of differentiation in neural crest derivatives entails grafting small fragments of a peripheral ganglion taken from a quail embryo into a younger chick embryo host. The transplantation has been performed either at the trunk (Le Lièvre *et al.*, 1980; Ayer-Le Lièvre and Le Douarin, 1982; Schweizer, Ayer-Le Lièvre and Le Douarin, 1983; Dupin, 1984) or the vagal (Fontaine-Pérus, Chanconie and Le Douarin, 1988) level of the host, at the time that crest cells start migrating (48 h and 36 h of incubation, respectively). The fate of the implanted cells can be followed via the quail nuclear marker, and information can be obtained concerning the extent to which crest-derived cells in diverse ganglia of different ages can contribute to embryonic structures such as cranial and spinal sensory ganglia, sympathetic chains, adrenal medulla, enteric plexuses, Schwann cells and connective tissue. The data obtained from these studies have provided evidence that not only are developmental potentialities of ganglion cells qualitatively restricted compared with those of neural crest cells, but the potencies that do remain are not uniformly distributed among the different types of ganglia.

(a) Presence of latent potentialities in peripheral ganglion cells

In these 'back-transplantation' studies the only crest-derived structures capable of colonizing sensory derivatives in the trunk are sensory ganglia themselves. Grafted autonomic ganglia contributed virtually no cells to host spinal ganglia whereas numerous cells from transplanted DRG were incorporated into these sensory structures where they differentiated into neurons and non-neuronal cells (Le Lièvre *et al.*, 1980). However, this phenomenon was observed only in grafts of sensory ganglia taken from donor embryos of less than 8 days of incubation. It was convincingly demonstrated that the ability of donor DRG to provide sensory neurons after back-transplantation was strictly correlated with the presence of mitotically active neuroblasts in the graft (Schweizer, Ayer-Le Lièvre and Le Douarin, 1983), suggesting strongly that postmitotic neurons are not involved in the process of differentiation occurring after transplantation.

In contrast to the strict confinement of sensory neuronal potentialities to sensory ganglia, precursors able to colonize and differentiate in a variety of 'autonomic' sites are widespread; when either autonomic (ciliary and sympathetic) or sensory (DRG and various cranial ganglia) derivatives were back-transplanted, graft-derived cells migrated to and differentiated in structures including the sympathetic ganglia, adrenal gland, ganglion of Remak (a parasympathetic structure specific to birds) and enteric plexuses (Le Douarin *et al.*, 1978; Le Lièvre *et al.*, 1980; Ayer-Le Lièvre and Le Douarin, 1982; Schweizer, Ayer-Le Lièvre and Le Douarin, 1983; Fontaine-Pérus, Chanconie and Le Douarin, 1988). This is consistent with the hypothesis formulated some years ago (Le Douarin, 1984, 1986) that sensory and autonomic lineages are segregated very early in development, and it also supports the idea that sensory ganglia normally develop from a mixed collection of progenitors of sensory and autonomic types. Exactly when the segregation occurs remains to be determined. Experiments involving the labelling of single cells in the dorsal neural tube *in vivo* (Bronner-Fraser and Fraser, 1989) revealed that, in the majority of embryos in which labelled cells were located in the spinal ganglia, no other peripheral sites were colonized, thus suggesting that progenitor cells with an exclusively sensory fate are present even before the neural crest is formed. On the other hand, Sieber-Blum (1989) applied an antibody directed against a sensory lineage-specific marker, SSEA-1, to cultures of isolated crest cells that had migrated from the neural tube *in vitro*, and concluded that dual sensory/autonomic potentialities were still present. It is probable, as suggested earlier, that the crucial event does not occur simultaneously in all precursors.

It is now apparent that a distinction has to be made between the 'autonomic-type' precursors of sympathetic derivatives and those of the enteric nervous system. Thus, all types of peripheral ganglia that have been studied contain cells that can become integrated into sympathetic ganglia and the adrenal medulla. Their differentiation into cells expressing a catecholaminergic phenotype, first identified by histofluorescence *in vivo* (Le Lièvre *et al.*, 1980), was confirmed and extensively studied *in vitro* in cultures of quail sensory ganglia (Xue, Smith and Le Douarin, 1985, 1987; Xue and Smith, 1988). In contrast, the only ganglia that are capable, after back-transplantation, of colonizing and differentiating in the gut are those that, like the enteric ganglia themselves, derive from the rostral (cranial or vagal) levels of the crest (e.g. ciliary, jugular-superior, petrosal, nodose). Sympathetic chain ganglia and DRG (which derive from the cervicothoracic crest) possess no 'enteric' potentialities (Le Lièvre *et al.*, 1980; Fontaine-Pérus, Chanconie and Le Douarin, 1988). A plausible explanation for these observations is that from the outset there is an unequal segregation of 'autonomic-sympathetic' and 'autonomic-enteric' precursors along the neural axis; this is in agreement with the conclusions drawn from a comparison of the respective differentiation capacities of cranial and trunk neural crest (section 4.5.1(a)).

There are several good reasons to believe that it is exclusively the non-neuronal population of peripheral ganglia that possesses autonomic potentialities. The back-transplantation of chimaeric nodose ganglia, in which either the non-neuronal cells (of neural crest origin) or the neurons (of placodal origin) were of quail type showed clearly that only the former migrated to and differentiated in the sympathetic ganglia and adrenal medulla (Ayer-Le Lièvre and Le Douarin, 1982); similar conclusions were reached concerning the contribution of nodose and petrosal ganglion cells to the intrinsic innervation of the gut (Fontaine-Pérus, Chanconie and Le Douarin, 1988). Furthermore, after grafts of ciliary ganglia in which the neurons had been labelled with ^{3}H-thymidine just prior to their ultimate division *in situ*, the great majority of neurons died shortly after the operation (Dupin, 1984). Finally, Xue, Smith and Le Douarin (1985) and Xue and Smith (1988) showed that the DRG cells capable of acquiring noradrenergic properties *in vitro* are recruited from a population of mitotically competent non-neuronal cells.

In addition to sensory and autonomic potentialities, a number of other types of developmental capabilities have been sought in neural crest derivatives. All ganglia tested in the back-transplantation paradigm were able to give rise to carotid body type I and II cells and Schwann cells along peripheral nerves in the cranial or trunk region. On the other hand, mesectodermal precursors were not found in any peripheral ganglia (Fontaine-Pérus, Chanconie and Le Douarin, 1988), although they remain until at least 3.5 days of incubation in the anterior branchial arches (Ciment and Weston, 1983, 1985). Melanocyte precursors are absent from branchial arches and persist in spinal ganglia until day 5 of incubation only (Cowell and Weston, 1970).

4.6 EXTRINSIC FACTORS INVOLVED IN THE SURVIVAL, PROLIFERATION AND DIFFERENTIATION OF NEURAL CREST CELLS

The embryonic microenvironment is important not only in conditioning the migration of crest cells from the summit of the neural tube; it is also believed to play key roles in promoting their survival, controlling their proliferation and triggering their differentiation. The evidence has come principally as a result of fairly straightforward experiments including prevention of normal tissue interactions in the embryo, association of neural crest with various embryonic tissues in organ culture, growth of neural crest in tissue culture in the presence of different cell types or of extracts prepared from them, and, more lately, systematic testing of a variety of known neurotrophic factors in model systems *in vivo* and *in vitro*.

Survival, proliferation and differentiation are phenomena that are often closely interrelated and it is not always obvious from experimentally obtained data which process is principally affected by a given factor. This is true *a fortiori* when one is dealing, not with purified molecules, but with cell-free extracts or conditioned media that may contain multiple 'activities'. Consequently, no attempt has been made to classify the observations cited below in terms of the mechanism of action of the factors under study.

4.6.1 Factors involved in the early development of spinal ganglia

One of the striking results of the back-transplantation experiments described in section 4.5.2(a) was the realization that sensory ganglion cell precursors have a remarkably limited topographical distribution in the developing embryo; they are found only in those ganglia (DRG and proximal cranial sensory ganglia) that develop in close proximity to the neural tube. Ablation of the neural tube shortly after cessation of crest cell migration prevented the development of the DRG, but not of the sympathetic ganglia (Teillet and Le Douarin, 1983). These observations led to the conjecture (Le Douarin, 1986) that progenitor cells of the sensory lineage are strictly dependent on a neural tube-derived factor that is diffusible over only a short distance. This dependence would be relatively short-lived, because axonal outgrowth to the periphery would rapidly provide access to other survival molecules, such as nerve growth factor (NGF), produced by the innervated targets. Sensory precursors migrating further afield (e.g. to the sites of sympathetic gangliogenesis) would rapidly perish for lack of the neural tube factor. In contrast, it is proposed that the survival of autonomic precursors is independent of this substance, meaning that they could break away from the neural tube with impunity.

This hypothesis has stood up well so far to experimental test. In an initial series of experiments, an inert barrier (silastic membrane) was inserted between the neural tube and the newly forming DRG in a young chick embryo. Thus separated from the neural tube, the presumptive ganglion cells, as predicted, died within 10 h, whereas cells that had migrated further ventrally aggregated normally into sympathetic ganglia. When an extract of embryonic neural tube was incorporated into the silastic membrane before its implantation, DRG cells were still found distal to the barrier 36 h after the operation and some had differentiated into neurons (Kalcheim and Le Douarin, 1986). Attempts were then made to identify the active agents. Extracts of other tissues, such as liver, had no positive effects on the survival of DRG precursors, nor had NGF or laminin. On the other hand, brain-derived neurotrophic factor (BDNF), when incorporated together with laminin in the silastic membrane, was able to rescue, albeit temporarily, cells in the DRG rudiments (Kalcheim *et al.*, 1987). BDNF was initially purified from pig brain on the basis of its ability to promote the survival of chick sensory neurons in culture (Barde, Edgar and Thoenen, 1982). Subsequently, it was shown that its administration to young embryos reduces markedly the degenerative events that normally occur during the development of spinal ganglia (Hofer and Barde, 1988). Likewise, addition of BDNF led to an up to six-fold increase in the number of neurons (many of which displayed substance P-like immunoreactivity) that developed in cultures of neural crest cells grown *in vitro* with adjacent somites (Kalcheim and Gendreau, 1988). However, it could not be determined whether the primary effect of the factor was on the differentiation of sensory neuron precursors, on the survival of differentiated neurons or on both.

In contrast to BDNF, NGF has apparently no influence on the survival and/or differentiation of neurons that arise in cultures of neural crest (Norr, 1973; Fauquet *et al.*, 1981; Ziller *et al.*, 1983; Kalcheim and Gendreau, 1988). On the other hand, basic fibroblast growth factor (bFGF), a polypeptide with well documented stimulatory effects on the survival and proliferation of glial cells (Raff *et al.*, 1978; Eccleston *et al.*, 1987; Unsicker *et al.*, 1987; Walicke, 1988), when associated with laminin, enhances significantly the survival of DRG precursors separated from the neural tube by a silastic membrane *in vivo*, and also increases the number of non-neuronal cells surviving in cultures of neural crest *in vitro* (Kalcheim, 1989). *In situ* studies provided reassuring evidence that bFGF is indeed present in the embryo in locations (i.e. central and peripheral nervous systems) and at stages appropriate for its postulated role in controlling survival and differentiation of neural crest-derived non-neuronal cells (Kalcheim and Neufeld, 1990). No mitogenic effect of bFGF was observed in avian neural crest cultures (Kalcheim, 1989). However, in cultures of neuroepithelium from mouse embryos, both basic and acidic FGF were found to stimulate cell survival and proliferation and also, at higher doses, to promote differentiation into neurons and glia (Murphy, Drago and Bartlett, 1990).

Goldstein, Teillet and Kalcheim (1990) convincingly demonstrated that the rostral sclerotome provides an environment that stimulates the multiplication of neural crest cell precursors of the DRG. After constructing chimaeric embryos containing compound rostral half-somites unilaterally (section 4.4.3), the authors compared the DRG on control and operated sides with respect to the volume of the ganglia, the number of cells and the proportion labelled after a short pulse of ^{3}H-thymidine. Within 1 day of the operation, all these parameters were increased by 40–50% in the ganglia that formed in contact with entirely rostral sclerotomal mesenchyme. However, since the study was performed at a stage when it is impossible to identify the different cell types in the ganglia, it could not be determined whether the mitogenic activity of the somite resulted in greater numbers of glial cells, neurons or both.

4.6.2 Factors affecting the phenotypic expression of neural crest cell progeny

The emergence of certain differentiated phenotypes is crucially dependent on interactions between neural crest cells and tissues that border their routes of migration or that constitute the environment in which they aggregate. A concrete, much studied example (see Le Douarin and Smith (1988) for references) is the neurochemical differentiation of the precursors of noradrenergic neurons. *In vivo*, catecholaminergic properties appear when, but not before, sympathoblasts assemble to form the primary sympathetic chains. Somites, ventral neural tube and notochord have all been implicated in triggering the expression of the catecholamine-related phenotype. In culture *in vitro*, the effect of these tissues can be mimicked by supplementing the medium with high concentrations of a soluble extract of chick embryo; under these conditions, catecholamine-containing cells differentiate after several days (Cohen, 1977; Howard and Bronner-Fraser, 1985; Ziller *et al.*, 1987). Relatively large amounts of the activity promoting noradrenergic differentiation are found in extracts of CNS and in neural tube-conditioned medium; the active molecule has not been identified, but has an M_r of less than 10000 (Howard and Bronner-Fraser, 1985, 1986).

Also studying the differentiation *de novo* of noradrenergic cells, not from neural crest but from the latent 'autonomic-sympathetic' precursors that are present in developing sensory ganglia (section 4.5.2(a)), Xue, Smith and Le Douarin (1985) showed that their expression of functional catecholamine-synthesizing enzymes *in vitro* also required the addition to the medium of chick embryo extract. In subsequent studies the same authors showed that physiological concentrations of insulin or a related polypeptide, insulin-like growth factor I, produced exactly the same differentiation-triggering effects (Xue, Le Douarin and Smith, 1988). Interestingly, in view of the fact that passage through several cycles of cell division appears to be an obligatory prerequisite for the differentiation of catecholaminergic precursors (Kahn and Sieber-Blum, 1983), insulin and the insulin-like growth factors are also potent mitogens for sympathetic neuroblasts in culture (DiCicco-Bloom and Black, 1988; DiCicco-Bloom, Townes-Anderson and Black, 1990). However, as in the case of many observations made in culture systems, the relevance of these effects to *in vivo* neurogenesis remains to be demonstrated.

Extracellular matrix components may also be of importance, not merely as substrates for migration, but as active participants in events leading to expression of differentiated phenotypes. Thus, fibronectin was found to have a highly positive effect on the development, from quail neural crest *in vitro*, of neuron-like cells expressing a variety of neuroactive substances (Sieber-Blum, Sieber and Yamada, 1981; Loring, Glimelius and Weston, 1982; Sieber-Blum, 1984). Again *in vitro*, reconstituted basement membranes were found to stimulate, strongly and specifically, the differentiation of catecholamine-containing cells and to inhibit the proliferation of other cell types (notably melanocytes) in the neural crest population (Maxwell and Forbes, 1987, 1990).

There is evidence from other culture studies of an inverse relationship between the differentiation of neural cells and of melanocytes (Vogel and Weston, 1988). Various soluble factors, including MSH (Satoh and Ide, 1987) and bFGF (Halaban *et al.*, 1988), can activate melanogenesis. However, an interesting series of experiments with amphibian and avian embryos suggests that extracellular matrix encountered by migrating crest cells may be directly responsible for the segregation of melanocytic and neural lineages. Perris, von Boxberg and Löfberg (1988), using an elegant methodological approach, implanted Nuclepore membranes into axolotl embryos. After 12h, the membranes, which had by then become coated with matrix materials, were removed, covered with isolated neural crest and incubated *in vitro* in a defined culture medium. Crest cells grown on membranes impregnated with subepidermal matrix differentiated into pigment cells, whereas on membranes coated with matrix material from the presumptive site of DRG formation, they developed into neurite-bearing, neurofilament-immunoreactive neurons. The authors suggested that differentiated phenotype expression might be governed in an instructive manner by local matrices. On the other hand, in an investigation of the migratory behaviour and developmental fate of avian quail neural crest cells cultured on fibronectin or laminin, Rogers, Bernard and Weston (1990) concluded that these components of the extracellular matrix control melanogenesis by modulating the patterns of cell dispersal. Rapid and extensive dispersal, promoted by fibronectin, resulted in significantly slower differentiation into melanocytes than did the rapid clustering provoked by laminin.

4.7 THE NEURAL CREST AND NEUROFIBROMATOSIS

The harmonious unfurling of the various steps of ontogeny that separate the neural crest from its many differentiated derivatives is the result of the complex interplay of diverse factors, intrinsic and extrinsic to crest cells. Consequently, developmental disorganization, such as may occur in neurofibromatosis, could theoretically be due to perturbances at one or more of several points. Clearly, neither the unquestionable origin in the neural crest of many of the cell types that are primarily concerned by neurofibromatosis, nor the occasional coexistence of this disorder with phaeochromocytomas or possibly neuroblastomas should be taken to imply that the dysregulation occurs exclusively, or even necessarily, at the level of the neural crest itself. Abnormal production of growth factors, cell surface molecules or components of the extracellular matrix that are indispensable for the normal development of crest derivatives could also, in principle, account for neurocristopathies.

Experimentally, it has proved possible to cause severe morphological anomalies, including defects of the nervous system, in Xenopus embryos by provoking the ectopic expression of N-cadherin (Detrick, Dickey and Kintner, 1990). A striking natural example of the consequences of an environmental deficiency on embryogenesis (migration, proliferation and/or differentiation) is provided by mutations at the steel (*Sl*) locus in the mouse; in mutant animals, development of three different, non-lineage-related cell populations (haematopoietic stem cells, primary germ cells and melanocytes) is impaired. The *Sl* locus has recently been shown to encode a novel stem cell growth factor (Zsebo *et al.*, 1990), which is expressed at sites of haematopoiesis and also by cells bordering the pathways of migration of primordial germ cells and melanocyte precursors (Matsui, Zsebo and Hogan, 1990). The growth factor is a ligand for c-*kit*, a tyrosine kinase receptor and product of the dominant white spotting (*W*) locus (Chabot *et al.*, 1988; Geissler, Ryan and Housman, 1988). Mutations at this locus affect the same cell types as those affected by mutations at the *Sl* locus.

The fact that neurofibromas can include cell types (e.g. endothelial, perineurial and mast cells) that do not originate from the neurectoderm suggests a mechanism that is not cell – or even lineage – autonomous but which involves extrinsic agents with a relatively broad spectrum of action. Extracts of neurofibromas contain a powerful mitogen for Schwann cells (Ratner, Bunge and Glaser, 1986) and human gliomas and meningiomas produce bFGF (Takahashi *et al.*, 1990) and may also contain additional angiogenic factors (Sheela, Riccardi and Ratner, 1990). However, no particular growth factor has yet been recognized as being the prime causal agent for any of the anomalies of neurofibromatosis (Riccardi, 1989). Likewise, it remains to be demonstrated that the abnormal expression of matrix or cell membrane molecules plays a role in the pathogenesis of the disease. It is nevertheless intriguing to learn that the huge neurofibromatosis gene contains, within an intron, three nested genes in opposing orientation (Viskochil *et al.*, 1990), one of which codes for a cell-adhesion glycoprotein on the surface of oligodendrocytes (Mikol, Gulcher and Stefansson, 1990). Although many shadowy points remain, the recent spectacular advances in its molecular biology (Buchberg *et al.*, 1990; Cawthon *et al.*, 1990; Viskochil *et al.*, 1990), hopefully foretoken rapid progress in our understanding of neurofibromatosis.

REFERENCES

Abo, I. and Balch, C.M. (1981) A differentiation antigen of human NK and K cells identified by a monoclonal antibody (HNK-1). *J. Immunol.*, **127**, 1024–9.

Anderson, D.J. (1989) The neural crest cell lineage problem: neuropoiesis? *Neuron*, **3**, 1–12.

Andrew, A. (1974) Further evidence that enterochromaffin cells are not derived from the neural crest. *J. Embryol. Exp. Morphol.*, **31**, 589–98.

Ayer-Le Lièvre, C.S. and Le Douarin, N.M. (1982) The early development of cranial sensory ganglia and the potentialities of their component cells studied in quail-chick chimaeras. *Dev. Biol.*, **94**, 291–310.

Balaban, E., Teillet, M.-A. and Le Douarin, N.M. (1988) Application of the quail-chick chimaera system to the study of brain development and behavior. *Science*, **241**, 1339–42.

Barald, K.F. (1988) Monoclonal antibodies made to chick mesencephalic neural crest cells and to ciliary ganglion neurons identify a common antigen of the neurons and a neural crest subpopulation. *J. Neurosci. Res.*, **21**, 107–18.

Barbu, M. *et al.* (1986) Heterogeneity in migrating neural crest cells revealed by a monoclonal antibody. *J. Neurosci.*, **6**, 2215–25.

Barde, Y.A., Edgar, D. and Thoenen, H. (1982) Purification of a new neurotrophic factor from mammalian brain. *EMBO J.*, **1**, 549–53.

Baroffio, A. and Blot, M. (1992) Statistical evidence for a random commitment of pluripotent cephalic neural crest cells. *J. Cell Sci.*, **103**, 581–7.

Baroffio, A., Dupin, E. and Le Douarin, N.M. (1988) Clone-forming ability and differentiation potential of migratory neural crest cells. *Proc. Natl. Acad. Sci. USA*, **85**, 5325–9.

Bolande, R.P. (1974) The neurocristopathies. A unifying concept of disease arising in neural crest maldevelopment. *Human Path.*, **5**, 409–29.

Boucaut, J.C. *et al.* (1984) Biologically active synthetic peptides as probes of embryonic development: a competitive peptide inhibitor of fibronectin function inhibits gastrulation in amphibian embryos and neural crest migration in avian embryos. *J. Cell Biol.*, **99**, 1822–30.

Bronner-Fraser, M. (1985) Alterations in neural crest migration by a monoclonal antibody that affects cell adhesion. *J. Cell Biol.*, **101**, 610–17.

Bronner-Fraser, M. (1986) Analysis of the early stages of trunk neural crest migration in avian embryos using monoclonal antibody HNK-1. *Dev. Biol.*, **115**, 44–55.

Bronner-Fraser, M. (1987) Perturbation of cranial neural crest migration by the HNK-1 antibody. *Dev. Biol.*, **123**, 321–31.

Bronner-Fraser, M. and Fraser, S. (1988) Cell lineage analysis shows multipotentiality of some avian neural crest cells. *Nature*, **335**, 161–4.

Bronner-Fraser, M. and Fraser, S. (1989) Developmental potential of avian trunk neural crest cells in situ. *Neuron*, **3**, 755–66.

Buchberg, A.M. *et al.* (1990) Sequence homology shared by neurofibromatosis type-1 gene and *IRA*-1 and *IRA*-2 negative regulators of the *RAS* cyclic AMP pathway. *Nature*, **347**, 291–4.

Bunge, M.B. *et al.* (1989) Perineurium originates from fibroblasts: demonstration *in vitro* with a retroviral marker. *Science*, **243**, 229–31.

Cawthon, R.M. *et al.* (1990) A major segment of the neurofibromatosis type 1 gene; cDNA sequence, genomic structure and point mutations. *Cell*, **62**, 193–201.

Chabot, B. *et al.* (1988) The proto-oncogene c-*kit* encoding a transmembrane tyrosine kinase receptor maps to the mouse *W* locus. *Nature*, **335**, 88–9.

Ciment, G. and Weston, J.A. (1982) Early appearance in neural crest and crest-derived cells of an antigenic determinant present in avian neurons. *Dev. Biol.*, **93**, 355–67.

Ciment, G. and Weston, J.A. (1983) Enteric neurogenesis by neural crest-derived branchial arch mesenchymal cells. *Nature*, **305**, 424–7.

Ciment, G. and Weston, J.A. (1985) Segregation of developmental abilities in neural crest-derived cells: identification of partially restricted intermediate cell types in branchial arches of avian embryos. *Dev. Biol.*, **111**, 73–83.

Cochard, P. and Coltey, P. (1983) Cholinergic traits in the neural crest: acetylcholinesterase in crest cells of the chick embryo. *Dev. Biol.*, **98**, 221–38.

Cohen, A. (1977) Independent expression of the noradrenergic phenotype by neural crest cells *in vitro*. *Proc. Natl. Acad. Sci. USA*, **74**, 2899–903.

Couly, G. and Le Douarin, N.M. (1985) Mapping of the early primordium in quail-chick chimaeras. I. Developmental relationships between placodes, facial ectoderm and prosencephalon. *Dev. Biol.*, **110**, 422–39.

Couly, G. and Le Douarin, N.M. (1987) Mapping of the early primordium in quail-chick chimaeras. II. The prosencephalic neural plate and neural folds: implications for the genesis of cephalic human congenital abnormalities. *Dev. Biol.*, **120**, 198–214.

Cowell, L.A. and Weston, J.A. (1970) An analysis of melanogenesis in cultured chick embryo spinal ganglia. *Dev. Biol.*, **122**, 670–97.

D'Amico-Martel, A. and Noden, D.M. (1983) Contribution of placodal and neural crest cells to avian peripheral ganglia. *Am. J. Anat.*, **166**, 445–68.

Derby, M.A. (1978) Analysis of glycosaminoglycans within the extracellular environments encountered by neural crest cells. *Dev. Biol.*, **66**, 321–36.

Detrick, R.J., Dickey, D. and Kintner, C.R. (1990) The effects of N-cadherin misexpression on morphogenesis in Xenopus embryos. *Neuron*, **4**, 493–506.

DiCicco-Bloom, E. and Black, I.B. (1988) Insulin growth factors regulate the mitotic cycle in cultured rat sympathetic neuroblasts. *Proc. Natl. Acad. Sci. USA*, **85**, 4066–70.

DiCicco-Bloom, E., Townes-Anderson, E. and Black, I.B. (1990) Neuroblast mitosis in dissociated cells: regulation and relationship to differentiation. *J. Cell Biol.*, **110**, 2073–86.

Duband, J.-L. and Thiery, J.P. (1990) Spatial and temporal distribution of vinculin and talin in migrating avian neural crest cells and their derivatives. *Development*, **108**, 421–33.

Duband, J.-L. *et al.* (1987) Adhesion molecules during somitogenesis in the avian embryo. *J. Cell Biol.*, **104**, 1361–74.

Dulac, C. *et al.* (1988) A surface protein expressed by avian myelinating and nonmyelinating Schwann cells but not by satellite or enteric glial cells. *Neuron*, **1**, 211–20.

Dupin, E. (1984) Cell division in the ciliary ganglion of quail embryos *in situ* and after back-transplantation into the neural crest migration pathways of chick embryos. *Dev. Biol.*, **105**, 288–99.

Dupin, E. *et al.* (1990) Schwann cell differentiation in clonal cultures of the neural crest, as evidenced by the anti-Schwann cell myelin protein monoclonal antibody. *Proc. Natl. Acad. Sci. USA*, **87**, 1119–23.

Eccleston, P.A. *et al.* (1984) Control of peripheral glial cell proliferation: a comparison of the division rates of enteric glia and Schwann cells and their response to mitogens. *Dev. Biol.*, **124**, 409–18.

Erickson, C.A., Loring, J.F. and Lester, S.M. (1989) Migratory pathways of HNK-1 immunoreactive neural crest cells in the rat embryo. *Dev. Biol.*, **134**, 112–18.

Fauquet, M. and Ziller, C. (1989) A monoclonal antibody directed against quail tyrosine hydroxylase: description and use in immunocytochemical studies on differentiating neural crest cells. *J. Histochem. Cytochem.*, **37**, 1197–205.

Fauquet, M. *et al.* (1981) Differentiation of autonomic neuron precursors *in vitro*: cholinergic and adrenergic traits in cultured neural crest cells. *J. Neurosci.*, **1**, 478–92.

Fontaine, J. and Le Douarin, N.M. (1977a) Do neural crest cells in the pancreas differentiate into somatostatin-containing cells? *Cell Tissue Res.*, **213**, 293–9.

Fontaine, J. and Le Douarin, N.M. (1977b) Analysis of endoderm formation in the avian blastoderm by the use of quail-chick chimaeras. The problem of the neurectodermal origin of the cells of the APUD series. *J. Embryol. Exp. Morphol.*, **41**, 209–22.

Fontaine, J., Le Lièvre, C. and Le Douarin, N.M. (1977) What is the developmental fate of the neural crest cells which migrate into the pancreas in the avian embryo? *Gener. Comp. Endocrinol.*, **33**, 394–404.

Fontaine–Pérus, J., Chanconie, M. and Le Douarin, N.M. (1988) Developmental potentialities in the non-neuronal population of quail sensory ganglia. *Dev. Biol.*, **128**, 359–75.

Garcia-Arraras, J.E. *et al.* (1986) Co-expression of somatostatin-like immunoreactivity and catecholaminergic properties in neural crest derivatives; comodulation of peptidergic and adrenergic differentiation in cultured neural crest. *Dev. Biol.*, **144**, 247–57.

Garcia-Arraras, J.E. *et al.* (1987) *In vivo* and *in vitro* expression of vasoactive intestinal polypeptide-like immunoreactivity by neural crest derivatives. *Dev. Brain Res.*, **33**, 255–65.

Geissler, E.N., Ryan, M.A. and Housman, D.E. (1988) The dominant white spotting (*W*) locus of the mouse encodes the *c-kit* proto-oncogene. *Cell*, **55**, 185–92.

Goldstein, R., Teillet, M.-A. and Kalcheim, C. (1990) The microenvironment created by grafting multiple rostral half-somites is mitogenic for neural crest cells. *Proc. Natl. Acad. Sci. USA*, **87**, 4476–80.

Halaban, R. *et al.* (1988) Basic fibroblast growth factor from human keratinocytes is a natural mitogen for melanocytes. *J. Cell Biol.*, **107**, 1611–19.

Harkin, J.C. (1986) Pathology of nerve sheath tumors. *Ann. N.Y. Acad. Sci.*, **486**, 147–54.

Hofer, M.M. and Barde, Y.A. (1988) Brain-derived neurotrophic factor prevents neuronal death *in vivo*. *Nature*, **331**, 261–2.

Hörstadius, S. (1950) *The Neural Crest: Its Properties and Derivatives in the Light of Experimental Research*. Oxford University Press, Oxford.

Howard, M.J. and Bronner-Fraser, M. (1985) Influence of neural tube-derived factors on differentiation of neural crest cells *in vitro*. I. Histochemical study on the appearance of adrenergic cells. *J. Neurosci.*, **5**, 3302–9.

Howard, M.J. and Bronner-Fraser, M. (1986) Neural tube-derived factors influence differentiation of neural crest cells *in vitro*: effects on activity of neurotransmitter biosynthetic enzymes. *Dev. Biol.*, **117**, 45–54.

Kahn, C.R. and Sieber-Blum, M. (1983) Cultured quail neural crest cells attain competence for terminal differentiation into melanocytes before competence to terminal differentiation into adrenergic neurons. *Dev. Biol.*, **95**, 232–8.

Kalcheim, C. (1989) Basic fibroblast growth factor stimulates survival of non-neuronal cells developing from trunk neural crest. *Dev. Biol.*, **134**, 1–10.

Kalcheim, C. and Gendreau, M. (1988) Brain-derived neurotrophic factor stimulates survival and neuronal differentiation in cultured avian neural crest. *Dev. Brain Res.*, **41**, 79–86.

Kalcheim, C. and Le Douarin, N.M. (1986) Requirement of a neural tube signal(s) for the differentiation of neural crest cells into dorsal root ganglia. *Dev. Biol.*, **116**, 451–66.

Kalcheim, C. and Neufeld, G. (1990) Expression of basic fibroblast growth factor in the nervous system of early avian embryos. *Development*, **109**, 203–15.

Kalcheim, C. and Teillet, M.-A. (1989) Consequences of somite manipulation on the pattern of dorsal root ganglion development. *Development*, **106**, 85–93.

Kalcheim, C. *et al.* (1987) *In vivo* effect of brain-derived neurotrophic factor on the survival of neural crest precursor cells of the dorsal root ganglia. *EMBO J.*, **6**, 2871–3.

Keynes, R.J. and Stern, C. (1984) Segmentation in the vertebrate nervous system. *Nature*, **310**, 786–9.

Kinutani, M. and Le Douarin, N.M. (1985) Avian spinal cord chimeras. I. Hatching ability and posthatching survival in homo- and heterospecific chimeras. *Dev. Biol.*, **111**, 243–55.

Lallier, T.E. and Bronner-Fraser, M. (1988) A spatial and temporal analysis of dorsal root and sympathetic ganglion formation in the avian embryo. *Dev. Biol.*, **127**, 99–112.

Layer, P.G., Alber, R. and Rathjen, F.G. (1988) Sequential activation of butyrylcholinesterase in rostral half somites and acetylcholinesterase in motoneurons and myotomes preceding growth of motor axons. *Development*, **102**, 387–96.

Le Douarin, N.M. (1969) Particularités du noyau interphasique chez la caille japonaise (*Coturnix coturnix japonica*). Utilisation de ces particularités comme 'marquage biologique' dans les recherches sur les interactions tissulaires et les migrations cellulaires au cours de l'ontogenèse. *Bull. Biol. Fr. Belg.*, **103**, 435–52.

Le Douarin, N.M. (1973) A Feulgen-positive nucleolus. *Exp. Cell Res.*, **77**, 459–68.

Le Douarin, N.M. (1982) *The Neural Crest*. Cambridge University Press.

Le Douarin, N.M. (1984) A model for cell line divergence in the ontogeny of the peripheral nervous system, in *Cellular and Molecular Biology of Neuronal Development* (ed. I. Black), Plenum Press, New York, pp. 3–28.

Le Douarin, N.M. (1986) Cell line segregation during peripheral nervous system ontogeny. *Science*, **231**, 1515–22.

Le Douarin, N.M. (1988) On the origin of pancreatic islet cells. *Cell*, **53**, 169–71.

Le Douarin, N.M. and Smith, J. (1988) Development of the peripheral nervous system: cell line segregation and chemical differentiation of neural crest cells, in *Handbook of Chemical Neuroanatomy, Vol. 6, The Peripheral Nervous System* (eds A. Björklund, T. Hökfelt and Ch. Owman), Elsevier, Amsterdam, pp. 1–50.

Le Douarin, N.M. and Teillet, M.-A. (1973) The migration of neural crest cells to the wall of the digestive tract in avian embryo. *J. Embryol. Exp. Morphol.*, **30**, 31–48.

Le Douarin, N.M. and Teillet, M.-A. (1974) Experimental analysis of the migration and differentiation of neuroblasts of the autonomic nervous system and of neurectodermal mesenchymal derivatives, using a biological cell marking technique. *Dev. Biol.*, **41**, 162–84.

Le Douarin, N.M. *et al.* (1978) Adrenergic differentiation of cells of the cholinergic ciliary and Remak ganglia in avian embryo following *in vivo* transplantation. *Proc. Natl. Acad. Sci. USA*, **75**, 2030–4.

Le Lièvre, C.S. and Le Douarin, N.M. (1975) Mesenchymal derivatives of the neural crest: analysis of chimaeric quail and chick embryos. *J. Embryol. Exp. Morphol.*, **34**, 125–54.

Le Lièvre, C.S. *et al.* (1980) Restriction of developmental capabilities in neural crest cell derivatives as tested by *in vivo* transplantation experiments. *Dev. Biol.*, **105**, 362–78.

Lewis, J. *et al.* (1981) Muscle nerve branches do not develop in chick wings devoid of muscle. *J. Embryol. Exp. Morphol.*, **64**, 211–32.

Loring, J.F. and Erickson, C.A. (1987) Neural crest cell migratory pathways in the trunk of the chick embryo. *Dev. Biol.*, **121**, 220–36.

Loring, J. Glimelius, B. and Weston, J.A. (1982) Extracellular matrix materials influence quail neural crest cell differentiation *in vitro*. *Dev. Biol.*, **90**, 165–74.

Luckenbill-Edds, L. and Carrington, J.L. (1988) Effect of hyaluronic acid on the emergence of neural crest cells from the neural tube of the quail. *Cell Tissue Res.*, **252**, 573–9.

Mackie, E.J. *et al.* (1988) The distribution of tenascin coincides with pathways of neural crest cell migration. *Development*, **102**, 237–50.

Matsui, Y., Zsebo, K.M. and Hogan, B.L.M. (1990) Embryonic expression of a haematopoietic growth factor encoded by the *Sl* locus and a ligand for c-*kit*. *Nature*, **347**, 667–9.

Maxwell, G.D. and Forbes, M.E. (1987) Exogenous basement-membrane-like matrix stimulates adrenergic development in avian neural crest cultures. *Development*, **101**, 767–76.

Maxwell, G.D. and Forbes, M.E. (1990) The phenotypic response of cultured quail trunk neural crest cells to a reconstituted basement-membrane-like matrix is specific. *Dev. Biol.*, **141**, 233–7.

Maxwell, G.D., Sietz, P.D. and Rafford, C.E. (1982) Synthesis and accumulation of putative neurotransmitters by cultured neural crest cells. *J. Neurosci.*, **2**, 879–88.

Maxwell, G.D., Sietz, P.D. and Jean, S. (1984) Somatostatin-like immunoreactivity in embryonic sympathetic ganglia. *J. Neurosci.*, **4**, 576–84.

Mikol, D.D., Gulcher, J.R. and Stefansson, K. (1990) The oligodendrocyte-myelin glycoprotein belongs to a distinct family of proteins and contains the HNK-1 carbohydrate. *J. Cell Biol.*, **110**, 471–80.

Murphy, M., Drago, J. and Bartlett, P.F. (1990) Fibroblast growth factor stimulates the proliferation and differentiation of neural precursor cells *in vitro*. *J. Neurosci. Res.*, **25**, 463–75.

Narayanan, C.H. and Narayanan, Y. (1978a) Determination of the embryonic origin of the mesencephalic nucleus of the trigeminal nerve in birds. *J. Embryol. Exp. Morphol.*, **43**, 85–105.

Narayanan, C.H. and Narayanan, Y. (1978b) On the origin of the ciliary ganglion in birds studied by the method of interspecific transplantation of embryonic brain regions between quail and chick. *J. Embryol. Exp. Morphol.*, **47**, 137–48.

Narayanan, C.H. and Narayanan, Y. (1980) Neural crest and placodal contributions in the development of the glossopharyngeal-vagal complex in the chick. *Anat. Rec.*, **196**, 71–82.

Newgreen, D.F. and Thiery, J. P. (1980) Fibronectin in early avian embryos: synthesis and distribution along migration pathways of neural crest cells. *Cell Tissue Res.*, **211**, 269–91.

Newgreen, D.F. *et al.* (1980) Differentiation of sympathetic and enteric neurons of the fowl embryo in grafts to the chorioallantoic membrane. *Cell Tissue Res.*, **208**, 1–19.

Newgreen, D.F., Scheel, M. and Kastner, V. (1986) Morphogenesis of sclerotome and neural crest in avian embryos. *In vivo* and *in vitro* studies on the role of notochordal extracellular material. *Cell Tissue Res.*, **244**, 299–313.

Newgreen, D.F., Powell, M.E. and Moser, B. (1990) Spatiotemporal changes in HNK-1/L2 glycoconjugates on avian embryo somite and neural crest cells. *Dev. Biol.*, **139**, 100–20.

Noden, D.M. (1978) The control of avian cephalic neural crest cytodifferentiation; II. Neural tissues. *Dev. Biol.*, **67**, 313–29.

Noden, D.M. (1987) Interactions between cephalic neural crest and mesodermal populations, in *Developmental and Evolutionary Aspects of the Neural Crest* (ed. P.F.A Maderson), Wiley Interscience, New York, pp. 89–119.

Norr, S.C. (1973) *In vitro* analysis of sympathetic neuron differentiation from chick neural crest cells. *Dev. Biol.*, **34**, 16–38.

Payette, R.F., Bennet, G.S. and Gershon, M.D. (1984) Neurofilament expression in vagal neural crest-derived precursors of enteric neurons. *Dev. Biol.*, **105**, 273–87.

Pearse, A.G.E. (1968) Common cytochemical properties of cells producing polypeptide hormones (the APUD series) and their relevance to thyroid and ultimobranchial C cells and calcitonin. *Proc. Roy. Soc. B*, **170**, 71-80.

Pearse, A.G.E. (1976) Peptides in brain and intestine. *Nature*, **262**, 92–4.

Perris, R., von Boxberg, Y. and Löfberg, J. (1988) Local embryonic matrices determine region-specific phenotypes in neural crest cells. *Science*, **241**, 86–9.

Pintar, J.E. (1978) Distribution and synthesis of glycosaminoglycans during quail neural crest morphogenesis. *Dev. Biol.*, **67**, 444–64.

Pratt, R.M., Larsen, M.A. and Johnston, M.C. (1975) Migration of cranial neural crest cells in a cell-free hyaluronate-rich matrix. *Dev. Biol.*, **44**, 298–305.

Raff, M. *et al.* (1978) Schwann cell growth factors. *Cell*, **15**, 813–22.

Ratner, N., Bunge, R.P. and Glaser, L. (1986) Schwann cell proliferation *in vitro*: an overview. *Ann. N.Y. Acad. Sci.*, **486**, 170–81.

Riccardi, V.M. (1989) Genetic alterations and growth factors in the pathogenesis of von Recklinghausen neurofibromatosis. *Neurofibromatosis*, **2**, 292–8.

Richardson, R.J., Hornbruch, A. and Wolpert, L. (1989) Pigment pattern expression in the plumage of the quail embryo and the quail-chick chimaera. *Development*, **107**, 805–18.

Rickmann, M., Fawcett, J.W. and Keynes, R.J. (1985) The migration of neural crest cells and the growth of motor axons through the rostral half of the chick somite. *J. Embryol. Exp. Morphol.*, **90**, 437–55.

Riopelle, R.J., McGarry, R.C. and Roder, J.C. (1986) Adhesion properties of a neuronal epitope recognised by the monoclonal antibody HNK-1. *Brain Res.*, **367**, 20–5.

Rogers, S.L., Bernard, L. and Weston, J.A. (1990) Substratum effects on cell dispersal, morphology and differentiation in cultures of avian neural crest cells. *Dev. Biol.*, **141**, 173–82.

Rovasio, R.A. *et al.* (1983) Neural crest cell migration: requirements for exogenous fibronectin and high cell density. *J. Cell Biol.*, **96**, 462–73.

Sadaghiani, B. and Vielkind, J.R. (1990) Distribution and migration pathways of

HNK1-immunoreactive neural crest cells in teleost fish embryos. *Development*, **110**, 197–209.

Satoh, M. and Ide, M. (1987) Melanocyte-stimulating hormone affects melanogenic differentiation of quail neural crest cells *in vitro*. *Dev. Biol.*, **119**, 579–86.

Schweizer, G., Ayer-Le Lièvre, C. and Le Douarin, N.M. (1983) Restrictions of developmental capacities in the dorsal root ganglia during the course of development. *Cell Diff.*, **13**, 191–200.

Serbedzija, G.N., Bronner-Fraser, M. and Fraser, S.E. (1989) A vital dye analysis of the timing and pathways of avian trunk neural crest cell migration. *Development*, **106**, 809–16.

Serbedzija, G.N., Fraser, S.E. and Bronner-Fraser, M. (1990) Pathways of trunk neural crest cell migration in the mouse embryo as revealed by vital dye labelling. *Development*, **108**, 605–12.

Sheela, S., Riccardi, V.M. and Ratner, N. (1990) Angiogenic and invasive properties of neurofibroma Schwann cells. *J. Cell Biol.*, **111**, 645–53.

Sieber-Blum, M. (1984) Fibronectin-regulated methionine enkephalin-like and somatostatin-like immunoreactivity in quail neural crest cell cultures. *Neuropeptides*, **4**, 457–66.

Sieber-Blum, M. (1989) Commitment of neural crest cells to the sensory neuron lineage. *Science*, 243, 1608–11.

Sieber-Blum, M. and Cohen, A.M. (1980) Clonal analysis of quail neural crest cells: they are pluripotent and differentiate *in vitro* in the absence of noncrest cells. *Dev. Biol.*, **80**, 96–106.

Sieber-Blum, M., Sieber, F. and Yamada, K.M. (1981) Cellular fibronectin promotes adrenergic differentiation of quail neural crest cells *in vitro*. *Exp. Cell Res.*, **133**, 285–95.

Smith, J., Cochard, P. and Le Douarin, N.M. (1977) Development of choline acetyltransferase and cholinesterase activities in enteric ganglia derived from presumptive adrenergic and cholinergic levels of the neural crest. *Cell Diff.*, **6**, 199–216.

Smith, J. *et al.* (1979) Acetylcholine synthesis by mesencephalic neural crest cells in the process of migration *in vivo*. *Nature*, **282**, 853–5.

Stern, C.D. and Keynes, R.J. (1987) Interactions between somite cells: the formation and maintenance of segment boundaries in the chick embryo. *Development*, **99**, 261–72.

Stern, C.D. *et al.* (1989) J1/tenascin-related molecules are not responsible for the segmented pattern of neural crest cells or motor axons in the chick embryo. *Development*, **107**, 309–19.

Takahashi, J.A. *et al.* (1990) Gene expression of fibroblast growth factors in human gliomas and meningiomas: demonstration of cellular source of basic fibroblast growth factor mRNA and peptide in tumour tissues. *Proc. Natl. Acad. Sci. USA*, **87**, 5710–14.

Tan, S.-S. *et al.* (1987) Asymmetric expression in somites of cytotactin and its proteoglycan ligand is correlated with neural crest cell distribution. *Proc. Natl. Acad. Sci. USA*, **84**, 7977–81.

Teillet, M.-A. and Le Douarin, N.M. (1983) Consequences of neural tube and notochord excision on the development of the peripheral nervous system in the chick embryo. *Dev. Biol.*, **98**, 192–211.

Teillet, M.-A., Kalcheim, C. and Le Douarin, N.M. (1987) Formation of the dorsal root ganglia in the avian embryo: segmental origin and migratory behavior of neural crest progenitor cells. *Dev. Biol.*, **120**, 329–47.

Thiery, J.P., Duband, J.-L. and Delouvée, A. (1982a) Pathways and mechanisms of avian neural crest migration and localisation. *Dev. Biol.*, **93**, 324–43.

Thiery, J.P. *et al.* (1982b) Cell adhesion molecules in early chick embryogenesis *Proc. Natl. Acad. Sci. USA*, **79**, 6737–41.

Tosney, K.W. (1978) The early migration of neural crest cells in the trunk region of the avian embryo: an electron microscopic study. *Dev. Biol.*, **62**, 317–33.

Tosney, K.W. (1988) Proximal tissues and patterned neurite outgrowth at lumbosacral levels of chick embryo: partial and complete deletion of the somite. *Dev. Biol.*, **127**, 266–86.

Tucker, G.C. *et al.* (1988) Expression of HNK-1/NC-1 epitope in early vertebrate neurogenesis. *Cell Tissue Res.*, **251**, 457–65.

Unsicker, K. *et al.* (1987) Astroglial and fibroblast growth factors have neurotrophic function for cultured peripheral and central nervous system neurons. *Proc. Natl. Acad. Sci. USA*, **84**, 5459–64.

Vincent, M. and Thiery, J.P. (1984) A cell surface marker for neural crest and placodal cells: further evolution in peripheral and central nervous system. *Dev. Biol.*, **103**, 468–81.

Vincent, M., Duband, J.-L. and Thiery, J.P. (1983) A cell surface determinant expressed early on migrating avian neural crest cells. *Dev. Brain Res.*, **9**, 235–8.

Viskochil, D. *et al.* (1990) Deletions and a translocation interrupt a cloned gene at the neurofibromatosis type 1 locus. *Cell*, **62**, 187–92.

Vogel, K.S. and Weston, J.A. (1988) A subpopulation of cultured neural crest cells has transient neurogenic potential. *Neuron*, **1**, 569–77.

Walicke, P.A. (1988) Basic and acidic fibroblast growth factors have trophic effects on neurons from multiple CNS regions. *J. Neurosci.*, **8**, 2618–28.

Wallace, M.R. *et al.* (1990) Type 1 neurofibromatosis gene: identification of a large transcript disrupted in three NF1 patients. *Science*, **249**, 181–6.

Weston, J.A. (1963) A radioautographic analysis of the migration and localisation of trunk neural crest cells in the chick. *Dev. Biol.*, **6**, 279–310.

Xue, Z.G. and Smith, J. (1988) High-affinity uptake of noradrenaline in quail dorsal root ganglion cells that express tyrosine hydroxylase immunoreactivity *in vitro*. *J. Neurosci.*, **8**, 806–13.

Xue, Z.G., Smith, J. and Le Douarin, N.M. (1985) Differentiation of catecholaminergic cells in cultures of avian sensory ganglia. *Proc. Natl. Acad. Sci. USA*, **82**, 8800–4.

Xue, Z.G., Smith, J. and Le Douarin, N.M. (1987) Developmental capacities of avian embryonic dorsal root ganglion cells: neuropeptides and tyrosine hydroxylase in dissociated cell cultures. *Dev. Brain Res.*, **34**, 99–109.

Xue, Z.G., Le Douarin, N.M. and Smith, J. (1988) Insulin and insulin-like growth factor-I can trigger the differentiation of catecholaminergic precursors in cultures of dorsal root ganglia. *Cell Differ. Dev.*, **25**, 1–10.

Ziller, C. *et al.* (1983) Early segregation of a neuronal precursor cell line in the neural crest as revealed by culture in a chemically defined medium. *Cell*, **32**, 627–38.

Ziller, C. *et al.* (1987) Cell lineages in peripheral nervous system ontogeny: medium-induced modulation of phenotypic expression in neural crest cultures. *Dev. Biol.*, **120**, 101–11.

Zsebo, K.M. *et al.* (1990) Stem cell factor is encoded at the *Sl* locus of the mouse and is the ligand for the c-*kit* tyrosine kinase receptor. *Cell*, **63**, 213–24.

5

Schwann cell biology

K.R. Jessen and R. Mirsky

5.1 INTRODUCTION

The ultimate understanding of neurofibromatosis will depend on knowing what controls the development, growth and maintenance of Schwann cells, which form the basis of neurofibromas. Axons in peripheral nerves are ensheathed by non-myelin- or myelin-forming Schwann cells. These two major variants of a single glial cell are quite different in size and structure and each expresses a characteristic set of proteins (for recent reviews see Bunge, Bunge and Eldridge, 1986; Bunge and Hopkins, 1990; Lemke, 1990; Mirsky and Jessen, 1990; Jessen and Mirsky, 1991; Gould *et al.*, 1991). They are thought to originate from a common embryonic Schwann cell. The development of this cell and the generation of the two mature Schwann cell types is critically dependent on axon-associated signals. Even in maturity these signals are required for the two cell types to retain their separate identities. In these cells, therefore, maintenance of differentiation and function depends on ongoing extrinsic signals to a much greater extent than it does in the Schwann cell counterparts in central fibre tracts, astrocytes and oligodendrocytes.

By far the best defined function of Schwann cells, as indeed of central glia, is the provision of myelin sheaths around the larger axons, which act to accelerate the conduction rate of action potentials. There is also evidence that Schwann cells provide guidance for regenerating axons, act as a source of growth factors for neurons and take part in the synthesis of the endoneurial extracellular matrix. It has also been suggested that they participate in the maintenance of ionic homeostasis in the microenvironment outside the axonal membrane. Furthermore, since Schwann cells have the capacity to express major histocompatibility complex (MHC) class II molecules and to present antigens to activated T cells, they are likely to take part in immune reactions in certain pathological conditions.

The parallels between Schwann cells and the glial cells of the central nervous system (CNS) have already been alluded to. They include similarities in molecular expression between myelin-forming Schwann cells and oligodendrocytes, and between non-myelin-forming Schwann cells and astrocytes, and common activities since central glia are likely to share with Schwann cells many of the functional properties mentioned above. Phenotypically the most striking similarity between central and peripheral glia is seen in the case of the enteric glial cells of the myenteric (Auerbach's) plexus. These cells are very similar to astrocytes in structure, relationship to connective tissue and neurons, and molecular expression. Other glial cells in the periphery include the satellite cells associated with the neuronal cell bodies of dorsal root sensory, sympathetic and many parasympathetic ganglia, the teloglia of somatic motor nerves and the specialized Schwann cells of Pacinian and Meissner's corpuscles.

Although all of these cells are closely related to Schwann cells of peripheral nerves they will not be dealt with further in this review. Our aim is to review recent work on the basic properties of normal Schwann cells. This should be helpful for understanding Schwann cell pathology in neurofibromatosis. Nevertheless, it should be made clear that the overwhelming majority of experimental studies have been carried out on rat rather than human cells and that it may not be justified to extrapolate in every case between the two species.

5.2 MOLECULAR COMPOSITION OF NON-MYELIN-FORMING AND MYELIN-FORMING SCHWANN CELLS *IN VIVO*

The molecular composition of Schwann cell myelin is well documented, and more recently the antigenic properties of both non-myelin- and myelin-forming Schwann cells have been comprehensively examined.

Non-myelin- and myelin-forming Schwann cells from several different species express the calcium-binding protein S100 both *in situ* and in culture (for a review see Mirsky and Jessen, 1990). Expression of this protein has been widely used to identify Schwann cells in human nerves and also to identify human Schwann cells in neurofibromas and in culture (Stefansson, Wollman and Moore, 1982; Scarpini *et al.*, 1986; Klingman and Hilt, 1988; Mata, Alessi and Fink, 1990). The S100 protein is also present in melanocytes, melanomas, some CNS glial cells and some neurons, so caution must be used in interpretation of results. Nevertheless, immunocytochemical labelling with antibodies to S100 is often a very convenient way of identifying Schwann cells.

Another important protein associated with Schwann cells is the low-affinity (p75) nerve growth factor (L-NGF) receptor. This can be recognized by two monoclonal antibodies, 192IgG (Chandler *et al.*, 1984;

Johnson, Taniuchi and DiStefano, 1988) or rat 217c (rat only) (Fields and Dammerman, 1985; Ferrari *et al.*, 1991). A study on L-NGF receptor expression in developing human nerves reported that non-myelinated femoral nerves from 13–14 week old fetuses were strongly positive for the L-NGF receptor but nerves at later developmental stages were not so strongly labelled. The decrease in receptor expression appeared to be temporally correlated with the onset of myelination (Scarpini *et al.*, 1988). *In vivo* L-NGF receptors have been reported to be absent from adult human nerves (Sobue *et al.*, 1988b) but are readily visualized immunohistochemically in nerves undergoing active axonal degeneration. Schwann cells in denervated nerves also expressed L-NGF receptors, whereas Schwann cells myelinating regenerating axons did not express these receptors. In rats, total receptor levels of L-NGF receptor in the sciatic nerve also decrease during the period of active myelination from the very high levels expressed during development (for a review see Johnson, Taniuchi and DiStefano, 1988). A recent study has shown that this down-regulation occurs to a much greater extent in Schwann cells of myelinated fibres than in Schwann cells of unmyelinated fibres since the L-NGF receptor continues to be expressed in adult non-myelin-forming Schwann cells at immunohistochemically detectable levels (Jessen *et al.*, 1990). It is therefore possible that in human nerves too, detectable levels of L-NGF receptor remain associated with Schwann cells of unmyelinated fibres. In culture both human and rat Schwann cells deprived of axonal contact up-regulate levels of L-NGF receptor protein and mRNA, and cultured Schwann cells from human neurofibromas also express L-NGF receptors (Pleasure *et al.*, 1986; DiStefano and Johnson, 1988; Scarpini *et al.*, 1988; Assouline and Pantazis, 1989). Treatment of cultured Schwann cells with agents that elevate intracellular cyclic AMP under conditions where DNA synthesis is suppressed, which mimics the effect of axonal *in vivo* signals (section 5.9), induces down-regulation of L-NGF receptors (Mokuno *et al.*, 1988; Morgan, Jessen and Mirsky, 1991). Thus, when Schwann cells are not in contact with axons, a situation found in some circumstances in neurofibromas, L-NGF receptor levels are high.

In mature nerves, myelin-forming Schwann cells of many species, including humans, express a set of proteins and mRNAs not expressed by non-myelin-forming Schwann cells. These include the major myelin glycoprotein P_0, myelin-associated glycoprotein (MAG), myelin basic protein (MBP), peripheral myelin protein (PMP) 22, the P_2 protein which is a lipid enzyme, and a 170kDa protein that is probably, though not certainly, confined to the myelin-forming phenotype (section 5.3) (Mirsky *et al.*, 1980; Trapp *et al.*, 1981; Trapp, Dubois-Dalcq and Quarles, 1984; Trapp and Quarles, 1984; Lemke and Axel, 1985; Martini and Schachner, 1986; Shuman, Hardy and Pleasure, 1986; Shuman *et al.*, 1988; Hahn *et al.*, 1987; Lemke, 1988; Lemke, Lamar and Patterson, 1988; Trapp,

Hauer and Lemke, 1988; Griffiths *et al.*, 1989; Spreyer *et al.*, 1991; Welcher *et al.*, 1991). In the rat, both myelin-forming and non-myelin-forming Schwann cells in Remak fibres express the glycolipids galactocerebroside and sulphatide (as detected by the 04 monoclonal antibody) (Jessen *et al.*, 1985; Jessen, Morgan and Mirsky, 1987; Mirsky *et al.*, 1990) and galactocerebroside has been found on the surface of human Schwann cells (Kennedy, Lisak and Raff, 1980; Scarpini *et al.*, 1988). Galactocerebroside, sulphatide and the myelin proteins disappear from the surface of Schwann cells in culture and are down-regulated in the distal stump of transected nerves. This suggests that the expression of all these molecules depends on axon-associated signals (Mirsky *et al.*, 1980, 1990; Mirsky and Jessen, 1990; Jessen and Mirsky, 1991).

In the rat at least, non-myelin-forming Schwann cells express a different set of proteins from myelin-forming Schwann cells. These include L-NGF receptors (see above), the cell-adhesion molecules N-CAM and L1 (Ng-CAM), a glial fibrillary acidic protein (GFAP)-like intermediate filament protein and two proteins recognized by rat-specific monoclonal antibodies, A5E3 and Ran-2 (Yen and Fields, 1981; Jessen and Mirsky, 1984; Jessen, Thorpe and Mirsky, 1984; Fields and Yen, 1985; Nieke and Schachner, 1985; Rieger *et al.*, 1985; Mirsky *et al.*, 1986; Jessen *et al.*, 1990).

The function of the proteins associated with the myelin sheath will be discussed in a later section. Much less is known about the functions of the protein markers associated with non-myelin-forming cells. There is direct evidence from tissue culture studies that the cell-adhesion molecules N-CAM and particularly L1 may be involved in axon–Schwann cell interactions in the premyelination stage (Seilheimer, Persohn and Schachner, 1989), but they could also be involved in the interaction between axons and Schwann cells in mature unmyelinated fibres since both the axons and Schwann cells in these fibres express these molecules *in situ* (Nieke and Schachner, 1985; Rieger *et al.*, 1985; Martini and Schachner, 1986; Mirsky *et al.*, 1986). The presence of L-NGF receptors on Schwann cells is intriguing. In cultured neonatal rat Schwann cells, most or all of these receptors are of the low-affinity type, whereas the biological actions of NGF are usually thought to require receptors of the high-affinity type (DiStefano and Johnson, 1988; Johnson, Taniuchi and DiStefano, 1988). It has been proposed that these receptors on Schwann cells could serve to hold NGF on the Schwann cell surface, and thus make the NGF available for uptake and transport by axons during periods of rapid axonal growth either during development or in regenerating nerves (Johnson, Taniuchi and DiStefano, 1988). It has also been reported that treatment with NGF up-regulates the level of surface L1 by about three times in cultured mouse Schwann cells (Seilheimer and Schachner, 1988). The function of the proteins A5E3 and Ran-2 associated with rat Schwann cells and of GFAP remain unknown.

Other proteins expressed by all Schwann cells *in vivo* or in culture include vimentin and laminin (Yen and Fields, 1981; Cornbrooks *et al.*, 1983; Mirsky and Jessen, 1990; Jessen and Mirsky, 1991). All Schwann cells in mature fibres are surrounded by a basal lamina and express the basal lamina components collagen type IV, entactin and heparan sulphate proteoglycan (Cornbrooks *et al.*, 1983; Bannerman *et al.*, 1986; Bunge, Bunge and Eldridge, 1986; Peltonen *et al.*, 1990). Recent reports suggest that the major type of laminin in peripheral nerves is of a relatively restricted subtype, called merosin (Leivo and Engvall, 1988; Leivo *et al.*, 1989a,b; Sanes *et al.*, 1990). The enzyme cyclic nucleotide phosphohydrolase (CNPase) is certainly present in myelin (section 5.3). It is likely to be expressed by non-myelin-forming Schwann cells as well since it is expressed by all Schwann cells in culture (Yoshino *et al.*, 1985; Trapp *et al.*, 1988).

5.3 THE MYELIN SHEATH

The myelin sheath consists of compacted layers of Schwann cell plasma membranes that wrap spirally around an axon. In the electron microscope myelin appears as a series of essentially concentric circles, consisting of the intraperiod line, which is formed by the apposition of the two external faces of the Schwann cell membranes, and the major dense line, which is formed by the apposition of the two cytoplasmic aspects of the membranes. *In vitro* observations suggest that the spiral arrangement of the membrane is formed as a result of the migration of the inner cytoplasmic lip of the spiral over the axonal surface (Bunge, Bunge and Bates, 1989). The number of spiral turns made in this way varies linearly with axon calibre, the largest axons having the thickest myelin sheaths (Friede, 1972). This implies the existence of a mechanism for tight regulation of the quantity of myelin synthesized, in addition to the axon-associated signals thought to trigger myelin formation (section 5.6).

The localization of the various myelin-forming proteins within the myelin-forming Schwann cell and their function in compaction and in interaction between axons and Schwann cells is gradually being clarified (Campagnoni, 1988; Lemke, 1988; Hudson, 1990). P_0 is the major protein of Schwann cell myelin (~50% of total protein). It is a transmembrane glycoprotein with an extracellular domain related to proteins of the immunoglobulin superfamily, which also includes cell-adhesion molecules such as N-CAM and L1 (Lemke and Axel, 1985; Lemke, Lamar and Patterson, 1988; Schachner, 1990). There is considerable evidence that possession of this type of domain makes it possible for molecules to bind to other molecules of the same type, i.e. to participate in homophilic interactions. Experimental evidence that P_0 can do so has recently been obtained from *in vitro* studies using P_0 gene transfection (D'Urso *et al.*,

1990; Filbin *et al.*, 1990). This, together with the presence of P_0 on the external side of the Schwann cell membrane, suggests that a major function of P_0 is compaction at the intraperiod line. In co-culture with neurons, Schwann cells infected with antisense P_0 mRNA do not make myelin (Owens and Boyd, 1991). Recent creation of a transgenic mouse in which P_0 has been knocked out suggests that deletion of this gene causes major upheavals, unsurprisingly, in myelin stability, but also leads eventually to death of some neurons (Giese *et al.*, 1992). The intracellular domain of P_0 shows similarities with MBP, which is responsible for compaction of the major dense line in oligodendrocyte myelin (Readhead *et al.*, 1987). In Schwann cells, however, MBP is present at relatively low levels and does not appear to be essential for compaction at the major dense line, since compaction of Schwann cell myelin is relatively unaffected in the *shiverer* mutant, which is deficient in MBP. It has therefore been suggested that P_0 is responsible for compaction not only of the intraperiod line, but also at the major dense line of Schwann cell myelin (Lemke, 1988). If this is true, then P_0 alone is responsible for functions that in oligodendrocyte myelin are carried out by several isoforms of MBP and proteolipid protein (PLP).

As mentioned above, MBP is less abundant in the myelin of Schwann cells than oligodendrocytes (~10% and 30% of total myelin proteins, respectively). It is present in several different isoforms generated by alternative splicing of a single gene transcript (Campagnoni, 1988). Whereas P_0 is synthesized in the rough endoplasmic reticulum and transported via the Golgi apparatus to insertion sites in the myelin membrane, the DNA sequences of two of the isoforms of MBP carry information that results in synthesis of MBP on free ribosomes at or near the sites of myelin assembly (Colman *et al.*, 1982; Staugaitis, Smith and Colman, 1990). MBP is an extrinsic membrane protein present on the cytoplasmic face of the bilayer and can be localized by immunohistochemistry to the major dense line (Omlin *et al.*, 1982). Studies on the *shiverer* mutation strongly suggest that MBP has a role in the compaction of oligodendrocyte myelin at the major dense line, but the significance of this protein in Schwann cells is less clear.

While P_0 and MBP are primarily present in compact myelin, MAG, P_2 and CNPase are enriched in other parts of the myelin-forming Schwann cell. MAG is an intrinsic membrane protein that exists in two isoforms, 67 and 72 kDa (Quarles, 1984; Lai *et al.*, 1987; Salzer, Holmes and Colman, 1987). The larger form is the major form in Schwann cells (Jessen and Mirsky, 1992). It belongs to the immunoglobulin superfamily like P_0, carries the HNK-1 carbohydrate epitope and shows particular sequence similarities with N-CAM. It is present at the initial stages of myelin formation (Martini and Schachner, 1986; Owens and Bunge, 1989; Owens *et al.*, 1990) and is found in mature Schwann cells in ad-axonal Schwann cell membranes but not in compact myelin (Trapp *et al.*, 1984; Martini and Schachner, 1986; Trapp, 1988). There is considerable evidence that MAG may act as a cell-adhesion molecule (Trapp and Quarles, 1984), mediating actions between axons and myelin-forming Schwann cells (Owens and Bunge, 1991).

The quantity of the small basic protein P_2 varies greatly between species and even within parts of the nervous system of a given species. It shows considerable sequence homology with a lipid transport protein in adipocytes and may thus have a similar function in Schwann cells (Trapp, Dubois-Dalcq and Quarles, 1984; Narayanan *et al.*, 1988).

CNPase is, like MBP, an extrinsic membrane protein (Vogel and Thompson, 1988). It is thought to be present in the major dense line of myelin but is also found in the cytoplasm, particularly in association with the cytoskeleton. Schwann cells contain significantly less CNPase than oligodendrocytes and the protein is also expressed outside the nervous system, e.g. in the thymus. PLP, which is considered to have a major role in compaction of the intraperiod line in oligodendrocyte myelin, is also expressed by Schwann cells, although it is not incorporated into Schwann cell myelin (Puckett *et al.*, 1987; Hudson, 1990; Ono *et al.*, 1990). The role of CNPase and PLP in Schwann cells is therefore still unclear.

5.4 SCHWANN CELL DEVELOPMENT

Morphological studies on the development of human peripheral nerves (Peters and Muir, 1959; Gamble and Breathnach, 1965; Gamble, 1966; Friede and Samorajski, 1968; Webster and Favilla, 1984) indicate that they develop in the same way as nerves from other mammalian species. From the earliest time that axons project out into the periphery from the spinal cord or sensory ganglia, they are accompanied by supporting cells that are the precursors of Schwann cells in mature peripheral nerves (Dahm and Landmesser, 1988). At a relatively early stage in development of human nerves, flattened Schwann cells at the periphery of the nerve surround groups of several hundred axons. As development proceeds the Schwann cells divide and invade the nerve, segregating the axons into smaller and smaller groups. Prior to myelination the larger axons segregate and lie isolated in troughs in the Schwann cell membrane while the cell at the same time envelops many smaller axons communally. At this stage the basal lamina starts to form. Subsequently the larger axons form a 1:1 relationship with single Schwann cells, which line up along the length of the axon. At this stage proliferation ceases and myelin sheaths, separated by nodes of Ranvier, form. Mature Remak fibres, in which several single unmyelinated axons are enclosed in individual furrows within the membrane of a single Schwann cell, develop after myelin formation is largely over (Diner, 1965; Webster and Favilla, 1984; Jessen *et al.*, 1985).

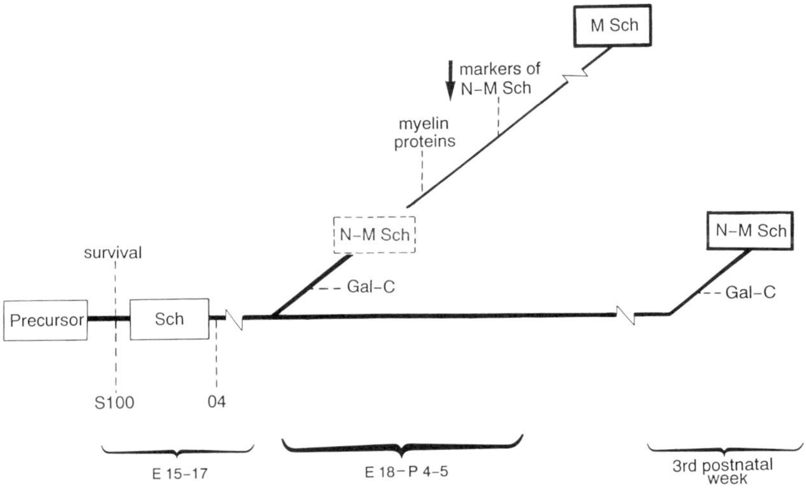

Figure 5.1 Development of the molecular phenotype of myelin-forming and non-myelin-forming Schwann cells from precursor cells in the rat sciatic nerve. Sch = Schwann cell; N-M Sch, in heavy box = mature non-myelin-forming Schwann cell; N-M Sch, in dashed box = cells with the molecular phenotype similar to mature non-myelin-forming cells, which will progress to myelination; M Sch = myelin-forming Schwann cell; Gal-C = galactocerebroside, indicates molecules that are down-regulated during differentiation of the Schwann cell along the myelin pathway. All other Schwann cell molecules or properties indicated are first seen at the time points indicated. Cells acquire the ability to survive alone in culture from embryo day 15 onwards; S100 first appears in Schwann cells between embryo days 15 and 16 and is present in 95% of Schwann cells at embryo day 18; 04 first appears shortly after S100 at embryo day 16 and is present in 95% of Schwann cells at embryo day 20; galactocerebroside first appears on cells in the myelin-forming pathway at embryo day 18 and the first P_0-positive cells are seen during the first postnatal day. By postnatal day 5 the first myelin-forming Schwann cells have down-regulated molecules such as GFAP, N-CAM, A5E3 and NGF receptors which are associated with non-myelin-forming Schwann cells. Cells in the non-myelin-forming pathway acquire Gal-C from the third postnatal week onwards without progressing to myelination. Differentiation of these cells is complete by the fifth to sixth postnatal weeks.

In the nerves innervating the rat hind limb, it is now possible to describe Schwann cell development from embryo day (E) 14 to maturity in terms of changes in the expression of a set of differentiation markers (Figure 5.1). Schwann cell precursors present in the nerves at E14–15 (section 5.5) give rise to S100 positive Schwann cells, first seen at E16. At E17 over 95% of cells dissociated from an excised sciatic nerve are S100 positive, the remaining cells being peri- or endoneurial fibroblastic cells. By E18 most Schwann cells also express the lipid antigen 04, which in the sciatic nerve is probably sulphatide. It first appears within the S100-positive cell population at E16, and by E20 95% of the S100-positive Schwann cells are also 04 positive (Mirsky *et al.*, 1990). At E18 it is possible to detect very low levels of the GFAP-like intermediate filament protein in some Schwann cells and by birth about half of the Schwann cells express immunohistochemically detectable GFAP. GFAP expression persists in mature non-myelin-forming cells. In the myelin-forming pathway this protein is only present transiently, however, since GFAP expression is suppressed soon after appearance of P_0. Schwann cells removed from axonal contact, e.g. in neuron-free cultures, continue to synthesize GFAP, and under these conditions GFAP reappears in cells that *in vivo* made myelin, showing that the suppression of GFAP expression during myelination is axon-dependent and reversible (Jessen *et al.*, 1990). Several other Schwann cell proteins, including L-NGF receptors, N-CAM and others, are regulated in a manner similar to that described here for GFAP (sections 5.2 and 5.6). Although Schwann cells are clearly capable of expressing GFAP in the absence of axonal contact, e.g. in neuron-free cultures, there is evidence that *in vivo* GFAP expression in mature non-myelin-forming cells is further up-regulated by contact with unmyelinated axons (Mokuno *et al.*, 1989; Neuberger and Cornbrooks, 1989; Jessen *et al.*, 1990). Galactocerebroside is first detectable at E18–19, and about half the Schwann cells express this lipid at birth (Mirsky *et al.*, 1980; Ranscht *et al.*, 1982; Jessen *et al.*, 1985). These cells will subsequently form myelin. Just prior to myelination, i.e. after acquisition of galactocerebroside but before significant expression of the major myelin protein P_0, the molecular phenotype of Schwann cells resembles that of mature non-myelin-forming Schwann cells, at least in the rat (Figure 5.1). These cells express L-NGF receptors, N-CAM, L1(Ng-CAM), A5E3 and Ran-2, in addition to S100, 04 and galactocerebroside. Furthermore, most of them transiently express GFAP as discussed above (Mirsky and Jessen, 1990; Jessen and Mirsky, 1991).

P_0 is first detectable at high levels during the first postnatal day when the first myelin wraps are also seen in the electron microscope (Brockes *et al.*, 1980; Mirsky *et al.*, 1980; Trapp *et al.*, 1981; Martini, Bollensen and Schachner, 1988). At a time when myelin-related differentiation has largely ceased, from the third postnatal week onwards, cells destined to differentiate into mature non-myelin-forming cells start to express galactocerebroside, and by the sixth postnatal week all Schwann cells in the nerve, both myelin-forming and non-myelin-forming, express galactocerebroside (Jessen *et al.*, 1985). It seems likely that a similar sequence of events occurs during the development of human Schwann cells since many of the same molecules are also present, although the detailed timing is unknown in most cases. It has been reported, however, that from approximately 7 weeks of embryonic age, S100 is expressed by Schwann cells associated with axons. In embryos younger than this, the

S100 labelling was much less consistent and appeared absent in many cells (Shearman and Franks, 1987).

5.5 SCHWANN CELL PRECURSORS

We have found that cells present in the rat sciatic nerve at E14 and E15 have two distinctly different properties from Schwann cells in older nerves. They do not express S100, although they are L-NGF-receptor positive, and they will not survive alone in culture in routine serum-containing media, although they can be rescued by conditioned medium from neurons. These cells have a characteristic flattened morphology *in vitro*, and already express most of the proteins that characterize non-myelin-forming Schwann cells in adult nerves. The main exception is GFAP, which appears later in Schwann cell development. They do not express the lipid antigen 04. In culture these cells can be distinguished from fibroblasts because they express L-NGF receptors, and all the evidence suggests that they are the precursors of the S100-positive Schwann cells that appear later in development (Jessen and Mirsky, 1991, 1992). Similar cells have been described in other systems, notably in cultures from quail neural crest but also in cultures from rat neural crest. Early studies by Holton and Weston (1982a,b) in quail used the acquisition of S100 to distinguish Schwann cells from non-neuronal precursor cells. Both their studies and those of Smith-Thomas and Fawcett (1989) and Smith-Thomas, Johnson and Fawcett (1990) suggest that the signal necessary for progression to S100-positive Schwann cells can be provided by neurons. If this turns out to be the case, this signalling would be unusual since it would bring about an irreversible change in Schwann cells (which remain S100-positive even when removed from axonal contact, although such cells may contain lower levels of the protein than those in contact with axons). In contrast, most of the known phenotypic changes induced by neuronal signals later in Schwann cell development are rapidly reversible (section 5.6).

5.6 CONTROL OF SCHWANN CELL PHENOTYPE

When regenerating axons from a myelinated nerve are anastomosed to the distal stump of a cut nerve that previously contained >99% unmyelinated fibres, the Schwann cells in the distal stump surround the large ingrowing axons and myelinate them in the normal way. On the basis of this type of experiment and many other related studies, it has become accepted that contact with appropriate axons provides a signal that induces the Schwann cells to form myelin (Bray, Rasminsky and Aguayo, 1981). What is appropriate in this context is, however, far from clear. Two main suggestions occur in the literature. Some authors have suggested that axon diameter is the crucial factor since only the larger axons will induce myelination, and therefore any axon that attains a certain critical diameter will induce synthesis of myelin components (Friede, 1972). Others have suggested that the larger axons possess specific signalling molecules that are not present on the smaller axons which interact with the Schwann cells and instruct them to make myelin (Bray, Rasminsky and Aguayo, 1981). It has also been suggested that Schwann cells can read not only axon diameter, but also the total axonal area contacted by the Schwann cell, cell length thus becoming an important factor in the induction of myelin synthesis (Griffin *et al.*, 1988). Various observations have been cited in support of these theories. Most recently it has been shown that enlargement of the target field of sympathetic neurons of the external carotid nerve is sufficient to induce the normally unmyelinated axons to become myelinated (Voyvoydic, 1989). Although these experiments were interpreted as supporting the importance of diameter in controlling myelination, it is in fact equally possible that increased neuronal growth leading to an increase in diameter above a critical size was accompanied by induction of expression of specific myelin signalling molecules in the cell membrane. So far all attempts to isolate molecules from neuronal membranes that will induce significant induction of myelination have been unsuccessful, but so have several attempts to induce myelination of synthetic fibres of appropriate diameter. Thus at present we do not know the nature of the major neuronal factors controlling myelination. Somewhat more is known about the intracellular signals in Schwann cells that are likely to be involved in Schwann cell development and differentiation (sections 5.8 and 5.9).

The two different Schwann cell phenotypes could be generated by induction of separate differentiation antigens in the two cell types. This seems unlikely in view of the fact that the phenotype of the mature non-myelin-forming Schwann cells is very similar to that of the premyelin Schwann cell just prior to acquisition of the myelin proteins (see above and Figure 5.1). The present evidence indicates that the two different phenotypes are in fact generated essentially through changes in protein expression in the myelin-forming pathway. These changes consist of up-regulation of the myelin proteins, followed shortly thereafter by down-regulation of expression of proteins like N-CAM, L1, L-NGF receptor and GFAP. These proteins are present in Schwann cells prior to myelination and are also characteristic of mature non-myelin-forming Schwann cells, although the level of L-NGF receptor on adult non-myelin-forming Schwann cells is probably lower than that on developing Schwann cells. Both the up-regulation and down-regulation are axon dependent and reversible, since Schwann cells deprived of axonal contact, either by dissociation and culture or by nerve transection *in vivo*, rapidly down-regulate expression of myelin genes and proteins (Mirsky *et al.*, 1980; Lemke and Chao, 1988; Martini and Schachner, 1988; Mokuno *et al.*, 1988; Trapp, Hauer and Lemke, 1988; Brunden, Windebank and Poduslo, 1990) and re-express L-NGF receptor protein and mRNA, N-CAM, A5E3 and GFAP (Nieke and Schachner, 1985; Rieger *et al.*, 1985; Jessen, Morgan and Mirsky, 1987; Taniuchi *et al.*, 1988; Jessen *et al.*, 1990; Mirsky and Jessen, 1990; Jessen and Mirsky, 1991). There is also evidence that axons regulate P_0 expression at both translational and post-translational levels (Brunden and Poduslo, 1987; Gupta, Poduslo and Mezet, 1988; Brunden, Windebank and Poduslo, 1990).

Like the L-NGF receptor, NGF is present in embryonic rat sciatic nerve and levels drop rapidly during the first 21 days of life (Heumann *et al.*, 1987a,b). NGF levels are also up-regulated in Schwann cells and fibroblasts distal to a crush or transection and, to a lesser extent, in Schwann cells grown in culture. The re-expression of NGF in fibroblastic (perineurial) cells but not Schwann cells *in vivo* is probably triggered indirectly by interleukin-1 (IL-1), which can be secreted by invading macrophages or under certain circumstances by the Schwann cells. The mechanism of up-regulation of NGF in Schwann cells is unknown (Heumann *et al.*, 1987a,b; Lindholm *et al.*, 1987; Bergsteinsdóttir *et al.*, 1991).

Although qualitative changes in protein expression appear to be confined to changes in the myelin-forming pathways, up-regulation of several lipid antigens including 04, galactocerebroside and the lipid antigens 08 and 09 occurs in both myelin- and non-myelin-forming Schwann cells during maturation. Like the proteins, however, levels of all of these lipids are rapidly down-regulated when Schwann cells are removed from axonal contact either by dissociation and culture or by nerve transection. Thus axons regulate the phenotype of both myelin-forming and non-myelin-forming cells (Eccleston *et al.*, 1987; Jessen, Morgan and Mirsky, 1987).

In most experimental situations, contact with axons appears to be necessary not only for induction of the myelin sheath but also for its maintenance. In the normal sympathetic ganglion of adult rats, however, some postganglionic axons normally possess a second myelin sheath. This sheath has lost contact with the axon after initial (presumably axon-dependent) myelin formation has occurred, and lies instead on the surface of another myelin-forming Schwann cell, still in axonal contact, from which it is separated by a basal lamina (Kidd and Heath, 1989a,b). This raises the possibility that under certain circumstances it may be possible to maintain a myelin sheath in the absence of axonal contact.

5.7 SCHWANN CELL CULTURES

Cell culture has proved an important tool in studies on Schwann cells. As will become clear in the following sections, a substantial amount of our knowledge about proliferation control, second messengers and differentiation, transmitter receptors and ion channels, the relationship between Schwann cells and the extracellular matrix (ECM) and the interaction between Schwann cells and the immune system, derive from *in vitro* studies.

Although most studies on the biology of Schwann cells have used Schwann cells from species other than humans, in recent years interest in Schwann cells from human nerves, both fetal and adult, has increased. Several different preparative methods have been described for obtaining cultures of purified human Schwann cells (Askanas *et al.*, 1980; Samuel *et al.*, 1987b; Scarpini *et al.*, 1988; Yong *et al.*, 1988; Assouline and Pantazis, 1989; Kim *et al.*, 1989). Most of these are based either on the dissociation procedure of Brockes, Field and Raff (1979), originally described for the purification of rat Schwann cells, or on explanting segments of nerve and allowing Schwann cells to grow out on to the culture dish. In some procedures the segment is re-explanted several times to ensure that highly purified cultures of Schwann cells are obtained before expansion with growth factors. The dissociation procedure involves enzymatic treatment of sciatic nerve segments, plating of single cells and subsequent elimination of fibroblastic cells by antimitotic agents, complement-mediated killing or a preplating step. It is more suited to cultures from fetal nerves, which contain little fibrous extracellular material, whereas the explant method is likely to give better results for adult nerves, which contain large amounts of collagen and other connective tissue. Purified Schwann cell cultures derived from dissociated or explanted dorsal root or superior cervical ganglia have been established by Wood (1976), and more recently methods have been described for the preparation of purified cultures of rat sensory neurons to which purified populations of both embryonic and adult Schwann cells can be added at will (Bunge, Bunge and Eldridge, 1986; Kuhlengel, Bunge and Bunge, 1990; Morrissey, Kleitman and Bunge, 1991). Recently, a method for selective culture of mitotically active human Schwann cells has been described (Rutkowski, Tennekoon and McGillicuddy, 1992).

In general the molecular properties of human Schwann cells are similar to those of Schwann cells from other species, and they seem to be under similar axonal control to Schwann cells from other species. Some reports do, however, suggest that their growth factor requirements may be somewhat different since doses of cAMP that stimulate rat Schwann cell proliferation inhibit proliferation of human Schwann cells in culture (Pleasure *et al.*, 1986). There are also conflicting reports about whether human Schwann cells can express MHC class II antigens in culture in the absence of added gamma-interferon (section 5.12).

5.8 REGULATION OF SCHWANN CELL PROLIFERATION

In mature normal nerves both non-myelin- and myelin-forming Schwann cells are mitotically quiescent. *In vivo*, proliferation of Schwann cells is seen principally under three different circumstances: during development, in damaged nerves as Schwann cells lose contact with axons, and during the generation of tumours. In none of these instances are the factors responsible for driving Schwann cell division known in molecular terms.

There is evidence from *in vitro* studies that Schwann cells secrete factors capable of stimulating their own division, and *in vivo* Schwann cells are in contact with at least two potential Schwann cell mitogens: laminin in the Schwann cell basal lamina, and the axolemmal surface. It may therefore be profitable to ask not only what drives Schwann cell division during development, injury and tumour formation, but also why Schwann cells gradually withdraw from the cell cycle as nerves develop and how Schwann cell division is prevented in normal nerves. There is in fact recent experimental evidence for the existence of factors that inhibit Schwann cell proliferation and it seems increasingly likely that Schwann cell division is regulated via interaction between positive and negative growth controls (Muir, Varon and Manthorpe, 1990; Muir and Manthorpe, 1992; Eccleston, Jessen and Mirsky, 1991).

Essentially all recent work in this field has been carried out *in vitro*, and mostly on cells derived from the rat sciatic nerve. Three identified polypeptides – transforming growth factor β (TGF-β), platelet derived growth factor (PDGF) and fibroblast growth factor (FGF) – in addition to impure preparations of glial growth factor (GGF) act as mitogens in rat Schwann cell cultures (Raff *et al.*, 1978; Brockes, Lemke and Balzer, 1980; Eccleston *et al.*, 1987, 1990; Ridley *et al.*, 1989; Davis and Stroobant, 1990; Kimura, Fischer and Schubert, 1990; Weinmaster and Lemke, 1990; Eccleston, 1992). Agents that elevate or mimic intracellular cyclic AMP (cAMP) synergize with these polypeptides further to promote Schwann cell DNA synthesis (Raff, Hornby-Smith and Brockes, 1978; Raff *et al.*, 1978). On the other hand, if experiments of this type are carried out in serum-free medium, it becomes clear that neither cAMP elevating agents nor growth factors stimulate DNA synthesis when applied singly. A combination of a cAMP-elevating agent and PDGF or FGF induces DNA synthesis, while a combination of cAMP and TGF-β is ineffective under these conditions (Stewart *et al.*, 1991). A combination of FGF or PDGF with TGF-β is, however, mitogenic, indicating that TGF-β can substitute for cAMP in the proliferation pathway (Schubert, 1992). Cyclic AMP elevating agents are also mitogenic in the presence of serum, presumably because they synergize with serum-derived growth factors.

These observations suggest that, in rat Schwann cells, activation of at least two intracellular pathways is required for stimulation of DNA synthesis, and also that serum-derived growth factors are not necessary for the synergy between cAMP or TGF-β and PDGF or FGF.

One explanation for the synergy between cAMP and growth factors is offered by the observation that elevation of cAMP levels enhances expression of PDGF receptors on Schwann cells (Weinmaster and Lemke, 1990). It is therefore possible that increased receptor expression leads to increased response to PDGF. If receptors for other mitogenic factors such as FGF are regulated in the same way, this mechanism could account for the synergy with cAMP. Schwann cells do, however, express PDGF receptors in the absence of cAMP elevation, and long-term Schwann cells with constitutively elevated cAMP levels, which respond to PDGF in the absence of other added factors, have similar numbers of receptors on their surfaces to short-term unstimulated Schwann cells (Eccleston *et al.*, 1990). The only other growth factor receptor known to be regulated by cAMP in Schwann cells is the low-affinity NGF receptor, which is down-regulated in response to cAMP elevation (Mokuno *et al.*, 1988; Morgan, Jessen and Mirsky, 1991).

One of the most potent mitogens for cultured rat Schwann cells is a factor associated with neuronal membranes that also causes mitosis in Schwann cells derived from human neurofibromas. This is likely to be a protein associated with a heparan sulphate on the axon surface (Sobue *et al.*, 1984, 1985; Ratner, Bunge and Glaser, 1985; Ratner *et al.*, 1988). It has been suggested that Schwann cell mitosis in response to axolemma is accompanied by enhanced inositol phospholipid metabolism and changes in intracellular pH (Saunders and DeVries, 1988; Saunders, Brandon and DeVries, 1989). Other Schwann cell mitogens appear to be secreted by the Schwann cells themselves, at least under culture conditions (Porter, Glaser and Bunge, 1987). One of these factors is PDGF but other factors are also present (Eccleston *et al.*, 1990; Eccleston, 1992). Components of the extracellular matrix, in particular laminin and fibronectin, also have the potential to promote Schwann cell proliferation. Both of these molecules synergize with autocrine Schwann cell growth factors (Porter *et al.*, 1986) and with factors that elevate cAMP. Plasminogen activators have also been reported to be mitogenic for rat Schwann cells (Baron van Evercooren *et al.*, 1987).

Long-term cultured rat Schwann cells lose growth control when they are cultured with a combination of GGF and forskolin and passaged repetitively over a period of weeks. The division rate of these cells in serum remains high long after mitogens have been removed. In fact, proliferation continues slowly even when the cells are deprived of serum; they presumably secrete autocrine proliferative factors (Porter *et al.*, 1986;

Porter, Glaser and Bunge, 1987). At least at early passage times, these long-term Schwann cells will myelinate axons present in the culture. When injected into a nerve these cells produced an encapsulated mass with the morphological characteristics of a Schwannoma (Langford, Porter and Bunge, 1988). Similar cells are also produced when the cultures are maintained without passage in serum-containing medium for several months. In the absence of axons, these cells gradually start secreting autocrine factors, including the BB form of PDGF (Eccleston *et al.*, 1990), which probably interacts with PDGF receptors on the Schwann cell surface. These cells also have constitutively elevated levels of cAMP (Stewart *et al.*, 1991).

There are very few studies on growth regulation in human Schwann cells. In Schwann cell cultures derived from normal human fetuses, GGF, PDGF, FGF and NGF have been reported to stimulate DNA synthesis in the presence of serum (Yong *et al.*, 1988). In Schwann-like cells cultured from dermal neurofibromas, GGF also stimulated DNA synthesis (Pleasure *et al.*, 1986; Sheela, Riccardi and Ratner, 1990). In a separate study, GGF-like activity was found in extracts from three out of three bilateral vestibular Schwannomas, five out of seven unilateral vestibular Schwannomas and two out of five neurofibromas (Brockes, Breakfield and Martuza, 1986). In contrast to rat Schwann cells, elevation of cAMP in serum-containing medium inhibited proliferation of Schwann-like cells derived from human neurofibromas (Pleasure *et al.*, 1985, 1986).

To understand the basis of Schwann cell proliferation in neurofibromas it will be of major interest to follow future developments stemming from the cloning of the neurofibromatosis 1 (NF1) gene (Ballester *et al.*, 1990; Martin *et al.*, 1990; Xu *et al.*, 1990). The gene product, called neurofibromin, appears to be generally expressed in normal cells, and neurofibromas result from an inactivating mutation. It is expressed at low levels in many cell types, but at high levels in non-myelin-forming Schwann cells, oligodendrocytes and neurons, including CNS neurons (Daston *et al.*, 1992). This is interesting in view of the mental retardation sometimes associated with neurofibromatosis. Sequence analysis indicates that the NF1 protein is related to the IRA1/2 proteins in yeast and GTPase activating proteins (GAP) in eukaryotic cells. These proteins bind to G proteins of the *ras* type, which are frequently intermediaries in division-promoting pathways. Since *ras* activity can be inhibited by interaction with GAP, inactivating mutations might be expected to accelerate proliferation. Two groups have recently shown that, like $p120^{GAP}$, neurofibromin interacts with $p21^{ras}$ (Basu *et al.*, 1992; DeClue *et al.*, 1992), a regulatory membrane protein that is likely to be involved in regulation of Schwann cell proliferation (Ridley *et al.*, 1988). It is particularly interesting that in malignant neurofibrosarcomas/Schwannomas derived from patients with neurofibromatosis, levels of neurofibromin are either low or not detectable at all. Perhaps as a consequence of this, levels of activated p21^{ras}, i.e. levels of p21^{ras} bound to GTP, are very much higher than normal, and it is suggested that this leads ultimately to tumour formation. As the levels of p120^{GAP}, the main protein interacting with p21^{ras} in many other cell types, are normal, these results also suggest that, in Schwann cells, neurofibromin and not p120^{GAP} may be the major protein responsible for controlling the levels of p21^{ras}-GTP (Basu *et al.*, 1992; DeClue *et al.*, 1992). Earlier experiments showed that in Schwann cells, cooperativity between v-*ras* and a nuclear oncogene was needed to promote cell division and transformation (Ridley *et al.*, 1988). This suggests that in addition to the loss of neurofibromin, other cellular changes are required for neurofibromas to form.

Another protein likely to be involved in Schwann cell proliferation is the p185^{neu} receptor, a member of the epidermal growth factor receptor family which has tyrosine kinase activity. A study on the expression of p185^{neu} mRNA and protein in the rat sciatic nerve reports that p185^{neu} is present in Schwann cells and that the levels of both protein and mRNA are much higher at birth than in adult nerves (Cohen *et al.*, 1992). After nerve transection, high levels of mRNA and protein are again seen in Schwann cells in the distal stump. Interestingly, levels of expression increase rather slowly and the amount of p185^{neu} mRNA continues to increase for at least 24 days after transection. Following transection, Schwann cells in the distal stump enter a transient proliferative phase with cell division peaking around the middle of the first week after the cut. High levels of Schwann cell proliferation do not therefore coincide with high levels of p185^{neu} mRNA expression in cut nerves. Nevertheless, a link between p185^{neu} and regulation of Schwann cell proliferation has been suspected for some time, as Schwannomas derived from ethylnitrosourea (ENU)-treated rats contain homozygous mutations in the transmembrane region of the *neu* gene (Perantoni *et al.*, 1987). This leads to increased tyrosine kinase activity (Bargmann and Weinberg, 1988). It has now been shown that cells containing a single mutant *neu* allele can be demonstrated in the trigeminal nerve of ENU-treated neonatal rats as soon as 7 days after treatment, whereas tumours normally develop after several months. These early mutant cells show higher proliferation rates within the nerve and the evidence suggests that transformation of the *neu* gene is an early event in the progression to tumorigenesis. The mutation appears to be cell-lineage specific as ENU-derived tumours from other cell types, including CNS tumours, do not show alterations in p185^{neu} (Nikitin *et al.*, 1991). These results can be related to the recent isolation and cloning of *neu* differentiation factor (NDF), a 44 kDa secreted glycoprotein that binds to the p185^{neu} receptor. This factor inhibits DNA synthesis and promotes differentiation in a mammary carcinoma line. It is suggested that mutations in p185^{neu} may lower binding of NDF to the p185^{neu} receptor, which could lead to loss of growth control (Peles *et al.*, 1992). It will clearly be of interest to determine whether NDF is involved in control of Schwann cell proliferation.

In addition to tumorigenesis, Wallerian degeneration resulting from nerve transection or crush represents another major situation in which proliferation of mature Schwann cells occurs. Both non-myelin- and myelin-forming Schwann cells in the distal stump enter a transient phase of proliferation (Clemence, Mirsky and Jessen, 1989), with a peak 2–4 days after nerve transection (Pellegrino *et al.*, 1986). The proliferative response is much lower in essentially unmyelinated nerves such as the cervical sympathetic trunk (Clemence, Mirsky and Jessen, 1989). One explanation for this would be that the proliferative response was positively related to the amount of myelin-breakdown products in the nerve. This idea has been advanced by DeVries and colleagues, who have shown that macrophages, which are known to invade degenerating nerves, produce mitogenic factor(s) for Schwann cells following lysosomal processing of myelin membranes (Baichwal, Bigbee and DeVries, 1988; Meador-Woodruff, Lewis and DeVries, 1984; Meador-Woodruff *et al.*, 1985). Other experiments show that both myelin breakdown and Schwann cell proliferation are markedly suppressed under conditions that do not allow macrophage invasion into the nerve (Beuche and Friede, 1985; Perry, Brown and Gordon, 1987; Lunn *et al.*, 1989). This is consistent with the notion of a causal relationship between macrophage invasion, myelin breakdown and Schwann cell proliferation during nerve degeneration.

Recently, several different lines of evidence have raised the possibility that, under normal conditions, Schwann cell proliferation may in part be held in check by the action of growth inhibitors. Rat Schwann cells show a marked suppression of DNA synthesis when co-cultured with purified neurons from the myenteric plexus, although their division rate is stimulated by co-culturing with dorsal root sensory or sympathetic neurons. The factor responsible for this effect has not been identified (Eccleston *et al.*, 1989a). Proliferation of Schwann cells is also inhibited by contact with type I collagen (Eccleston *et al.*, 1989c). Interferon-gamma acts as an effective suppressor of DNA synthesis in Schwann cells stimulated to divide by cAMP elevation (Eccleston *et al.*, 1989b). This is relevant in view of the observation that peripheral neurons contain interferon-like immunoreactivity (Ljungdahl *et al.*, 1989) and the indirect evidence that cAMP may be elevated in Schwann cells *in vivo* (section 5.9). Schwann cell proliferation is also inhibited by gangliosides (Sobue *et al.*, 1988a). Perhaps most interesting is the evidence that Schwann cells secrete proteins that inhibit their own growth (Muir, Varon and Manthorpe, 1990; Eccleston *et al.*, 1991; Muir and Manthorpe, 1992).

Thus, growth regulation by extrinsic factors such as soluble peptides, axon-associated factors, matrix constituents and macrophage derived molecules may, in Schwann cells, be superimposed on an interplay between positive and negative autocrine control loops. There is clearly a long way to go before regulation of Schwann cell proliferation is fully understood.

5.9 CYCLIC AMP AND SCHWANN CELL DIFFERENTIATION

In 1984 Sobue and Pleasure observed that when Schwann cells in culture were treated with cAMP analogues they could be induced to express galactocerebroside on their surfaces. This was the first indication that raised intracellular levels of cAMP might be involved in Schwann cell differentiation. Since that time, elevation of intracellular cAMP has been shown to induce many other phenotypic changes in Schwann cells. These include the expansion and flattening of the Schwann cells to form large membranous expansions (Sobue, Shuman and Pleasure, 1986; Morgan, Jessen and Mirsky, 1991), the induction of a 170 kDa protein (Shuman *et al.*, 1988), which may be identical to the recently cloned Schwann cell membrane glycoprotein (SAG) described by Dierperink *et al.* (1992), the induction of the myelin-specific protein P_0 and its mRNA and the induction of the mRNA for MBP (Lemke and Chao, 1988), the induction of the suppressed cAMP-inducible POU (SCIP) gene which is a POU-domain transcription regulation factor (Monuki *et al.*, 1989), and the induction of the 04 lipid antigen (Mirsky *et al.*, 1990). Synthesis of basal lamina components is also increased by elevation of cAMP levels (Baron van Evercooren *et al.*, 1986).

Some of these differentiation events, like 04 induction, are associated *in vivo* with early Schwann cell development, while others, such as induction of the myelin proteins, are associated with later development. Some, like 04, galactocerebroside and basal lamina formation, are associated with both myelin-forming and non-myelin-forming Schwann cells, while others, such as induction of the myelin proteins, are associated with myelin-forming Schwann cells only. It is, however, significant that all of these events are associated with axon-associated signals *in vivo*. Many gene regulatory proteins have cAMP responsive elements in the promoter regions of their genes, and cAMP is known to up-regulate expression of the SCIP gene, activated in Schwann cells relatively early in development before the onset of myelination, and which may in turn have effects on later genes, including P_0, which, at least in transfected cells, it represses (Monuki *et al.*, 1990; He *et al.*, 1991). There are also reports that in other systems cAMP can act as an intermediary between ligand–receptor interactions at the cell surface and changes in gene activity (Dumont, Jauniaux and Roger, 1989). It is therefore possible that a crucial part of axon–Schwann cell signalling *in vivo* operates through elevation of cAMP in Schwann cells.

The observation that elevation of cAMP promotes a significant number of events that *in vivo* are axon-dependent and associated with Schwann cell differentiation, raises the possibility that a single axon-related signalling mechanism operating by raising cAMP levels drives much of Schwann cell differentiation. This would include 04 expression and galactocerebroside synthesis in both myelin-forming and non-myelin-forming cells, and myelin induction and suppression of proteins such as the L-NGF receptor and N-CAM in myelin-forming cells only. The axon-associated signal in question should be present at a relatively early stage of development, i.e. from E16–17 onwards, and be associated with axons of all calibres. Both of these features distinguish this proposal from the alternative proposal (section 5.6) that cAMP is the second messenger of a specific myelination signal, associated only with larger-calibre axons.

The proposal that cAMP elevation acts *in vivo* as a general Schwann cell differentiation signal, inducing events that during development occur over a period of many days, raises the question of timing. For instance, what is the timing mechanism that allows cAMP elevation to induce 04 expression at E16 but delays P_0 expression in response to the same signal to the first postnatal day, i.e. by 4–5 days? In principle, this could be achieved by an intrinsically programmed change in those factors that

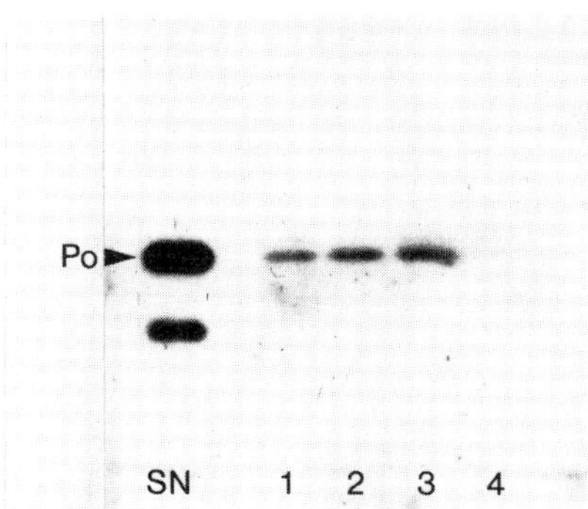

Figure 5.2 Immunoblot of P_0 induction in Schwann cells. SN: Extract of 5-day-old rat sciatic nerve, 25 μg loaded. Lanes 1–3: Extracts from dissociated Schwann cell cultures from 5-day-old rat sciatic nerve treated with agents that elevate or mimic cAMP. Lane 1: cAMP analogues; lane 2: cholera toxin, lane 3: forskolin, lane 4: no treatment, 31 μg of extract loaded in each lane. Note that at the P_0 position (arrowed) an immunoreactive band is visible in the sciatic nerve lane and in each of lanes 1–3, but not in lane 4 (control). In the sciatic nerve extract a lower breakdown product of P_0 is also visible. (Source: Morgan, Jessen and Mirsky, 1991.)

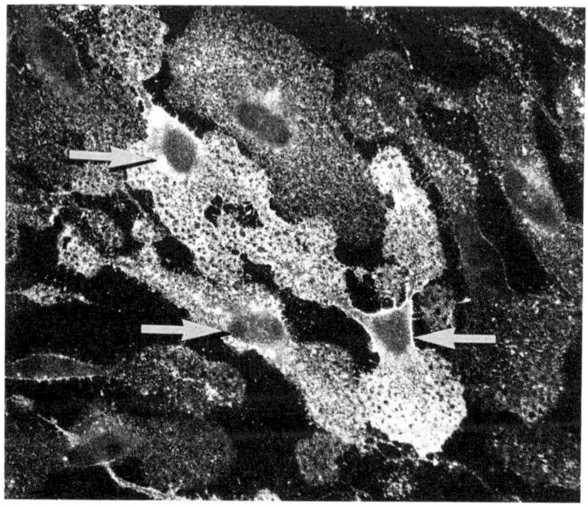

Figure 5.3 Induction of P_0 in Schwann cells treated with cholera toxin. P_0-positive Schwann cells cultured from 5-day-old rat sciatic nerve. Cells were cultured on a laminin substrate and treated with cholera toxin, and labelled with P_0 antibodies after 3 days of treatment. Cells were viewed with fluorescein optics to visualize P_0. Note the flattened shape of the Schwann cells and the P_0 immunofluorescence distributed throughout the whole area of each cell. Nuclei of three intensely P_0-positive cells are indicated by arrows. (Source: L. Morgan.)

determine the intracellular translation of the cAMP signal. We have, at present, no evidence for such a mechanism.

There is, however, an alternative way in which the translation of the cAMP signal can be switched to induce early Schwann cell differentiation, i.e. 04 expression, on the one hand, or to induce a later developmental stage, i.e. P_0 expression, on the other. We have found that this can be achieved by regulation of Schwann cell proliferation (Morgan, Jessen and Mirsky, 1991). As mentioned earlier (section 5.8), when cAMP is elevated in Schwann cells cultured in the presence of serum or growth factors, they respond by proliferation, whereas this response is essentially absent in serum-free media. We can therefore examine the effects on Schwann cells of elevating cAMP under proliferating and non-proliferating conditions. We find that individual Schwann cells that are proliferating will express the early antigen 04 in response to cAMP elevation whereas quiescent Schwann cells show a different response. In these cells a marked increase in size and flattening is seen with induction of large amounts of P_0 protein, which can be visualized immunohistochemically or in immunoblots (Figures 5.2 and 5.3). Cells in which the P_0 is most strongly induced also down-regulate the proteins N-CAM, L-NGF receptor, GFAP and A5E3. All of these changes mimic events that occur during *in vivo* maturation of Schwann cells (see section 5.4 on cessation of proliferation before myelin synthesis *in vivo*). Thus 04, but not myelination, is induced, as *in vivo*, in a proliferating cell population, while in non-dividing cells P_0 is induced and N-CAM, L-NGF receptor, GFAP and A5E3 are down-regulated. We therefore suggest that, *in vivo*, cAMP elevation, presumably induced by axon-associated factors, acts as a primary signal that triggers 04 expression and synergizes with growth factors to drive Schwann cell proliferation in the premyelination period. Withdrawal from the cell cycle, first seen in Schwann cells around birth, acts as a secondary signal, which, when superimposed on elevated cAMP levels, triggers myelination (Figure 5.4) (Mirsky and Jessen, 1990; Jessen and Mirsky, 1991; Morgan, Jessen and Mirsky, 1991). Inhibition of Schwann cell division *in vivo*, about which little is known, could be brought about by either withdrawal of growth factors, down-regulation of growth factor receptors, uncoupling of these receptors from intracellular signals that cause mitosis, or active inhibitory factors (section 5.8).

The hypothesis outlined above does not explain the generation of non-myelin-forming cells. It is possible that the degree of cAMP elevation in individual cells determines whether it forms myelin or not when it is withdrawn from the cell cycle. This could differ between cells associated with the larger axons and those associated with the smaller axons. There

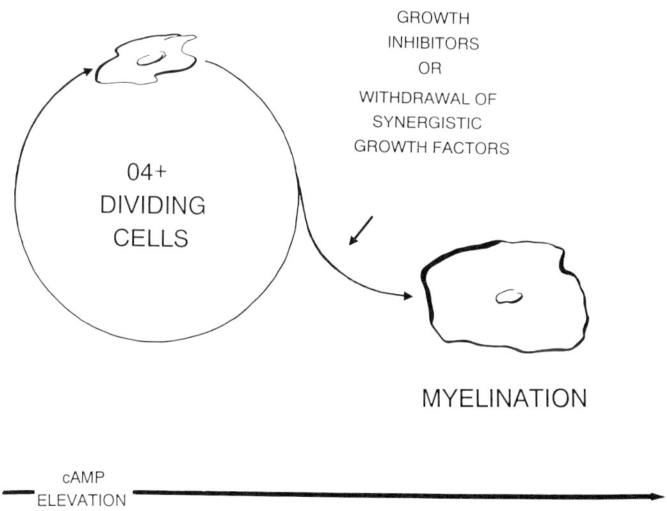

Figure 5.4 The proliferative state may control the response to cAMP *in vivo*. It is envisaged that axon-dependent elevation of cAMP induces early differentiation (04 expression) under conditions in which cAMP simultaneously synergizes with growth factors to promote Schwann cell proliferation. Withdrawal from the cell cycle (brought about as indicated via other mechanisms) triggers myelination, since in quiescent cells the ongoing cAMP elevation induces myelination.

is no evidence for or against this idea. An alternative possibility is that the structural polarization of the Schwann cell generated by the flattening of the cell between the basal lamina and the axon is a prerequisite for the induction of myelination in a galactocerebroside-positive cell. There are several precedents for polarization inducing differentiation (for discussion in the context of Schwann cells see Bunge, Bunge and Eldridge, 1986). In Schwann cells this polarization would be most effectively achieved in a cell associated with a single axon with a diameter that was large with respect to the size of the Schwann cell. This proposal has the merit of incorporating recent work on cAMP and Schwann cell differentiation and earlier suggestions that axon diameter is a crucial factor in myelin induction (section 5.6).

5.10 ION CHANNELS AND NEUROTRANSMITTER RECEPTORS IN SCHWANN CELLS

Schwann cells and other glia have ion channels and neurotransmitter receptors which have similar characteristics to those found in neurons (for reviews see Barres, Chun and Corey, 1990; Bevan, 1990). Most of the investigations on the properties of these ion channels and receptors have been carried out on cultured Schwann cells, but some workers, notably Chiu and associates, have also used nerve preparations that reflect *in situ* characteristics. In view of the marked alterations in the molecular phenotype of Schwann cells that occur when these cells are dissociated from the nerve and taken into culture (section 5.6), caution must be used in extrapolating the results obtained from cultured Schwann cells to intact nerves. Clearly, channels and receptors identified in Schwann cells in culture show that they can be expressed under appropriate conditions, but they do not show which proteins the Schwann cells actually express when in contact with axons in the intact animal.

5.10.1 Ion channels

Patch clamp electrodes, which measure ion currents, and microelectrodes, which are often used to record changes in membrane potential, have both been used to investigate the properties of ion channels in Schwann cells. In cultured Schwann cells at least four distinct ion channels can be distinguished, two selective for potassium ions, one selective for sodium ions and one permeable to chloride ions (Chiu, Shrager and Ritchie, 1984; Konishi, 1989; Howe and Ritchie, 1988; Shrager, Chiu and Ritchie, 1985; Hoppe, Kettenmann and Verkhratsky, 1990). The two distinctive channels permeable to potassium ions can be distinguished on the basis of their speed of inactivation and in their differential sensitivities to tetraethylammonium (TEA) ions and 4-aminopyridine (4-AP), and which channel is expressed seems to depend to some extent on the animal species from which the Schwann cells are derived (Howe and Ritchie, 1988; Konishi, 1989). The first channel, found predominantly in rabbit Schwann cells, is a voltage-gated channel which is opened when the membrane is depolarized to >–40 mV, is blocked most effectively by TEA, and is normally only slowly inactivated and shows delayed rectification. The second, which predominates in rat and human Schwann cells, is also voltage sensitive, activated at more negative potentials, blocked most effectively by 4-AP and is inactivated within milliseconds. Channels with the same kinetic characteristics and conductances as both these channels exist in neurons. Neurons generally possess more different types of K^+ channels than glial cells, some of which are regulated by Ca^{++} concentration. These Ca^{++} dependent K^+ channels have not been found in cultured Schwann cells (Shrager, Chiu and Ritchie, 1985; Hoppe, Kettenmann and Verkhratsky, 1990). Schwann cells from several different species, including humans, possess tetrodotoxin-sensitive voltage-gated Na^+ channels of a type similar to those found in neurons (Chiu, Shrager and Ritchie, 1984; Shrager, Chiu and Ritchie, 1985; Howe and Ritchie, 1990). These channels become active when the membrane is depolarized to between –30 and –40 mV and are blocked by tetrodotoxin. They are rapidly activated and inactivated. Rabbit Schwann cells also possess channels selectively permeable to chloride ions, which are activated at positive membrane potentials (Howe and Ritchie, 1988).

In situ, Chiu (1987) has reported that Schwann cells associated with axons in unmyelinated fibres have different channel properties from those associated with myelinated fibres. His interpretation of his results on myelin-forming Schwann cells has been challenged by Howe and Ritchie (1990), on the basis that the capacitance of the myelin membrane itself is so large that it would mask measurement of currents resulting from rapidly activating and inactivating channels even if they were present. With that caveat in mind, it is possible to state that non-myelin-forming Schwann cells in intact nerve possess sodium channels of a tetrodotoxin-sensitive type and that denervation causes a decrease in the total Na^+ current flowing, presumably reflecting a decrease in the number of Na^+ channels in these cells once denervated. Outward currents, probably due to K^+, can also be recorded from non-myelin-forming Schwann cells and these do not change on denervation (Chiu, 1988, 1991). In contrast, no Na^+ currents were recorded from myelin-forming Schwann cells (but see criticism above) and on denervation these cells showed a measurable inward Na^+ current, suggesting that up-regulation of this channel occurs on denervation of myelin-forming Schwann cells.

During development, it appears that early in myelination (rat postnatal day 1), myelin-forming Schwann cells, which are making their first myelin wraps at this time, have two types of K^+ channels. The first channel is an inwardly rectifying channel that is open at the resting membrane potential (–80 mV), and the second has the same characteristics as the TEA-sensitive, slowly inactivating voltage-gated channel described above in cultured Schwann cells. Neither of these channels is measurable as myelin formation proceeds, but again this could be due to technical reasons rather than because of down-regulation of channel expression (Wilson and Chiu, 1990). It has been proposed that the TEA-sensitive channels could be involved in Schwann cell proliferation in the denervated distal stump of intact nerves, since TEA, which blocks the channels, inhibits Schwann cell proliferation in cultured nerve segments (Chiu and Wilson, 1989).

5.10.2 Neurotransmitter receptors

These have been extensively studied in cultured astrocytes (for reviews see Bevan, 1990; Wilkin, Marriot and Cholewinski, 1990), but much less extensively in Schwann cells. In general, the function of these receptors on glial cells is little understood but their presence suggests a more complex interaction between neurons and glia than was at one time envisaged.

Schwann cells in culture express β_1-adrenergic receptors and vasoactive intestinal peptide (VIP) receptors, both of which transiently elevate intracellular cAMP levels (Yasuda *et al.*, 1988). Despite this, neither of these compounds cause proliferation of Schwann cells (Davis and Stroobant, 1990).

Receptor autoradiography studies on mixed cultures of cells derived from heart atria, show that some, but not all, S100-positive cells (either Schwann cells or satellite cells) associated with the intrinsic ganglia of the heart have neuropeptide Y (NPY) receptors and receptors for the peptide secretin (James *et al.*, 1990).

5.11 SCHWANN CELLS AND THE EXTRACELLULAR MATRIX

Both non-myelin-forming Schwann cells and myelin-forming Schwann cells are surrounded by a basal lamina. Outside this lies the endoneurium containing fibroblasts, collagen fibrils, fibronectin and presumably other general constituents of the extracellular matrix (ECM) (Palm and Furcht, 1983; Thomas and Ochoa, 1984).

It is now clear that the Schwann cells themselves are able to synthesize and secrete many of the matrix components and assemble their own basal lamina in the absence of endoneurial fibroblasts (Bunge, Bunge and

Eldridge, 1986). Furthermore there are many instances where impairment in basal lamina formation correlates with failure of Schwann cells to achieve a mature relationship with axons and elaborate a myelin sheath. This may indicate a causal relationship, i.e. that the assembly of their own basal lamina is a necessary prerequisite for the Schwann cells to achieve further maturation, including myelination (Bunge, Bunge and Eldridge, 1986; Eldridge *et al.*, 1987; Eldridge, Bunge and Bunge, 1989).

The Schwann cell basal lamina contains general basal lamina components including laminin, type IV collagen, entactin and heparan sulphate proteoglycan (Shelleswell *et al.*, 1979; Sanes, 1982; Palm and Furcht, 1983; Tohyama and Ide, 1984; Bannerman *et al.*, 1986; Bunge, Bunge and Eldridge, 1986). There is also evidence that the Schwann cell basal lamina contains molecules that have a more restricted distribution, including type V and type VI collagens, antigens present on skeletal muscle basal lamina, and merosin, a molecule closely related to laminin B chains, which is the main form of laminin found in peripheral nerve (Sanes and Chiu, 1983; Leivo and Engvall, 1988; Peltonen *et al.*, 1990; Sanes *et al.*, 1990). In the developing mouse sciatic nerve, laminin is present not only in the basement membrane, but is also associated with the Schwann cell membrane, unmyelinated axons and collagen fibrils in the endoneurial space (Küecherer-Ehret *et al.*, 1990).

Basal lamina that is apparently normal in morphology and molecular content can be assembled around Schwann cells in co-cultures of neurons and Schwann cells containing virtually no fibroblasts. Under these conditions the Schwann cells secrete several ECM components into the culture medium including laminin and collagen types I, III and IV (Bunge *et al.*, 1983; Carey *et al.*, 1983). Secretion of collagen types I and III is consistent with the observation that collagen fibrils can be seen by electron microscopy in the vicinity of Schwann cells in these co-cultures (Bunge *et al.*, 1980). Further evidence that Schwann cells can synthesize ECM material, including collagen types I, III, IV and V, and laminin A and B1 chains comes from experiments on normal cultures of human Schwann cells and Schwann cells derived from cutaneous neurofibromas (Jakkola *et al.*, 1989; Peltonen *et al.*, 1990).

While the ability of Schwann cells to synthesize ECM components is no longer in doubt, much remains to be learned about the regulation of this activity. Regulation of basal lamina synthesis and assembly is a particularly important question in view of the correlation between basal lamina formation and Schwann cell differentiation mentioned earlier. *In vitro* studies have shown that purified Schwann cells do not assemble basal lamina, while basal lamina is formed around axon–Schwann cell units in co-cultures of neurons and Schwann cells. The axonal control of basal lamina formation evident in this type of experiment may in part take place via control of type IV collagen secretion, since the amount of type IV collagen secreted by purified Schwann cells is considerably lower than that secreted in the presence of neurons (Carey *et al.*, 1983). It has now been shown that other factors can substitute for axons to induce Schwann cell basal lamina formation. Basal lamina is formed around Schwann cells in aneural tubes inserted into transected nerves (Ikeda *et al.*, 1989) and by Schwann cells *in vitro* grown in close proximity to fibroblasts (Bunge and Wood, 1989). Expression of basal lamina components by cultured Schwann cells, in particular collagen type IV, is also up-regulated by agents that elevate or mimic intracellular cAMP and by vitamin C (Baron van Evercooren *et al.*, 1986; Eldridge *et al.*, 1987).

There are several circumstances *in vitro* and at least one *in vivo* condition seen in the dystrophic mouse in which failure to myelinate correlates with failure to assemble normal basal lamina. That is to say, whenever a Schwann cell forms a normal myelin sheath it is also covered by basal lamina, and the basal lamina on Schwann cells that associate with axons but fail to ensheath them is either abnormal or absent (for review see Bunge, Bunge and Eldridge, 1986). The notion that the failure to myelinate is caused by the failure to assemble basal lamina is supported by experiments in which addition of exogenous basal lamina-like material induced myelin formation by Schwann cells under conditions in which they were unable to manufacture their own basal lamina (Carey, Todd and Rafferty, 1986).

5.12 INTERACTION OF SCHWANN CELLS WITH CELLS OF THE IMMUNE SYSTEM

In common with several other cell types, both rat and human Schwann cells can be induced to express MHC class II molecules in response to treatment with gamma-interferon (Samuel *et al.*, 1987a,b; Armati, Pollard and Gatenby, 1990). In the rat, Schwann cells in normal nerves are MHC class II negative (Samuel *et al.*, 1987a). Whether human Schwann cells normally express MHC class II molecules in the absence of disease is more controversial. In normal peripheral human nerves it appears that Schwann cells are in general MHC class II negative (Pollard *et al.*, 1986; Scarpini *et al.*, 1990). Positive Schwann cells have, however, been identified by immunohistochemical methods in postmortem or biopsy material from human peripheral ganglia and nerve roots taken from subjects without identified peripheral nerve disease (De Martini *et al.*, 1989; Esiri and Reading, 1989). Several reports indicate that cultured human Schwann cells are MHC class II negative, whereas other groups report that many Schwann cells in cultures from both fetal and adult nerves express MHC class II antigens without prior exposure to gamma-interferon, and that the number of MHC class II positive cells increases with time in culture (Kim *et al.*, 1989; Scarpini *et al.*, 1990). The reason for this discrepancy is at present unclear.

There are several reports of MHC class II expression that appears to be associated with Schwann cells in human peripheral nerves that have been injured or damaged. Since much of this work is done on tissue sections it is difficult to be absolutely sure that the MHC class II expression is actually associated with the Schwann cells and not with other cells, invading or otherwise, found in the endoneurial space (Cadoni, Zicca and Mancardi, 1986; Pollard *et al.*, 1986; Scarpini *et al.*, 1990).

The fact that Schwann cells do become MHC class II positive under certain conditions suggests that they have the potential to become involved as antigen-presenting cells in activation of the immune response, since it is generally assumed that MHC class II positive cells are capable of presenting antigens to activated T lymphocytes. Several studies on cultured rat Schwann cells show that MHC class II positive Schwann cells support proliferation of activated T cells or T cell lines, which is indicative of antigen presentation, and present autoantigens such as MBP and P_2 protein and foreign antigens such as *Mycobacterium leprae* (Wekerle *et al.*, 1986; Kingston *et al.*, 1989; Argall *et al.*, 1992a,b). Exogenously added gamma-interferon is not necessary for the response, since MHC class II antigens are induced when Schwann cells are incubated with activated T cells and antigen alone; this induction is mediated by gamma-interferon and tumour necrosis factor, presumably secreted by the T cells themselves. It has also been shown that some Schwann cells in rat sciatic nerves injected with gamma-interferon or *M. leprae* are MHC class II positive when examined using teased nerve preparations, 1 week after injection (Bergsteinsdóttir, Kingston and Jessen, 1992). More myelin-forming Schwann cells than non-myelin-forming Schwann cells become MHC class II positive in these experiments, suggesting that the two cell types may not have identical responses to antigens or cytokines. Other studies show that guinea pig nerves examined 5 weeks after injection of *M. leprae* contain MHC class II positive cells which, when examined at the electron microscope level, have the characteristics of macrophages, the Schwann cells being negative (Cowley *et al.*, 1989). One interpretation of this observation is that the Schwann cell response is of relatively short duration unless a chronic injury or infection is established. In addition to expression of class II molecules, antigen-presenting cells normally secrete IL-1, which is essential for T cell activation. It has recently been shown that rat Schwann cells in culture produce IL-1 activity in response to bacterial antigens and that this can be demonstrated both in a bioassay and immunohistochemically within the Schwann cells (Bergsteinsdóttir *et al.*, 1991).

Human Schwann cells in peripheral nerves have also been reported to have Fc gamma receptors and receptors for the C3b/C4b complement components. Although both of these receptors were detectable immunohistochemically in nerve fibres at 10 weeks of gestation, functional Fc receptor activity was not detected until just before the onset of myelination (18–19 weeks) and functional C3b/C4b receptor activity was only found after myelination had occurred. In culture both of these receptors disappeared from Schwann cells (Vedeler *et al.*, 1990).

In summary, it appears that Schwann cells not only have many of the properties of antigen-presenting cells, but also possess receptors for immunoglobulins and components of the complement pathway. It therefore seems very likely that under certain conditions, together with professional antigen-presenting cells such as macrophages, they may participate in immune responses in peripheral nerves.

ACKNOWLEDGEMENTS

We would like to thank all the past and present members of our laboratory for their contribution to many of the experiments described here. The work has been supported by grants from the Medical Research Council of Great Britain, Action Research, the Wellcome Trust and the Multiple Sclerosis Society of Great Britain and Northern Ireland.

REFERENCES

Argall, K.G., Armati, P.J., Pollard, J.D. *et al.* (1992a) Interactions between $CD4^+$ T-cells and rat Schwann cells *in vitro*. 1. Antigen presentation by Lewis rat Schwann cells to P_2-specific $CD4^+$ T-cell lines. *J. Neuroimmunol.*, **40**, 1–18.

Argall, K.G., Armati, P.J., Pollard, J.D. and Bonner, J. (1992b) Interactions between $CD4^+$ T-cells and rat Schwann cells *in vitro*. 2. Cytotoxic effects of P_2-specific $CD4^+$ T-cell lines on Lewis rat Schwann cells. *J. Neuroimmunol.*, **40**, 19–30.

Armati, P.J., Pollard, J.D. and Gatenby, P. (1990) Rat and human Schwann cells *in vitro* can synthesize and express MHC molecules. *Muscle Nerve*, **13**, 106–16.

Askanas, V., Engel, W.K., Dalakas, M.C. *et al.* (1980) Human Schwann cells in tissue culture: histochemical and ultrastructural studies. *Arch. Neurol.*, **37**, 329–37.

Assouline, J.G. and Pantazis, N.J. (1989) Localisation of the nerve growth factor receptor on fetal human Schwann cells in culture. *Exp. Cell Res.*, **182**, 499–512.

Baichwal, R.R., Bigbee, J.W. and DeVries, G.H. (1988) Macrophage-mediated myelin-related mitogenic factor for cultured Schwann cells. *Proc. Natl. Acad. Sci. USA*, **85**, 1701–5.

Ballester, R., Marchuk, D., Boguski, M. *et al.* (1990) The *NF1* locus encodes a protein functionally related to mammalian GAP and yeast *IRA* proteins. *Cell*, **63**, 85–9.

Bannerman, P.G.C., Mirsky, R.M., Jessen, K.R. *et al.* (1986) Light microscopic immunolocalization of laminin, type IV collagen, nidogen, heparan sulphate proteoglycan and fibronectin in the enteric nervous system. *J. Neurocytol.*, **15**, 733–43.

Bargmann, C.I. and Weinberg, R.A. (1988) Oncogenic activation of the *neu*-encoded receptor protein by point mutation and deletion. *EMBO J.*, **7**, 2043–52.

Baron van Evercooren, A., Gansmüller, A., Gumpel, M. *et al.* (1986) Schwann cell differentiation *in vitro*: Extracellular matrix deposition and interaction. *Dev. Neurosci.*, **8**, 182–96.

Baron van Evercooren, A., Leprince, P., Rogister, B. *et al.* (1987) Plasminogen activators in developing peripheral nervous system, cellular origin and mitogenic effect. *Brain Res.*, **433**, 101–8.

Barres, B.A., Chun, L.L.Y. and Corey, D.P. (1990) Ion channels in vertebrate glia. *Ann. Rev. Neurosci.*, **13**, 441–74.

Basu, T.N., Gutmann, D.H., Fletcher, J.A. *et al.* (1992) Aberrant regulation of *ras* proteins in malignant tumour cells from type 1 neurofibromatosis patients. *Nature*, **356**, 713–15.

Bergsteinsdóttir, K., Kingston, A., Mirsky, R. and Jessen, K.R. (1991) Rat Schwann cells produce interleukin-1. *J. Neuroimmunol.*, **34**, 15–23.

Bergsteinsdóttir, K., Kingston, A. and Jessen, K.R. (1992) Rat Schwann cells can be induced to express major histocompatibility complex class II molecules *in vivo*. *J. Neurocytol.*, **21**, 382–90.

Bevan, S. (1990) Ion channels and neurotransmitter receptors in glia. *Semin. Neurosci.*, **2**, 467–81.

Beuche, W. and Friede, R.L. (1985) A quantitative assessment of myelin sheaths in the peripheral nerves of dystrophic, quaking and trembler mutants. *Acta Neuropathol. (Berl)*, **66**, 275–303.

Bray, G.M., Rasminsky, M. and Aguayo, A. (1981) Interactions between axons and their sheath cells. *Ann. Rev. Neurosci.*, **4**, 127–62.

Brockes, J.P., Fields, K.L. and Raff, M.C. (1979) Studies on cultured rat Schwann cells. I. Establishment of purified populations from cultures of peripheral nerve. *Brain Res.*, **165**, 105–18.

Brockes, J.P., Lemke, G.E. and Balzer, D.R. (1980) Purification and preliminary characterization of glial growth factor from bovine pituitary. *J. Biol. Chem.*, **255**, 8374–7.

Brockes, J.P., Raff, M.C., Nishiguchi, D.J. and Winter, J. (1980) Studies on cultured rat Schwann cells, III. Assays for peripheral myelin proteins. *J. Neurocytol.*, **9**, 67–77.

Brockes, J.P., Breakfield, X.O. and Martuza, R.L. (1986) Glial growth factor-like activity in Schwann cell tumors. *Ann. Neurol.*, **20**, 317–22.

Brunden, K.R. and Poduslo, J.F. (1987) Lysosomal delivery of the major myelin glycoprotein in the absence of myelin assembly: posttranslational regulation of the level of expression of P_0 by Schwann cells. *J. Cell Biol.*, **104**, 661–9.

Brunden, K.R., Windebank, A.J. and Poduslo, J.F. (1990) Role of axons in the regulation of P_0 biosynthesis by Schwann cells. *J. Neurosci. Res.*, **26**, 135–43.

Bunge, M.B. and Wood, P.M. (1989) Basal lamina deposition on Schwann cells cultured with fibroblasts in the absence of neurons. *Soc. Neurosci. Abst.*, **15**, 689.

Bunge, R.P. and Hopkins, J.M. (1990) The role of peripheral and central glia in neural regeneration in vertebrates. *Semin. Neurosci.*, **2**, 509–18.

Bunge, M.B., Williams, A.K., Wood, P.M. *et al.* (1980) Comparison of nerve cell and nerve cell plus Schwann cell cultures with particular emphasis on basal lamina and collagen formation. *J. Cell Biol.*, **84**, 184–202.

Bunge, M.B., Bunge, R.P., Carey, D.J. *et al.* (1983) Axonal and non-axonal influences on Schwann cell development, in *Developing and Regenerating Vertebrate Nervous Systems* (eds P.W. Coates, R.R. Markwald and A.D. Kenny), Liss, New York, pp. 71–105.

Bunge, R.P., Bunge, M.B. and Eldridge, C.F. (1986) Linkage between axonal ensheathment and basal lamina production by Schwann cells. *Ann. Rev. Neurosci.*, **9**, 305–28.

Bunge, R.P., Bunge, M.B. and Bates, M. (1989) Movements of the Schwann cell nucleus implicate progression of the inner (axon-related) Schwann cell process during myelination, *J. Cell Biol.*, **109**, 273–84.

Cadoni, A., Zicca, A. and Mancardi, G.L. (1986) Schwann cell expression of HLA-DR antigen in peripheral neuropathies. *Lancet*, **8518**, 1282–3.

Campagnoni, A.T. (1988) Molecular biology of myelin proteins from the nervous system. *J. Neurochem.*, **51**, 1–14.

Carey, D.J., Eldridge, C.F., Cornbrooks, C.J. *et al.* (1983) Biosynthesis of type IV collagen by cultured rat Schwann cells. *J. Cell Biol.*, **97**, 473–9.

Carey, D.J., Todd, M.S. and Rafferty, C.M. (1986) Schwann cell myelination: induction by exogenous basement membrane-like extracellular matrix. *J. Cell Biol.*, **102**, 2254–63.

Chandler, C.E., Parsons, L.M., Hosang, M. and Shooter, E.M. (1984) A monoclonal antibody modulates the interaction of nerve growth factor with PC12 cells. *J. Biol. Chem.*, **259**, 6882–9.

Chiu, S.Y. (1987) Sodium currents in axon associated Schwann cells from adult rabbits. *J. Physiol.*, **386**, 181–203.

Chiu, S.Y. (1988) Changes in excitable properties in Schwann cells of adult rabbit sciatic nerves following nerve transection. *J. Physiol.*, **396**, 173–88.

Chiu, S.Y. (1991) Functions and distribution of voltage-gated sodium and potassium channels in mammalian Schwann cells. *Glia*, **4**, 541–58.

Chiu, S.Y. and Wilson, G.F. (1989) The role of potassium channels in Schwann cell proliferation in Wallerian degeneration of explant rabbit sciatic nerves. *J. Physiol.*, **408**, 199–222.

Chiu, S.Y., Shrager, P. and Ritchie, J.M. (1984) Neuronal type sodium and potassium channels in rabbit cultured Schwann cells. *Nature*, **311**, 156–7.

Clemence, A., Mirsky, R. and Jessen, K.R. (1989) Non-myelin-forming Schwann cells proliferate rapidly during Wallerian degeneration in the rat sciatic nerve. *J. Neurocytol.*, **18**, 185–92.

Cohen, J.A., Yachnis, A.T., Arai, M. *et al.* (1992) Expression of the *neu* proto-oncogene by Schwann cells during peripheral nerve development and Wallerian degeneration. *J. Neurosci. Res.*, **31**, 622–34.

Colman, D.R., Kreibich, G., Frey, A.B. and Sabatini, D.D. (1982) Synthesis and incorporation of myelin polypeptides into CNS myelin. *J. Cell Biol.*, **95**, 598–608.

Cornbrooks, C.J., Carey, D.J., McDonald, J.A. *et al.* (1983) *In vivo* and *in vitro* observations on laminin production by Schwann cells. *Proc. Natl. Acad. Sci. USA*, **80**, 3850–4.

Cowley, S.A., Butter, C., Gschmeissner, S.E. *et al.* (1989) An immunoelectronmicroscopical study of the expression of major histocompatibility complex (MHC) class II antigens in guinea pig sciatic nerves following induction of intraneural myobacterial granulomas. *J. Neuroimmunol.*, **23**, 223–31.

Dahm, L.M. and Landmesser, L. (1988) The regulation of intramuscular nerve branching during normal development and following activity blockade. *Dev. Biol.*, **130**, 621–44.

Daston, M.M., Scable, H., Nordlund, M. *et al.* (1992) The protein product of the neurofibromatosis type 1 gene is expressed at highest abundance in neurons, Schwann cells, and oligodendrocytes. *Neuron*, **8**, 415–28.

Davis, J.B. and Stroobant, P. (1990) Platelet-derived growth factors and fibroblast growth factors are mitogens for rat Schwann cells. *J. Cell. Biol.*, **110**, 1353–60.

DeClue, J.E., Papageorge, A.G., Fletcher, J.A. *et al.* (1992) Abnormal regulation of mammalian $p21^{ras}$ contributes to malignant tumor growth in von Recklinghausen (type 1) neurofibromatosis. *Cell*, **69**, 265–73.

De Martini, I., Bianchini, D., Schenone, A. *et al.* (1989) Class II antigen expression on human cultured Schwann cells from patients with Charcot-Marie-Tooth disease. *Neurosci. Lett.*, **100**, 331–4.

Dieperink, M.E., O'Neill, A., Magnoni, G. *et al.* (1992) SAG: a Schwann cell membrane glycoprotein. *J. Neurosci.*, **12**, 2177–85.

Diner, O. (1965) Les cellules de Schwann en mitose et leurs rapports avec les axones au cours du developpement du nerf sciatique chez le rat. *C.R. Acad. Sci.*, **261**, 1731–4.

DiStefano, D.S. and Johnson, E.M. (1988) Nerve growth factor receptors on cultured rat Schwann cells. *J. Neurosci.*, **8**, 231–41.

Dumont, J.E., Jauniaux, J.-C. and Roger, J.P. (1989) The cyclic AMP mediated stimulation of cell proliferation. *TIBS*, **14**, 67–71.

D'Urso, D., Brophy, P.J., Staugaitis, S.M. *et al.* (1990) Protein zero of peripheral nerve myelin: biosynthesis, membrane insertion, and evidence for homotypic interaction. *Neuron*, **4**, 449–60.

Eccleston, P.A. (1992) Regulation of Schwann cell proliferation: mechanisms involved in peripheral nerve development. *Exp. Cell. Res.*, **199**, 1–9.

Eccleston, P.A., Jessen, K.R. and Mirsky, R. (1987) Control of peripheral glial cell proliferation: a comparison of the division rates of enteric glial and Schwann cells and their response to mitogens. *Dev. Biol.*, **124**, 409–17.

Eccleston, P.A., Mirsky, R., Jessen, K.R. *et al.* (1987) Postnatal development of rat peripheral nerves: an immunohistochemical study of membrane lipids common to non-myelin forming Schwann cells, myelin forming Schwann cells and oligodendrocytes. *Dev. Brain Res.*, **35**, 249–56.

Eccleston, P.A., Bannerman, P.G.C., Pleasure, D.E. *et al.* (1989a) Control of peripheral glial cell proliferation: enteric neurons exert an inhibitory influence. *Development*, **107**, 107–12.

Eccleston, P.A., Jessen, K.R. and Mirsky, R. (1989b) Transforming growth factor-β and gamma-interferon have dual effects on growth of peripheral glia. *J. Neurosci. Res.*, **24**, 530–42.

Eccleston, P.A., Mirsky, R. and Jessen, K.R. (1989c) Type I collagen preparations inhibit DNA synthesis in glial cells of the peripheral nervous system. *Exptl. Cell Res.*, **182**, 173–85.

Eccleston, P.A., Collarini, E.J., Mirsky, R. *et al.* (1990) Schwann cells secrete a PDGF-like factor: evidence for an autocrine growth mechanism. *Eur. J. Neurosci.*, **2**, 985–92.

Eccleston, P.A., Jessen, K.R. and Mirsky, R. (1991) Spontaneous Schwann cell immortalization *in vitro*: short-term cultured Schwann cells secrete inhibitory activity. *Development*, **112**, 33–42.

Eldridge, C.F., Bunge, M.B., Bunge, R.P. and Wood, P.M. (1987) Differentiation of axon-related Schwann cells *in vitro*. I. Ascorbic acid regulates basal lamina assembly and myelin formation. *J. Cell Biol.*, **105**, 1023–34.

Eldridge, C.F., Bunge, M.B. and Bunge, R.P. (1989) Differentiation of axon-related Schwann cells *in vitro*: II. Control of myelin formation by basal lamina. *J. Neurosci.*, **9**, 625–38.

Esiri, M.M. and Reading, M.C. (1989) Macrophages, lymphocytes and major histocompatibility complex (HLA) class II antigens in adult human sensory and sympathetic ganglia. *J. Neuroimmunol.*, **28**, 187–93.

Ferrari, G., Fabris, M., Polato, P. *et al.* (1991) Rat NGF receptor is recognised by the tumour-associated monoclonal antibody 217c. *Exp. Neurol.*, **112**, 183–94.

Fields, K.L. and Dammerman, M. (1985) A monoclonal antibody equivalent to anti-rat neural antigen-1 as a marker for Schwann cells. *Neuroscience*, **15**, 877–86.

Fields, K.L. and Yen, S. (1985) A subset of Schwann cells in peripheral nerves contain a 50-kDa protein antigenically related to astrocyte intermediate filaments. *J. Neuroimmunol.*, **8**, 311–30.

Filbin, M.T., Walsh, F.J., Trapp, B.D. *et al.* (1990) The role of myelin P_0 protein as a homophilic adhesion molecule. *Nature*, **344**, 871–2.

Friede, R.L. (1972) Control of myelin formation by axon caliber (with a model of the control mechanism). *J. Comp. Neurol.*, **144**, 233–52.

Friede, R.L. and Samorajski, T. (1968) Myelin formation in the sciatic nerve of the rat. *J. Neuropathol. Exp. Neurol.*, **27**, 546–70.

Gamble, H.J. (1966) Further electron microscope studies of human foetal peripheral nerves. *J. Anat.*, **100**, 487–502.

Gamble, H.J. and Breathnach, A.S. (1965) An electron microscope study of human foetal peripheral nerves. *J. Anat.*, **99**, 573–84.

Giese, K.P., Martini, R., Lemke, G. *et al.* (1992) Mouse P_0 gene disruption leads to hypomyelination, abnormal expression of recognition molecules, and degeneration of myelin and axons. *Cell*, **71**, 565–76.

Gould, R.M., Mirsky, R., Jessen, K.R. and Tennekoon, G.I. (1991) The cell of Schwann, in *Myelin: Biology and Chemistry* (ed. R. Martenson), CRC Press, Boca Raton.

Griffin, J.W., Rosenfeld, J., Hoffman, P.N. *et al.* (1988) The axonal cytoskeleton: influences on nerve fibre form and Schwann cell behavior, in *Intrinsic Determinants of Neuronal Form and Function* (eds R.J. Lasek and M.M. Black), Alan R. Liss, New York, pp. 403–39.

Griffiths, I.R., Mitchell, L.S., McPhilemy, K. *et al.* (1989) Expression of myelin protein genes in Schwann cells. *J. Neurocytol.*, **18**, 345–52.

Gupta, S.K., Poduslo, J.F. and Mezet, C. (1988) Temporal changes in P_0 and MBP gene expression after crush-injury of the adult peripheral nerve. *Brain Res.*, **464**, 133–41.

Hahn, A.F., Whitaker, J.N., Kachar, B. and Webster, H. de F. (1987) P_2, P_1 and P_0 myelin expression in developing rat sixth nerve: a quantitative immunocytochemical study. *J. Comp. Neurol.*, **260**, 501–12.

He, X., Gerrero, R., Simmons, D.M. *et al.* (1991) Tst-1, a member of the POU domain gene family, binds the promoter of the gene encoding the cell surface adhesion molecule P_0. *Mol. Cell. Biol.*, **11**, 1739–44.

Heumann, R., Korsching, S., Bandtlow, C. and Thoenen, H. (1987a) Changes in nerve growth factor synthesis in non-neuronal cells in response to sciatic nerve transection. *J. Cell Biol.*, **104**, 1623–31.

Heumann, R., Lindholm, D., Bandtlow, C. *et al.* (1987b) Differential regulation of mRNA encoding nerve growth factor and its receptor in macrophages. *Proc. Natl. Acad. Sci. USA*, **84**, 8735–9.

Holton, B. and Weston, J.A. (1982a) Analysis of glial cell differentiation in peripheral nervous tissue I. S100. Accumulation in quail embryo spinal ganglion cultures. *Dev. Biol.*, **89**, 64–71.

Holton, B. and Weston, J.A. (1982b) Analysis of glial cell differentiation in peripheral nervous tissue II. Neurons promote S100 synthesis by purified glial precursor cell populations. *Dev. Biol.*, **89**, 72–81.

Hoppe, D., Kettenmann, H. and Verkhratsky, A.N. (1990) Single potassium channel properties in mouse cultured Schwann cells. *Pflugers Arch.*, **415**, R17.

Howe, J.R. and Ritchie, J.M. (1988) Two types of potassium channels in rabbit cultured Schwann cell. *Proc. R. Soc. Lond. B*, **235**, 19–27.

Howe, J.R. and Ritchie, J.M. (1990) Sodium currents in Schwann cells from myelinated and non-myelinated nerves of neonatal and adult rabbits. *J. Physiol.*, **425**, 169–210.

Hudson, L.D. (1990) The molecular biology of myelin proteins. *Semin. Neurosci.*, **2**, 483–96.

Ikeda, K., Oda, Y., Tomita, K. *et al.* (1989) Isolated Schwann cells can synthesize basement membrane *in vivo*. *J. Elect. Microsc.*, **38**, 230–4.

Jaakkola, S., Peltonen, J., Riccardi, V. *et al.* (1989) Type I neurofibromatosis: selective expression of extracellular matrix genes by Schwann cells, perineurial cells and fibroblasts in mixed cultures. *J. Clin. Invest.*, **84**, 253–61.

James, S., Hassall, C.J.S., Polak, J.M. and Burnstock, G. (1990) Visualisation of specific binding sites for atrial naturetic peptide on neuronal cells of cultured rat sympathetic ganglia. *Cell Tiss. Res.*, **259**, 129–37.

Jessen, K.R. and Mirsky, R. (1984) Non-myelin-forming Schwann cells coexpress surface proteins and intermediate filaments not found in myelin forming cells: a study of Ran-2, A5E3 antigen and glial fibrillary acidic protein. *J. Neurocytol.*, **13**, 923–34.

Jessen, K.R. and Mirsky, R. (1991) Schwann cell precursors and their development. *Glia*, **4**, 9–18.

Jessen, K.R. and Mirsky, R. (1992) Schwann cells: early lineage, regulation of proliferation and control of myelin formation. *Curr. Opin. Neurobiol.*, **2**, 575–81.

Jessen, K.R., Thorpe, R. and Mirsky, R. (1984) Molecular identity, distribution and heterogeneity of glial fibrillary acidic protein: an immunoblotting and immunohistochemical study of Schwann cells, satellite cells, enteric glia and astrocytes. *J. Neurocytol.*, **13**, 187–200.

Jessen, K.R., Morgan, L., Brammer, M. and Mirsky, R. (1985) Galactocerebroside is expressed by non-myelin-forming Schwann cells *in situ*, *J. Cell Biol.*, **101**, 1135–43.

Jessen, K.R., Mirsky, R. and Morgan, L. (1987) Myelinated, but not unmyelinated axons reversibly down-regulate N-CAM in Schwann cells. *J. Neurocytol.*, **16**, 689–700.

Jessen, K.R., Morgan, L. and Mirsky, R. (1987) Axonal signals regulate the differentiation of non-myelin-forming Schwann cells: an immunohistochemical study of galactocerebroside in transected and regenerating nerves. *J. Neurosci.*, **7**, 3362–9.

Jessen, K.R., Morgan, L., Stewart, H.J.S. and Mirsky, R. (1990) Three markers of adult non-myelin-forming Schwann cells, 217c(Ran-1), A5E3 and GFAP: development and regulation by neuron–Schwann cell interactions. *Development*, **109**, 91–103.

Johnson, E.M., Jr, Taniuchi, M. and DiStefano, P.S. (1988) Expression and possible function of nerve growth factor receptors on Schwann cells. *Trends Neurosci.*, **11**, 299–304.

Kennedy, P.G., Lisak, R.P. and Raff, M.C. (1980) Cell type-specific markers for human glial and neuronal cells in culture. *Lab. Invest.*, **43**, 342–51.

Kidd, G.J. and Heath, J.W. (1989a) Double myelination of axons in the sympathetic nervous system of the mouse. I. Ultrastructural features and distribution. *J. Neurocytol.*, **17**, 245–61.

Kidd, G.J. and Heath, J.W. (1989b) Double myelination of axons in the sympathetic nervous system of the mouse. II. Mechanisms of formation. *J. Neurocytol.*, **17**, 263–76.

Kim, S.U., Yong, V.W., Watabe, K. and Shin, D.H. (1989) Human fetal Schwann cells in culture. *J. Neurosci. Res.*, **22**, 50–9.

Kimura, H., Fischer, W.H. and Schubert, D. (1990) Structure, expression and function of a Schwannoma-derived growth factor. *Nature*, **348**, 257–60.

Kingston, A., Bergsteinsdóttir, K., Jessen, K.R. *et al.* (1989) Schwann cells co-cultured with stimulated T cells and antigen express major histocompatibility complex (MHC) class II determinants without interferon-gamma pretreatment: synergistic effects of interferon-gamma and tumor necrosis factor on MHC class II induction. *Eur. J. Immunol.*, **19**, 177–83.

Klingman, D. and Hilt, D.C. (1988) The S100 protein family. *Trends Biochem. Sci.*, **13**, 437–43.

Konishi, T. (1989) Voltage-dependent potassium channels in cultured mammalian Schwann cells. *Brain Res.*, **499**, 273–80.

Küecherer-Ehret, A., Graeber, M.B., Edgar, D. *et al.* (1990) Immunoelectron microscopic localization of laminin in normal and regenerating mouse sciatic nerve. *J. Neurocytol.*, **19**, 111–26.

Kuhlengel, K.R., Bunge, M.B. and Bunge, R.P. (1990) Implantation of cultured sensory neurons and Schwann cells into lesioned neonatal rat spinal cord. I. Methods for preparing implants from dissociated cells. *J. Comp. Neurol.*, **293**, 63–73.

Lai, C., Brow, M.A., Nave, K.-A. *et al.* (1987) Two forms of IB236/myelin-associated glycoprotein, a cell-adhesion molecule for postnatal neural development are produced by alternative splicing. *Proc. Natl. Acad. Sci. USA*, **84**, 4337–42.

Langford, L.A., Porter, S. and Bunge, R.P. (1988) Immortalized rat Schwann cells produce tumors *in vivo*. *J. Neurocytol.*, **17**, 521–9.

Leivo, I. and Engvall, E. (1988) Merosin, a protein specific for basement membranes of Schwann cells, striated muscle, and trophoblast, is expressed late in nerve and muscle development. *Proc. Natl. Acad. Sci. USA*, **85**, 1544–8.

Leivo, I., Laurila, P., Wahlstrom, T. and Engvall, E. (1989a) Expression of merosin, a tissue specific basement membrane protein, in the intermediate trophoblast cells of choriocarcinoma and placenta. *Lab. Invest.*, **60**, 783–90.

Leivo, I., Engvall, E., Laurila, P. and Miettinen, M. (1989b) Distribution of merosin, a laminin-related tissue-specific basement membrane protein, in human Schwann cell neoplasms. *Lab. Invest.*, **61**, 426–32.

Lemke, G. (1988) Unwrapping the genes of myelin. *Neuron*, **1**, 533–43.

Lemke, G. (1990) Glial growth factors. *Semin. Neurosci.*, **2**, 437–43.

Lemke, G. and Axel, R. (1985) Isolation and sequence of a major cDNA encoding the major structural protein of peripheral nerve. *Cell*, **40**, 501–8.

Lemke, G. and Chao, M. (1988) Axons regulate Schwann cell expression of the major myelin and NGF receptor genes. *Development*, **102**, 499–504.

Lemke, G., Lamar, E. and Patterson, J. (1988) Isolation and analysis of the gene encoding peripheral myelin protein zero. *Neuron*, **1**, 1–11.

Lindholm, D., Heumann, R., Meyer, M. and Thoenen, H. (1987) Interleukin -1 regulates synthesis of nerve growth factor in non-neuronal cells of rat sciatic nerve. *Nature*, **330**, 658–9.

Ljungdahl, A., Olsen, T., Van der Meide, P.H. and Höjeberg, B. (1989) Interferon-gamma-like activity in certain neurons of the central and peripheral nervous system. *J. Neurosci. Res.*, **245**, 451–6.

Lunn, E.R., Perry, V.H., Brown, M.C. *et al.* (1989) Absence of Wallerian degeneration does not hinder regeneration in peripheral nerve. *Eur. J. Neurosci.*, **1**, 27–33.

Martin, G.A., Viskochil, D., Bollag, G. *et al.* (1990) The GAP-related domain of the neurofibromatosis type 1 gene product interacts with *ras* p21. *Cell*, **63**, 843–9.

Martini, R. and Schachner, M. (1986) Immunoelectronmicroscopic localization of neural cell adhesion molecules (L1, N-CAM and MAG) and their shared carbohydrate epitope and myelin basic protein in developing sciatic nerve. *J. Cell Biol.*, **103**, 2439–48.

Martini, R. and Schachner, M. (1988) Immunoelectronmicroscopic localisation of neural cell adhesion molecules (L1, N-CAM and myelin-associated glycoprotein) in regenerating adult mouse sciatic nerve. *J. Cell Biol.*, **106**, 1735–46.

Martini, R., Bollensen, E. and Schachner, M. (1988) Immunocytological localization of the major peripheral nervous system glycoprotein P_0 and the L2/HNK-1 and L3 carbohydrate structures in developing and adult mouse sciatic nerve. *Dev. Biol.*, **129**, 330–8.

Mata, M., Alessi, D. and Fink, D.J. (1990) S100 is preferentially distributed in myelin-forming Schwann cells. *J. Neurocytol.*, **19**, 432–42.

Meador-Woodruff, J.H., Lewis, B.L. and DeVries, G.H. (1984) Cyclic AMP and calcium as potential mediators of stimulation of cultured Schwann cell proliferation by axolemma-enriched and myelin-enriched membrane fractions. *Biochem. Biophys. Res. Commun.*, **122**, 373–80.

Meador-Woodruff, J.H., Yoshino, J.E., Bigbee, J.W. *et al.* (1985) Differential proliferation responses of cultured Schwann cells to axolemma and myelin-enriched fractions. II. Morphological studies. *J. Neurocytol.*, **14**, 619–35.

Mirsky, R. and Jessen, K.R. (1990) Schwann cell development and the regulation of myelination. *Semin. Neurosci.*, **2**, 423–36.

Mirsky, R., Winter, J., Abney, E.R. *et al.* (1980) Myelin-specific proteins and glycolipids in rat Schwann cells and oligodendrocytes in culture. *J. Cell Biol.*, **84**, 483–94.

Mirsky, R., Jessen, K.R., Schachner, M. and Goridis, C. (1986) Distribution of the adhesion molecules N-CAM and L1 on peripheral neurons and glia in adult rats. *J. Neurocytol.*, **15**, 799–815.

Mirsky, R., Dubois, C., Morgan, L. and Jessen, K.R. (1990) Prenatal Schwann cell development: appearance of 04 differentiation antigen in rat embryo sciatic nerve and its regulation by axon–Schwann cell signals. *Development*, **109**, 105–16.

Mokuno, K., Sobue, G., Reddy, V.R. *et al.* (1988) Regulation of Schwann cell nerve growth factor receptor by cyclic adenosine 3′,5′-mono-phosphate, *J. Neurosci. Res.*, **21**, 465–72.

Mokuno, K., Kamholz, J., Behrman, T. *et al.* (1989) Neuronal modulation of Schwann cell glial fibrillary acidic protein (GFAP). *J. Neurosci. Res.*, **23**, 396–405.

Monuki, E.S., Weinmaster, G., Kuhn, R. and Lemke, G. (1989) SCIP: a glial POU domain gene regulated by cyclic AMP. *Neuron*, **3**, 783–93.

Monuki, E.S., Kuhn, R., Weinmaster, G. *et al.* (1990) Expression and activity of the POU transcription factor SCIP. *Science*, **249**, 1300–3.

Morgan, L., Jessen, K.R. and Mirsky, R. (1991) The effects of cyclic AMP on differentiation of cultured Schwann cells: progression from an early phenotype (04^+) to a myelin phenotype (P_0^+, $GFAP^-$, $N\text{-}CAM^+$, NGF-receptor$^-$) depends on growth inhibition. *J. Cell Biol.*, **112**, 457–67.

Morrissey, T.K., Kleitman, N. and Bunge, R.P. (1991) Isolation and functional characterization of Schwann cells derived from adult peripheral nerve. *J. Neurosci.*, **11**, 2433–42.

Muir, D. and Manthorpe, M. (1992) Stromelysin generates a fibronectin fragment that inhibits Schwann cell proliferation. *J. Cell Biol.*, **116**, 177–85.

Muir, D., Varon, S. and Manthorpe, M. (1990) Schwann cell proliferation *in vitro* is under negative autocrine control. *J. Cell Biol.*, **111**, 2663–71.

Narayanan, V., Barbosa, E., Reed, R. and Tennekon, G. (1988) Characterization of a cloned cDNA encoding rabbit myelin P2. *J. Biol. Chem.*, **263**, 8332–7.

Neuberger, T.J. and Cornbrooks, C.J. (1989) Transient modulation of Schwann cell antigens after peripheral nerve transection and subsequent regeneration. *J. Neurocytol.*, **18**, 695–710.

Nieke, J. and Schachner, M. (1985) Expression of the neural cell adhesion molecules L1 and N-CAM and their common carbohydrate epitope L2-HNK-1 during development and after transection of adult mouse sciatic nerve. *Differentiation*, **30**, 141–51.

Nikitin, A.Y., Ballering. L.A.P., Lyons, J. and Rajewsky, M.F. (1991) Early mutation of the *neu* (erbB-2) gene during ethylnitrosourea-induced oncogenesis in the rat Schwann cell lineage. *Proc. Natl. Acad. Sci. USA*, **88**, 9939–43.

Omlin, F.X., Webster, H. de F., Palkovits, C.G. and Cohen, S.R. (1982) Immunocytochemical localization of basic protein in major dense line regions of central and peripheral myelin. *J. Cell Biol.*, **95**, 242–8.

Ono, K., Friedrich, V., Hudson, L. *et al.* (1990) The unexpected expression of the major CNS protein, proteolipid protein, in Schwann cells *in vivo* and *in vitro*. *Neurol. Neurobiol.*, **53**, 201–8.

Owens, G.C. and Boyd, C.J. (1991) Expressing antisense P_0 mRNA in Schwann cells perturbs myelination. *Development*, **112**, 639–49.

Owens, G.C. and Bunge, R.P. (1989) Evidence for an early role for myelin associated glycoprotein in the process of myelination. *Glia*, **2**, 119–28.

Owens, G.C. and Bunge, R.P. (1991) Schwann cells infected with a recombinant retrovirus expressing myelin-associated glycoprotein antisense RNA do not form myelin. *Neuron*, **7**, 565–75.

Owens, G.C., Boyd, C.J., Bunge, R.P. and Salzer, J.L. (1990) Expression of recombinant myelin-associated glycoprotein in primary Schwann cells promotes the initial investment of axons by myelinating Schwann cells. *J. Cell. Biol.*, **111**, 1171–80.

Palm, S.L. and Furcht, L.T. (1983) Production of laminin and fibronectin by Schwannoma cells: cell protein interactions *in vitro* and protein localisation in peripheral nerve *in vivo*. *J. Cell Biol.*, **96**, 1218–26.

Peles, E., Bacus, S.S., Koski, R.A. *et al.* (1992) Isolation of the *neu*/HER-2 stimulatory ligand: a 44kd glycoprotein that induces differentiation of mammary tumor cells. *Cell*, **69**, 205–16.

Pellegrino, R.G., Politis, M.J., Ritchie, J.M. and Spencer, P.S. (1986) Events in degenerating rat peripheral nerve: induction of Schwann cell S phase and its relation to nerve fiber degeneration. *J. Neurocytol.*, **15**, 17–28.

Peltonen, J., Jaakkola, S., Hsiao, L.L. *et al.* (1990) Type IV collagen. *In situ* hybridizations and immunohistochemistry reveal abundant mRNA and protein levels in human neurofibroma, Schwannoma and normal peripheral nerve tissues. *Lab. Invest.*, **62**, 487–92.

Perantoni, A.O., Rice, J.M., Reed, C.D. *et al.* (1987) Activated *neu* oncogene sequences in primary tumours of the peripheral nervous system induced in rats by transplacental exposure to ethylnitrosourea. *Proc. Natl. Acad. Sci. USA.*, **84**, 6317–21.

Perry, V.H., Brown, M.C. and Gordon, S. (1987) The macrophage response to central and peripheral nerve injury. *J. Exp. Med.*, **165**, 1218–23.

Peters, A. and Muir, A.R. (1959) The relationship between axons and Schwann cells during development of peripheral nerves in the rat. *Q.J. Exp. Physiol.*, **44**, 117–30.

Pleasure, D., Kreider, B., Shuman, S. and Sobue, G. (1985) Tissue culture studies of Schwann cell proliferation and differentiation. *Dev. Neurosci.*, **7**, 364–73.

Pleasure, D., Kreider, B., Sobue, G. *et al.* (1986) Schwann-like cells cultured from human dermal neurofibromas. Immunohistological identification and response to Schwann cell mitogens. *Ann. N.Y. Acad. Sci.*, **486**, 227–40.

Pollard, J.D., McCombe, P.A., Baverstock, J. *et al.* (1986) Class II antigen expression and T lymphocyte subsets in chronic inflammatory demyelinating neuropathy. *J. Neuroimmunol.*, **13**, 123–34.

Porter, S., Clark, M.B., Glaser, L. and Bunge, R.P. (1986) Schwann cells stimulated to proliferate in the absence of neurons retain full functional capacity. *J. Neurosci.*, **6**, 3070-8.

Porter, S., Glaser, L. and Bunge, R.P. (1987) Release of autocrine growth factor by primary and immortalized Schwann cells. *Proc. Natl. Acad. Sci. USA*, **84**, 7768–72.

Puckett, C., Hudson, L., Ono, K. *et al.* (1987) Myelin-specific proteolipid protein is expressed in myelinating Schwann cells but is not incorporated into myelin sheaths. *J. Neurosci. Res.*, **18**, 511–18.

Quarles, R.H. (1984) Myelin-associated glycoprotein in development and disease. *Dev. Neurosci.*, **6**, 285–303.

Raff, M.C., Abney, E., Brockes, J.P. and Hornby-Smith, A. (1978a) Schwann cell growth factors. *Cell*, **15**, 813–22.

Raff, M.C., Hornby-Smith, A. and Brockes, J.P. (1978b) Cyclic AMP as a mitogenic signal for cultured rat Schwann cells. *Nature*, **273**, 672–3.

Ranscht, B., Clapshaw, P.A., Price, J. *et al.* (1982) Development of oligodendrocytes and Schwann cells studied with a monoclonal antibody against galactocerebroside. *Proc. Natl. Acad. Sci. USA*, **79**, 2709–13.

Ratner, N., Bunge, R.P. and Glaser, L. (1985) A neuronal heparan sulfate proteoglycan is required for dorsal root ganglion neuron stimulation of Schwann cell proliferation. *J. Cell. Biol.*, **101**, 744–54.

Ratner, N., Hong, D., Lieberman, M.A. *et al.* (1988) The neuronal cell-surface molecule mitogenic for Schwann cells is a heparin binding protein. *Proc. Natl. Acad. Sci. USA*, **85**, 6992–6.

Readhead, C., Popko, B., Takahashi, N. *et al.* (1987) Expression of a myelin basic protein gene in transgenic shiverer mice: correction of the dismyelinating phenotype. *Cell*, **48**, 703–12.

Ridley, A.J., Paterson, H.F., Noble, M. and Land, H. (1988) *Ras*-mediated cell cycle arrest is altered by nuclear oncogenes to induce Schwann cell transformation. *EMBO J.*, **7**, 1635–45.

Ridley, A.J., Davis, J.B., Stroobant, P. and Land, H. (1989) Transforming growth factors – β1 and β2 are mitogens for rat Schwann cells. *J. Cell Biol.*, **109**, 3419–24.

Rieger, F., Daniloff, J.K., Pincon-Raymond, M. *et al.* (1985) Neuronal cell adhesion molecules and cytotactin and co-localized at the node of Ranvier. *J. Cell. Biol.*, **103**, 379–91.

Rutkowski, J.L., Tennekoon, G.I. and McGillicuddy, J.E. (1992) Selective culture of mitotically active human Schwann cells from adult sural nerves. *Ann. Neurol.*, **31**, 580–6.

Salzer, J.L., Holmes, W.P. and Colman, D.R. (1987) The amino acid sequences of the myelin-associated glycoproteins: homology to the immunoglobulin gene superfamily. *J. Cell Biol.*, **104**, 957–65.

Samuel, N.M., Jessen, K.R., Grange, J.M. and Mirsky, R. (1987a) Gamma interferon, but not *Mycobacterium leprae*, induces major histocompatibility class II antigens on cultured rat Schwann cells. *J. Neurocytol.*, **16**, 281–7.

Samuel, N.M., Mirsky, R., Grange, J.M. and Jessen, K.R. (1987b) Expression of major histocompatibility complex class I and class II antigens in human Schwann cell cultures and effects of infection with *Mycobacterium leprae*. *Clin. Exp. Immunol.*, **68**, 500–9.

Sanes, J. (1982) Laminin, fibronectin and collagen in synaptic and extrasynaptic portions of muscle fibre basement membrane. *J. Cell Biol.*, **93**, 442–51.

Sanes, J.R. and Chiu, A.Y. (1983) The basal lamina of the neuromuscular junction. *Cold Spring Harbor Symp. Quant. Biol.*, **48**, 667–78.

Sanes, J.R., Engvall, E., Butkowski, R. and Hunter, D.D. (1990) Molecular heterogeneity of basal laminae: isoforms of laminin and collagen IV at the neuromuscular junction and elsewhere. *J. Cell Biol.*, **111**, 1685–99.

Saunders, R.D. and DeVries, G.H. (1988) Schwann cell proliferation is accompanied by enhanced inositol phospholipid metabolism. *J. Neurochem.*, **50**, 876–82.

Saunders, R.D., Brandon, Y.W. and DeVries, G.H. (1989) Role of intracellular pH in the axolemma- and myelin-induced proliferation of Schwann cells. *J. Neurochem.*, **52**, 1576–81.

Scarpini, E., Meda, G., Baron, P. *et al.* (1986) S-100 protein and laminin: immunocytochemical markers for human Schwann cells *in vitro*. *Exp. Neurol.*, **93**, 77–83.

Scarpini, E., Ross, A.H., Rosen, J.L. *et al.* (1988) Expression of nerve growth factor receptor during human peripheral nerve development. *Dev. Biol.*, **125**, 301–10.

Scarpini, E., Lisak, R.P., Beretta, S. *et al.* (1990) Quantitative assessment of class II molecules in normal and pathological nerves. Immunocytochemical studies *in vivo* and in tissue culture. *Brain*, **113**, 659–75.

Schachner, M. (1990) Novel functional implication of glial recognition molecules. *Semin. Neurosci.*, **2**, 497–508.

Schubert, D. (1992) Synergistic interactions between transforming growth factor beta and fibroblast growth factor regulate Schwann cell mitosis. *J. Neurobiol.*, **23**, 143–8.

Seilheimer, B. and Schachner, M. (1988) Studies of adhesion molecules mediating interactions between cells of peripheral nervous system indicate a major role for L1 in mediating sensory neurone growth on Schwann cells in culture. *J. Cell Biol.*, **107**, 341–51.

Seilheimer, B., Persohn, E. and Schachner, M. (1989) Neural cell adhesion molecule expression is regulated by Schwann cell–neuron interactions in culture. *J. Cell Biol.*, **108**, 1909–15.

Shearman, J.D. and Franks, A.J. (1987) S100 protein in Schwann cells of the developing human peripheral nerve: an immunohistochemical study. *Cell Tiss. Res.*, **249**, 459–63.

Sheela, S., Riccardi, V.M. and Ratner, N. (1990) Schwann cells in neurofibromas show premalignant properties. *J. Cell Biol.*, **111**, 645–54.

Shelleswell, G.B., Restall, D.J., Duance, V.C. and Bailey, A.J. (1979) Identification and differential distribution of collagen types in the central and peripheral nervous systems. *FEBS Lett.*, **106**, 305–8.

Shrager, P., Chiu, S.Y. and Ritchie, J.M. (1985) Voltage dependent sodium and potassium channels in mammalian cultured Schwann cells. *Proc. Natl. Acad. Sci. USA*, **82**, 948–52.

Shuman, S., Hardy, M. and Pleasure, D. (1986) Immunochemical characterization of peripheral nervous system myelin 170000 M_r glycoprotein. *J. Neurochem.*, **35**, 1183–9; *J. Neurochem.*, **50**, 190–4 (1988).

Shuman, S., Hardy, M., Shobue, G. and Pleasure, D. (1988) A cyclic AMP analogue induces synthesis of a myelin-specific glycoprotein by cultured Schwann cells. *J. Neurochem.*, **50**, 190–4.

Smith-Thomas, L.C. and Fawcett, J. W. (1989) Expression of Schwann cell markers by mammalian neural crest cells *in vitro*. *Development*, **105**, 251–62.

Smith-Thomas, L.C., Johnson, A.R. and Fawcett, J.W. (1990) The effects of retinal neurons on neural crest differentiation into Schwann cells. *Development*, **109**, 925–34.

Sobue, G. and Pleasure, D. (1984) Schwann cell galactocerebroside induced by derivatives of adenosine 3′,5′-monophosphate. *Science*, **224**, 72–4.

Sobue, G., Brown, M.J., Kim, S.U. and Pleasure, D. (1984) Axolemma is a mitogen for human Schwann cells. *Ann. Neurol.*, **15**, 449–52.

Sobue, G., Sonnenfeld, K., Rubenstein, A.E. and Pleasure, D. (1985) Tissue culture studies of neurofibromatosis: effects of axolemmal fragments and cyclic adenosine 3′,5′-monophosphate analogues on proliferation of Schwann-like and fibroblast-like neurofibroma cells. *Ann. Neurol.*, **18**, 68–73.

Sobue, G., Shuman, S. and Pleasure, D. (1986) Schwann cell responses to cyclic AMP: proliferation, change in shape, and appearance of surface galactocerebroside. *Brain Res.*, **362**, 23–32.

Sobue, G., Taki, T., Yasuda, T. and Mitsuma, T. (1988a) Gangliosides modulate Schwann cell proliferation and morphology. *Brain Res.*, **474**, 289–95.

Sobue, G., Yasuda, T., Mitsuma, T. *et al.* (1988b) Expression of nerve growth factor receptor in human peripheral neuropathies. *Ann. Neurol.*, **24**, 64–72.

Spreyer, P., Kuhn, G., Hanemann, C.O. *et al.* (1991) Axon-regulated expression of a Schwann cell transcript that is homologous to a 'growth arrest-specific' gene. *EMBO J.*, **10**, 3661–8.

Staugaitis, S.M., Smith, P.R. and Colman, D.R. (1990) Expression of myelin basic protein isoforms in nonglial cells. *J. Cell. Biol.*, **110**, 1719–27.

Stefansson, K., Wollman, R.L. and Moore, B.W. (1982) Distribution of S-100 protein outside the central nervous system. *Brain Res.*, **234**, 309–17.

Stewart, H.J.S., Eccleston, P.A., Jessen, K.R. and Mirsky, R. (1991) The interaction between cAMP elevation, identified growth factors and serum components in regulating Schwann cell growth. *J. Neurosci. Res.*, **30**, 346–52.

Taniuchi, M., Clark, H.B., Schweitzer, J.B. and Johnson, E.M. (1988) Expression of nerve growth factor receptors by Schwann cells of axotomized peripheral nerves: ultrastructural location, suppression by axonal contact and binding properties. *J. Neurosci.*, **664**, 681.

Thomas, P.K. and Ochoa, J. (1984) Microscopic anatomy of peripheral nerve fibers, in *Peripheral Neuropathy*, 2nd edn (eds P.J. Dyck, P.K. Thomas, E.H. Lambert and R.P. Bunge), W.B. Saunders, Philadelphia, pp. 39–96.

Tohyama, K. and Ide, C. (1984) The localisation of laminin and fibronectin on the Schwann cell basal lamina. *Arch. Histol. Jpn.*, **47**, 519–32.

Trapp, B.D. (1988) Distribution of the myelin-associated glycoprotein and P_0 during compaction in quaking mouse peripheral nerve. *J. Cell Biol.*, **107**, 675–85.

Trapp, B.D. and Quarles, R.H. (1984) Immunocytochemical localization of the myelin-associated glycoprotein – fact or artifact. *J. Neuroimmunol.*, **6**, 231–49.

Trapp, B.D., Itoyama, Y., Sternberger, N.H. *et al.* (1981) Immunocytochemical localization of P_0 protein in Golgi complex membranes and myelin of developing rat Schwann cells. *J. Cell Biol.*, **90**, 1–6.

Trapp, B.D., Dubois-Dalcq, M. and Quarles, R.H. (1984) Ultrastructural localization of P_2 protein in actively myelinating Schwann cells. *J. Neurochem.*, **43**, 944–8.

Trapp, B.D., Bernier, L., Andrews, S.B. and Colman, D.R. (1988) Cellular and subcellular distribution of 2′,3′-cyclic nucleotide 3′-phosphodiesterase and its mRNA in the rat central nervous system. *J. Neurochem.*, **51**, 859–68.

Trapp, B.D., Hauer, P. and Lemke, G. (1988) Axonal regulation of myelin protein mRNA levels in actively myelinating Schwann cells. *J. Neurosci.*, **8**, 3515–21.

Vedeler, C.A., Scarpini, E., Beretta, S. *et al.* (1990) The ontogenesis of Fc gamma receptors and complement receptors CR1 in human peripheral nerve. *Acta Neuropathol. (Berl.)*, **80**, 35–40.

Vogel, U.S. and Thompson, R.J. (1988) Molecular structure, localization and possible functions of the myelin-associated enzyme 2′3′-cyclic-nucleotide 3′-phosphodiesterase. *J. Neurochem.*, **50**, 1667–77.

Voyvodic, J.T. (1989) Target size regulates calibre and myelination of sympathetic axons. *Nature*, **342**, 430–3.

Webster, H. de F. and Favilla, J.T. (1984) Development of peripheral nerve fibres, in *Peripheral Neuropathy*, 2nd edn (eds P.J. Dyck, P.K. Thomas, E.H. Lambert and R. Bunge), W.B. Saunders, Philadelphia, pp. 329–59.

Weinmaster, G. and Lemke, G. (1990) Cell-specific cyclic-AMP-mediated induction of the PDGF receptor. *EMBO J.*, **9**, 915–20.

Wekerle, H., Schwab, M., Linington, C. and Meyerman, R. (1986) Antigen presentation in the peripheral nervous system: Schwann cells present endogenous myelin autoantigens to lymphocytes. *Eur. J. Immunol.*, **16**, 1551–7.

Wilkin, G.P., Marriott, D.R. and Cholewinski, A.J. (1990) Astrocyte heterogeneity. *Trends Neurosci.*, **13**, 43–5.

Wilson, G.F. and Chiu, S.Y. (1990) Potassium channel regulation in Schwann cells during early myelinogenesis. *J. Neurosci.*, **10**, 1615–25.

Wood, P.M. (1976) Separation of functional Schwann cells and neurons from normal peripheral nerve tissue. *Brain Res.*, **115**, 361–75.

Xu, G., Lin, B., Tanaka, K. *et al.* (1990) The catalytic domain of the neurofibromatosis type 1 gene product stimulates *ras* GTPase and complements *ira* mutants of *S. cerevisiae*. *Cell*, **63**, 835–41.

Yasuda, T., Sobue, G., Mitsuma, T. and Takahashi, A. (1988) Peptidergic and adrenergic regulation of the intracellular 3′,5′-cyclic adenosine monophosphate content in cultured rat Schwann cells. *J. Neurol. Sci.*, **88**, 315–25.

Yen, S. and Fields, K.L. (1981) Antibodies to neurofilament, glial filament and fibroblast intermediate proteins bind to different cell types of the nervous system. *J. Cell Biol.*, **88**, 115–26.

Yong, V.W., Kim, S.U., Kim, M.W. and Shin, D.H. (1988) Growth factors for human glial cells in culture. *Glia*, **1**, 113–23.

Yoshino, J., Dinneen, M.P., Sprinkle, T.J. and DeVries, G.H. (1985) Localisation of 2′,3′-cyclic nucleotide 3′-phosphodiesterase on cultured Schwann cells. *Brain Res.*, **325**, 199–203.

6

Pathology of neurofibromatosis 1 and 2

O.D. Wiestler and H. Radner

6.1 INTRODUCTION

The neurofibromatoses are hereditary cancer-prone disorders that involve a variety of tissues and cell types including the skin, central and peripheral nervous systems, iris and skeletal system. Some of the manifestations represent true neoplastic lesions, others are of dysplastic or malformative origin. On the basis of clinical and genetic studies, at least two distinct forms of neurofibromatosis have been identified (Chapter 1). Neurofibromatosis 1 (NF1) is characterized by predominant manifestations in the skin, i.e. café au lait spots, axillary freckling, multiple neurofibromas and Lisch nodules of the iris. Several laboratories have recently succeeded in identifying and cloning the NF1 gene on the long arm of chromosome 17. The NF1 gene encodes a large protein with sequence homology to the *ras* oncogene-associated family of GTPase activating proteins (Xu *et al.*, 1990).

Neurofibromatosis 2 (NF2) is much less common and presents with bilateral vestibular Schwannomas, multiple Schwannomas and neurofibromas of the peripheral and spinal nerves, meningiomas and gliomas. The genetic locus affected in NF2 has been mapped to the long arm of chromosome 22 (Seizinger, Martuza and Gusella, 1986; Seizinger *et al.*, 1987a). In addition to these established entities, several variant forms of neurofibromatosis have been described, most of which appear to be associated with NF1. This chapter summarizes histopathological features of the common manifestations of NF1 and NF2. Preference will be given to lesions of the skin and of the central and peripheral nervous system.

6.2 NEUROFIBROMATOSIS 1

Manifestations frequently associated with NF1 include neurofibromas, pigmented lesions of the skin, hamartomas of the iris (Lisch nodules),

Table 6.1 Characteristic features of dermal and plexiform neurofibromas

	Dermal neurofibroma	*Plexiform neurofibroma*
Location	Superficial (dermis), not associated with major nerves	Subcutaneous or visceral, associated with major nerves
Number	Multiple	Single
Age at onset	Puberty	Usually pre-pubertal
Progression to neurofibrosarcoma	No	5%
Regional hypertrophy	Absent	Common
Local pigmentation	Absent	Common

optic nerve gliomas, skeletal lesions and microscopic alterations of the cerebral cortex (Chapter 7).

6.2.1 Neurofibroma

Neurofibromas are spindle cell tumours that originate from a peripheral nerve sheath. This neurofibroma neoplasm was originally described by the German pathologist Friedrich Daniel von Recklinghausen (von Recklinghausen, 1882), who also identified neurofibromas as the hallmark of a disorder that was later referred to as von Recklinghausen's neurofibromatosis. The presence of multiple dermal neurofibromas is considered an important diagnostic criterion for NF1 (Riccardi, 1981). Whether solitary neurofibromas represent a *forme fruste* of NF1 remains to be determined by molecular analysis with genetic markers for the NF1 gene. Neurofibromas represent the most common manifestation of NF1; when located in the dermis, these tumours can grow to large lumpy masses. Two variants of neurofibroma are observed in NF1, i.e. dermal and plexiform neurofibroma (Table 6.1). Dermal neurofibromas in NF1 are characterized by their superficial location and occurrence in large numbers. These tumours originate from terminal nerve branches in the skin and are not associated with major peripheral nerve trunks. In contrast, the plexiform neurofibroma frequently originates from subcutaneous or visceral peripheral nerves and may cause a fusiform appearance in the affected nerve (Kleihues *et al.*, 1988). The histogenesis of this tumour is still controversial because neurofibromas contain a mixture of Schwann cells and perineurial fibroblasts.

(a) Dermal neurofibroma

Macroscopically, the dermal neurofibroma presents as a soft, yellowish-grey nodular or pedunculated mass (Bouldin, 1990). The tumour is well

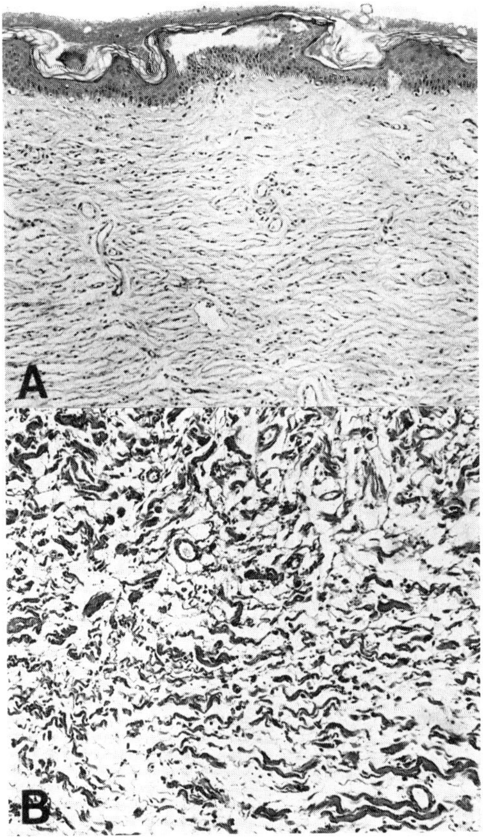

Figure 6.1 Histopathological appearance of the dermal neurofibroma. (A) Spindle cell neoplasm of low cellularity. H & E, × 80. (B) High power view of the tumour with characteristic cell processes. Masson trichrome stain, × 175.

circumscribed but not encapsulated. Histopathologically, dermal neurofibromas are characterized by an extrafascicular proliferation of a loose population of spindle-shaped cells with delicate processes (Figure 6.1). Some common features include the formation of collagen fibres and myxoid degeneration. The mitotic activity is low. This tumour may show a diffuse appearance but without evidence of an aggressive invasion of the adjacent tissues. In contrast to Schwannomas, nuclear palisading is uncommon, but structures resembling tactile corpuscles may be found (Smith and Bhawan, 1980). Mast cells are usually scattered throughout the tumour tissue. Although the terminal nerve branch from which the dermal neurofibroma originates can frequently not be identified, special stains may reveal occasional axons within the tumour. The overlying epidermis may be thin but is otherwise unaffected. In contrast to the plexiform neurofibroma, malignant progression of dermal neurofibromas is extremely uncommon.

(b) Nodular neurofibroma

Nodular neurofibromas may be present along the course of peripheral nerves and major nerve trunks. They are discrete tumours that do not merge into the surrounding tissue, and are not associated with surrounding connective tissue hypertrophy.

(c) Plexiform neurofibroma

Plexiform neurofibromas are almost exclusively associated with neurofibromatosis (Harkin, 1980). These neoplasms frequently exhibit a marked intrafascicular growth along major peripheral nerves, spinal nerve roots and in the retroperitoneal and mediastinal compartments (Rubenstein, 1986). The plexiform neurofibroma can involve long segments of a nerve and in some instances even extend into the spinal cord (Harkin, 1980). Many of these neoplasms originate from major nerve plexuses and major peripheral nerves, including retroperitoneal and gastrointestinal nerve fascicles (Weller and Cervós-Navarro, 1977). Plexiform neurofibromas may also involve cranial nerves or spinal nerve roots (Russell and Rubinstein, 1977; Weller and Cervós-Navarro, 1977).

Plexiform neurofibromas may be fairly discrete nodular tumours along a nerve or nerve root, or diffuse tumours. These diffuse tumours may be associated with diffuse hypertrophy of the surrounding connective tissue and other structures. The fascicular organization of the affected nerve segment is maintained and individual fascicles may become enlarged by the intrafascicular neoplasm to such an extent that they acquire features of a nerve plexus (hence the term plexiform neurofibroma) (Bouldin, 1990). Plexiform neurofibromas have the potential for malignant progression into neurofibrosarcomas.

The tumour is generally soft and grey in colour without haemorrhage or significant degenerative changes (Bouldin, 1990). Microscopically, plexiform neurofibromas present as moderately cellular spindle cell neoplasms. The tumour cells are embedded in an abundant extracellular myxoid matrix, which often contains numerous mast cells. The tumour cells are frequently associated with bundles of collagen thus distorting the neural appearance of the neoplasm (Figure 6.2). Nuclear palisading is uncommon but structures resembling tactile corpuscles (Smith and Bhawan, 1980; Watabe *et al.*, 1983) may occasionally be found (Russell and Rubinstein, 1977). Components with microscopic features of Schwannomas can sometimes be encountered in these neurofibromas (see below).

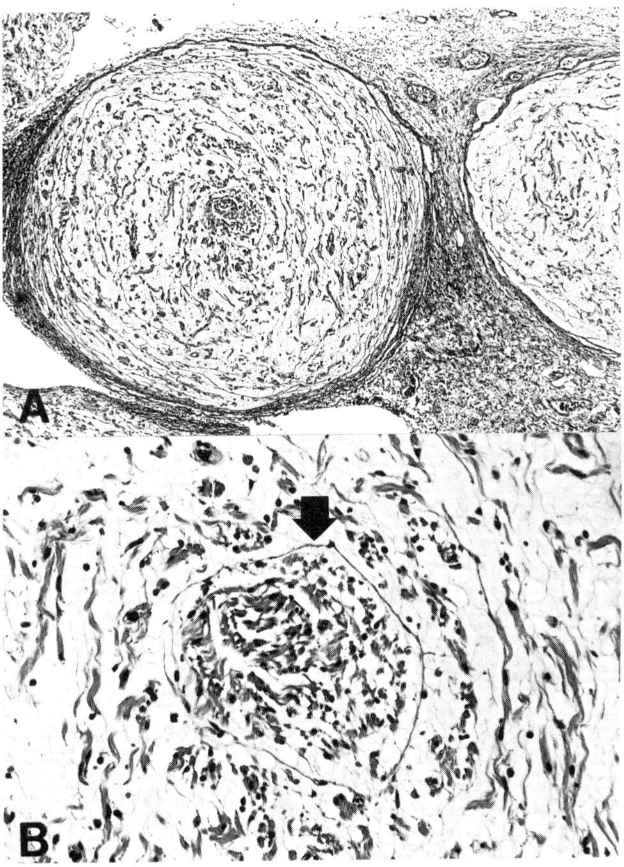

Figure 6.2 Histopathological appearance of the plexiform neurofibroma. Intrafascicular growth of the tumour cells leads to a marked swelling and expansion of the nerve. Pre-existing nerve fascicles are detectable in the centre of the tumour (arrow in B). (A) Masson trichrome stain, × 50; (B) Masson trichrome stain, × 200.

In plexiform neurofibromas with a prominent intrafascicular growth pattern, residual nerve fibres are often concentrated in the centre of the affected fascicles (Figure 6.2b; Bouldin, 1990).

Ultrastructurally, neurofibromas show a mixture of Schwann cells and perineurial fibroblasts. Compared with Schwannomas, these neoplasms usually exhibit significant amounts of extracellular collagen as well as myelinated and unmyelinated axons (Sian and Ryan, 1981). Occasional 'onion bulb' architectures may be found (Asbury and Johnson, 1978). The Schwann cell component of the tumour can be identified immunohistochemically using antibodies to the Ca^{2+}-binding protein S100 (Stefansson, Wollmann and Jerkovic, 1982; Kleihues, Kiessling and Janzer, 1987).

Antibodies to the intermediate filament protein vimentin will bind to both cell types in the tumour.

In addition to the classical dermal and plexiform neurofibromas, less common variants of this tumour have been described such as a melanotic neurofibroma, a pseudo-tactile-corpuscle neurofibroma and the epitheloid neurofibroma (Kleihues *et al.* 1988).

Because of the potential overlap in the histopathological appearance of these neoplasms and solitary Schwannomas and their common Schwann cell component, several authors have suggested that solitary neurofibromas and solitary Schwannomas should be considered as one clinical entity (Das Gupta *et al.*, 1969). However, the close association between plexiform neurofibromas and NF1, the potential of plexiform neurofibromas for malignant progression, the distinctive histopathological features and recent genetic data all justify a clear-cut distinction between these neoplasms (Enzinger and Weiss, 1988).

The differential diagnosis of neurofibromas includes Schwannoma, dermal leiomyoma, dermatofibroma and neural nevus (Bouldin, 1990).

6.2.2 Neurofibrosarcoma

Plexiform neurofibromas have the potential for malignant progression to neurofibrosarcoma (Plate 1). Less than 5% of NF1 patients develop neurofibrosarcomas. Owing to their aggressive growth and metastatic behaviour, these neoplasms constitute a major life-threatening complication in NF1. In an autopsy study of neurofibromatosis patients, Rubinstein (1986) identified neurofibrosarcoma as the major cause of death in six out of 11 cases of NF1. Recent molecular genetic data suggest that inactivation of the *p53* tumour suppressor gene is a critical factor in the sarcomatous progression of neurofibromas (Menon *et al.*, 1990). In most instances, malignant progression of the fibroblast component appears to be responsible for the development of neurofibrosarcomas. The morphological appearance is that of a malignant spindle cell neoplasm that may be difficult to distinguish from other sarcomas such as fibrosarcoma, malignant fibrous histiocytoma and leiomyosarcoma (Figure 6.3). Immunohistochemical reactions with antibodies to cell- and tissue-specific marker antigens can aid in the differential diagnosis of these sarcomas. Particularly useful are antibodies to S100 protein for identification of Schwann cells, antibodies to smooth muscle actin and desmin as markers for leiomyosarcoma, and desmin and myoglobin for rhabdomyosarcoma. Malignant fibrous histiocytoma may show a strong immunoreactivity for histiocytic antigens including lysozyme, α_1-antichymotrypsin and α_1-antitrypsin. The immunohistochemical profiles of benign and malignant tumours of the nerve sheaths and of other

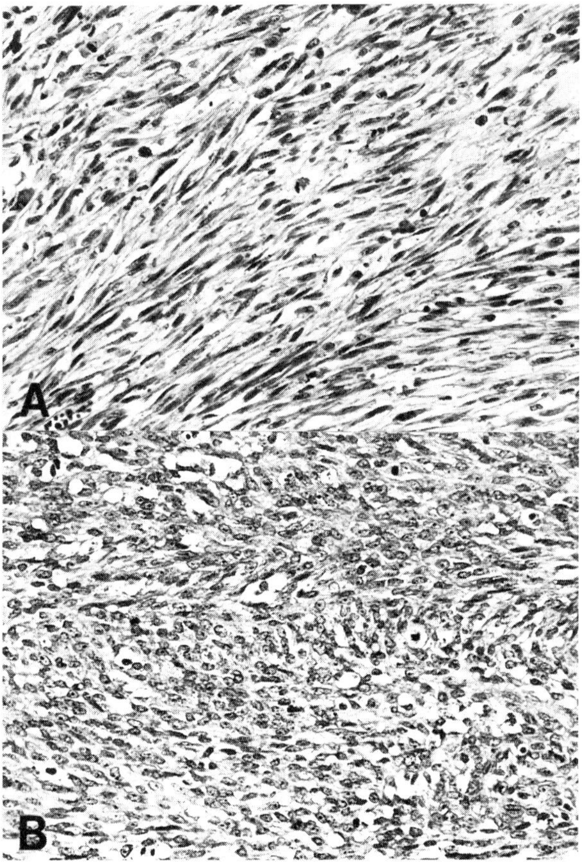

Figure 6.3 Microscopic appearance of neurofibrosarcoma (malignant peripheral nerve sheath tumour). (A) Spindle cell neoplasm with cellular and nuclear polymorphism and increased mitotic activity. H & E, × 200. (B) Epithelioid variant of a malignant peripheral nerve sheath tumour with numerous mitotic figures. Masson trichrome stain, × 200.

spindle cell neoplasms are summarized in Table 6.2. A comprehensive review of immunohistochemical reagents and techniques can be found in DeLellis (1988) and Kleihues, Kiessling and Janzer (1987).

A particular differential diagnostic problem can arise in distinguishing neurofibrosarcoma and malignant Schwannoma, both of which originate from components of the peripheral nerve sheath. The detection of S100 protein is of limited use in this situation because malignant Schwannomas tend to lose expression of this marker antigen. Several authors have therefore suggested classifying both tumours as a common entity. The recently revised version of the World Health Organization (WHO)

Table 6.2 Immunohistochemical profile of nerve sheath tumours and other spindle cell neoplasms

Tumour	*Vimentin*	*Keratin*	*S100*	*Leu 7*	*Muscle actin*	*Desmin*	*Myoglobin*	*α_1-ACT*	*α_1-AT*
Neurofibroma	+	–	+	+	–	–	–	–	–
Schwannoma	+	–	+	+	–	–	–	–	–
Malignant Schwannoma	+	–	(+)	+	–	–	–	–	–
Meningioma	+	(+)	–	–	–	–	–	–	–
Malignant meningioma	+	(+)	–	–	–	–	–	–	–
Melanoma	+	–	+	–	–	–	–	–	–
Malignant fibrous histiocytoma	+	–	–	–	–	–	–	+	+
Fibrosarcoma	+	–	–	–	–	–	–	–	–
Liposarcoma	+	–	+	–	–	–	–	–	–
Leiomyosarcoma	+	–	(+)	(+)	+	+	–	–	–
Rhabdomyosarcoma	+	–	(+)	(+)	+	+	+	–	–
Spindle cell carcinoma	–	+	–	–	–	–	–	–	–

Leu 7, antibody to a carbohydrate moiety expressed in haematopoietic and neural cells.
α_1-ACT = alpha$_1$-antichymotrypsin; α_1-AT = alpha$_1$-antitrypsin.
+, regularly expressed; (+), occasionally expressed; –, not expressed.

classification of nervous system tumours (Kleihues, Burger and Scheithauer, 1993) has introduced the diagnostic term 'malignant peripheral nerve sheath tumour (MPNST)' for both neurofibrosarcoma and malignant Schwannoma. Rare epitheloid and melanotic variants of MPNST have also been described (Figure 6.3b).

6.2.3 Schwannomas

Schwannomas are solid neoplasms originating from Schwann cells of the peripheral nervous system. Bilateral Schwannomas of the eighth cranial nerve and multiple Schwannomas of spinal nerve roots are diagnostic of NF2. A detailed description of these tumours will therefore be given in the section on NF2. In NF1, Schwannomas are reported at very low incidence (Enzinger and Weiss, 1988). Rather than involving cranial nerves or spinal nerve trunks, Schwannomas tend to develop in distal segments of peripheral nerves. Mixed neoplasms with components of both Schwannoma and neurofibroma are not uncommon in neurofibromatosis patients. We have also observed such tumours in several patients with NF2.

6.2.4 Café au lait macules

Pigmented lesions of the skin are a hallmark of NF1 (Kanter *et al.*, 1980; Rubinstein, 1986). The presence of at least six café au lait macules (CAL) over 15 mm at their maximum diameter is one of the criteria for establishing the diagnosis of NF1 in postpubertal patients (National Institutes of Health, 1987). Although characteristically associated with NF1, CAL are not specific for it. Occasional CAL occur in as many as 60% of NF2 patients (Eldridge, 1981) and about 10% of the normal population. CAL represent dysplastic melanocytic lesions without a potential for neoplastic transformation. Microscopically, CAL present as focal hyperpigmentation in the basal layer of an otherwise normal epidermis (Enzinger and Weiss, 1988). Pigmented axillary freckles have the same histopathological appearance.

6.2.5 Skeletal lesions

Sphenoid wing dysplasia and congenital bowing and thinning of long cortical bones have frequently been described in NF1 patients. In a systematic study of 250 neurofibromatosis patients, Rubenstein *et al.* (1984) found major orthopaedic problems in 6.8% of patients. These manifestations may cause exophthalmos, fractures of the long bones and pseudoarthrosis (Rubenstein, 1986). Histopathologically, affected bones show non-specific changes.

6.2.6 Hamartomas of the iris (Lisch nodules)

Lisch nodules represent small pigmented hamartomas of the iris. These hamartomas were first described by Waardenburg in 1918 and examined histopathologically by Goldstein and Wexler in 1930. However, the association with NF1 was noted by Lisch in 1937. Multiple Lisch nodules are considered a diagnostic hallmark of NF1 (Flueler, Boltshauser and Kilchhofer, 1986). In a prospective study on 77 patients with NF1, Lewis and Riccardi (1981) described iris nodules in 92% of patients aged 6 years or older. In younger children, the incidence was only 19%. Similar figures were recently reported by Lubs *et al.* (1991) who found Lisch nodules in all 65 NF1 patients above the age of 21 years.

Despite the common occurrence of Lisch nodules, there are only few reports documenting characteristic morphological features (Goldstein and Wexler, 1930; Wolter and Butler, 1963). They present as well circumscribed nodules arising anywhere on the surface of the iris. There is great variation in the extent of pigmentation and the size of these lesions. Histopathologically, Lisch nodules are composed of pigmented spindle cells. The melanocytic nature of these cells was confirmed by electron microscopic studies, which demonstrated melanosomes in many of the cells (Perry and Font, 1982). These nodules are considered melanocytic hamartomas without evidence for malignant progression into malignant melanoma. The differential diagnosis of Lisch nodules includes intrastromal nevi of the iris (Lewis and Riccardi, 1981), melanoma of the iris and neurofibroma (Wolter, 1969); however, these are not common manifestations of NF1 (Perry and Font, 1982).

6.2.7 Pilocytic astrocytoma of the optic nerve (optic pathway glioma)

A variety of gliomas have been reported in patients with NF1 (Rubinstein, 1986). The most frequently encountered central nervous system (CNS) tumours in these patients are optic nerve gliomas, which may develop as unilateral or bilateral neoplasms (Davis, 1940; Borit and Richardson, 1982; Lewis *et al.*, 1984; Ilgren, Kinnier-Wilson and Stiller, 1985). Hemispheric, cerebellar and brain stem astrocytomas (Ilgren, Kinnier-Wilson and Stiller, 1985) and glioblastomas (Manuelidis and Solitare, 1971) have occasionally been reported in NF1 (Hochstrasser, Boltshauser and Valavanis, 1988). The incidence of pilocytic astrocytomas of the optic nerve in NF1 patients appears to be in the order of 5–15% (Duffner and Cohen, 1988; Packer *et al.*, 1988). Compared with sporadic optic pathway gliomas, the tumours found in NF1 patients are highly variable in their biological behaviour. This observation has caused a debate on the nature of these neoplasms. While most authors regard these tumours as true neoplastic lesions, some investigators have proposed a hamartomatous nature in those cases that did not show evidence of progression over long observation periods (Borit and Richardson, 1982; Rubinstein, 1986). However, optic pathway gliomas may also show a rapid clinical course and aggressive behaviour. A biological basis for these remarkable differences in growth potential remains obscure.

Optic pathway gliomas can be localized in the orbit, along the optic nerves or in the optic chiasm where they may induce a diencephalic syndrome. Macroscopically, some optic gliomas present as circumscribed solid masses whereas others lead to a diffuse extension of the affected nerve segment. The characteristic histopathological appearance is that of a pilocytic astrocytoma with bipolar tumour cells, Rosenthal fibres and protein droplets (Plate 2). Vascular proliferations can occur, but significant mitotic activity and areas of necrosis are absent. A microcystic tumour matrix and pseudofascicular growth pattern are frequently observed. In contrast to sporadic pilocytic astrocytomas of the optic nerve with predominant intraneural growth of the nerve, optic gliomas in NF1 patients may show a circumferential perineurial pattern of infiltration in the subarachnoid space around the optic nerve. Such differences in the growth behaviour between sporadic and NF1 associated pilocytic astrocytomas have been stressed by Stern, DiGiacinto and Housepian (1979). The immunocytochemical demonstration of glial fibrillary acidic protein (GFAP) confirms the astrocytic nature of these neoplasms (Plate 2b). A strong reaction is usually detectable in tumour cell processes, Rosenthal fibres and protein droplets. Anaplastic variants of optic nerve gliomas are rare.

6.2.8 Malformative lesions in NF1

In a detailed microscopic study of the brain, Rosman and Pearce (1967) discovered abnormalities in the cortical architecture of all 10 patients diagnosed with NF1. Similar changes could not be found in the brain of five normal individuals. This indicates that these changes may represent a common manifestation of NF1. Pathological findings included random orientation of neurons, disarray of cortical lamination and neuronal heterotopias in the molecular and subcortical white matter. It was proposed that these abnormalities may define a morphological substrate for the mental deficiency that is frequently encountered in neurofibromatosis. Careful analysis of the neocortex in the NF2 patients included in the series of Wiestler *et al.* (1989) did not reveal disturbances in the neuronal morphology and cortical cytoarchitecture despite the presence of abundant dysplastic glial foci.

In a comprehensive autopsy study of 11 NF1 patients, Rubinstein (1986) identified focal proliferations of fibrillary subependymal glia with the development of well-defined nodules or fingerlike projections at various levels of the ventricular cavities in three of these cases. The histological features of these glial foci are indistinguishable from those of small subependymal pilocytic astrocytomas. Subependymal gliofibrillary nodules have been associated with aqueduct stenosis in NF1. Sixteen examples in which aqueductal stenosis, presumed to be due to similar polypoid ependymal granulations, resulted in hydrocephalus have recently been reviewed by Horwich, Riccardi and Francke (1983). A circumscribed hyperplastic gliosis was observed in NF1 patients with cerebral infarcts suggesting that astrocytes in these patients are prone to a pronounced proliferative reaction (Rubinstein, 1986). However, a progression of such hyperplastic lesions into macroscopic astrocytomas has not been documented. Another manifestation of this proliferative potential is the appearance of circumscribed areas of fibrillary gliosis in the cerebellum and adjacent leptomeninges, which have also been referred to as meningioencephalic cerebellar gliosis or localized cerebellar dysplasia (Walker, 1941; Rubinstein, 1986).

In occasional cases of NF1, micronodular vascular proliferations in the nervous system (Rubinstein, 1986) and visceral organs (Reubi, 1944; Feyrter, 1949; Mikuz, Weiser and Propst, 1975) can be a prominent feature (vascular neurofibromatosis). Several forms of vascular hyperplastic lesions in neurofibromatosis have been described (Reubi, 1944; Feyrter, 1949; Mikuz, Weiser and Propst, 1975). The adventitial nodular form, with endothelial proliferation within the vasa vasorum of small-calibre arteries, results in the development of glomerulus-like foci in the perivascular space. Another form largely consists of cellular hyperplasia of the intimal and muscular medial elements of arterioles. There is some dispute as to the histogenesis of these vascular alterations, some of which have been attributed to endothelial cells and others to smooth muscle cells or perineurial cells in the vascular walls. The similarity of some of these lesions to the glomeruloid foci of vascular endothelial proliferation found in malignant gliomas suggests an endothelial origin (Rubinstein, 1986). Malformative CNS lesions can be summarized as:

- abnormal architecture of cerebral cortex
- neuronal heterotopia
- hypertrophic gliosis of optic nerve
- hyperplastic proliferative gliosis
- subependymal gliofibrillary nodules
- meningoencephalic cerebellar gliosis
- micronodular vascular proliferations
- hydromyelia.

6.3 NEUROFIBROMATOSIS 2

In 1822, Wishart described a young patient with multiple tumours of the dura and cranial nerves including bilateral tumours of the eighth nerve. The combination of multiple meningiomas and Schwannomas has been recognized as the central form of neurofibromatosis, now called NF2 (Gardner and Frazier, 1930; Worster-Drought, Dickson and McMenemey, 1937; Gardner and Turner, 1940; Lichtenstein, 1949; Rubinstein, 1963; Rodriguez and Berthrong, 1966; Moyes, 1968; Alliez, Masse and Alliez, 1975; Riccardi and Mulvihill, 1981; Riccardi and Eichner, 1986; Rubenstein, 1986; Martuza and Eldridge, 1988). On the basis of genetic linkage studies, the central form of neurofibromatosis can now be distinguished from NF1. The gene affected in NF1 was mapped to the long arm of chromosome 17 and appears to act in a dominant fashion (Barker *et al.*, 1987; Seizinger *et al.*, 1987b). A genetic marker on the long arm of chromosome 22 segregates with NF2 (Wertelecki *et al.*, 1988). A loss of constitutional heterozygosity for the chromosome 22 locus in tumours and the observation of deletions affecting this chromosomal region in these patients indicate a recessive mutation of a tumour-suppressor gene as the underlying molecular defect in this disorder (Seizinger, Martuza and Gusella, 1986; Seizinger *et al.*, 1987a). Gusella and coworkers have recently succeeded in identifying this gene (Trofatter *et al.*, 1993). The great majority of neoplasms in NF2 are derived from Schwann cells of the cranial nerves and spinal nerve roots and from meningothelial cells. In addition to intracranial and intraspinal Schwannomas and meningiomas, the spectrum of neoplastic lesions in NF2 includes astrocytomas, intramedullary ependymomas and neurofibromas.

The clinical manifestations of NF2 are described in Chapter 18. Malformative CNS lesions are as follows:

- glial microhamartomas
- meningioangiomatosis of the brain
- fibrous gliosis in the molecular layer of the cerebellum
- ependymal ectopias
- intramedullary Schwannosis
- marginal gliosis of the spinal cord
- syringomyelia
- hydromyelia
- Chiari malformation of medulla and sacral spina bifida
- disorganization of cortical neurons
- Schwannosis of spinal blood vessels (angioneuromatosis).

6.3.1 Schwannomas

Schwannomas are neoplasms derived from Schwann cells of the peripheral nervous system. Alternative terms for these tumours include neurinoma, neurilemmoma and neuroma. Bilateral vestibular Schwannomas are the hallmark of NF2, and therefore NF2 used to be referred to as bilateral acoustic neurofibromatosis (Plate 3a). In a study of 250 neurofibromatosis patients at the Mount Sinai Hospital, acoustic Schwannomas were found in five cases, all of which were classified as NF2 (Rubenstein *et al.*, 1984). Rubinstein (1986) published an autopsy study of eight patients with bilateral vestibular Schwannomas.

Vestibular Schwannomas usually arise in the nerve segment between the glial–Schwann cell junction and the labyrinth (Stewart, Liland and Schuknecht, 1975). For unknown reasons, the vestibular branch of the eighth nerve is more frequently the site of origin than the cochlear branch (Stewart, Liland and Schuknecht, 1975). The Schwann cell ensheathment of the eighth nerve does not commence until the nerve is either near the internal auditory meatus or within the internal auditory canal. Most Schwannomas are therefore located at the meatus or within the canal (Bridger and Farkashidy, 1980). The tumour grows slowly, and usually enlarges the meatus. Taking the course of least resistance it grows medially into the cerebellopontine angle rather than laterally within the internal auditory canal (Bouldin, 1990). The eighth cranial nerve is progressively compressed and destroyed by the tumour. As the tumour enlarges, it may also compress one or more of the adjacent cranial nerves (V, VII, IX, X, XI), the brain stem and the cerebellum (Bouldin, 1990). The enlarging mass eventually leads to increased intracranial pressure, hydrocephalus and cerebellar herniation (Bouldin, 1990). Tumours of such large size are now uncommon owing to the improvement of functional auditory tests (Bouldin, 1990) and neuroimaging techniques. Currently, the brain stem auditory-evoked response (BAER) allows detection of small tumours in the internal auditory meatus (Hart, Gardner and Howieson, 1983). Occasionally, Schwannomas may also arise on other cranial nerves, especially on the fifth cranial nerve (Evans *et al.*, 1992). These tumours never originate from the first or second cranial nerve, which represent CNS tissue and do not contain Schwann cells.

Intraspinal Schwannomas are intradural, extramedullary tumours usually arising from the posterior spinal roots (Bouldin, 1990). In some instances, the neoplasm may extend through the intervertebral foramen. About 5% of NF2 patients present with numerous spinal Schwannomas (Plate 4). In some instances, the extent of tumour burden increases towards the caudal end of the cord (Plate 3b).

Peripheral Schwannomas may arise on any peripheral nerve. They are found at all ages and there is no sex predilection (Russell and Rubinstein, 1989). Most commonly, the tumours develop in major peripheral nerves of the extremities, the posterior mediastinum or the retroperitoneum. Intradermal Schwannomas are rare (Harkin and Reed, 1969).

The great majority of solitary Schwannomas are not associated with

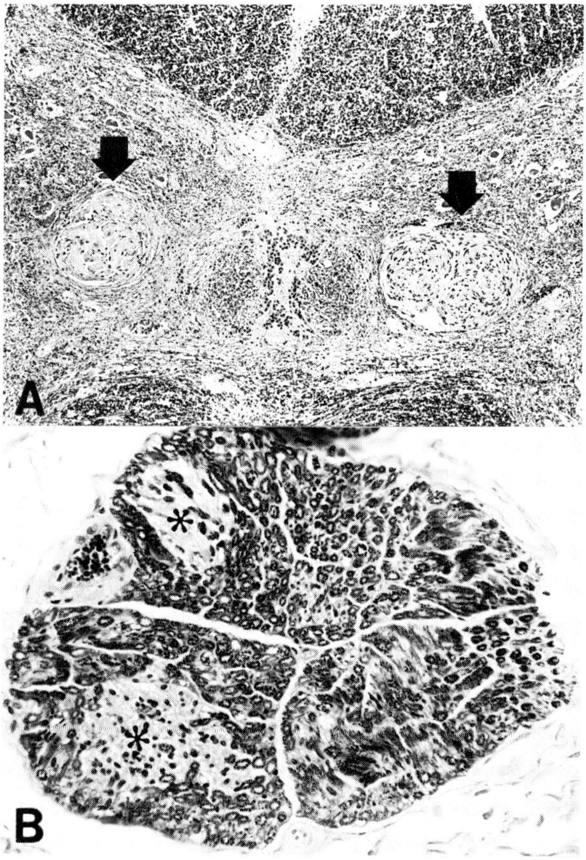

Figure 6.4 Microscopic foci of proliferated Schwann cells (Schwannosis) in the spinal grey matter (a, arrows) and in a spinal nerve root (b, asterisks) of a patient with NF2. (a) Luxol-Nissl stain, × 63; (b) Luxol-Nissl stain, × 175.

neurofibromatosis. Multiple tumours should, however, always raise suspicion of neurofibromatosis. Bilateral acoustic Schwannomas and multiple Schwannomas of spinal nerve roots are the major manifestations of NF2. In NF2 patients, Schwannomas may develop at unusual sites such as the spinal cord or cerebrum.

In addition to macroscopic tumours, the peripheral nerves of NF2 patients contain numerous microscopic foci of Schwann cell proliferation (Figure 6.4). These foci most likely represent precursor lesions with a potential for progression into Schwannomas.

Grossly, Schwannomas present as encapsulated tumours ranging in diameter from a few millimetres to several centimetres. Very rarely, peripheral Schwannomas may show a plexiform or multinodular growth pattern (Iwashita and Enjoji, 1987). The nerve of origin can often be identified in the capsule of the neoplasm (Bouldin, 1990). The surface is usually firm and the tissue has a white or yellowish colour. Microscopically, fusiform cells predominate in these tumours (Kleihues *et al.*, 1988). Generally, there is a fibrous capsule beyond which branches of the corresponding nerve may be found (Kleihues *et al.*, 1988). Many Schwannomas show a biphasic histopathological growth pattern. One architecture, designated Antoni type A, is produced by interwoven fascicles of elongated cells with conspicuous spindle-shaped nuclei that frequently exhibit palisading and contribute to the formation of Verocay bodies (Plate 3c). The stroma is acidophilic and finely fibrillar. Occasionally, the spindle cells form whorls resembling those found in meningiomas, or isolated wavy fascicles similar to those occurring in neurofibromas (Bouldin, 1990). A second growth pattern (Antoni type B) is characterized by a reticular, microcystic appearance, lower cellularity and regressive changes including fatty degeneration and accumulation of macrophages. Degenerative changes are common in Schwannomas and include foci of foamy cells, recent haemorrhage, macrophages, cysts, lymphocytic or plasmacytic infiltrates, zones of dense fibrosis and hyalinized blood vessels ('ancient' Schwannoma). Metaplastic foci of bone and cartilage are occasionally present (Bouldin, 1990). Rarely, focal glandular differentiation (Woodruff, 1976) or melanin pigment produced by neoplastic Schwann cells can be found (Lowman and Livolsi, 1980). Hyalinization of blood vessel walls is common in Schwannomas, but other vascular changes may also be observed (Bouldin, 1990). Some tumours contain prominent vascular channels reminiscent of an angioma (Gruskin and Carberry, 1979). Pleomorphic and hyperchromatic changes of nuclei are common in Schwannomas, as are foci of hypercellularity. However, these features are not indicative of malignancy. Mitotic figures are uncommon and their presence should raise concerns about malignancy (Bouldin, 1990). Reticulin fibres are abundant, separating individual cells and running parallel with the long axis of a cell. Such fibres are most easily found in Antoni A areas and only variably in Antoni B tissue.

Immunohistochemical reactions can be useful to distinguish Schwannomas from other spindle cell neoplasms. The Ca^{2+}-binding protein S100 is strongly expressed in normal and neoplastic Schwann cells. The lack of S100 expression should always cast doubt on the Schwann cell origin of a neoplasm, although highly anaplastic Schwannomas tend to lose immunoreactivity for S100 protein. The distinction of other spindle cell tumours may require immunohistochemical reactions with antibodies to cell type-specific antigens such as S100 protein, desmin, α-actin and histiocytic proteins. Leu-7 antigen and vimentin can be demonstrated in most Schwannomas (Weiss, Langloss and Enzinger, 1983; Gould *et al.*, 1986; Johnson, Glick and Davis, 1988;

Kawahara *et al.*, 1988). Occasional Schwannomas contain cells with immunoreactive GFAP (Bouldin, 1990).

Ultrastructurally, neoplastic Schwann cells display a distinct basal lamina, long cytoplasmic processes and rare intercellular junctions (Erlandson and Woodruff, 1982; Sian and Ryan, 1981). In the Antoni A areas, the attenuated Schwann cell processes interdigitate and occasionally form mesaxon-like structures that wrap around other Schwann cell processes (Bouldin, 1990).

The differential diagnosis of cerebellopontine angle tumours includes Schwannoma, meningioma and astrocytoma. A pilocytic astrocytoma of the cerebellum or an astrocytoma of the brain stem may grow into the cerebellopontine angle and mimic a Schwannoma. Histopathologically, the distinction of fibroblastic meningioma and Schwannoma can be difficult, and may require the use of immunocytochemical techniques. Strong expression of S100 protein favours the diagnosis of a Schwannoma in such cases.

A peripheral Schwannoma must be distinguished from a leiomyoma, well-differentiated leiomyosarcoma and neurofibroma (Bouldin, 1990). The smooth muscle tumours are characterized by their immunoreactivity for smooth muscle α-actin and desmin. Neurofibromas do not exhibit Antoni A and B patterns, are not encapsulated and contain occasional axons. However, NF1 and NF2 patients may develop mixed neoplasms with Schwannoma and neurofibroma components.

The malignant progression of Schwannomas in NF2 is a rare event, since individual patients have large numbers of these tumours which do not become malignant. Among six autopsy cases of NF2, we have observed one patient who died from a metastasizing mediastinal Schwannoma.

6.3.2 Meningioma

Intracranial meningiomas can be observed in a high percentage of patients with NF2. In our own autopsy series of six NF2 cases, meningiomas were invariably present. Most of these patients present with multiple meningiomas that sometimes only affect one hemisphere of the brain. Grossly and microscopically, there are no significant differences compared with sporadic meningiomas. Among the variants of this tumour, the meningothelial type of meningioma is most common. The neoplasm shows syncytia, whorls and occasionally psammoma bodies. We have not observed anaplastic meningiomas in our material. In some instances, meningiomas may be associated with meningioangiomatosis (see below). Rubinstein (1986) reported a rather high incidence of choroid plexus meningiomas in NF2.

6.3.3 Gliomas

The spectrum of glial tumours in NF2 includes pilocytic astrocytomas of the brain and spinal cord (Plate 4), as well as cerebral and spinal ependymomas. Most of these neoplasms are morphologically benign and not distinguishable from their sporadic counterparts. Pilocytic astrocytomas of the optic nerves, optic chiasm and optic tracts, which frequently develop in NF1, are not usually seen in NF2.

6.3.4 Glial microhamartomas

In a detailed postmortem examination of the brain in six cases of NF2, we have observed disseminated clusters of immature neuroectodermal cells in the grey matter of the cerebral cortex and basal ganglia (Figure 6.5). On the basis of their morphology and immunoreactivity, these clusters have been tentatively designated glial microhamartomas (Wiestler *et al.*, 1989). While in some cases only occasional small clusters were noticed, others exhibited numerous confluent lesions. The cells, although often polymorphic and multinucleated, did not show mitotic activity or a tendency for neoplastic transformation. To determine the histogenesis of these foci, extensive immunocytochemical reactions were carried out with antibodies to a variety of glial, neuronal, epithelial, endothelial, mesenchymal, myogenic, melanocytic and haematopoietic antigens. With the exception of S100 protein, no immunoreactivity was detectable. S100 protein was consistently expressed in these foci, irrespective of their size, location or degree of polymorphism (Plate 3). The Ca^{2+}-binding protein S100 has been found in a variety of cell types including astrocytes, oligodendrocytes, ependymal cells, Schwann cells, Langerhans cells and haematopoietic cells (Kahn *et al.*, 1982; Takahashi *et al.*, 1984; Donato, 1986; Schwechheimer, 1986; Kleihues, Kiessling and Janzer, 1987). The immunohistochemical expression pattern does not, therefore, allow for an unequivocal identification of the affected cell type. Russell and Rubinstein (1989) favoured an astrocytic origin for these dysplastic glial cells despite the occasional appearance of rod-shaped and spherical blepharoblasts. The expression of S100 protein in the absence of GFAP immunoreactivity, which has been reported in glial hamartomas (Kleihues, Kiessling and Janzer, 1987), would be compatible with a hamartomatous origin of these dysplastic glial cells in NF2. Considering the marked susceptibility to neoplastic transformation of the neuroectodermal cells in NF2, the possibility that dysplastic glial cells might represent preneoplastic or neoplastic astrocytes was also considered. However, none of the numerous microhamartomas had reached a macroscopic size, showed evidence of mitotic activity or showed detectable signs of spontaneous regression. It therefore appears unlikely that

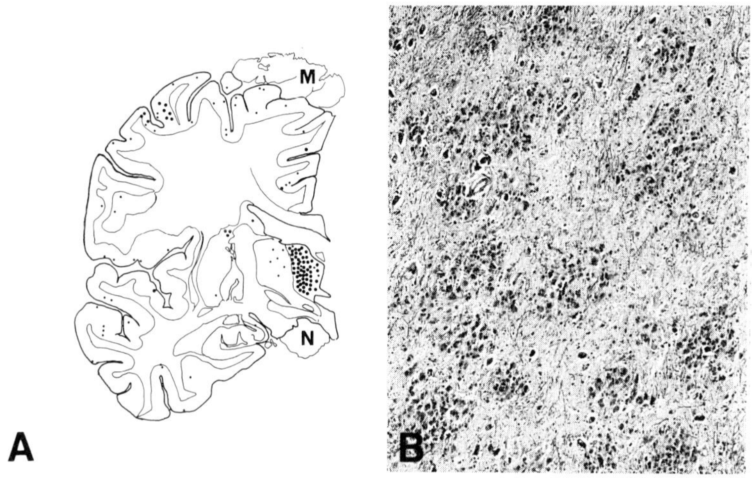

Figure 6.5 (A) Distribution of glial microhamartomas in the left cerebral hemisphere of a patient with NF2. Note the clustering of hamartomas in the thalamus. (B) Higher power view of the thalamus in this patient. Luxol-Nissl stain, × 50. M = parasagittal meningioma; N = Schwannoma of the third cranial nerve.

these foci bear a significant potential for neoplastic transformation. Although we did not systematically analyse the CNS of patients with NF1, our data strongly suggest that these microhamartomas constitute a morphological hallmark of NF2.

6.3.5 Meningioangiomatosis

Meningioangiomatosis represents a composite lesion with a meningothelial and a vascular component. This lesion is usually localized in the cerebral cortex, but may also occur in the thalamus or mesencephalon. The meningothelial component exhibits features of a meningioma, including whorl formations and psammoma bodies; the vascular portion is characterized by dysplastic angiomatous vessels with hyalinized walls (Figure 6.6). A detailed microscopic examination often reveals an additional glial component, which has led some authors to use the term angioreticuloglioma for this manifestation of NF2. Although meningioangiomatosis has been reported adjacent to meningiomas, the available data suggest a dysplastic/hamartomatous rather than a neoplastic nature of this lesion. Multiple foci of meningioangiomatosis can be detected in the brain of some patients. In Rubinstein's postmortem series, meningioangiomatosis was detectable in four out of 11 NF2 cases. Although characteristically associated with NF2, meningioangiomatosis

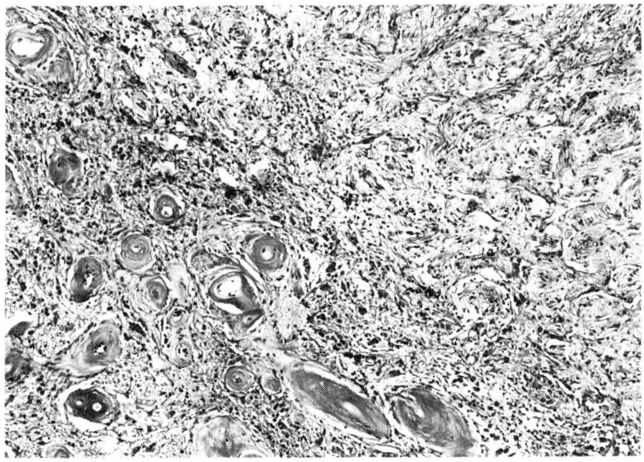

Figure 6.6 Meningioangiomatosis in NF2. This is a combined hamartomatous lesion with hyalinized, dysplastic blood vessels, numerous reticulin fibres and clusters of meningothelial cells. H & E, × 50.

has in rare instances been described in the absence of other manifestations of the disease (Kasantikul and Brown, 1981; Halper, Scheithauer and Okazaki, 1985).

In addition to these common CNS malformations, several other malformative lesions have been described in the brain and spinal cord of NF2 patients. Ectopic foci of ependymal cells are often seen in the spinal cord. In some instances, ependymal ectopias can be associated with spinal ependymomas (Rubinstein, 1986). Syringomyelia and hydromyelia are occasional findings in NF2 patients, but may develop secondary to spinal neoplasms. The cerebellar cortex may exhibit dysplastic areas of fibrous gliosis. It remains to be elucidated if these hamartomas are caused by the abnormal NF2 gene or if they represent secondary changes.

6.3.6 Other malformative CNS lesions in NF2

In a comprehensive neuropathological study (22 cases) of malformative CNS alterations in neurofibromatosis (11 central, 11 peripheral) presented by Rubinstein (1963, 1986), NF2 was shown frequently to be associated with hamartomatous lesions, many of which appear to be specific for this disorder. Such malformative lesions may involve a variety of cell types, including Schwann cells, meningothelial, endothelial, astrocytic and ependymal cells (Rubinstein, 1986). Occasionally, a close topographical relationship can be found between microscopic dysplastic lesions and macroscopic CNS tumours (Rubinstein, 1986). In addition to the glial microhamartomas described above, intramedullary Schwannosis, meningioangiomatosis and ependymal ectopias are a frequent finding in NF2 (Rubinstein, 1963, 1972; Russell and Rubinstein, 1989).

The term intramedullary Schwannosis has been applied to microscopic foci of Schwann cells in the spinal cord. In many cases, these foci originate in the vicinity of the superficial posterior horn where Schwann cells and reticulin fibres enter the neural parenchyma. Circumscribed Schwannosis may also be observed in the grey matter of the spinal cord adjacent to the central canal (Figure 6.4a). Schwannosis can occur as an isolated lesion or in association with glial or Schwann cell neoplasms. The biological nature of these foci is controversial. A dysplastic origin has been proposed by some authors, whereas others favour reactive Schwann cell proliferation as the pathogenetic mechanism. Histopathologically, areas of intramedullary Schwannosis are virtually indistinguishable from the numerous clusters of atypical Schwann cells found in the spinal roots and peripheral nerves of NF2 patients, indicating that they constitute the same type of lesion. The occasional association with macroscopic Schwannomas suggests a preneoplastic potential of these foci. Schwannosis originating from the perivascular connective tissue in the spinal cord is sometimes referred to as angioneuromatosis (Russell and Rubinstein, 1989).

REFERENCES

Alliez, J., Masse, J.-L. and Alliez, B. (1975) Tumeurs bilatérales de l'acoustique et maladie de Recklinghausen observées dans plusieurs générations. *Rev. Neurol.*, **131**, 545–58.

Asbury, A.K. and Johnson, P.C. (1978) *Pathology of Peripheral Nerve*, W.B. Saunders, Philadelphia.

Barker, D. *et al.* (1987) Gene for von Recklinghausen neurofibromatosis is in the pericentromeric region of chromosome 17. *Science*, **236**, 1100–2.

Borit, A. and Richardson, E.P., Jr (1982) The biological and clinical behaviour of pilocytic astrocytomas of the optic pathways. *Brain*, **105**, 161–87.

Bouldin, T.W. (1990) Nerve biopsy, in *Diagnostic Neuropathology*, vol. II (eds J. Garcia *et al.*), Fields & Wood, pp. 175–92.

Bridger, M.W. and Farkashidy, J. (1980) The distribution of neuroglia and schwann cells in the 8th nerve of man. *J. Laryngol. Otol.*, **94**, 1353–62.

Das Gupta, T.K. *et al.* (1969) Benign solitary schwannomas (neurilemomas). *Cancer*, **24**, 355–66.

Davis, F.A. (1940) Primary tumors of the optic nerve (a phenomenon of Recklinghausen's disease). A clinical and pathologic study with a report of four cases and a review of the literature. *Arch. Ophthalmol. New. Ser.*, **23**, 735–821, 957–1018.

DeLellis, R.A. (1988) *Advances in Immunohistochemistry*, Raven Press, New York.

Donato, R. (1986) S-100 proteins. *Cell Calcium*, **7**, 123–45.

Duffner, P.K. and Cohen, M.E. (1988) Isolated optic nerve gliomas in children with and without neurofibromatosis. *Neurofibromatosis*, **1**, 201–11.

Eldridge, R. (1981) Central neurofibromatosis with bilateral acoustic neuroma. *Adv. Neurol.*, **9**, 57–65.

Enzinger, F.M. and Weiss, S.W. (1988) *Soft Tissue Tumors*, 2nd edn, C.V. Mosby, St Louis.

Erlandson, R.A. and Woodruff, J.M. (1982) Peripheral nerve sheath tumors: an electron microscopic study of 43 cases. *Cancer*, **49**, 273–87.

Evans, D.G.R. *et al.* (1992) A clinical study of type 2 neurofibromatosis. *Quart. J. Med.*, **304**, 613–18.

Feyrter, F. (1949) Über die vasculäre Neurofibromatose, nach Untersuchungen am menschlichen Magen-Darmschlauch. *Virchows Arch.*, **317**, 221–65.

Flueler, U., Boltshauser, E. and Kilchhofer, A. (1986) Iris hamartomata as diagnostic criterion in neurofibromatosis. *Neuropediatrics*, **17**, 183–5.

Gardner, W.J. and Frazier, C.H. (1930) Bilateral acoustic neurofibromas: a clinical study and field survey of a family of five generations with bilateral deafness in thirty eight members. *Arch. Neurol. Psychiatry*, **23**, 266–302.

Gardner, W.J. and Turner, O. (1940) Bilateral acoustic neurofibromas. Further clinical and pathologic data on hereditary deafness and Recklinghausen's disease. *Arch. Neurol. Psychiatry*, **44**, 76–99.

Goldstein, I. and Wexler, D. (1930) Melanosis uveae and melanoma of the iris in neurofibromatosis (Recklinghausen). *Arch Ophthalmol.*, **3**, 288–96.

Gould, V.E. *et al.* (1986) The intermediate filament complement of the spectrum of nerve sheath neoplasms. *Lab. Invest.*, **55**, 463–74.

Gruskin, P. and Carberry, J.N. (1979) Pathology of acoustic tumors, in *Acoustic Tumors*, vol. 1 (eds W.F. House and C.M. Luetje), Baltimore, University Park Press, pp. 85–148.

Halper, J., Scheithauer, B.W. and Okazaki, H. (1985) Meningioangiomatosis: report of three cases with associated Alzheimer's neurofibrillary change. *Lab Invest.*, **52**, 27A.

Harkin, J.C. (1980) Differential diagnosis of peripheral nerve tumors, in *Management of Peripheral Nerve Problems* (ed. G.E. Omer and M. Spinner), W.B. Saunders, Philadelphia, pp. 657–68.

Harkin, J.C. and Reed, R.J. (1969) *Tumors of the Peripheral Nervous System*, Armed Forces Institute of Pathology, Bethesda.

Hart, R.C., Gardner, D.P. and Howieson, J. (1983) Acoustic tumors: atypical features and recent diagnostic tests. *Neurology*, **33**, 211–21.

Hochstrasser, H., Boltshauser, E. and Valavanis, A. (1988) Brain tumors in children with von Recklinghausen neurofibromatosis. *Neurofibromatosis*, **1**, 233–9.

Horwich, A., Riccardi, V.M. and Francke, U. (1983) Aqueductal stenosis leading to hydrocephalus – an unusual manifestation of neurofibromatosis. *Am. H. Med. Genet.*, **14**, 577–81.

Ilgren, E.B., Kinnier-Wilson, L.M. and Stiller, C.A. (1985) Gliomas in neurofibromatosis: a series of 89 cases with evidence for enhanced malignancy in associated cerebellar astrocytomas, in *Pathology Annual*, Part 1, Vol. 20 (eds S.C. Sommers, P.P. Rosen and R.E. Fechner), Appleton-Century-Crofts, Norwalk, Conn, pp. 331–58.

Iwashita, T. and Enjoji, M. (1987) Plexiform neurilemmoma: a clinicopathological and immunohistochemical analysis of 23 tumours from 20 patients. *Virchows Archiv A*, **411**, 305–9.

Johnson, M.D., Glick, A.D. and Davis, B.W. (1988) Immunohistochemical evaluation of Leu-7, myelin basic-protein, S 100-protein, glial-fibrillary acidic-protein, and LN3 immunoreactivity in nerve sheath tumors and sarcomas. *Arch. Pathol. Lab. Med.*, **112**, 155–60.

Kahn, H.J. *et al.* (1982) Role of antibody S-100 protein in diagnostic pathology. *Am J. Clin. Pathol.*, **79**, 341–7.

Kanter, W.R. *et al.* (1980) Central neurofibromatosis with bilateral acoustic neuroma: genetic, clinical and biochemical distinctions from peripheral neurofibromatosis. *Neurology*, **30**, 851–9.

Kasantikul, V. and Brown, W.J. (1981) Meningioangiomatosis in the absence of von Recklinghausen's disease. *Surg. Neurol.*, **15**, 71–5.

Kawahara, E. *et al.* (1988) Expression of glial fibrillary acidic protein (GFAP), vimentin, S-100 protein, and neurofilament in 38 schwannomas and 18 neurofibromas. *Am. J. Surg. Path.*, **12**, 115–20.

Kleihues, P., Kiessling, M. and Janzer, R.C. (1987) Morphological markers in neuro-oncology. *Curr. Top. Pathol.*, **77**, 307–38.

Kleihues, P. *et al.* (1988) *Tumoren des Nervensystems. Standardisierte Nomenklatur, Biologisches Verhalten und klinisch-pathologische Definitionen*, Springer-Verlag, Berlin, Heidelberg.

Kleihues, P., Burger, P.C. and Scheithauer, B.W. (1993) *Histological Typing of Tumours of the Central Nervous System*, 2nd edn, Berlin, Heidelberg, Springer-Verlag.

Lewis, R.A. and Riccardi, V.M. (1981) Von Recklinghausen neurofibromatosis. Incidence of iris hamartomata. *Ophthalmology*, **88**(4), 348–54.

Lewis, R.A. *et al.* (1984) Von Recklinghausen neurofibromatosis. II. Incidence of optic gliomata. *Ophthalmologica*, **91**, 929–35.

Lichtenstein, B.W. (1949) Neurofibromatosis (von Recklinghausen's disease of the nervous system). *Arch. Neurol. Psychiatry*, **62**, 822–39.

Lisch, K. (1937) Über Beteiligung der Augen, insbesondere das Vorkommen von Irisknötchen bei der Neurofibromatose (Recklinghausen). *Z. Augenheilkd.*, **93**, 137–43.

Lowman, R.M. and Livolsi, V.A. (1980) Pigmented (melanotic) schwannomas of the spinal cord. *Cancer*, **46**, 391–7.

Lubs, M.-L. E. *et al.* (1991) Lisch nodules in neurofibromatosis type 1. *New Engl. J. Med.*, **324**, 1264–6.

Manuelidis, E.E. and Solitare, G.B. (1971) Glioblastoma multiforme, in *Pathology of the Nervous System*, 2nd edn (ed. J. Minckler), McGraw-Hill. New York, pp. 2026–71.

Martuza, R.L. and Eldridge, R. (1988) Neurofibromatosis 2 (bilateral acoustic neurofibromatosis). *N. Engl. J. Med.*, **318**, 684–8.

Menon, A.G. *et al.* (1990) Chromosome 17p deletions and p53 gene mutations associated with the formation of malignant neurofibrosarcomas in von Recklinghausen neurofibromatosis. *Proc. Natl. Acad. Sci. USA*, **87**, 5435–9.

Mikuz, G., Weiser, G. and Propst, A. (1975) Vascular neurofibromatosis. *Pathol. Microbiol.*, **43**, 195–8.

Moyes, P.D. (1968) Familial bilateral acoustic neuroma affecting 14 members from four generations. *J. Neurosurg.*, **29**, 78–82.

National Institutes of Health (1987) Neurofibromatosis. *National Institutes of Health Consensus Development Conference Statement*, **6**, 12.

Packer, R.J. *et al.* (1988) Intracranial visual pathway gliomas in children with neurofibromatosis. *Neurofibromatosis*, **1**, 212–22.

Perry, H.D. and Font, R.L. (1982) Iris nodules in von Recklinghausen's neurofibromatosis. Electron microscopic confirmation of their melanocytic origin. *Arch. Ophthalmol.*, **100**, 1635–40.

Reubi, F. (1944) Les vaisseaux et les glandes endocrines dans la neurofibromatose. *Schweiz. Z. Pathol. Bakteriol.*, **7**, 168–236.

Riccardi, V.M. (1981) Von Recklinghausen neurofibromatosis. *N. Engl. J. Med.*, **305**, 1617–26.

Riccardi, V.M. and Mulvihill, J.J. (1981) Neurofibromatosis (von Recklinghausen disease). Genetics, cell biology, and biochemistry, Vol. 29, in

Advances in Neurology (eds V.M. Riccardi and J.J. Mulvihill), Raven Press, New York.

Riccardi, V.M. and Eichner, J.E. (eds) (1986) *Neurofibromatosis. Phenotype, Natural History and Pathogenesis,* Johns Hopkins University Press, Baltimore.

Rodriguez, H.A. and Berthrong, M. (1966) Multiple primary intracranial tumors in von Recklinghausen's neurofibromatosis. *Arch. Neurol.*, **14**, 467–75.

Rosman, N.P. and Pearce, J. (1967) The brain in multiple neurofibromatosis (von Recklinghausen's disease): a suggested neuropathological basis for the associated mental defect. *Brain,* **90**, 829–37.

Rubenstein, A.E. (1986) Neurofibromatosis. A review of the clinical problem, in *Neurofibromatosis,* vol. 486 (ed. A.E. Rubenstein, R.P. Bunge and D.E. Housman), New York Academy of Sciences, New York, pp. 1–13.

Rubenstein, A.E. *et al.* (1984) Neurological complications in 250 cases of neurofibromatosis. *Ann. Neurol.*, **16**(1), 133.

Rubinstein, L.J. (1963) Tumeurs et hamartomes dans la neurofibromatose centrale, in *Les Phakomatoses Cérébrales* (ed. L. Michaux and M. Feld), SPEI Editeurs, Paris, France, pp. 427–51.

Rubinstein, L.J. (1972) Tumors of the central nervous system, in *Atlas of Tumor Pathology,* 2nd series, fascicle 6, Armed Forces Institute of Pathology, Washington, D.C.

Rubinstein, L.J. (1986) The malformative central nervous system lesions in the central and peripheral forms of neurofibromatosis. A neuropathological study of 22 cases, in *Neurofibromatosis,* vol. 486 (eds A.E. Rubenstein, R.P. Bunge and D.E. Housman), New York Academy of Sciences, New York, pp. 14–29.

Russell, D.S. and Rubinstein, L.J. (1977) *Pathology of Tumours of the Nervous System,* 4th edn, Edward Arnold, London.

Russell, D.S. and Rubinstein, L.J. (1989) *Pathology of Tumours of the Nervous System,* 5th edn, Edward Arnold, London, pp. 766–808.

Schwechheimer, K. (1986) Nervale Tumormarker (neural tumor markers). *Verh. Dtsch. Ges. Pathol.*, **70**, 82–103.

Seizinger, B.R., Martuza, R.L. and Gusella, J.F. (1986) Loss of genes on chromosome 22 in tumorigenesis of human acoustic neuroma. *Nature,* **322**, 644–7.

Seizinger, B.R. *et al.* (1987a) Common pathogenetic mechanism of three tumor types in bilateral acoustic neurofibromatosis. *Science,* **236**, 317–19.

Seizinger, B.R. *et al.* (1987b) Genetic linkage of von Recklinghausen neurofibromatosis to the nerve growth factor receptor gene. *Cell,* **49**, 589–94.

Sian, C.S. and Ryan, S.F. (1981) The ultrastructure of neurilemmoma with emphasis on Antoni B tissue. *Hum. Pathol.*, **12**, 145–60.

Smith, T.W. and Bhawan, J. (1980) Tactile-like structures in neurofibromas: an ultrastructural study. *Acta Neuropathol.* (Berlin), **50**, 233–6.

Stefansson, K., Wollmann, R. and Jerkovic, M. (1982) S-100 protein in soft-tissue tumors derived from Schwann cells and melanocytes. *Am. J. Pathol.*, **106**, 261–8.

Stern, J., DiGiacinto, G.V. and Housepian, E.M. (1979) Neurofibromatosis and optic glioma: clinical and morphological correlations. *Neurosurgery,* **4**, 524–8.

Stewart, T.J., Liland, J. and Schuknecht, H.G. (1975) Occult schwannomas of the vestibular nerve. *Arch. Otolaryngol.*, **101**, 91–5.

Takahashi, K. *et al.* (1984) Immunohistochemical study on the distribution of a and b subunits of S-100 protein in human neoplasm and normal tissues. *Virchows Arch. [B],* **45**, 385–96.

Trofatter, J.A. *et al.* (1993) A novel moisein-, erzin- radixin-like gene is a candidate for the neurofibromatosis 2 tumour suppressor. *Cell,* **2**, 791–800.

von Recklinghausen, F. (1882) Über die multiplen Fibrome der Haut und ihre

Beziehung zu den multiplen Neuromen, in *Virchow Festschrift*. A, Hirschwald, Berlin.

Waardenburg, P.J. (1918) Heterochrome en melanosis. *Ned. Tijdschr. Geneeskd*, **2**, 1453–5.

Walker, A.E. (1941) Astrocytosis arachnoideae cerebelli. A rare manifestation of von Recklinghausen's neurofibromatosis. *Arch. Neurol. Psychiatry*, **45**, 520–32.

Watabe, K. *et al.* (1983) Tactile-like corpuscles in neurofibromas: immunohistochemical demonstration of S-100 protein. *Acta Neuropathol.*, **61**, 173–7.

Weiss, S.W., Langloss, J.M. and Enzinger, F.M. (1983) Value of S-100 protein in the diagnosis of soft tissue tumors with particular reference to benign and malignant Schwann cell tumors. *Lab. Invest.*, **49**, 299–308.

Weller, R.O. and Cervós-Navarro, J. (1977) *Pathology of Peripheral Nerves*, Butterworths, London.

Wertelecki, W. *et al.* (1988) Neurofibromatosis 2: clinical and linkage studies of a large kindred. *N. Engl. J. Med.*, **319**, 278–83.

Wiestler, O.D. *et al.* (1989) Distribution and immunoreactivity of cerebral micro-hamartomas in bilateral acoustic neurofibromatosis (neurofibromatosis 2). *Acta Neuropathol.*, **79**, 137–43.

Wishart, J.H. (1822) Case of tumours in the skull, dura mater and brain. *Edinburgh Med. Surg. J.*, **18**, 393–7.

Wolter, J.R. and Butler, R.G. (1963) Pigment spots of the iris and ectropion uveae with glaucoma in neurofibromatosis. *Am. J. Ophthalmol.*, **56**, 964–73.

Woodruff, J.M. (1976) Peripheral nerve tumors showing glandular differentiation (glandular schwannomas). *Cancer*, **37**, 2399–413.

Worster-Drought, C., Dickson, W.E.C. and McMenemey, W.H. (1937) Multiple meningeal and perineurial tumors with analogous changes in the glia and ependyma (neurofibroblastomatosis). *Brain*, **60**, 85–117.

Xu, G. *et al.* (1990) The neurofibromatosis type 1 gene encodes a protein related to GAP. *Cell*, **62**, 599–608.

7

Neurofibromatosis 1: a clinical and genetic overview

S.M. Huson

7.1 INTRODUCTION

Neurofibromatosis 1 (NF1) is one of the commonest autosomal dominant disorders in man with an estimated birth incidence of 1 in 2500 to 3300 (Crowe, Schull and Neel, 1956; Huson *et al.*, 1989). The major features of the disease are café au lait spots, peripheral neurofibromas and Lisch nodules (pigmented iris hamartomas). The morbidity and mortality caused by NF1 are largely dictated by the occurrence of complications, which are numerous and can involve any of the body systems (Table 7.1). Whether or not complications will occur cannot be predicted, even within families. At the present time there is no specific preventative treatment for any of the disease features.

7.2 DISEASE PREVALENCE

Although major prevalence studies have only been undertaken in populations of Caucasian origin, the medical literature contains case reports from all parts of the world. There is nothing to suggest that the prevalence of NF1 is not similar throughout the world, except in certain populations where other effects may have increased prevalence (Fuller, Cox and Gardner, 1989). I undertook a population-based study of NF1 in southeast Wales (Huson, Harper and Compston, 1988; Huson *et al.*, 1989) and found a prevalence between 1 in 4150 to 4950 or approximately 20 per 100 000 of population. Case ascertainment included exhaustive searches of medical records from hospitals within the study area and contacts with general practitioners and hospital consultants. When possible I confirmed the diagnosis by personal examination. Despite this I probably did not ascertain those affected children who were new mutations and had no complications. I have taken this possible under-ascertainment into

Table 7.1 Clinical features of NF1

Major defining features
Café au lait spots ± axillary freckling
Peripheral neurofibromas
Lisch nodules

Minor disease features
Macrocephaly
Short stature

Complications (by body system)
(a) *Nervous system*
Plexiform neurofibromas
Intellectual handicap
Coordination problems
Spinal neurofibromas
Peripheral nerve malignancy
Gliomas (particularly optic nerve)
Aqueduct stenosis
Epilepsy
Hypsarrhythmia
(b) *Skeletal*
Scoliosis
Vertebral scalloping
Lateral thoracic meningocele
Lambdoid suture defects
Pseudoarthrosis of distal long bones
(c) *Genitourinary*
Neurofibromas
Pelvic rhabdomyosarcoma
(d) *Endocrine*

Duodenal carcinoid
(e) *Cardiovascular*
Hypertension
Renal artery stenosis
Intracranial artery stenosis
(f) *Respiratory*
Neurofibromas of oral cavity, larynx, mediastinum
(g) *Gastrointestinal*
Visceral neurofibromas
(h) *Haematopoietic*
Atypical forms of childhood leukaemia
(i) *Skin*
Juvenile xanthogranuloma

account in estimating the upper range of prevalence. The results of the five other surveys are summarized in Table 7.2.

Three of the four most recent surveys, which used similar methods, showed prevalence rates within the same range. However, a study in New Zealand (Fuller, Cox and Gardner, 1989) showed a higher prevalence, which the authors believed to be due to studying a small population. Their patients were descended from a small group of ancestors with a disproportionate number of NF1 heterozygotes, who passed the gene onto several offspring. If only six or seven of the recent founders of the larger families had not lived in Dunedin, the prevalence of NF1 would have been similar to other studies. A Russian study (Sergeyev, 1975) relied on detection of café au lait spots in a population study of 16 year olds undergoing premilitary examination. Those with a significant number of lesions were referred for the survey. Although this method should have identified all males in this age group, irrespective of state of health, the prevalence discovered was low, suggesting a significant underestimation.

The only way of obtaining the true birth incidence of NF1 would be to follow a cohort of children from birth, which has not been done. Several of the large studies have estimated birth incidence as shown in Table 7.2. The difference between birth incidence and prevalence suggests that patients with NF1 die prematurely. All the studies that analysed prevalence in relation to age showed a decreased prevalence in the older age groups (Samuelsson and Axelsson, 1981; Huson, Harper and Compston, 1988; Fuller, Cox and Gardner 1989; Clementi *et al.*, 1990).

7.3 CLINICAL FEATURES

7.3.1 Major defining features

Café au lait spots, peripheral neurofibromas and Lisch nodules are the features of NF1 that consistently develop in the majority of affected individuals. They form the basis of the National Institutes of Health (NIH) diagnostic criteria other than complications relatively specific to NF1 (Table 1.2).

(a) Café au lait spots and freckling

Café au lait spots are not unique to NF1 sufferers. Crowe and Schull (1953) reported that 690 of 6853 (10.1%) institutionalized patients with no other features of NF1 had up to five café au lait spots; the majority (684/690) had one to three lesions, four had four lesions and only two had five lesions. Burwell, James and Johnston (1982) reported that 25.3% of 732 children aged 4–11 years had one to three lesions, and Kopf *et al.* (1985) observed

Table 7.2 Summary of estimates of prevalence and mutation rate for NF1

Study (year, country)	*Method of ascertainment*	*Prevalence*	*Estimated birth incidence*	*Mutation rate (method)*
Crowe, Schull and Neel (1956, USA)	Surveys of general hospital admissions and state mental institutions	–	1/2500–3300	$1.4–2.6 \times 10^{-4}$ (direct) $0.7–0.9 \times 10^{-4}$ (indirect) $f = 0.53$
Sergeyev (1975, USSR)	Population sample of 16-year-old youths	1/7800	–	$4.4–4.9 \times 10^{-5}$ (direct)
Samuelsson and Axelsson (1981, Sweden)	Population based	1/4600	–	4.3×10^{-5} (direct)
Huson *et al.* (1989, UK)	Population based	1/4150–4950	1/2558	$3.07–5.01 \times 10^{-5}$ (direct) $6.62–10.36 \times 10^{-5}$ (indirect) $f = 0.47$
Fuller, Cox and Gardner (1989, New Zealand)	Population based	1/2062–2190	–	–
Clementi *et al.* (1990, Italy)	Population based	1/6711	1/4292[a]	6.5×10^{-5} (direct)

[a] I have taken the disease incidence given in this paper for the 0–9 year group to represent an estimate of birth incidence.

the same number in 13.8% of patients attending a private dermatology clinic. Clinically, there are no differences between the café au lait spots in NF1 patients and those in the general population; it is the increased number that is significant. Based on their study, Crowe and Schull (1953) concluded that the presence of six or more café au lait spots of a significant diameter (>1.5 cm) should lead to the presumptive diagnosis of NF1 even in the absence of a family history. This conclusion has stood up remarkably well to the test of time and is the experience of others who have examined large numbers of patients (Huson, Harper and Compston, 1988; Riccardi, 1992). As with any other 'rule' in clinical medicine, there are occasional exceptions and some affected individuals have only four or five café au lait spots; these are usually older people with other disease features. The number of café au lait spots decreases with age (Crowe, Schull and Neel, 1956; Huson, Harper and Compston, 1988; Riccardi, 1992). In assessing young patients with only one or two café au lait spots in association with a few peripheral nerve tumours, the clinician should consider the possible diagnosis of neurofibromatosis 2 (NF2), the other well-defined form of neurofibromatosis.

Café au lait spots are the first manifestations of the disease and may be present at birth. They increase in number throughout childhood, but appear to stop increasing or even decrease in adulthood. In my study (Huson, Harper and Compston, 1988), parents had noted café au lait spots for the first time within the first year of life (82%) and by the age of 4 years in all affected children. In the few individuals at risk that I have followed prospectively from birth, the majority who turned out to be affected had some café au lait spots, but not necessarily six or more, by the age of 1 year.

Café au lait spots vary in diameter from 0.5 to 50 cm or more, but the majority are less than 10 cm. They usually have smooth contours, but some, particularly the larger ones, have irregular outlines. Their colour intensity varies with background skin pigmentation. In children with very pale complexions, café au lait spots may be very difficult to recognize and are best assessed with an ultraviolet lamp. Figure 7.1 shows typical café au lait spots in a young child. Various investigators have examined café au lait spots in NF1 to look for features specific to the disease. Benedict *et al.* (1968) reported that the café au lait spots of patients with NF1 showed large numbers of giant pigment macules (now termed melanin macroglobules); they were also present, though less frequent, in normal skin. Melanin macroglobules are not specific to NF1, being occasionally found in normal people and more frequently in other disorders including Albright's syndrome, Leopard syndrome and xeroderma pigmentosum (Fitzpatrick and Martuza, 1986). To discover whether melanin macroglobules could be used as a diagnostic marker for NF1, Martuza *et al.* (1985) undertook a light microscope study of café au

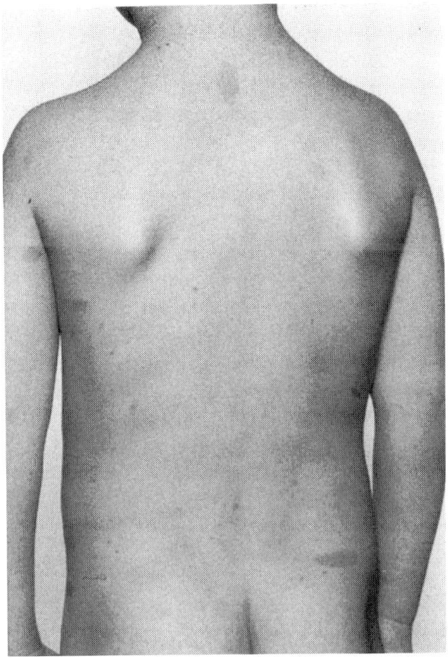

Figure 7.1 Typical appearance of café au lait spots in a child. (Reproduced from *Clinical Neurology* by permission of Churchill Livingstone.)

lait spots in NF1 sufferers and normal individuals. The café au lait spots in NF1 had significantly more melanin macroglobules than those in normal subjects. However, all the NF1 patients were at least 16 years of age, when other NF1 features are usually present. Riccardi (1992) reported that café au lait spots from two children with NF1 showed only occasional melanin macroglobules. Melanin macroglobules probably increase with age and are not a useful diagnostic marker of NF1 in young children, the time when such a marker is most needed.

The other characteristic pigmentation, which appears to be unique to NF1, is freckling in the axilla, and other sites of skin apposition. Crowe (1964) first described axillary freckling in NF1. Riccardi, in various publications summarized in his book (Riccardi, 1992), has drawn attention to freckling in other areas, particularly the base of the neck, groins and submammary regions in women. In obese people with NF1, freckles can be seen between skin folds. In some patients with NF1 there seems to be no demarcation in the zones of freckling between these areas, and the patients have small freckles all over the trunk and proximal extremities. The freckles resemble café au lait spots, and are 1–3 mm in diameter and histologically similar (Johnson and Charneco, 1970; Figure 7.2). They appear after the café au lait spots; the youngest patient with axillary

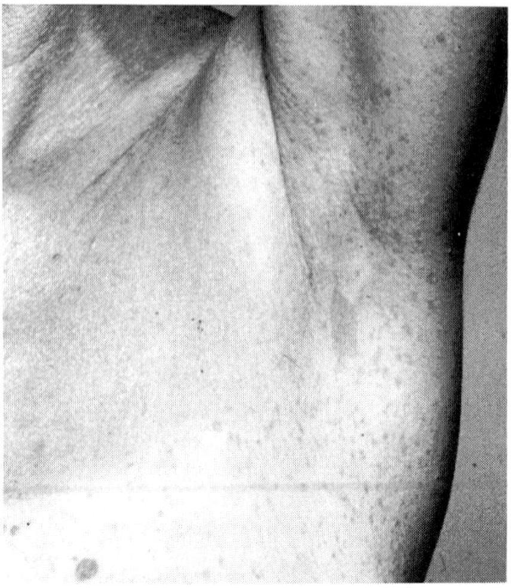

Figure 7.2 Axillary freckling.

freckling in my population study was 3 years of age. Freckling was present in the axilla in 67% and in the inguinal region in 44% of my patients. Twenty-nine per cent of women aged more than 20 years had submammary freckling (Huson, Harper and Compston, 1988). Total 'trunk freckling' seemed less frequent, but the exact number was not documented. All forms of skin crease freckling were most prevalent in young adults (Table 7.3).

Table 7.3 Percentage of patients with each of the major defining features by age in the southeast Wales study

Age (years)	*Number of cases*	*Café au lait spots (%)*	*Axillary freckling (%)*	*Cutaneous neurofibromas (%)*	*Lisch nodules (%)*
0–5	7	100	14	0	66
6–10	14	100	50	14	82
11–15	21	100	62	33	71
16–20	14	93	86	93	100
21–30	28	93	75	100	90
31–40	26	89	92	100	96
41–50	13	62	77	100	88
51–60	13	77	69	100	100
61–70	13	62	62	100	88
71–85	6	0	67	100	100

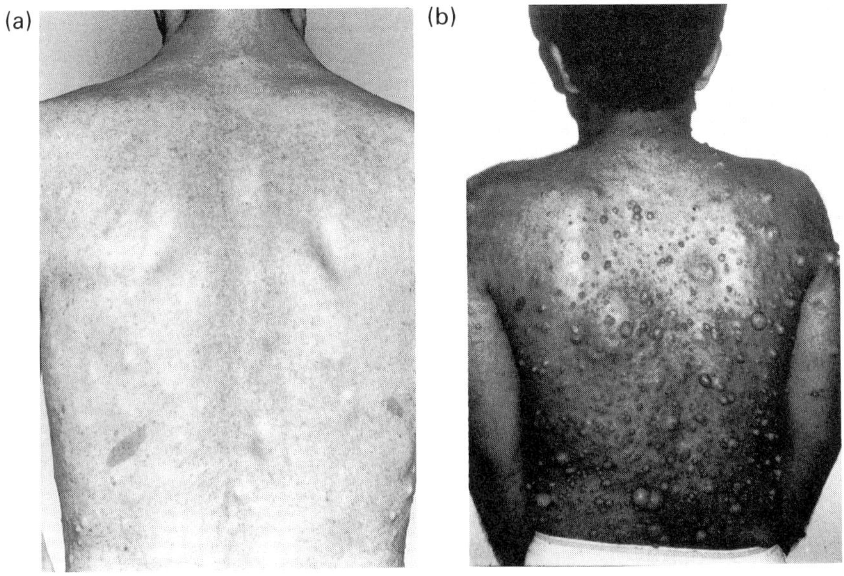

Figure 7.3 Dermal neurofibromas: the number of these lesions is very variable (a) A 42-year-old man with an 'average' number of neurofibromas. (Reproduced from Huson, Harper and Compston (1988) by permission of Oxford University Press.) (b) A severely affected 31-year-old man.

(b) Peripheral neurofibromas

On clinical assessment, I distinguish dermal and nodular peripheral neurofibromas. Dermal neurofibromas lie within the dermis and epidermis, move passively with the skin, and are present in most adults with NF1. The majority are discrete nodules with a characteristic violaceous colour, feel soft, almost gelatinous and vary from 0.1 cm to several centimetres in diameter. In older patients and in those with very numerous lesions, some usually become papillomatous and larger. Figure 7.3 shows their typical appearance. Dermal neurofibromas are found mainly on the trunk and are only present in large numbers on exposed areas of the body in more severe cases. Only 18% of my patients had obvious lesions on the head and neck.

Dermal neurofibromas develop after the café au lait spots. My youngest patient with dermal neurofibromas was 7 years of age. The number of neurofibromas is only roughly proportional to age. Severely and mildly affected cases can be seen in all age groups from the teens onwards. In my population study all the adults over the age of 20 years had dermal neurofibromas. However, some older people satisfy the diagnostic criteria for NF1 but do not have dermal neurofibromas even at quite an advanced age. These people seem to be the exception rather than the rule. With the increasing awareness of NF1 I am being referred an increasing but small number of at-risk relatives who just have pigmentary changes even in adult life. There seems to be no way to predict who will develop many unsightly neurofibromas and who very few.

Dermal neurofibromas are the only one of the major disease features to cause symptoms or morbidity. A small but significant group of patients complain of pruritus overlying the lesions (21% of cases in the author's study); the lesions are rarely painful. Although most patients with NF1 seem to come to terms with their lesions, some are persistently distressed by their appearance. Women with NF1 often comment that their neurofibromas increase in size and number during pregnancy. Some observe that there is partial regression after delivery of the baby. In my series, 33% of parous women commented on an exacerbation during pregnancy. Dermal neurofibromas rarely, if at all, undergo sarcomatous change, but it is sensible to remove rapidly enlarging painful lesions. Haemorrhage into a neurofibroma may cause sudden painful enlargement (Francis and Mackie, 1987; Poston *et al.*, 1990).

Nodular neurofibromas develop in a minority of NF1 patients. They arise from the major peripheral nerve trunks and have a much firmer consistency and more defined margins than dermal neurofibromas. I think about 5% of NF1 patients have nodular neurofibromas, but no-one has recorded them systematically. When present, they may give rise to neurological symptoms, which rarely occur with true dermal lesions. Pressure on nodular neurofibromas may give rise to paraesthesiae. Removal of nodular neurofibromas is more difficult than for dermal neurofibromas because of major nerve trunk involvement, and requires the expertise of a surgeon experienced in peripheral nerve surgery.

Plexiform neurofibromas, which are diffuse tumours associated with hypertrophy of surrounding tissue, occur in about a third of patients and are described in section 7.3.3.

(c) Lisch nodules

Lisch nodules are harmless iris hamartomas (Chapter 10). Because of their development during childhood (Table 7.3), after the café au lait spots but before peripheral neurofibromas, Lisch nodules are useful for confirming the diagnosis in children with no family history and only multiple café au lait spots. They are also useful in distinguishing the different forms of neurofibromatosis (Chapters 1 and 19).

(d) Age of appearance of major defining features

Table 7.3 shows the percentage of patients in my Welsh series with each of the three major defining features and axillary freckling at different ages. The only group where definite diagnosis can be difficult is the children with multiple café au lait spots, no family history and no other disease features. Even in the absence of Lisch nodules, follow-up studies of cohorts of children with this presentation show that the majority of them eventually satisfy the diagnostic criteria for NF1 (Pollak *et al.*, 1992; Korf, 1992).

7.3.2 Minor disease features

Included as minor disease features are those that occur in quite a high proportion of NF1 patients but are not so specific to NF1 that they can be used as a diagnostic criterion. None of them are associated with significant morbidity.

(a) *Macrocephaly*

Large heads, or macrocephaly, are now a well-recognized feature of NF1 (Chapter 8) and occurred in 45% of my Welsh population (Huson, Harper and Compston, 1988).

(b) *Short stature*

Riccardi (1981) first reported that a significant proportion of NF1 patients have short stature. Follow-up studies of his patients have confirmed this (Riccardi, 1992). In my Welsh series (Huson, 1989), after excluding those with skeletal complications of the disease and identified unrelated causes of short stature, 31.5% (39/124) individuals were at or below the third centile for height. The heights of affected individuals were converted to standard deviation scores (SDS), using the data of Tanner and Whitehouse (1976), by the formula:

$$\mathrm{SDS} = \frac{X - X_1}{\mathrm{SD}}$$

where X is the patient's height, X_1 the population mean for that age and SD the population standard deviation. The SDS for affected individuals was -1.20 ± 1.07 and for normal siblings -0.12 ± 1.02 ($p = 0.001$ by unpaired *t*-testing). There was no significant difference between sexes. These results imply that affected males are 8 cm under expected height and females 7.62 cm, purely on the basis of having NF1. Two of the patients in the study population had had full endocrinological investigations for short stature and no abnormalities were detected. Occasional patients with short stature and NF1 have growth disturbance as a result of pituitary/hypothalamic involvement from an optic chiasm tumour. These cases are exceptional. The cause of short stature in the majority of NF1 patients is unknown.

(c) Less well-defined minor disease features

A number of additional features have been observed by clinicians who assess a large number of NF1 patients. Although their significance is uncertain, their description should stimulate future systematic study and may offer clues to the function of the NF1 gene.

In one study, Campbell de Morgan spots or angiomas were more frequent in NF1. These are cherry or ruby in colour, round or oval in shape and 1 mm to at most a few millimetres in diameter. They are slightly raised from the skin and are most common on the trunk, abdomen and thighs. They do not cause symptoms and become more frequent with age, so that they have also been called senile angiomas (also cherry or ruby angiomas). Wertelecki *et al.* (1988) counted the number of Campbell de Morgan spots in NF1 patients, a cohort of unaffected relatives and in unrelated US Caucasians. The NF1 patients had significantly more lesions at all ages than either of the control groups. Wertelecki *et al.* (1988) speculated that in the general population the appearance of Campbell de Morgan spots is age related and that in NF1, whatever mechanism prevents them occurring earlier in the normal population, is disturbed. Their distribution was similar to that of café au lait spots and dermal neurofibromas, i.e. predominantly on the trunk and proximal extremities. Since these are warmer parts of the body, their appearance might be related to temperature. I have not noted Campbell de Morgan spots as a major feature in any of my patients. However, Wertelecki considered five such spots as significant and this might be missed on routine examination. Campbell de Morgan spots need to be assessed in other large NF1 populations.

Some clinicians have commented that the general appearance of NF1 patients is somewhat abnormal and question whether NF1 is associated with facial dysmorphism in addition to that caused by some disease complications. These features, like the other minor disease features, are not specific for NF1 and, unlike height and head circumference, are difficult to measure objectively.

The combination of short stature, macrocephaly and slight clumsiness no doubt contributes to an overall NF1 phenotype in some affected individuals. Some children with NF1 also have facial dysmorphic features which form a recurring pattern. This has led some authors to suggest that there may be a specific NF1 facial phenotype. I find that these features are similar to those seen in mild Noonan's syndrome, with slight ptosis, mild hypertelorism, down-slanting palpebral fissures and posteriorly rotated ears. Because some of my own patients with these features have an affected parent or sibling without them, I do not believe that this is part of a specific neurofibromatosis–Noonan phenotype as Opitz and Weaver (1985) suggested, but that in some cases NF1 is associated with these features as part of the disease process. Kaplan and Rosenblatt (1985), reporting patients with NF1 and some Noonan facial features, drew similar conclusions. Pectus excavatum is another dysmorphic feature seen in NF1 and Noonan's syndrome, and was present in 31% (209/675) of Riccardi's patients (1992).

Another general feature of NF1 patients observed by myself and others (J.G. Hall, personal communication, 1989; Riccardi, 1992) is generalized skin hyperpigmentation, underlying the more intense café au lait spots. Evidence that this is one of the effects of the NF1 gene itself comes from some of my series of patients with segmental NF (unpublished data). In the affected areas of skin, the whole segment is darker in colour than the rest of the body, with the NF1 features superimposed within the darker segment.

Finally I and others (Riccardi, 1992) have noted possible effects of the NF1 gene on connective tissue. The faces of some NF1 patients look prematurely old; the darker skin colour may contribute to this, but the skin also seems excessively lax. In addition, craniofacial surgeons (M. Poole, personal observation, 1992) are often disappointed with the outcome of surgery in NF1 and feel that this is partly related to a generalized connective tissue abnormality, rather than the specific local lesion that had precipitated surgery.

7.3.3 Complications of NF1

(a) Overview of frequency of complications

If the NF1 phenotype simply consisted of the features described so far in this chapter, the appearance of the skin would be regarded as distressing by some affected individuals, but otherwise the disease would not be considered a major problem. The complications make NF1 a disease with significant morbidity and mortality. The complications only occur in a proportion of individuals and their occurrence cannot be predicted, even within families, so that NF1 is an extremely difficult disease for patients to accept and for doctors to manage. Achieving the balance between appropriate disease monitoring and creating unnecessary anxiety is difficult for the physician to achieve. This situation was compounded by the fact that until relatively recently we had no accurate data about the frequency of complications. Even now we have limited information about the natural history of NF1. For example, does the occurrence of any one complication in childhood predict that another will develop later?

Table 7.4 Prevalence of selected major disease complications in large surveys of NF1

	Borberg (1951)	*Crowe, Schull and Neel (1956)*	*Brasfield and Das Gupta (1972)*	*Carey, Laub and Hall (1979)*	*Samuelsson (1981)*	*Riccardi (1992)*	*Huson, Harper and Compston (1988)*
Method of case ascertainment	Hospital records	Hospital records and family studies	Hospital records	Genetic clinic records	Population based	Cases referred to special interest clinic	Population based
Diagnostic criteria adequate for excluding other forms of neurofibromatosis	Probably	No	Criteria not stated	No	NF2, yes; other forms, no	Yes	Yes
Number of cases	84	223	110	131	74	953	135
Age range	All ages	All ages	All ages	All ages	Adults only	All ages	All ages
Prevalence of complication (%)							
Plexiform neurofibroma	16	16	NS	NS	22	39	32
CNS tumours	10	3	8	7[a]	0	15[b]	2
Vestibular Schwannoma	1	5	0	NS[a]	0	0	0
Peripheral nerve malignancy	1	2	29	0	3	4	2

NS = not stated
[a] Probably includes one case of NF2.
[b] All optic pathway gliomas, two-thirds of which were asymptomatic.

I define a complication of NF1 as any condition that occurs at an increased frequency in patients with the disease compared with the general population. Some of the complications are relatively specific to NF1 such as sphenoid wing dysplasia. Others are seen as isolated problems in the general population (e.g. scoliosis and the malignancies related to NF1), and here the question is whether there is actually an increased frequency in NF1 patients and if so how great is the increase. Purists may argue that some of the things that I describe as disease complications would be better classified as disease associations (e.g. juvenile xanthogranulomas), but such a distinction complicates the issue unnecessarily.

From an historical perspective, clinical reports of complications affecting most of the body systems began to appear in the literature soon after NF1 was recognized as a distinct entity (von Recklinghausen, 1882). The multiplicity of reports made it obvious that some conditions occurred with an increased frequency in NF1 patients. As Dr Mulvihill points out in Chapter 12, the problem is that case reports do not provide a denominator that permits quantification of the risk of a particular complication developing in an individual.

The first large clinical studies of NF1 of Borberg (1951) and Crowe, Schull and Neel (1956) identified the spectrum and frequency of disease complications. Since that time there have been five further major studies (Brasfield and Das Gupta, 1972; Carey, Laub and Hall, 1979; Samuelsson, 1981; Riccardi and Eichner, 1986; Huson, Harper and Compston, 1988; Riccardi, 1992). Table 7.4 shows the frequency of selected complications in these studies. Comparison of the studies highlights some of the problems with these cross-sectional studies in describing the true frequency of complications. In some of the studies no distinction was made between NF1 and other forms of neurofibromatosis (Crowe, Schull and Neel, 1956; Carey, Laub and Hall, 1979; Samuelsson, 1981). The frequency found for the occurrence of vestibular Schwannoma highlights this particular problem. The study of Crowe, Schull and Neel is often cited as showing that 5% of patients with NF1 developed vestibular Schwannomas. When their data are reviewed, none of the patients with definite vestibular Schwannoma would satisfy the NIH diagnostic criteria for NF1 and all probably had NF2. The other major problem with some of the studies is that as the samples were not population-based, the frequency of complications may represent an overestimate, resulting from referral of more severely affected cases to specialists (Borberg, 1951; Brasfield and Das Gupta, 1972; Carey, Laub and Hall, 1979; Riccardi, 1992). This is best exemplified by the frequency of peripheral nerve malignancy of 29% in the study of Brasfield and Das Gupta. This very high figure is explained by the fact that one of the two hospitals from which they obtained their patients was a specialist cancer hospital. I was aware of these problems when embarking on my study in southeast

Table 7.5 Frequency of NF1 complications in 135 cases ascertained through the author's population-based study in southeast Wales (Huson, Harper and Compston, 1988; Huson, Compston and Harper, 1989; Huson, 1989)

Complication	*Number (%) of all cases <18 years of age (n = 39, unless stated)*	*Number (%) of cases ≥ 18 years of age (n = 96, unless stated)*	*Percentage frequency of complications overall*
Plexiform neurofibromas			
All lesions	17 (43.6)	23/86 (26.7)	30.0
Large lesions of head and neck	3 (7.7)	1/86 (1.2)	3.0
Limb/trunk lesions associated with significant skin/bone hypertrophy	2 (5.1)	5/86 (5.8)	5.6
Education			
Special school education	1/34 (2.9)	12/90 (13.3)	10.5
Remedial class education	8/34 (23.5)	13/90 (14.4)	16.9
Normal education, specific learning difficulties	2/34 (5.9)	5/90 (5.6)	5.6
Epilepsy			
No known cause	2 (5.1)	4 (4.2)	4.4
Secondary to disease complications	0	3 (3.1)	2.2
Hypsarrhythmia	1 (2.6)	1 (1.0)	1.5
Symptomatic CNS tumours (including optic glioma)	2 (5.1)	2–3/138 (1.5–2.2)	1.5–2.2
Spinal neurofibromas	0	2 (2.1)	1.5
Acoustic neuroma	0	0	0
Aqueduct stenosis	0	2 (2.1)	1.5
Meningioangiomatosis[a]	0	1 (1.0)	0.7
Malignancy secondary to NF1 (peripheral nerve tumours, pelvic rhabdomyosarcoma)	0	4/138 (2.9)	2.9
Scoliosis			
Requiring surgery	1 (2.6)	5 (5.2)	4.4
Less severe	1 (2.6)	6 (6.3)	5.2

Table 7.5 Continued

Complication	*Number (%) of all cases <18 years of age (n = 39, unless stated)*	*Number (%) of cases ⩾ 18 years of age (n = 96, unless stated)*	*Percentage frequency of complications overall*
Pseudoarthrosis of tibia and fibula			
Resulting in non-union and eventual below-knee amputation	1 (2.6)	2 (2.1)	2.2
Less severe forms	1 (2.6)	1 (1.0)	1.5
Lambdoid suture defect	0	1 (1.0)	0.7
Gastrointestinal neurofibromas	1 (2.6)	2 (2.1)	2.2
Renal artery stenosis	0	2 (2.1)	1.5
Phaeochromocytoma	0	1 (1.0)	0.7
Duodenal carcinoid	0	2 (2.1)	1.5
Delayed puberty (no underlying cause)[b]	–	2 (2.1)	1.5
Congenital glaucoma	0	1 (1.0)	0.7
Juvenile xanthogranuloma	1 (2.6)	0	0.7
Complications (which would have been symptomatic) not seen in study population but definitely associated with NF1			
Sphenoid wing dysplasia			
Atypical forms of childhood leukaemia		Presumed frequency ⩽1%	
Cerebrovascular disease			

[a] Diagnosis of NF1 now uncertain.
[b] Possibility incidence not increased above general population.

Wales, and, although I admit to bias (!), my study is the only one so far that clearly distinguishes NF1 from other forms of neurofibromatosis and tried to assess an unbiased population. Even then it has to be acknowledged that mildly affected individuals would have been easily missed. The only way to establish the true frequency of complications in NF1 would be to follow populations of NF1 patients and their offspring for a number of years.

Table 7.5 shows the frequency of all the complications found in the southeast Wales population. The disease complications not seen in the study population, which would have been symptomatic if present, are also listed; their presumed frequency is equal to or less than 1%. In addition, other complications are relatively specific to NF1 but asymptomatic, and would not have been detected by my study, which relied on clinical symptoms. These include scalloping of the lumbar vertebrae and anterior spinal meningoceles. Riccardi (1992) reported vertebral scalloping in 10% (41/404) of patients who had had lumbar spine radiographs. In one of my patients dural ectasia caused vertebral scalloping and symptomatic nerve root compression. The frequency of anterior spinal meningoceles is unknown but they rarely cause symptomatic root or cord compression.

Since my previous report, I have decided that two possible complications should be deleted. The first concerns possible abnormalities of sexual development. The frequency of delayed puberty in my series was within the normal limits for the general population. Riccardi (1992), in his most recent review, reported premature puberty in several patients but always secondary to CNS complications. He concluded that premature or delayed puberty is not definitely associated with NF1. Secondly, in my original series I reported a case of NF1 with meningioangiomatosis. On reviewing the literature in preparing for this book, I realized that most previous cases of meningioangiomatosis had occurred in cases of NF2 not NF1. My patient was 53 years of age when assessed, had 16 café au lait spots, no abnormal freckling and approximately 50 dermal neurofibromas; Lisch nodules were not sought. He had had a previous cervical spine neurofibroma removed, but had no clinical evidence of vestibular Schwannomas. His father was said by the family to have had café au lait spots and skin tumours but no other disease complications. Although this patient satisfied the diagnostic criteria for NF1, the fact he had a cervical neurofibroma and meningioangiomatosis raises the possibility of one of the more unusual forms of neurofibromatosis.

(b) Some clinical complications (not specifically discussed elsewhere)

Plexiform neurofibromas

In the older NF1 literature, the descriptive terms of elephantiasis neuromatosa or fibroma pendulum were used to describe very large plexiform neurofibromas (Borberg, 1951; Crowe, Schull and Neel, 1956). Plexiform neurofibromas are distinct clinically and pathologically from dermal neurofibromas. They usually present as large subcutaneous swellings (diffuse plexiform neurofibromas) with ill-defined margins varying from a few centimetres in diameter to those involving a whole area of the body (Figure 7.4). Their consistency is usually soft, although occasionally hypertrophied nerve trunks can be palpated within the mass. The skin overlying the lesion is often abnormal (23 out of 45 of the

(a)

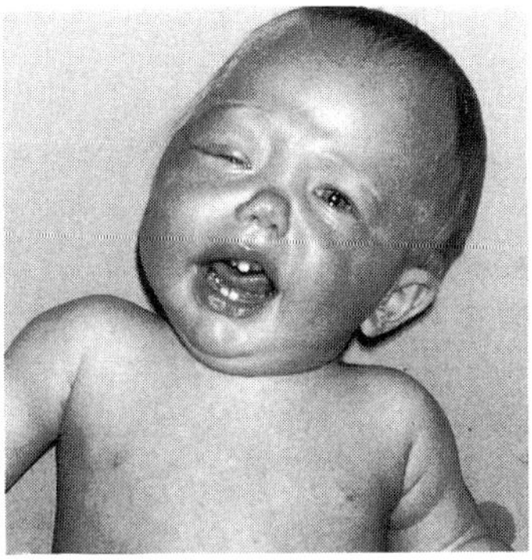

(b)

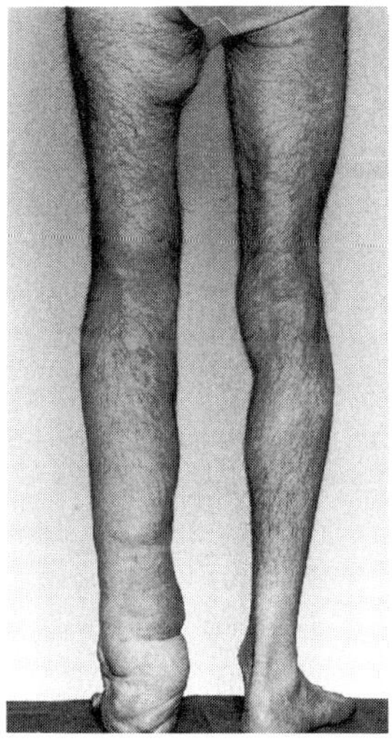

(c)

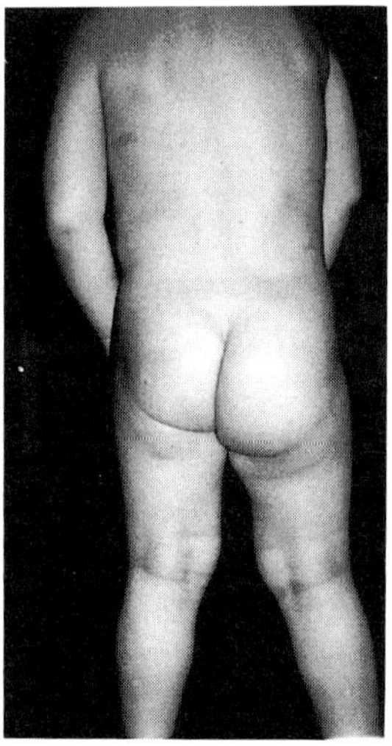

Figure 7.4 Plexiform neurofibromas. (a) Facial plexiform neurofibroma in a 2-month-old girl (used with permission). (b) Plexiform neurofibroma of left leg, associated with limb overgrowth, in a 38-year-old man. He had required epiphyseal plating of the tibia to prevent further overgrowth as a teenager. (c) Plexiform neurofibroma causing localized buttock overgrowth in a 3-year-old child.

lesions in my series) owing to a combination of hypertrophy, café au lait pigmentation or hypertrichosis. The age at which these lesions appear is also quite different from dermal neurofibromas. The largest, most significant plexiform neurofibromas are all probably obvious on careful clinical examination within the first year or two of life. In my series (Huson, Harper and Compston, 1988) 16 of the 40 cases with plexiform neurofibromas were aged less than 14 years; in eight of these individuals the lesion had been noted within the first year of life. All the large facial lesions were present within the first year.

In the Welsh study, plexiform neurofibromas were most frequent on the trunk (20 out of 45 lesions) followed by the limbs (17/45) and head and neck (8/45). They were rarely symptomatic, but their cosmetic burden was considerable. The specific features associated with plexiform neurofibromas in the region of the eye are discussed in Chapters 10 and 14. Plexiform neurofibromas on a limb may cause hypertrophy of that limb (Chapter 11). The lesions that I have seen on the trunk rarely cause symptoms, but if particularly large may need recurrent surgery to contain their size. Plexiform neurofibromas arising on the buttock or perineum need to be monitored carefully. I have seen several cases where the cutaneous signs indicated a relatively small lesion, but there was extensive internal growth eventually causing ureteric obstruction. Perineal plexiform neurofibromas in young girls with NF1 have occasionally caused sexual ambiguity (Griebel *et al.*, 1991). Plexiform neurofibromas in the neck can be particularly troublesome. I know of two unreported cases in which children were born with obvious neck swellings resulting from diffuse plexiform neurofibromas. If they continue to grow aggressively they can cause respiratory failure and death (Apter *et al.*, 1975; Kimmellman, 1979). Plexiform neurofibromas in the neck involving the cervical spine can erode and deform the vertebrae and compromise the spinal cord (Chapter 8).

In some patients, the plexiform neurofibromas do not present as diffuse subcutaneous swellings. The nerve trunks develop multiple nodular neurofibromas that seem to run into one another, as described by Drs Wiestler and Radner in Chapter 6. Riccardi (1992) describes these as nodular plexiform neurofibromas. Their age at onset is not known definitely; the two patients I have seen became symptomatic in their teens. They are much less frequent than the diffuse plexiform neurofibromas: in the Welsh series, none of the patients had a nodular plexiform neurofibroma. This is the kind of lesion that Smith illustrated so beautifully in his nineteenth century description of the disease (Chapter 1, Figure 1.4b). These tumours involve the peripheral nerve trunks and, in my experience, cause pain much more frequently than diffuse plexiform neurofibromas. It is difficult to remove nodular plexiform neurofibromas surgically without leaving neurological deficit. Plexiform neurofibromas may undergo malignant change as reviewed in section 7.5.

Juvenile xanthogranulomas

Juvenile xanthogranulomas developing in NF1 are clinically and histologically similar to those developing in the general population (Cooper *et al.*, 1984). They present within the first year or two of life as papules or small nodules, usually less than 1 cm in diameter. The lesions usually develop on the head, trunk or extremities and may be single, but are usually multiple. They tend to regress with age. In themselves the xanthogranulomas do not cause significant morbidity, but there is a possible increase in juvenile myeloid leukaemia in children with NF1 and these lesions (Cooper *et al.*, 1984). This connection is reviewed by Drs Viskochil and Carey in Chapter 19. Although the chance of developing myeloid leukaemia, even with xanthogranulomas, is extremely small in NF1, it is prudent to follow children with NF1 and xanthogranuloma more closely during early childhood.

7.3.4 The association of NF1 with other genetic diseases

The NF1 literature includes frequent reports of the coincidental occurrence of NF1 and another genetic disease in one or more family members. These reports may give clues to the gene localization of one of the diseases and to the pathogenesis of the conditions if the phenotypes are altered by their co-existence.

My original research was intended to discover whether the gene for NF1 was on chromosome 19 because of the apparent co-segregation of NF1 and myotonic dystrophy in two families (Ichikawa *et al.*, 1981; Rivas and DiLiberti, 1984). My study showed no evidence of linkage with chromosome 19 markers (Huson *et al.*, 1986) and there was no evidence of any alteration in the phenotype of either disease. Reports of other neurogenetic diseases, particularly hamartomatoses, co-existing with NF1 are particularly frequent. These include tuberous sclerosis (Schull and Crowe, 1953) and von Hippel Lindau disease (Tishler, 1975; Thomas, Schwartz and Gragoudas, 1978). The association with peroneal muscular atrophy may be due in part to the occurrence of neurofibromatou neuropathy (Chapter 8).

A list of all the reported disease associations would need a dedicated chapter. None of the other reports have either given a clue to a gene localization or contributed to understanding the disease pathogenesis of NF1.

7.4 DIFFERENTIAL DIAGNOSIS OF NF1

In the introduction to their classical book, Crowe, Schull and Neel (1956) stated:

> There is much in the literature which suggests the diagnosis of neurofibromatosis is frequently beclouded with uncertainty. Our experience would indicate otherwise.

I have certainly found that the clinical diagnosis of NF1 is usually straightforward. The most common pitfall is distinguishing other forms of neurofibromatosis. It is unusual to see patients with NF1 misdiagnosed as having NF2, but patients with NF2 or one of the rarer forms have often been told originally that they have NF1. The clinical features of NF2 are

Table 7.6 Alternative diagnoses made in 23 out of 119 index referred cases as having NF1 in the study of Huson, Harper and Compston (1988)

Alternative diagnoses	*Number of cases*
Diagnosis	
Multiple lipomas	11
Melanocytic naevi (i.e. not café au lait spots)	1
Steatocystoma multiplex	1
Leopard syndrome	1
Rheumatoid arthritis (nodular)	1
Multiple spinal Schwannomas	1
Other forms of NF	
NF2	1
'Segmental NF' – plexiform NF of left sciatic nerve	1
? 'Late onset' NF – six peripheral neurofibromas, no other features	1
Café au lait pigmentation only	
Mental retardation; three large areas of atypical pigmentation	1
Less than six café au lait spots ($n = 4$, 2 and 1)	3

discussed in Chapter 18 and other forms of neurofibromatosis, including Watson syndrome, in Chapter 19.

There are a number of conditions with which NF1 is occasionally confused. In my Welsh study, 19% (23/119) of the original index cases were found not to have NF1 after further assessment. The alternative diagnoses are summarized in Table 7.6. Sixteen individuals had other diagnoses and three other forms of neurofibromatosis. A further four either had café au lait spots within the limits of the normal population (three cases) or atypical café au lait pigmentation and severe mental retardation for which the cause was not established (one case). One further child 10 months old (not listed in the table) was excluded from the study because her parents were unaffected, and she had no disease features except for 14 café au lait spots. She has gone on to develop other features of NF1. It is hoped with increasing awareness of the different forms of neurofibromatosis that the level of misdiagnosis will gradually decrease. It is disappointing that in the first 2 years of the Oxford neurofibromatosis clinic, 10 out of 120 patients (8%) referred as having NF1 were rediagnosed after assessment at the clinic (four had segmental

NF, one scoliosis with only one café au lait spot, two urticaria pigmentosa, two infantile myofibromatosis and one multiple lipomas). The conditions that can be confused with NF1 are reviewed below; apart from multiple lipomatosis, they are all very rare conditions. Other genetic conditions such as multiple endocrine neoplasia syndromes (Thakker and Ponder, 1988) may have overlapping features (e.g. in type 2B, phaeochromocytomas and the mucosal neuromas), but are not difficult to distinguish clinically. They may share some interesting pathogenetic mechanisms.

7.4.1 Differential diagnosis: conditions with abnormal skin pigmentation

(a) McCune–Albright's syndrome

Patients with this syndrome have areas of café au lait pigmentation in association with polyostotic fibrous dysplasia and sexual precocity (Smith, 1982). The café au lait pigmentation in McCune–Albright's syndrome tends to cover larger areas of the body than in NF1. The borders tend to be more jagged than in NF1 and were compared with the 'coast of Maine' by Albright *et al.* (1937). The smooth borders in NF1 have been compared with the 'coast of California'. Although these distinctions are generally true, the café au lait spots in NF1 can have jagged edges and therefore one cannot rely on the border shape of the pigmentation as a distinguishing feature (Benedict *et al.*, 1968). The café au lait patches in McCune-Albright's syndrome tend to have a mosaic segmental distribution: they do not cross the midline and tend to be unilateral in a given body area. There is a 3:2 female to male sex preponderance, and all reported cases have been sporadic. Because of the distribution of the skin pigmentation and its sporadic occurrence, it was suggested that affected individuals are mosaics as a result of an early postzygotic somatic mutation (Happle, 1987). The hyperfunction of multiple endocrine tissues in the syndrome involves cells that respond to extracellular signals through activation of the hormone-sensitive adenylate cyclase system, the membrane-bound enzyme system that catalyses the formation of the intracellular second messenger cyclic AMP (cAMP). It has now been shown (Weinstein *et al.*, 1991) that patients with the syndrome have mutations within exon 8 of the $G_s\alpha$ gene. This results in increased cAMP formation. Furthermore, in each patient the proportion of cells affected varied from tissue to tissue.

(b) Multiple lentigenes (Leopard) syndrome

This syndrome was first reported by Gorlin, Anderson and Blaw (1969). They used the acronym LEOPARD to denote the clinical features:

(a) (b) (c)

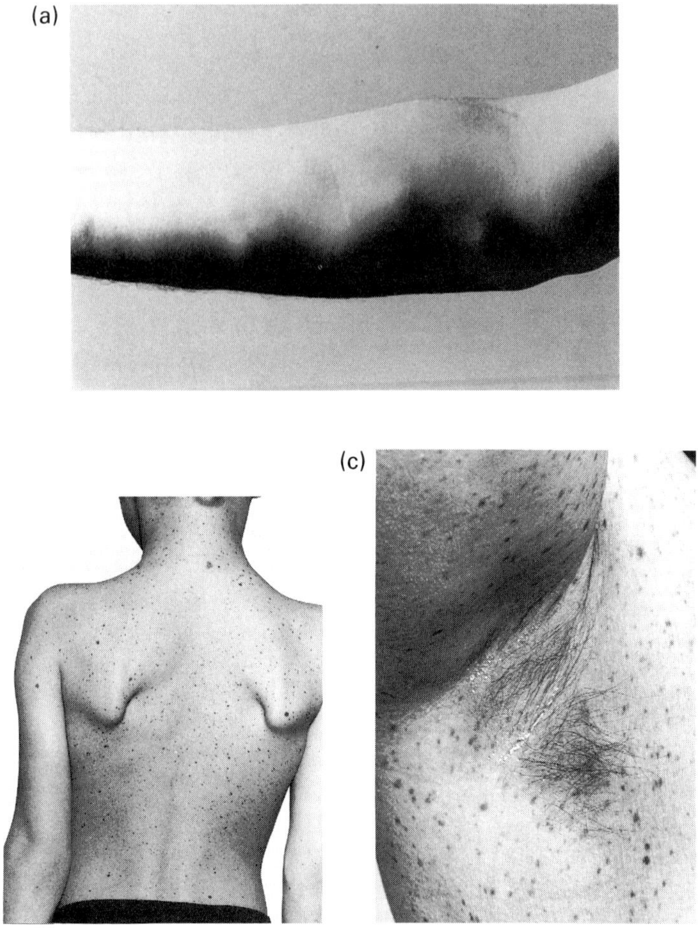

Figure 7.5 Differential diagnosis of NF1. (a) Multiple lipomatosis: multiple subcutaneous swellings of the forearm. (b) Leopard syndrome: typical appearance of lentigenes; lentigenes in the axilla can be labelled as axillary freckling and the patient misdiagnosed as having NF1 (c).

Lentigenes, **E**KG abnormalities, **O**cular hypertelorism, **P**ulmonic stenosis, **A**bnormalities of genitalia, **R**etardation of growth and **D**eafness. Inheritance is autosomal dominant with wide variation in expression (Smith, 1982).

The confusion with NF1 occasionally arises because of the lentigenes (Figure 7.5). These are darker than the abnormal pigmentation in NF1, of smaller diameter (1–5 mm) and can be slightly raised from the skin. The lentigenes occur particularly on the neck and trunk, including in the axillae. I have seen two cases misdiagnosed as NF1 and reported to have axillary freckling.

(c) Bannayan–Riley–Ruvalcaba syndrome

Cohen (1989) suggested that three formerly recognized syndromes probably represented one disease entity. The principal features are macrocephaly and subcutaneous tumours, which are either lipomas or haemangiomas. The confusion with NF1 arises because some affected individuals have café au lait spots; in males, pigmented macules on the glans and shaft of the penis are characteristic (Cohen, 1989). Although most reported cases have been isolated, there have been several with parent to child transmission, making autosomal dominant inheritance with variable expression likely.

Korf (1992) stresses the importance of examining the parents of isolated cases of possible NF1 because the disease features of the other rarer syndromes may be more obvious in adults. In his series, three of the 41 children referred as having NF1 had alternative diagnoses. The diagnoses were McCune–Albright's syndrome, Leopard syndrome and Bannayan–Riley–Ruvalcaba syndrome; in the latter two, an affected parent with obvious disease features helped secure the diagnosis.

(d) Urticaria pigmentosa

Although to the experienced eye the lesions in this condition are distinct from café au lait spots, it is included as I have seen three children (including one sib pair) misdiagnosed as having NF1. The characteristic lesions are orange-brown in colour and may be slightly raised; they vary in size from approximately 2 to 20 mm. Trauma to the lesions, e.g. scraping them with a blunt object, produces erythema and oedema (Dariers sign). Most cases have been isolated and familial cases are rare. Both dominant and recessive inheritance has been postulated (Shaw, 1968; McKusick, 1990).

7.4.2 Differential diagnosis: conditions with cutaneous/subcutaneous swelling

(a) Multiple lipomas

Benign lipomas, like neurofibromas, can arise as isolated lesions in the general population. When multiple they may be due to the autosomal dominant condition multiple lipomatosis (McKusick, 1989), which is by far the most common of the conditions confused with NF1. Lipomas present as subcutaneous swellings, which are much firmer on palpation than dermal neurofibromas, but may be confused with nodular neurofibromas (Figure 7.5). Lipomas are well-defined lesions and there is no involvement of the overlying skin. The most useful clinical differentiation is that nodular neurofibromas may be painful; patients complain that when they hit the lesions they develop acute paraesthesiae and this is seen on palpation of the lesions. Nodular neurofibromas are also limited in distribution to the course of the peripheral nerves to which they are tethered. Lipomas are rarely painful and patients usually present because of concern over an enlarging asymptomatic lump. When multiple, lipomas tend to be on the limbs (distal forearms and thighs) and abdomen. Apart from occasional involvement of the gastrointestinal tract, there are no other disease features in multiple lipomatosis.

(b) Proteus syndrome

The differential diagnosis of Proteus syndrome is discussed by Dr Clark in Chapter 17. In nearly a decade of assessing individuals with regard to a diagnosis of NF1, I have only seen one child for whom an initial diagnosis of Proteus syndrome was made. The diagnosis had been suggested at the age of 18 months on the basis of unilateral lower limb hypertrophy and swelling of the foot. On the sole of the foot the swelling had a moccasin-type appearance as described in Proteus syndrome. The child had no other features noted on initial examination, but had extremely pale skin. It was only when her multiple café au lait spots became more obvious and vertebral scalloping was noted on spinal radiographs that NF1 was correctly diagnosed. When I saw her at the age of 3 years, the café au lait spots were still difficult to see by naked eye examination. The appearance of the sole resembled that in Proteus syndrome, so that very rarely diffuse plexiform neurofibromas may resemble the swellings in Proteus syndrome.

(c) Congenital generalized fibromatosis

This condition is also referred to as juvenile or infantile myofibromatosis (McKusick, 1990). It is characterized by multiple fibroblastic tumours involving skin, striated muscles, bones and viscera. The lesions are often present at birth and more may develop in early childhood. After this, the tumours undergo spontaneous regression. However, children with visceral involvement can have a poor prognosis because of local effects of the tumours. Although there are no associated pigmentary changes, NF1 had been the initial diagnosis in all five of the cases reported by Baird and Worth (1976). Inheritance is autosomal recessive (McKusick, 1990).

(d) Steatocystoma multiplex

This is a rare autosomal dominant disorder (McKusick, 1990) in which patients develop painless cutaneous swellings from childhood, which increase in number throughout life. The swellings are found mainly on the trunk and limbs. The lesions have a yellowish coloration, a firm consistency and on biopsy show disordered sebaceous gland elements. The lesions rarely cause symptoms, but in the one family who consulted me, the lesions tended to become infected quite frequently.

7.5 NATURAL HISTORY OF NF1

Because the morbidity and mortality of NF1 are largely dictated by the occurrence of its complications, all the problems related to complication frequency estimates reviewed by myself above and Dr Mulvihill in his chapter on malignancy apply to discussions about natural history. The best follow-up epidemiological data available on NF1 patients at this time are those from the 39-year follow-up of cases identified by Borberg in 1951, undertaken by Sorensen, Mulvihill and Nielsen (1986). Survival rates to June 1983 of patients who were alive on 1 January 1944 were lower than the year, age and sex specific death rates of the general population. Mortality was increased among probands, especially females, compared with affected relatives; female relatives had a survival rate just below that of the general population. Borberg's probands had been originally identified through hospital inpatient records and the authors concluded that patients requiring admission to hospital had a poor prognosis, whereas incidentally diagnosed relatives had a considerably better outcome. This study also showed that NF1 patients with one malignancy (including CNS tumours and phaeochromocytoma) had an increased risk of developing a second malignancy, which occurred in 16 out of 70 patients (23%). A second cancer develops in only 4% of persons with malignancy in the general population (Storm *et al.*, 1985).

Riccardi (1992) has recently reported an update on his large series of patients. Thirty-nine of the 947 patients evaluated as part of his neurofibromatosis research programme (Riccardi, 1992) have died during the follow-up period; in 28 cases the cause was related to NF1. The marked difference between this and the proportion of deaths related to NF1 in the Welsh study was probably due to ascertainment bias in a specialist neurofibromatosis clinic population. Neurofibrosarcoma was the cause of death in 17 of Riccardi's patients, with a mean age at death of 31.12 years. In 14 of the 17 patients, the malignancy arose in a pre-existing plexiform neurofibroma. Of the remaining 11 patients, five died of complications related to paraspinal neurofibromas; three from complications of diffuse plexiform neurofibromas; and single patients from an astrocytoma, metastatic carcinoid tumour and complications of childhood-onset renovascular hypertension.

Samuelsson, Zoller and Erdheim (1992) presented preliminary data on a 12-year follow-up of the Gothenburg cohort. Twenty-three patients had died during the follow-up period, showing increased mortality compared

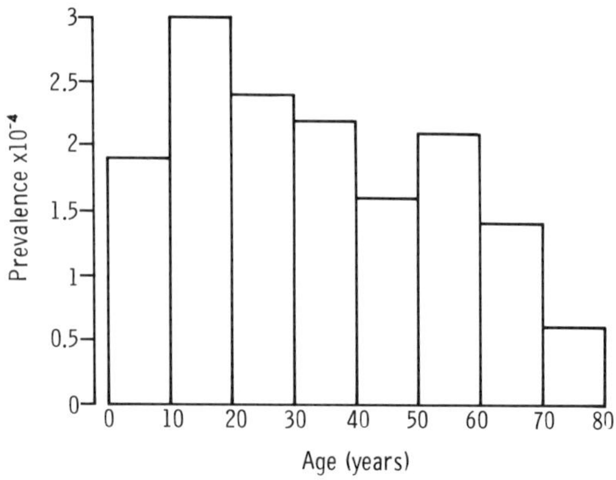

Figure 7.6 Difference in the estimated prevalence of NF1 with age. (Reproduced from Huson, Harper and Compston (1988) by permission of Oxford University Press.)

with the general Swedish population ($p < 0.001$); the causes of death were not given in their abstract. Eighteen of 74 adults had malignant tumours, more than expected in the population at large judged by information from the Swedish Cancer Registry for comparison ($p < 0.01$). Three of these malignancies were neurofibrosarcomas.

In my own study (Huson, Harper and Compston, 1988), the contribution of NF1 to mortality was assessed in two ways. Firstly, it was indirectly estimated from the variation in disease prevalence with age (Figure 7.6). The decrease in prevalence from the second decade onwards cannot be accounted for solely by under-ascertainment. The low prevalence in those aged under 10 years is probably explained by under-ascertainment of sporadically affected children without complications. The mortality attributable to NF1 was also assessed by looking at the cause of death in 25 deceased affected relatives. Death was definitely attributable to NF1 in six cases (24%). The causes of death were pelvic rhabdomyosarcomas in two children aged 6 months and 2 years; a frontal astrocytoma in a 32 year old; neurofibrosarcoma in a 24 year old; obstructive hydrocephalus following removal of a neurofibroma at C1–2 in a 51 year old; and acute left ventricular failure and haemorrhage into an undiagnosed phaeochromocytoma in a 54 year old. A further patient had died from a subarachnoid haemorrhage secondary to hypertension of unknown aetiology, and this may have been NF1 related. Follow-up monitoring of the Welsh cohort is in progress (the author in collaboration with Dr J. Sampson and Dr I. Cordeiro).

The question parents of children with NF1 most frequently ask is 'how many cutaneous neurofibromas will develop and what complications will

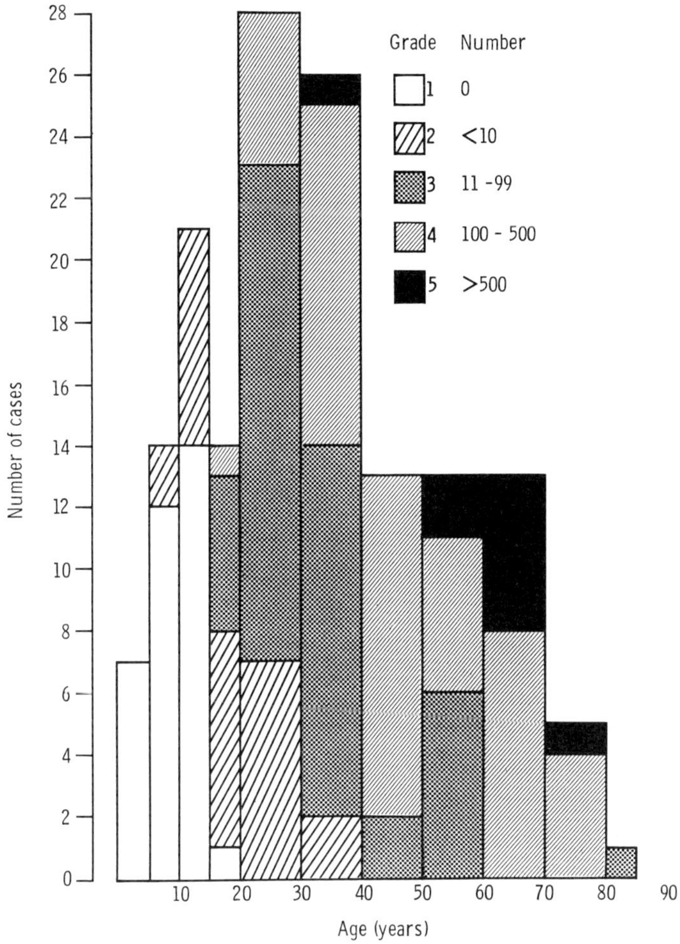

Figure 7.7 Comparison of the number of dermal neurofibromas with age. Each patient ($n = 155$) was given a grade reflecting the number of lesions. (Reproduced from Huson, Harper and Compston (1988) by permission of Oxford University Press.)

arise?'. Both questions are almost impossible to answer accurately from the data available at the present time. Cross-sectional studies of patients of different ages show that the number of neurofibromas is roughly proportional to age (Figure 7.7). Within a given age group, however, one sees people with multiple neurofibromas and others with very few. There are no prospective data available on how and when neurofibromas develop in different individuals and so we have no way of knowing whether predictions about future development can be based, for example, on the number present in late teens.

With regard to the occurrence of complications, there are no known factors that predict that any complication will definitely occur in a given patient. We know of one or two factors that increase the risk of a given complication occurring, but we do not know the exact risk to a given individual. Although we know that most sarcomas occur in pre-existing plexiform lesions, the risk to a given individual with a plexiform lesion of developing a sarcoma is unknown. Similarly, an increased risk of second tumours was identified by Sorensen *et al.* (1986), we do not know whether this will include children who are identified as having asymptomatic optic gliomas on routine magnetic resonance imaging (MRI) scans. Riccardi in his studies adopted a system for grading overall disease severity. The classification is as follows (from Riccardi and Kleiner, 1977).

- Minimal (grade 1) – café au lait spots only, or café au lait spots and only a limited number of dermal neurofibromas without cosmetic or functional significance.
- Mild (grade 2) – dermal neurofibromas in large numbers, and/or with limited specific adverse consequences on a cosmetic or functional level (e.g. on the face, in an intertriginous zone), and asymptomatic intraosseous lesions.
- Moderate (grade 3) – dermal neurofibromas in large numbers, visceral (e.g. gastrointestinal) neurofibromas, skeletal problems (e.g. pseudoarthrosis or scoliosis), relatively well-controlled seizures, modest local hypertrophy.
- Severe (grade 4) – problems leading to major health impairment, often requiring surgical intervention, including intracranial and spinal tumours, malignant Schwannomas, neurofibrosarcomas, phaeochromocytomas, uncontrolled seizures, mental retardation, hydrocephalus and progressive or diffuse hypertrophic growth.

Using these severity grades in his follow-up work, Riccardi (1992) has developed probability curves for the age-related risk of a patient being in a particular grade. Although these studies have given important insights into the natural history of NF1, I feel that the grading system has certain drawbacks. It may be better to treat separately the occurrence of neurofibromas (the only major defining feature to cause significant morbidity) and complications. Most complications are not progressive: they are either present or not present. Easton *et al.* (1993) suggest that the occurrence of each complication is probably influenced by different modifying factors (section 7.6.5).

In conclusion, there remain many unanswered questions about natural history, which can only be addressed by large follow-up studies, ideally in populations with near total ascertainment. It is important to develop relatively uniform ways of assessing and grading NF1 so that data from individual studies can be pooled. The impact of different methods of disease monitoring should also become apparent from such studies. To this end, the sponsorship by the National Neurofibromatosis Foundation of the development of an international neurofibromatosis clinical database by Friedmann, Birch and Greene (1993) is to be applauded.

7.6 GENETIC ASPECTS

7.6.1 Inheritance

All the major surveys of NF1 (Table 7.1; Riccardi and Lewis, 1988) have confirmed that the inheritance of NF1 is autosomal dominant as originally suggested by Preiser and Davenport (1918). It is not yet established whether NF1 is a true dominant disorder, i.e. whether heterozygotes and homozygotes display the same phenotype. The penetrance of the NF1 gene is virtually 100% by the age of 5 years, when affected individuals will have developed café au lait spots (Huson, Compston and Harper, 1989). I am aware of only three examples of apparent non-penetrance of NF1 in the medical literature (Spence *et al.*, 1983, 1986).

7.6.2 Gonadal and gonosomal mosaicism

Although once the disease is established within a family all affected individuals satisfy the diagnostic criteria for NF1, there is a small but significant literature of limited disease manifestations in parents of children who apparently presented as the first case of NF1 in the family. In some dominant conditions, such as tuberous sclerosis, apparently normal parents having more than one affected child is a well-recognized phenomenon (Osborne, Fryer and Webb, 1991) and is presumed to be due to germline mosaicism. In NF1 there have only been two families in which two affected children have been born to normal parents (Riccardi and Lewis, 1988). These could simply have occurred by chance and may not represent germline mosaicism. In the same paper, Riccardi and Lewis (1988) reported two families in which one parent appeared to have limited expression of the NF1 gene. In one, a mother of two affected sons had bilateral Lisch nodules as her only disease manifestation, and in the other the father of an affected son had a cervical Schwannoma and two peripheral neurofibromas. There have been other similar reports. Rubenstein *et al.* (1983) reported two further families. In one, a father and daughter both appear to have segmental NF, and in the other the father of a boy with NF1 had six neurofibromas and a café au lait spot on his left flank. Boltshauser, Stocker and Mackler (1989) reported a further case in which a father with right upper segment cutaneous changes had a daughter with classical NF1. I have seen two examples of this (both unpublished); in one the father of an affected daughter had unilateral axillary freckling, in the other the mother had left upper quadrant cutaneous changes and an affected daughter.

The parents in these cases are probably examples of gonosomal mosaics for the *NF1* gene (i.e. they have both somatic and gonadal involvement); experimental work in the mouse and the available evidence in man suggest that the primitive ectoderm is multipotential (Gardner, 1983). A single mutation of the *NF1* gene at this stage of development could therefore result in limited disease manifestations and gonadal involvement. From the clinical viewpoint these cases emphasize the importance of examining both the skin and irides of parents and siblings of apparently isolated cases. It is also important to realize that even though the segment of the body affected in segmental NF is distant from the gonads, there can be gonadal involvement. Therefore, it is difficult fully to reassure individuals with apparent segmental NF that there is no risk of NF1 occurring in their offspring, although with the available information it is impossible to quantify this risk accurately.

7.6.3 Mutation: rate and mechanism

In all the major surveys of NF1, approximately half the cases represent the first person with NF1 in their family and are assumed to represent new gene mutations. NF1 has one of the highest mutation rates in man; the estimates of mutation rate are summarized in Table 7.2. The reason for this high mutation rate and the mechanism of mutation are unknown. Advanced paternal age is associated with new mutations in some disorders (e.g. haemophilia A and Lesch-Nyhan syndrome on the X chromosome, achondroplasia and Apert syndrome are examples of autosomal disorders). This phenomenon is most easily explained if new mutations occur at mitosis in a spermatogonial stem cell which undergoes asymmetric division, one daughter persisting as the stem cell. In this way, the stem cell population can accumulate mutations with time. Paternal origin of the mutations is explained because only the male stem cells, and not oogonia, undergo mitotic divisions after birth (Vogel and Motulsky, 1986). In NF1, however, there is little evidence for an advanced paternal age effect. A parental age effect on mutation can be examined by two methods. An indirect method is to look at the birth order of sporadic cases of a genetic condition to see if they are born later in the sibship than expected; if a birth order effect is identified, it does not of course indicate the reason why. A direct method to look for a parental age effect is to compare the parents' ages of sporadic cases of a condition with those of parents in the general population having children in the same year. If no appropriate general population data exist, other comparisons are possible, such as comparing the parental ages of sporadic and familial cases.

Five studies have looked at birth order and/or parental age effect in

NF1. My studies (Huson *et al.*, 1989) and those of Samuelsson and Axelsson (1981) showed no birth order or parental age effect; Clementi *et al.* (1990) examined only for a parental age effect and did not identify one. Sergeyev (1975) pooled data from his own and three previous studies to analyse birth order in 193 sibships, and although none of the studies when analysed individually showed a significant birth order effect, the pooled data did. Affected individuals were born later than normal sibs both when whole sibships ($p = 0.004$) and sibships without the last sib ($p = 0.03$) were analysed. The 56 cases in Sergeyev's personal study also showed a weak paternal age increase over population controls (1.99 years, $p = 0.03$). In their study, Riccardi and colleagues (1984) studied the parental age at birth of a much larger number of NF1 new mutations. They found the paternal age to be raised by 3.15 years ($n = 187$, $p < 0.001$) and maternal age by 1.39 years ($n = 171$, $p < 0.001$). Further analysis showed that the increase in maternal age was accounted for solely by the increase in paternal age but not *vice versa*.

The reason for the discrepancy in findings between the different studies is not obvious. In my own study, the birth order data on the small number in the study ($n = 33$, $p = 0.08$) suggested that had a larger number of families been studied, a significant effect may have been seen. With the parental age data, however, there was no suggestion at all of an effect. One possible explanation for the different results is ascertainment bias in the population studied by Riccardi *et al.* (1984). The cases analysed were drawn from a population referred to a special interest clinic and it may be that older parents of new mutations are more likely to seek specialist referral, resulting in a biased sample. Overall, one must conclude that if an increased parental age effect does exist for NF1, it is small when compared with that in other disorders such as achondroplasia or Apert syndrome.

The lack of a paternal age effect might suggest a meiotic origin of most NF1 mutations. However, molecular studies have shown that most mutations arise on the paternally derived chromosome 17 (Jadayel *et al.*, 1990; Stephens *et al.*, 1992). As the recombination frequency in the region of the *NF1* locus is greater in females than males, a meiotic origin would be expected to give a bias towards mutation in the maternally derived chromosome 17, not the paternally derived chromosome. As there is also equal transmission of the NF1 gene through the male and female germlines in established families, there is no suggestion that selection against mutations carried on maternally derived chromosomes explains for the paternal origin of new mutations. The situation is similar for retinoblastoma. Both diseases show a predominance of paternal new mutations with little or no paternal age effect (Dryja *et al.*, 1989). Jadayel *et al.* (1990) concluded that most *NF1* mutations arise either at mitosis in a cell that is not a self-renewing stem cell, or independently of mitosis, for example in mature sperm. Paternal chromosomes are more susceptible to this mutation than are maternal chromosomes, for reasons that are unclear. They suggested that the differences in methylation of paternal and maternal germ cells that are believed to be associated with genomic imprinting could be a possible mechanism.

7.6.4 Genetic fitness

Since the mutation rate is high and the prevalence of NF1 is not increasing, the genetic fitness of NF1 sufferers must be reduced. Genetic fitness in NF1 has been analysed by three studies (Crowe, Schull and Neel, 1956; Samuelsson and Akesson, 1988; Huson *et al.*, 1989). All three studies have shown a reduction in relative fertility. In my own studies, the overall fitness was just below half that of the general population, being lower in men (0.31) than women (0.60). These results are remarkably similar to those of Crowe, Schull and Neel (1956) who found an overall fitness of 0.53 (male 0.41 and female 0.75). Samuelsson and Akesson (1988) gave an overall relative fertility of 0.78, and although they commented that the effect is more marked in males than females, they did not give sex-specific figures. The reduction of fitness in NF1 cannot be explained solely by severe intellectual handicap or disease complications causing severe morbidity or mortality before adulthood, since these are infrequent. Crowe, Schull and Neel (1956) showed that failure to marry contributes significantly to decreased genetic fitness in NF1, but even the married people still showed a reduction (0.80). The reasons for this are not clear, but there is no evidence for pregnancy wastage, so the explanation may be an overall reduction in fecundity.

7.6.5 Variability of gene expression

All of the major NF1 surveys that have specifically addressed this issue have found that the severity of NF1 is extremely variable within families (Riccardi, Kleiner and Lubs, 1979; Carey, Laub and Hall, 1979; Huson, Compston and Harper, 1989). Variability affects both the major defining features and the occurrence of complications. The reason for the variability is unknown. Possibilities include the effect of modifying genes, environmental factors, chance or a combination of these.

As identical twins have the same genetic make-up, they are a good starting point for studying the genetic component of NF1 variability. In Table 7.7, I have summarized the clinical features of the 19 pairs of identical twins I found in the English and German literature, and added an unpublished pair of my own. Brady (1962) cites a further four pairs, which were not included because of lack of detail. Extra details of the twins in the study of Easton *et al.* (1993) were provided by Mrs M. Ponder.

Table 7.7 Disease features in 19 identical; twin pairs with NF1

Authors	*Sex of twins*	*Age at time of report (years)*	*Confirmation of monozygosity*	*Family history of NF1*	*Concordance for disease features*	
					CAL spots and dermal NFs	*Complications*
Akesson, Axelsson & Samuelsson (1983)	Female	24	No information on placenta; identical HLA and blood grouping	No	In number	Both had learning difficulties. One had a plexiform NF of the neck; the other an NFS of the right leg (13 years)
Atlas *et al*. (1988)	Male	21	No information	No	No information	Both had agenesis of corpus callosum (N.B. this is not a recognized NF1 complication) and multiple spinal NFs.
Bauer, Lubs and Lubs (1988)	Male	7	Monochorionic placenta; identical red cell types	No	In number	Both had learning difficulties but only one had a mesenteric plexiform NF
Borberg (1951)	Female	37	No information	Yes	Skin of one twin said to be almost exact mirror image of other	Both had intellectual handicap

Table 7.7 Continued

Authors	*Sex of twins*	*Age at time of report (years)*	*Confirmation of monozygosity*	*Family history of NF1*	*Concordance for disease features*	
					CAL spots and dermal NFs	*Complications*
Brady (1962)	Male	7	Single chorion and amnion	Yes	No information	Both had subependymal spongioblastomas of IVth ventricle; one had optic nerve glioma at autopsy; not clear whether other had detailed optic nerve examination
Crawford and Buckler (1983)	Male	7,13[a]	Single chorion and DNA typing	No	In number	Both had optic chiasm gliomas and needed remedial school education
Diekmann, Hüther and Pfeiffer (1967)	Female	6	Blood groups	Yes	No information	Only one twin had plexiform NF of head and ear
Dresner and Montgomery (1949)	Female	13	Single placenta	Yes	Skin changes almost identical in number and distribution (both CAL and dermal NF)	Both had optic chiasm glioma
Easton *et al*. (1993)	Female	14	DNA typing	Yes	In number	Both had scoliosis; only one had a plexiform NF

Table 7.7 Continued

Authors	*Sex of twins*	*Age at time of report (years)*	*Confirmation of monozygosity*	*Family history of NF1*	*Concordance for disease features*	
					CAL spots and dermal NFs	*Complications*
Easton *et al.* (1993)	Male	14	DNA typing	Yes	In number	Both had scoliosis; only one had a plexiform NF
Easton *et al.* (1993)	Female	26	DNA typing	No	In number	Both had scoliosis and epilepsy
Easton *et al.* (1993)	Female	29	DNA typing	Yes	In number	Both had epilepsy
Easton *et al.* (1993)	Female	35	DNA typing	Yes	In number	Only one had a plexiform NF
Huson (unpublished)	Female	23	Clinical appearance	Uncertain, mother unaffected, not in contact with father for many years	Comparison not possible	One twin seen at 23 years, 4 years after her identical twin died of an NFS. This had arisen in a pre-existing nodular NF. Both twins had had several nodular NFs removed
Kleinhans and Mühlenstadt (1981)	Female	18	No information	Yes	No information	One had plexiform NF in the pelvic area (subject of the paper). The other had 'neurofibromatosis involving the nervus trigeminus'; I presume this refers to a facial plexiform NF

Table 7.7 Continued

Authors	*Sex of twins*	*Age at time of report (years)*	*Confirmation of monozygosity*	*Family history of NF1*	*Concordance for disease features*	
					CAL spots and dermal NFs	*Complications*
Loftis (1940)	Female	42	No information	No	In number	Both had 'low average intelligence'; one had tumour on vocal cord but no details given
Pascual-Castroviejo *et al.* (1988)	Female	15	Single placenta	Yes	No information	One had glioma of left optic nerve; other of right optic nerve and chiasm; both had aqueduct stenosis
Riccardi, Kleiner and Lubs (1979)	Female	6	Single chorion and amnion	No	No concordance	One had optic chiasm enlargement and hydrocephalus (cause uncertain); other no symptoms but no neuroimaging
Troch (1953)	Female	?	Single chorion and amnion	Yes	Described as similar	One twin had epilepsy; cardiazol stimulation provoked a grand mal seizure in the other
Vaughn, Bachman and Sommer (1981)	Female	4	Identical HLA and blood groups	No	Described as similar	One twin had optic glioma (aged 2 years); other had normal CT scan at 4 years

[a] Update on these twins by personal communication from M. Ponder who examined them at 13 years of age for the study reported by Easton *et al.* (1993).
CAL = café au lait spot; NF = neurofibroma; NFS = neurofibrosarcoma.

It is important to note that the twins reported by Crawford and Buckler (1983; Buckler, personal communication, 1992) were reported independently by Cartwright (1982). This does not seem to have been appreciated in previous summaries of identical twins with NF1 (Bauer, Lubs and Lubs, 1988).

With regard to two of the major defining features, café au lait spots and dermal neurofibromas, in the 13 pairs where the skin appearance is specifically described all except the pair reported by Riccardi, Kleiner and Lubs (1979) had similar numbers of lesions, but they were not usually in the same site. With regard to disease complications, six out of seven pairs were discordant for plexiform neurofibromas and only one pair were concordant, but the lesions were at very different sites (pelvis and face). Two pairs were discordant for development of neurofibrosarcoma at the time of reporting, the tumours having developed in the affected twin 11 and 4 years previously. For optic gliomas, three pairs were concordant and three discordant, although in two of these it is difficult to know from the report whether an asymptomatic lesion was adequately excluded. Five pairs were concordant for learning difficulties; three for epilepsy (although in one pair one of the twins became symptomatic only after cardiazol stimulation); two for scoliosis and single pairs for aqueduct stenosis, a fourth ventricle subependymal spongioblastoma, multiple spinal neurofibromas and agenesis of the corpus callosum. From these reports one must conclude disease expression in NF1 is not entirely genetically controlled. For café au lait spots and dermal neurofibromas, it seems that where they appear is a random event, although there is considerable genetic influence on the number of lesions developing. For some disease complications there seems to be a strong genetic influence (e.g. learning disability) whereas the development of plexiform neurofibromas must be influenced by other factors as well.

With regard to NF1 variability in extended families, most clinical studies have based their findings on a relatively subjective assessment with no formal statistical analysis of the degree of similarity. Easton *et al.* (1993) have recently analysed the variation and expression in NF1 more objectively. They examined 175 individuals in 48 NF1 families, including six monozygotic (MZ) twin pairs (Table 7.7; five previously unpublished pairs and the twin pair reported by both Cartwright (1982) and Crawford and Buckler (1983)). They looked at the number of café au lait spots and dermal neurofibromas in each individual and correlated them within families. Both showed the highest correlation in identical twins, with significant but lower correlation in first-degree relatives and even lower correlation between more distant relatives. The high correlation in MZ twins suggests a strong genetic component in variation of expression; however, the low correlation between more distant relatives suggests that the *NF1* mutation itself plays only a minor role.

The study looked at intrafamilial correlation of five disease complications: plexiform neurofibromas, optic gliomas, scoliosis, epilepsy and intellectual handicap (defined as need for referral for remedial education). In the MZ twins the only complication showing discordance was plexiform neurofibromas (three out of three pairs were discordant); the twin pairs were concordant for the remaining complications (optic gliomas, one pair; scoliosis, three pairs; epilepsy, two pairs; and need for remedial education, one pair). In the family studies all complications except plexiform neurofibromas showed significant familial clustering. The familial effects for these complications were also consistent with polygenic effects, although the data were insufficient to rule out other models such as a significant effect of different *NF1* mutations. There was no evidence that any of the complications tended to occur more commonly together in affected individuals. Therefore, the degree of expression of *NF1* is largely determined by other modifying loci, and these modifying genes vary from one disease feature to another.

Factors other than modifying genes may play a part. The importance of the effect of genomic imprinting (Hall, 1990) on the expression of genetic disease is becoming increasingly appreciated. If this was significant in NF1, one would expect increased disease severity in the offspring of the parent of a particular sex. If genomic imprinting was important only in certain disease complications, these features would always arise when the gene was inherited from a parent of a particular sex. A possible maternal effect on severity of NF1 was first suggested by Miller and Hall in 1978. Studying 62 cases aged less than 18 years, ascertained from the records of a children's orthopaedic and university hospital, they found an increased severity in children born to affected mothers compared with those having affected fathers or with new mutations. Three subsequent reports (Carey, Laub and Hall, 1979; Riccardi and Wald, 1987; Huson *et al.*, 1989) have not confirmed this effect in a combined total of 443 NF1 sufferers. The study of Riccardi and Wald (1987) also found no disease feature with an abnormal distribution related to the sex of the affected parent. It must be concluded that there is no maternal effect on disease severity.

7.6.6 Genotype–phenotype correlation

The chromosomal localization and subsequent cloning of the *NF1* gene (Chapter 2) provided the basic tools by which some of the unanswered questions about the genetic basis of NF1 could be addressed. The starting point in understanding variation in gene expression is to see if there is any correlation between specific gene mutations and disease features. The paucity of mutations identifiable in large series of NF1 patients with available technology (Upadhyaya *et al.*, 1992) means there has been little progress in this area to date. The recent formation of an international NF1 mutation consortium by the National Neurofibromatosis Foundation is an important step in ensuring data from as many patients as possible are available for comparison. The work of Easton *et al.* (1993) reviewed above predicts that NF1 genotype and phenotype will not be closely correlated because of the role of modifying genes. The identification of such genes will require complex gene mapping studies in groups of families with apparent clustering of a given complication. This endeavour will require international collaboration of clinicians and scientists as such families are relatively uncommon.

ACKNOWLEDGEMENTS

The author is grateful to Maggie Ponder for her help in compiling Table 7.7, to Marquella Kallimassia for assistance in German translation and to many clinical colleagues and families for their assistance.

REFERENCES

Akesson, H.O., Axelsson, R. and Samuelsson, B. (1983) Neurofibromatosis in monoz. twins: a case report. *Acta Genet. Med. Gemellol*, **32**, 245–9.

Albright, F., Butler, A.M., Hampton, A.O. and Smith, P. (1937) Syndrome characterized by osteitis fibrosa disseminata, areas of pigmentation and endocrine dysfunction, with precocious puberty in females. Report of five cases. *N. Engl. J. Med.*, **216**, 727–46.

Apter, N., Chemke, J., Hurwitz, N. and Levin, S. (1975) Neonatal neurofibromatosis: unusual manifestations with malignant clinical course. *Clin. Genet.*, **7**, 388–93.

Atlas, S.W., Zimmermann, R.A., Bruce, D. *et al.* (1988) Neurofibromatosis and agenesis of the corpus callosum in identical twins: MR diagnosis. *Am. J. Neuroradiol.*, **9**, 598–601.

Baird, P.A. and Worth, A.J. (1976) Congenital generalized fibromatosis: an autosomal recessive condition? *Clin. Genet.*, **9**, 488–94.

Bauer, M., Lubs, H. and Lubs, M.L. (1988) Variable expressivity of von Recklinghausen neurofibromatosis (NF1) in identical twins. *Neurofibromatosis*, **1**, 323–9.

Benedict, P.H., Szabo, G., Fitzpatrick, T.B. and Sinesi, S.J. (1968) Melanotic macules in Albright's syndrome and in neurofibromatosis. *JAMA*, **205**, 72–80.

Boltshauser, E., Stocker, H. and Mackler, M. (1989) Neurofibromatosis type 1 in a child of a parent with segmental neurofibromatosis. *Neurofibromatosis*, **2**, 244–5.

Borberg, A. (1951) Clinical and genetic investigations into tuberous sclerosis and Recklinghausen's neurofibromatosis. *Acta Psychiatr. Neurol.* (suppl.), **71**, 1–239.

Brady, W.T. (1962) Brain stem gliomas causing hydrocephalus in twins with von Recklinghausen's disease. *J. Neuropath. Exp. Neurol.*, **2**, 555–65.

Brasfield, R.D. and Das Gupta, T.K. (1972) Von Recklinghausen's disease: a clinicopathological study. *Ann. Surg.*, **175**, 86–104.

Burwell, R.G., James, N.J. and Johnston, D.I. (1982) Café-au-lait spots in schoolchildren. *Arch. Dis. Child.*, **57**, 631–2.

Carey, J.C., Laub, J.M. and Hall, B.D. (1979) Penetrance and variability of neurofibromatosis: a genetic study of 60 families. *Birth Defects*, **15**(5B), 271–81.

Cartwright, S.C. (1982) Concordant optic glioma in a pair of monozygotic twins with neurofibromatosis. *Clin. Pediatr. (Phila.)*, **11**(4), 236–8.

Clementi, M., Barbujani, C., Turolla, L. and Tenconi, R. (1990) Neurofibromatosis 1: a maximum likelihood estimation of mutation rate. *Hum. Genet*, **84**, 116–18.

Cohen, M., Jr (1989) A comprehensive and critical assessment of overgrowth and overgrowth syndromes. Bannayan-Riley-Ruvalcaba syndrome. *Adv. Hum. Genet.*, **18**, 236–47.

Cooper, P.H., Frierson, H.F., Kayne, A.L. and Sabio, H. (1984) Association of juvenile xanthogranuloma with juvenile myeloid leukaemia. *Arch. Dermatol.*, **120**, 371–5.

Crawford, M.J. and Buckler, M.J.H. (1983) Optic gliomata affecting twins with neurofibromatosis. *Dev. Med. Child. Neurol.*, **25**, 370–3.

Crowe, F.W. (1964) Axillary freckling as a diagnostic aid in neurofibromatosis. *Ann. Intern. Med.*, **61**, 1142–3.

Crowe, F.W. and Schull, W.J. (1953) Diagnostic importance of the café au lait spot in neurofibromatosis. *Arch. Intern. Med.*, **91**, 758–66.

Crowe, F.W., Schull, W.J. and Neel, J.V. (1956) *A Clinical, Pathological and Genetic Study of Multiple Neurofibromatosis*, Charles C. Thomas, Springfield, Illinois.

Diekmann, L., Hüther, W. and Pfeiffer, R.A. (1967) Ungewöhnliche Erscheinungsformen der Neurofibromatose (von Recklinghausensche Krankheit) im Kindesaltes. *Ztschr. Kinderh.*, **101**, 191–222.

Dresner, E. and Montgomery, D.A.D. (1949) Primary optic atrophy in von Recklinghausen's disease (multiple neurofibromatosis). *Q. J. Med.*, **18**, 93–104.

Dryja, T.P., Mukai, S., Petersen, R. *et al.* (1989) Parental origin of mutations of the retinoblastoma gene. *Nature*, **339**, 556–8.

Easton, D.F., Ponder, M.A., Huson, S.M. and Ponder, B.A.J. (1993) An analysis of variation in expression of NF1: evidence for modifying genes. *Am. J. Hum. Genet.*, **53**, 305–13.

Fitzpatrick, T.B. and Martuza, R.L. (1986) Clinical diagnosis of von Recklinghausen's neurofibromatosis. *Ann. N.Y. Acad. Sci.*, **486**, 383–5.

Francis, D.M.A. and Mackie, W. (1987) Life-threatening haemorrhage in patients with neurofibromatosis. *Aust. N.Z. J. Surg.*, **57**, 679–82.

Friedmann, J., Birch, P., Green, C. and the NNFF International Database Participants (1993) National Neurofibromatosis Foundation international database. *Am. J. Med. Genet.*, **45**, 397–9.

Fuller, L.C., Cox, B. and Gardner, R.J.M. (1989) Prevalence of von Recklinghausen neurofibromatosis in Dunedin, New Zealand. *Neurofibromatosis*, **2**, 278–83.

Gardner, R.L. (1983) Cell lineage and cell commitment in the early mammalian embryo, in *The Biological Basis of Reproductive and Developmental Medicine* (ed. J.B. Warshaw), Elsevier, Amsterdam, pp. 31–41.

Gorlin, R.J., Anderson, R.C. and Blaw, M. (1969) Multiple lentigines syndrome. *Am. J. Dis. Child.*, **117**, 652–62.

Griebel, M.L., Redman, J.F., Kemp, S.F. and Elders, M.J. (1991) Hypertrophy of clitoral hood: presenting sign of neurofibromatosis in female child. *Urology*, **37**, 337–9.

Hall, J.G. (1990) Genomic imprinting: review and relevance to genetic diseases. *Am. J. Hum. Genet.*, **46**, 857–73.

Happle, R. (1987) Lethal genes surviving by mosaicism: a possible explanation for sporadic birth defects involving the skin. *J. Am. Acad. Dermatol.*, **16**, 899–906.

Huson, S.M. (1989) Clinical and genetic studies of von Recklinghausen neurofibromatosis. MD thesis, University of Edinburgh.

Huson, S.M., Meredith, A.L., Sarfarazi, M. *et al.* (1986) Linkage analysis of peripheral neurofibromatosis (von Recklinghausen disease) and chromosome 19 markers linked to myotonic dystrophy. *J. Med. Genet.*, **23**, 55–7.

Huson, S.M., Harper, P.S. and Compston, D.A.S. (1988) Von Recklinghausen neurofibromatosis: a clinical and population study in South East Wales. *Brain*, **111**, 1355–81.

Huson, S.M., Clark, D., Compston, D.A.S. and Harper, P.S. (1989) A genetic study of von Recklinghausen neurofibromatosis in South East Wales. I: Prevalence, fitness, mutation rate and effect of parental transmission on severity. *J. Med. Genet.*, **26**, 704–11.

Huson, S.M., Compston, D.A.S. and Harper, P.S. (1989) A genetic study of von Recklinghausen neurofibromatosis in South East Wales. II: Guidelines for genetic counselling. *J. Med. Genet.*, **26**, 712–21.

Ichikawa, K., Crosley, C.J., Culebras, A. and Weitkamp, L. (1981) Coincidence of neurofibromatosis and myotonic dystrophy in a kindred. *J. Med. Genet.*, **18**, 134–8.

Jadayel, D., Fain, P., Upadhyaya, M. *et al.* (1990) Paternal origin of new mutations in von Recklinghausen neurofibromatosis. *Nature*, **343**, 558–9.

Johnson, B.L. and Charneco, D.L. (1970) Café au lait spots in neurofibromatosis and in normal individuals. *Arch. Dermatol.*, **102**, 442–6.

Kaplan, M.S. and Rosenblatt, B. (1985) A distinctive facial appearance in neurofibromatosis von Recklinghausen. *Am. J. Med. Genet.*, **21**, 463–70.

Kimmellman, C.P. (1979) Otolaryngolic aspects of neurofibromatosis. *Arch. Otolarygol.*, **105**, 732–6.

Kleinhans, G. and Mühlenstadt, D. (1981) Neurofibromatosis involving urinary bladder and vesic-vaginal septum. *Urology*, **20**, 215–17.

Kopf, A.W., Levine, L.J., Rigel, D.S. *et al.* (1985) Prevalence of congenital-nevus-like nevi, nevi spilli, and café-au-lait spots. *Arch. Dermatol.*, **121**, 766–9.

Korf, B.R. (1992) Diagnostic outcome in children with multiple café-au-lait spots. *Pediatrics*, **90**, 924–7.

Loftis, E.L. (1940) Reckinghausen's disease in identical twins. *Arch. Dermatol.*, **42**, 657.

Martuza, R.L., Philippe, I., Fitzpatrick, T.B. *et al.* (1985) Melanin macroglobules as a cellular marker of neurofibromatosis: a quantitative study. *J. Invest. Dermatol.*, **85**, 347–50.

McKusick, V.A. (1990) *Mendelian Inheritance in Man*, 10th edn, Johns Hopkins University Press, Baltimore.

Miller, M. and Hall, J.G. (1978) Possible maternal effect on severity of neurofibromatosis. *Lancet*, **ii**, 1071–3.

NIH Consensus Development Conference Statement (1988) Neurofibromatosis. *Arch. Neurol.*, **45**, 575–8.

Opitz, J.M. and Weaver, D.D. (1985) Editorial comment: The neurofibromatosis–Noonan syndrome. *Am. J. Med. Genet.*, **21**, 477–90.

Osborne, J., Fryer, A. and Webb, D. (1991) Epidemiology of tuberous sclerosis. *Ann. N.Y. Acad. Sci.*, **615**, 125–7.

Pascual-Castroviejo, I., Verdu, A., Roman, M. *et al.* (1988) Optic glioma with progressive occlusion of the aqueduct of sylvius in monozygotic twins with neurofibromatosis. *Brain Dev.*, **10**, 24–9.

Pollak, J., Landau, K., Kuenzle, C. *et al.* (1992) Diagnose der Neurofibromatose 1 im Vorschulalter. *Schweiz. Med. Wschr.*, **122** (suppl. 47), 7.

Poston, G.J., Grace, P.A., Venn, G. and Spencer, J. (1990) Recurrent near-fatal haemorrhage in von Recklinghausen's disease. *Br. J. Clin. Pract.*, **44**, 755–6.

Preiser, S.A. and Davenport, C.B. (1918) Multiple neurofibromatosis (von Recklinghausen's disease) and its inheritance. *Am. J. Med. Sci.*, **156**, 507–41.

Riccardi, V.M. (1981) Von Recklinghausen neurofibromatosis. *N. Engl. J. Med.*, **305**, 1617–27.

Riccardi, V.M. (1992) *Neurofibromatosis: Phenotype, Natural History and Pathogenesis*, 2nd edn, Johns Hopkins University Press, Baltimore.

Riccardi, V.M. and Eichner, T.E. (1986) *Neurofibromatosis: Phenotype, Natural History and Pathogenesis*, Johns Hopkins University Press, Baltimore.

Riccardi, V.M., and Kleiner, B. (1977) Neurofibromatosis: a neoplastic birth defect with two age peaks of severity. *Birth Defects*, **13**(3C), 131–8.

Riccardi, V.M. and Lewis, R.A. (1988) Penetrance of von Recklinghausen neurofibromatosis: a distinction between predecessors and descendants. *Am. J. Hum. Genet.*, **42**, 284–9.

Riccardi, V.M. and Wald, J.S. (1987) Discounting an adverse maternal effect on severity of neurofibromatosis. *Pediatrics*, **79**, 386–93.

Riccardi, V.M., Kleiner, B. and Lubs, M.L. (1979) Neurofibromatosis: variable expression is not intrinsic to the mutant gene. *Birth Defects*, **15**, 283–9.

Riccardi, V.M., Dobson, C.E., Chakraborty, R. and Bontke, C. (1984) The pathophysiology of neurofibromatosis: IX. Paternal age as a factor in the origin of new mutations. *Am. J. Med. Genet.*, **18**, 169–76.

Rivas, M.L. and DiLiberti, J.H. (1984) Genetic linkage between myotonic dystrophy and neurofibromatosis. *Birth Defects*, **20**, 570–1.

Rubenstein, A.E., Bader, J.L., Aron, A.A. and Wallace, S. (1983) Familial transmission of segmental neurofibromatosis. *Neurology*, **33** (suppl. 2), 76.

Samuelsson, B. (1981) Neurofibromatosis (von Recklinghausen's disease): a clinical/psychiatric and genetic study, MD Thesis, University of Goteborg, Sweden.

Samuelsson, B. and Akesson, H.O. (1988) Relative fertility and mutation rate in neurofibromatosis. *Hereditas*, **108**, 169–71.

Samuelsson, B. and Axelsson, R. (1981) Neurofibromatosis. A clinical and genetic study of 96 cases in Gothenburg, Sweden. *Acta Derm. Venereol.* [*Suppl.*], (*Stockh.*), **95**, 67–71.

Samuelsson, G., Zoller, M. and Erdheim, I. (1992) Manifestations of NF1 in a Swedish cohort followed for 12 years. NNFF International Neurofibromatosis Symposium, Vienna.

Schull, W.J. and Crowe, F.W. (1953) Neurocutaneous syndromes in the M. kindred. *Neurology*, **3**, 904–9.

Sergeyev, A.S. (1975) On the mutation rate of neurofibromatosis. *Hum. Genet.*, **28**, 129–38.

Shaw, J.M. (1968) Genetic aspects of urticaria pigmentosa. *Arch. Derm.*, **97**, 137–8.

Smith, D.W. (1982) *Recognisable Patterns of Human Malformation*, W.B. Saunders, Philadelphia.

Sorensen, S.A., Mulvihill, J.T. and Nielsen, A. (1986) Longterm follow up of von Recklinghausen neurofibromatosis: survival and malignant neoplasms. *N. Engl. J. Med.*, **314**, 1010–15.

Spence, M.A., Bader, J.L., Parry, D.M. *et al.* (1983) Linkage analysis of neurofibromatosis (von Recklinghausen disease). *J. Med. Genet.*, **20**, 334–7.

Spence, M.A., Parry, D.M., Bader, J.L. *et al.* (1986) Genetic linkage analysis of neurofibromatosis. *Ann. N.Y. Acad. Sci.*, **486**, 287–92.

Stephens, K., Kayes, L., Riccardi, V.M. *et al.* (1992) Preferential mutation of the neurofibromatosis type 1 gene in paternally-derived chromosomes. *Hum. Genet.*, **88**, 279–82.

Storm, H.H., Jensen, O.M., Ewertz, M. *et al.* (1985) Summary: multiple primary cancers in Denmark, 1943–80. *Nat. Cancer Inst. Monogr.*, **68**, 411–30.

Tanner, J.M. and Whitehouse, R.H. (1976) Clinical longitudinal standards for height, weight, height velocity, weight velocity and stages of puberty. *Arch. Dis. Child.*, **51**, 170–9.

Thakker, R.V. and Ponder, B.A.J. (1988) Multiple endocrine neoplasia. *Clin. Endocrinol. Metab.*, **2**(4), 1031–67.

Thomas, J.V., Schwartz, P.L. and Gragoudas, E.S. (1978) Von Hippel's disease in association with von Recklinghausen's neurofibromatosis. *Br. J. Ophthalmol.*, **62**, 604–8.

Troch, C. (1953) Neurofibromatose chez des jumelles univitellines dont l'une avec épilepsie clinique: remarques éléctroencephalographiques. *Acta Neurol. Psychiatr. Belg.*, **53**, 393.

Tishler, P.V. (1975) A family with coexistent von Recklinghausen's neurofibromatosis and von Hippel Lindau's disease. *Neurology*, **25**, 840–4.

Upadhyaya, M., Shen, M., Cherryson, A. *et al.* (1992) Analysis of mutations at the neurofibromatosis 1 (NF1) locus. *Hum. Mol. Genet.*, **1**, 735–40.

Vaughn, A.J., Bachman, D. and Sommer, A. (1981) Neurofibromatosis in monozygotic twins: a case report of spontaneous mutation. *Am. J. Med. Genet.*, **8**, 155–8.

Vogel, F. and Motulsky, A.G. (1986) *Human Genetics*, 2nd edn., Springer, Berlin.

von Recklinghausen, F.D. (1882) *Ueber die multiplen fibrome der Haut und ihre Beziehung zu den multiplen Neuromen*, Hirschwald, Berlin.

Weinstein, L.S., Shenker, A., Gejman, P.V. *et al.* (1991) Activating mutations of the stimulatory G protein in the McCune–Albright syndrome. *N. Engl. J. Med.*, **325**, 1688–95.

Wertelecki, W., Superneau, D.W., Forehand, L.W. and Hoff, E.T. (1988) Angiomas and von Recklinghausen neurofibromatosis. *Neurofibromatosis*, **1**, 137–45.

8

Neurological complications of neurofibromatosis 1

R.A.C. Hughes

8.1 INTRODUCTION

Neurological complications of neurofibromatosis 1 (NF1) derive not only from the neurofibromas themselves, but also from central nervous system (CNS) malformations and tumours, and the secondary complications resulting from deformities of the skull and skeleton. The neurological problems that have been considered part of the NF1 phenotype are listed in Tables 8.1 and 8.2. Intellectual handicap is more extensively discussed in Chapter 9, and ocular manifestations including optic gliomas in Chapter 10. The temptation to accept every neurological occurrence in a patient with NF1 as part of the disease has to be avoided: there is no *a priori* reason why patients with NF1 should be more or less liable to neurological complaints that affect the rest of the population. For instance, two of the first 103 patients in our series had multiple sclerosis, but this will not lead me to propose anything more than selection bias in a neurologist's practice. The reported occurrence of NF1 and myotonic dystrophy is probably merely another coincidence (Duquenne *et al.*, 1990). In the ensuing chapter the strength of the association with each manifestation will be considered, the presenting features described and optimal management discussed.

8.2 INTELLECTUAL HANDICAP

Mental retardation, usually only mild or moderate, has been discovered in about a quarter of patients with NF1. There were reports of a few cases of severe mental retardation in early series. Modern series have reported intellectual handicap or learning disability in about 30% of patients. The most accurate figure is probably provided by the southeast Wales population-based study in which 10% of 124 cases required or had

Table 8.1 Neurological complications of NF1

Cerebral
- Mental retardation
- Macrocephaly
- Epilepsy
- Cerebral tumours
- Aqueduct stenosis
- Sphenoid wing dysplasia
- Occlusive vascular disease
- Hypertensive vascular disease

Cranial nerve
- Optic nerve glioma
- Cranial nerve neurofibromas

Spinal canal
- Spinal root neurofibroma
- Intraspinal tumour
- Lateral thoracic meningocele
- Kyphoscoliosis

Peripheral nerves
- Neurofibroma
- Plexiform neurofibroma
- Malignant Schwannoma/neurofibrosarcoma
- Peroneal muscular atrophy

Psychiatric consequences

Table 8.2 Percentage of patients with neurological complications in selected large series of patients with NF1

	Rubenstein (1986)	*Ferner and Hughes (unpublished)*	*Huson, Harper and Compston (1988)*
Total number of patients	250	103	96
Learning difficulties/mental retardation	12	34/8	27
Epilepsy	4	1	8
Cerebral/brain stem glioma (not optic pathway)	2	3	0
Optic glioma	2	4	0
Vestibular Schwannoma	–	0	0
Spinal canal neurofibroma	6	1	2
Aqueduct stenosis	1	1	2
Kyphoscoliosis requiring surgery	–	–	5
Sphenoid wing dysplasia	1	1	–

required special schooling and 17% remedial education (Huson, Harper and Compston, 1988). This high frequency of intellectual impairment has been further investigated in our own study of a population in southeast London, which will be described in the next chapter. Suffice it to say at this point that the intellectual impairment presents in childhood as learning difficulties and is non-progressive. The learning difficulties cannot be accounted for by rare CNS complications such as tumours, hydrocephalus or epilepsy. There is also no association between macrocephaly and intellectual impairment. It is possible that learning difficulties are related to subtle abnormalities of the architecture of the cerebral cortex, which were described by Rosman and Pearce (1967).

8.3 MACROCEPHALY

Weichert *et al.* (1973), having encountered two children with neurofibromatosis and large heads, identified macrocranium on skull radiographs of 75% of a hospital-based series of 24 children with neurofibromatosis. Since then, macrocephaly has become recognized as a feature of NF1 (Riccardi, 1981). This has been confirmed in population studies. In Huson's population-based series (Huson, Harper and Compston, 1988), 45% of 115 cases had a head circumference at or above the 97th centile compared with 15% of 40 siblings ($p = 0.001$). Cases known to have hydrocephalus or plexiform neurofibromas, which would have affected the measurement, were excluded. Similarly in our southeast London series, 58% of 103 cases had head circumferences above the 98th percentile compared with 30% of age-matched controls (Ferner and Hughes, in preparation). In making these comparisons it has been important to use contemporary controls because average head circumference has become larger since publication of the latest available centile charts. In a radiographic study, cranial volumes above the 95th percentile were identified in 44% of 52 patients but in none of 26 patients with tuberous sclerosis, another phakomatosis (Holt and Kuhns, 1976). The occurrence of macrocephaly was not related to the known presence of a cerebral tumour or hydrocephalus in that series, and air encephalograms showed relatively normal ventricular size in the four cases with the largest heads. In our series, cases with large heads were investigated by magnetic resonance imaging (MRI) and the enlargement was due to apparent enlargement of the whole brain and not to hydrocephalus.

Although large heads in patients with NF1 are usually due to macrocephaly, the finding of an increasing head circumference in children, or of a large head with other signs and symptoms, should lead to consideration of hydrocephalus as a result of either a tumour of the third ventricle or posterior fossa, or aqueduct stenosis, or cerebellar ectopia, all of which have been associated with NF1 (see below).

8.4 EPILEPSY

Most reviewers have unquestioningly accepted that epilepsy is more common in NF1 than the general population (Riccardi, 1981; Rubenstein *et al.*, 1981). Riccardi (1981) reported that 'at least 4' of 139 patients from a hospital-based series had documented seizures not due to intracranial mass lesions. This frequency is only marginally greater than the point prevalence of epilepsy in the Western world, which ranges from 0.15 to 3 per 100, and the lifetime prevalence, which has been estimated to lie between 2 and 5 per 100 (Shorvon, 1990). The apparently increased frequency could be accounted for by the inevitable selection bias imposed by a hospital-based study. In our neurologically biased study, 11.7% of 103 cases had epilepsy (Ferner and Hughes, unpublished data). Attempted population-based studies have reported epilepsy in 3% of 74 cases (Samuelsson, 1981) and 8% of 96 cases. In the second of these series, four of the eight cases had structural causes for their epilepsy and four did not (Huson, Harper and Compston, 1988). Two of these cases had hypsarrhythmia, and four similar cases were encountered by Riccardi and Eichner (1986). Hypsarrhythmia may therefore be a genuine, albeit rare, association with NF1; it is a common and characteristic feature of tuberous sclerosis. Epilepsy in general is a common manifestation of gross disorders of neuronal migration, including diffuse neuronal heterotopias (Editorial, 1990).

The overall conclusion from these series is that NF1 carries a small increased risk of epilepsy, from about 2–5% in the normal population to just over 5%. This is only partly accounted for by the recognized macroscopic abnormalities such as tumours, hydrocephalus or infarcts. The residual increase in risk may be accounted for by the microscopic abnormalities of cortical architecture described by Rosman and Pearce (1967) as the basis for mental retardation. Such an increase in prevalence of epilepsy as does exist could therefore be explained by focal or multifocal abnormalities without invoking a hypothesis of generalized lowering of seizure threshold.

8.5 HEADACHE

It has been claimed that headache is more common in NF1 patients attending a special clinic than in the general population (Riccardi, 1981). However, an increased frequency of headache has not been stressed in reviews by other authorities (Rubenstein *et al.*, 1981) and was not noted as a special feature in the population study of Huson, Harper and Compston

(1988). Patients with NF1 will be at least as liable to tension headache, and probably migraine, as non-affected individuals in whom the prevalence of migraine ranges from 1–19% of men to 3–29% of women (Blau, 1987). In our series, two of 103 patients and one of 103 control subjects had migraine (Hughes and Ferner, unpublished data). Rare patients with cerebral tumours, uncompensated hydrocephalus, malignant plexiform neurofibromas affecting the scalp and phaeochromocytoma may have headache as part of their clinical picture. In a unique case, episodic facial pain, ptosis and lacrimation in a 3½-year-old girl, resembling migrainous neuralgia, was attributed to a supraclinoid internal carotid artery stenosis (Levisohn, Mikhael and Rothman, 1978). Patients with NF1 may also have headache as a result of anxiety or depression associated with their disease.

8.6 CEREBRAL TUMOURS

8.6.1 Introduction

At the back of the minds of many patients with headache, and their physicians, is the concern about a cerebral tumour. This concern has been unnecessarily exaggerated in NF1 by previous confusion between NF2, in which CNS tumours are indeed common, and NF1, in which they are rare. This confusion reduces the usefulness of earlier reviews (Canale and Bebin, 1972).

8.6.2 Optic gliomas

Optic gliomas, discussed in detail in Chapter 10, are the only CNS tumours with a markedly increased frequency in NF1. Subclinical tumours occurred in 15% of patients in one hospital-based series submitted to imaging studies (Lewis and Riccardi, 1981), and symptomatic tumours were known to be present in 1.5% of patients in a population study (Huson, Harper and Compston, 1988). When the tumours do produce symptoms they usually do so in children by causing non-paralytic squint with amblyopia or unilateral proptosis. They may be suspected in patients with NF1 with otherwise unexplained reduction in visual acuity or optic atrophy. They are usually extremely indolent tumours, not progressing over many years, or never progressing, but about 5% of tumours eventually extend into the chiasm (Alvord and Lofton, 1988; North American Study Group for Optic Glioma, 1989) and then either into the contralateral optic nerve or posteriorly along the optic tract into the cerebral hemisphere (Figure 8.1). The differential diagnosis from meningioma, investigation with computed tomography (CT) and MRI and conservative approach to management of optic gliomas are described in

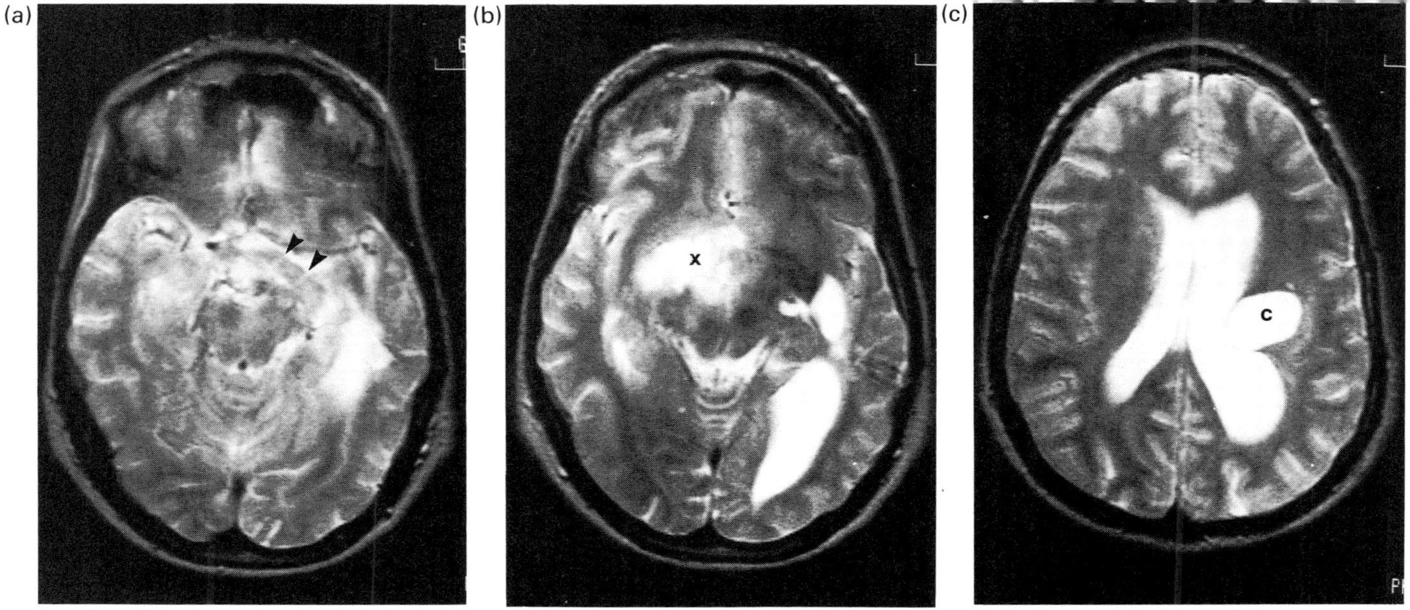

Figure 8.1 T2-weighted axial images (SE TR 192/TE 100) from a man aged 22 years showing the late stages of a chiasmal glioma, which has spread back into both cerebral hemispheres. The tumour presented at age 2 years as a suprasellar cyst causing a right homonymous hemianopia and hemiparesis. Following aspiration of the cyst and irradiation, the patient's condition remained stable until 3 months before these scans were performed, when he became drowsy. Despite further radiotherapy he gradually deteriorated and died 18 months later. (a) The chiasm is thickened and there is a thickening of the left optic tract (arrowheads) leading back to an extensive area of altered signal in the deep part of the left temporal lobe. (b) Extensive altered signal and swelling in the right basal ganglia and medial temporal lobe (x). The lateral part of the left basal ganglia deep to the insular cortex contains a partly cystic, partly solid area of altered signal (c). The cystic component extends superiorly to lie lateral to and indent the left lateral ventricle. (Scans provided by Dr J. Bingham and Dr T. Cox, Philip Harris Nuclear Magnetic Resonance Unit, UMDS, Guy's Hospital, and reproduced with their permission.)

Chapter 10. The rare tumours that spread posteriorly gradually produce contralateral hemisensory impairment and hemiparesis from involvement of the thalamus and internal capsule. Obstruction of the foramen of Magendie or the third ventricle may also produce hydrocephalus with headache and drowsiness. This clinical progression is rare and takes place over years so that judging the efficacy of treatment regimens is difficult. In individual cases, needle biopsy of deeply situated tumour tissue may be possible and space-occupying cysts can sometimes be drained with benefit. It is our practice to offer radiotherapy when there is clinical and radiological evidence of progression. Symptomatic hydrocephalus will require insertion of a shunt.

8.6.3 Other CNS tumours

There is a widespread presumption that CNS tumours, apart from optic gliomas, are more common in NF1 than in the rest of the population, which has been perpetuated in the most recent reviews (Mulvihill *et al.*, 1990). Although anecdotal case reports of cerebral, brain stem and spinal cord tumours testify to this association, the older literature is contaminated by inclusion of NF2 cases in which CNS gliomas and meningiomas, sometimes multiple, are common. For instance, of four autopsy cases reported by Horie *et al.* (1974), one must be discounted because the clinical history indicated a diagnosis of NF2. However, the other three patients probably did have NF1, and also had cerebral tumours, consisting of a grade 1 astrocytoma in the basal ganglia and temporal lobe, an occipital glioblastoma multiforme and a grade 3 astrocytoma at the cervico-medullary junction. Similarly, in a French series of six cases of neurofibromatosis, four had NF2 associated with meningiomas and two had NF1, one with a glioma in the medulla and one with a frontal glioma (Wertheimer *et al.*, 1957). It was series like these that gave rise to the impression that neurofibromatosis is associated with meningiomas. While there is a clear association between NF2 and meningioma, there is scant evidence of an increased incidence of meningioma in NF1 (Tada *et al.*, 1988; Eljamel and Foy, 1989).

Recent large series include few cases of glioma in NF1 outside the visual pathway or meningiomas. For instance, in a Swiss hospital-based series of 133 children, there were 20 optic pathway gliomas and only five gliomas in other parts of the brain (Hochstrasser, Boltshauser and Valavanis, 1988). Huson, Harper and Compston (1988) found no gliomas in their population study of 135 cases apart from two with symptomatic optic glioma, although one relative with NF1 living outside the study area had died from a frontal astrocytoma and another with an uncertain diagnosis of NF1 had died from a cerebellar astrocytoma. In our own neurologically biased series of 103 patients, there were four patients with an optic glioma and three with a cerebral glioma. In another neurologically based series of 250 patients, there were two astrocytomas, three 'other glial tumours' and three meningiomas (Rubenstein, 1986). Even in that series there remains a possible confusion with NF2 as there were five patients with vestibular Schwannoma, which is exceedingly rare in NF1 (see below). Since neurologists only encounter primary CNS tumours in 2–3% of their NF1 patients, the incidence of glioma in NF1 is at most four times greater than that in the general population of the UK, in which 0.7% of deaths are caused by malignant brain tumours (Office of Population Censuses and Surveys, 1987). Useful data about the prevalence, sites and possible special features of CNS tumours in NF1 are difficult to glean from the literature. Ilgren, Kinnier-Wilson and Stiller (1985) collected information on 68 children from a British national cancer registry and added information on 19 other patients, including adults from specialist centres. Although NF2 was not specifically excluded, vestibular Schwannomas are not mentioned in the lists of associated neoplasms in any of the cases, so most of the patients probably had NF1. The cases included 43 optic gliomas, 17 cerebellar tumours, 11 third ventricle tumours, 11 cerebral gliomas, four brain stem gliomas and three spinal cord tumours. Pathological aspects of these tumours are described in Chapter 6.

Cerebellar tumours, to judge by anecdotal reports and series in the literature, occur next in frequency to optic gliomas. They present with headache, vomiting and features of raised intracranial pressure together with ataxia, disequilibrium, head tilt and other features of a posterior fossa lesion. MRI scans are better than CT scans for imaging posterior fossa tumours. In our series (Ferner *et al.*, 1993) a small asymptomatic space-occupying lesion, probably a low-grade glioma, was revealed in one cerebellar hemisphere by MRI scanning (Figure 8.2). The cerebellar tumours in the series of Ilgren, Kinnier-Wilson and Stiller (1985) included 15 astrocytomas and two ependymomas, but medulloblastomas were not represented. Half the astrocytomas were considered malignant on histological grounds, a significantly higher proportion than in their contemporary series of non-NF1 cerebellar astrocytomas. The discovery of asymptomatic gliomas on MRI scans, such as that in Figure 8.2, casts doubt on the idea that cerebellar astrocytomas in NF1 are necessarily more malignant than usual.

Cerebral gliomas were frequently reported in association with neurofibromatosis in the older literature, which did not clearly distinguish NF1 and NF2. For instance, nine cases of cerebral tumour were discovered in a series of 110 patients by Brasfield and Das Gupta (1972) and other series and reports are discussed by Ilgren, Kinnier-Wilson and Stiller (1985). In general, few special clinical or pathological features have been noted that would distinguish the gliomas of patients with NF1 from those of the rest of the population. Gliomas may occur at a younger age than expected.

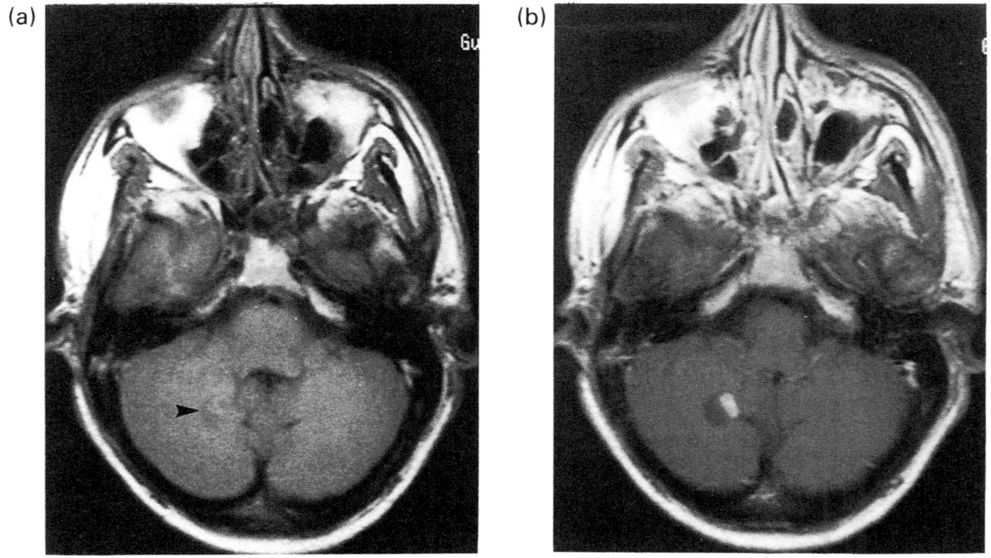

Figure 8.2 T1-weighted axial scans (SE TR 500/TE 20) of the posterior fossa of a man aged 21 years with NF1 showing an abnormality considered to be a low-grade glioma or hamartoma in the right cerebellar hemisphere. The main clinical complaint was of abnormally aggressive behaviour. Examination was normal apart from mild nerve deafness in the right ear, which cannot be accounted for by this lesion. (a) Small, rounded area of low signal intensity in the inferior part of the right cerebellar hemisphere (arrowhead). (b) After intravenous gadolinium-DTPA there is enhancement of the medial part of the abnormality, which is probably a glioma or hamartoma. This had not changed over 2 years. There were also areas of altered signal in the left globus pallidus, right cerebral peduncle and right parietal lobe. (Scans provided by Dr J. Bingham and Dr T. Cox, Philip Harris Nuclear Magnetic Resonance Unit, UMDS, Guy's Hospital, and reproduced with their permission.)

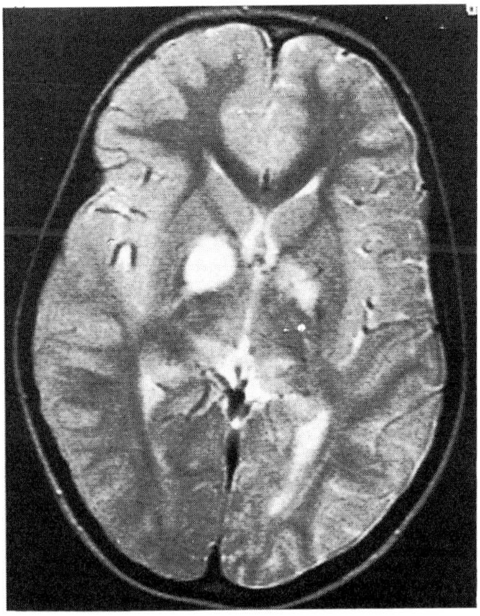

Figure 8.3 T2-weighted axial image (SE TR 2059/TE 90) showing asymptomatic abnormalities in a girl aged 11 years with NF1. There is increased signal in the globus pallidus on both sides, especially the right. The ventricles are of normal size. (Scan provided by Dr J. Bingham and Dr T. Cox, Philip Harris Nuclear Magnetic Resonance Unit, UMDS, Guy's Hospital, and reproduced with their permission.)

Multicentric gliomas have been described in several instances (Wertheimer *et al.*, 1957; Scharenberg, 1971; Horie *et al.*, 1974) and may be unusually common. Gliomas may also arise at unusual sites, one of which is around the third ventricle, where Ilgren, Kinnier-Wilson and Stiller (1985) reported 11 astrocytomas infiltrating the hypothalamus or thalamus. In one case a separate optic glioma was discovered at postmortem examination, an example of multicentric glioma formation. Some, but not all, of the children who develop precocious puberty have tumours of the optic pathway which may be responsible for abnormal activation of the hypothalamo-pituitary-adrenal axis (Laue *et al.*, 1985) (Chapter 13). MRI studies have often revealed extensive abnormalities, especially in the basal ganglia, whose pathology is uncertain (Figure 8.3). Although they resemble gliomas, they are usually asymptomatic and have not progressed over the few years that MRI has been available.

Five children with brain stem gliomas were reported whose clinical course was more insidious than is usual for gliomas in this situation in non-neurofibromatosis subjects (Milstein *et al.*, 1989). In addition, irradiation induced protracted improvement, which is also unusual. The brain stem is one of the regions where extensive abnormalities may be

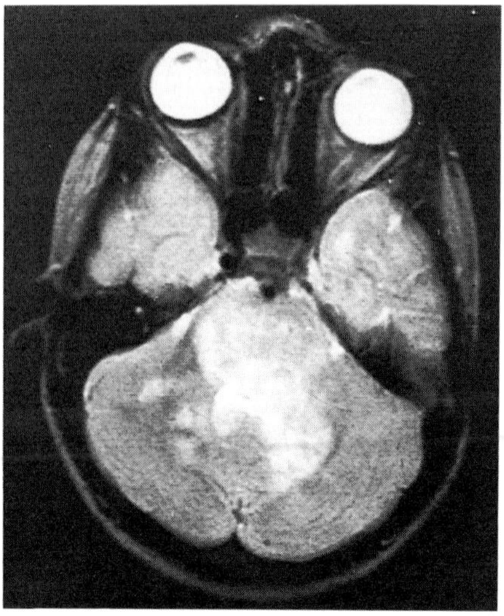

Figure 8.4 T2-weighted axial image (SE TR 2059/TE 90) showing an asymptomatic abnormality in the brain stem of a girl aged 11 years with NF1 (same patient as in Figure 8.3). There is increased signal in the pons and both middle cerebellar peduncles, especially the left, with swelling causing distortion of the contour of the pons and displacing the fourth ventricle from its anterior left lateral aspect. This appearance was unchanged from 9 months earlier. This is probably a low-grade glioma or hamartoma. (Scan provided by Dr J. Bingham and Dr T. Cox, Philip Harris Nuclear Magnetic Resonance Unit, UMDS, Guy's Hospital, and reproduced with their permission.)

detected by MRI in the absence of neurological deficit (Figure 8.4); in one of our cases such a lesion displaced the fourth ventricle in such a way as to suggest an intrinsic tumour (Figure 8.5). The lesion was not associated with any neurological symptoms or deficit and had not changed 1 year later, but a low-grade brain stem glioma is the most likely diagnosis.

Spinal cord tumours have also occasionally been reported in association with NF1, although they are more common in NF2. They usually present with a gradually progressive paraparesis, impairment of pain and temperature sensation, and reflex loss at the level of the tumour indicating an intrinsic cord tumour. They have to be distinguished from compression of the cord by a spinal root neurofibroma and from syringomyelia (which was reported to be a rare complication of neurofibromatosis in the older literature); MRI is the best method of making the distinction. Treatment of intrinsic cord tumours is difficult. They may only be slowly progressive and best left alone, but the usual practice is to confirm the diagnosis by neurosurgical biopsy and offer irradiation, which may arrest progression and sometimes produces improvement. In

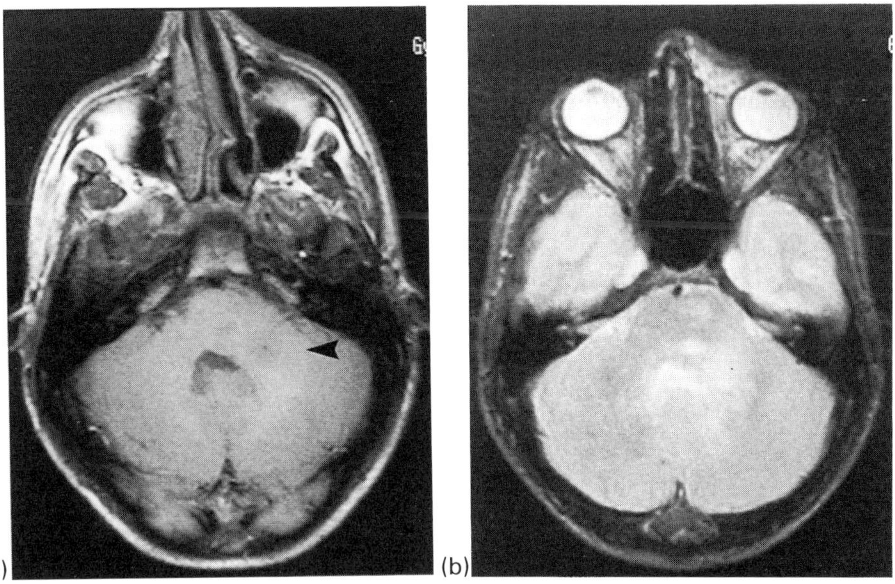

Figure 8.5 Abnormality in the pons of a man aged 19 years with a history of learning difficulties and clumsiness at school, whose only neurological abnormality was mild incoordination of the right upper limb. (a) T1-weighted axial image (SE TR 450/TE 30). There is swelling of the left brachium pontis (arrowhead) with distortion of the fourth ventricle. (b) T2-weighted axial image (SE TR 2000/TE 80). Increased signal in the left brachium pontis with swelling causing distortion of the fourth ventricle is seen. There were no associated symptoms or signs and 9 months later the appearances were unchanged. This is probably a low-grade glioma or hamartoma. (Scans provided by Dr J. Bingham and Dr T. Cox, Philip Harris Nuclear Magnetic Resonance Unit, UMDS, Guy's Hospital, and reproduced with their permission.)

the series of Ilgren, Kinnier-Wilson and Stiller (1985) there were three intrinsic cord tumours, including a low-grade astrocytoma, an unspecified ependymoma and an unspecified glioma.

8.7 INCREASED-INTENSITY LESIONS ON T2-WEIGHTED MRI BRAIN SCANS

Increased-intensity lesions are commonly found on T2-weighted MRI brain scans even in asymptomatic patients with NF1. They may be more common in children and young adults and occur especially in the basal ganglia and brain stem. Ferner *et al.* (1993) found such lesions in 13 of 38 patients. The pathological correlation of these lesions has not yet been made. Some lesions show radiological evidence of displacing neighbouring structures, and enhancement after intravenous injection of contrast medium. Such lesions may be low-grade gliomas, whereas non-space-occupying lesions that do not enhance are more likely to be areas of non-proliferative dysplasia. As discussed in Chapter 9, these abnormal lesions are not related to the occurrence of mental handicap in NF1.

8.8 VESTIBULAR SCHWANNOMA

Although the eighth cranial nerve is a site of predilection for the growth of solitary Schwannomas in the general population, and the hallmark of NF2 is bilateral vestibular Schwannomas, there is no evidence that the incidence of vestibular Schwannomas is increased in NF1. There are no reports of vestibular Schwannomas in any of the recent population studies in which NF1 has been clearly distinguished from NF2. Nevertheless, there was an increased prevalence of deafness in a hospital-based series of patients with NF1: 45 (65%) of 69 patients had some deficit on a test of pure tone thresholds, and the deficit was severe in eight patients. The cause of these abnormalities was not identified, but auditory brain stem evoked responses were abnormal in 33% of 51 patients, often showing a delay in central conduction time (Pikus, 1990). Rare cases of conductive deafness as a result of neurofibromas occluding the external auditory meatus have been reported (McKennan, 1991).

8.9 AQUEDUCT STENOSIS

Hydrocephalus due to aqueduct stenosis is a rare, but probably genuine, association with NF1. In some cases the pathological basis consists of focal proliferation of subependymal glial cells around the aqueduct; such collections of cells have been compared to fibrillary astrocytic gliomas, but do not behave in a progressive manner. Three examples were described in one neuropathological series of 11 cases, only two of which caused hydrocephalus (Rubinstein, 1986). At least 25 examples of aqueduct stenosis without tumours have been reported in NF1 (Horwich, Riccardi and Francke, 1983; Riviello *et al.*, 1988; Senveli *et al.*, 1989). Symptomatic hydrocephalus will require management by shunting, usually with a ventriculo-peritoneal shunt, but sometimes by third ventriculostomy (Senveli *et al.*, 1989). Modern imaging techniques may reveal arrested hydrocephalus which does not require treatment. MRI scans are superior to CT scans for demonstrating posterior fossa tumours. One case of a tiny pilocytic astrocytoma arising from the aqueduct and causing hydrocephalus has been reported (Hosoda *et al.*, 1986).

Two cases of NF1 have been reported in association with hydrocephalus due to the Chiari I malformation (abnormally low placement of the cerebellar tonsils causing obstruction of the outflow of the fourth ventricle) (Afifi *et al.*, 1988). Only one other report of Chiari I malformation (without hydrocephalus) has appeared (Hornstein and Borchers, 1989). This association is certainly rare and might be coincidental.

8.10 CEREBROVASCULAR DISEASE

Three cases of stenosis or occlusion of the supraclinoid portion of the internal carotid artery were reported by Hilal *et al.* (1971); all three had optic gliomas and two had received radiotherapy, which can itself cause arterial occlusion. By 1988, Sobata, Ohkuma and Suzuki (1988) were able to review 37 similar cases, including one of their own, of which only four had received radiotherapy and only eight had tumours, showing that stenosis/occlusion can occur independently of either. Stenosis/occlusion has usually been identified following the development of a stroke in childhood. However, it was once found on investigation of a migrainous neuralgia-like syndrome (Levisohn, Mikhael and Rothman, 1978), and was sometimes an incidental finding during investigation of some other problem. Most cases have affected the internal carotid artery, usually the supraclinoid portion just beyond the origin of the ophthalmic artery, or the proximal portions of the anterior and middle cerebral arteries (Chono *et al.*, 1985). Rarely the posterior cerebral or vertebral arteries have been affected (Taboada *et al.*, 1979). Multiple arteries are often involved (Sasaki *et al.*, 1984). The usual radiological appearance is of a smooth constriction or occlusion of the supraclinoid portion of the internal carotid artery with the formation of an extensive collateral pseudoangiomatous capillary network. When intra-arterial contrast medium is injected, this network fills, resembling the puff of smoke from the top of a Japanese volcano, named Moya Moya, and therefore called the Moya Moya syndrome. Although superficial temporal–middle cerebral artery anastomosis has been tried in adult patients with the Moya Moya syndrome who do not have NF1, there is no evidence that the procedure is helpful and it would be technically more difficult in children. Management has therefore been conservative.

Ten cases of cerebral aneurysm in association with NF1 have been reported, half having presented with subarachnoid haemorrhage and half with a miscellany of symptoms, sometimes as an incidental finding (Sobata, Ohkuma and Suzuki, 1988). Four of these 10 cases also had internal carotid stenosis and the pathogenesis of the aneurysms may be related to the known abnormalities of blood vessels in NF1 rather than being the usual type of berry aneurysm encountered in the general population. Increased flow in collateral arteries associated with an occlusion may encourage aneurysm formation. A unique asymptomatic aneurysmal dilatation of the petrous carotid artery was recently reported (Frank, Brown and Wilson, 1989). Three patients with large arteriovenous fistulae, two affecting the vertebral arteries and one affecting the internal maxillary artery (Deans *et al.*, 1982), have been reported in NF1. Another patient had an intrasellar cavernous haemangioma (Mitsuhashi *et al.*, 1991).

Reports of an increased prevalence of cerebrovascular disease in NF1 (Riccardi, 1981) have to be carefully interpreted since cerebrovascular disease is common in the community at large. The incidence of atherothrombotic brain infarctions in a follow-up study in Framingham, Massachusetts was 1/1000 for ages 35–64 years and 5/1000 for males and 4/1000 for females aged 65 years and over (Wolf *et al.*, 1987). Accordingly, reports of the occurrence of stroke in hospital-based series of patients with stroke cannot by themselves be taken as evidence of cerebrovascular pathology. Patients with NF1 are at increased risk of hypertension, which is a risk factor for stroke owing to both cerebral infarction and cerebral haemorrhage. Treatment of hypertension should reduce the risk of stroke from these causes. Rapid lowering of the blood pressure is dangerous in patients who have a cerebral circulation compromised by internal carotid stenosis or occlusion (Pellock *et al.*, 1980). Therefore the clinical history and examination should be reviewed for evidence of cerebral ischaemia before embarking on antihypertensive treatment. Where doubt exists, a CT scan should be undertaken seeking evidence of cerebral atrophy, which is usually evident in the Moya Moya syndrome, and consideration should be given to investigating the cerebral circulation by contrast radiography or non-invasive ultrasound techniques.

8.11 INTRASPINAL NEUROFIBROMAS

Spinal root neurofibromas may compress the spinal cord or the spinal root on which they are growing. They characteristically form dumb-bell tumours that may compress both the spinal cord and the spinal root and enlarge the affected intravertebral foramen. Compression of the spinal cord usually presents with weakness of the limbs and impairment of sensation below the level of the lesion. The initial symptoms and signs may be asymmetrical producing a partial Brown–Sequard syndrome with ipsilateral pyramidal signs and impairment of light touch, position, and vibration sensation, and contralateral impairment of pain and temperature sensation. Urinary retention or incontinence may occur, but usually relatively late compared with intrinsic cord tumours, in which they may occur early (see below). Pain at the level of the tumour is common, and may be severe radicular pain aggravated by coughing, and (unlike an intervertebral disc protrusion) worsened by lying down. These tumours usually enlarge slowly and steadily, and once they have begun to produce symptoms of cord compression, they should be removed surgically as soon as possible because the compressed spinal cord is at risk of

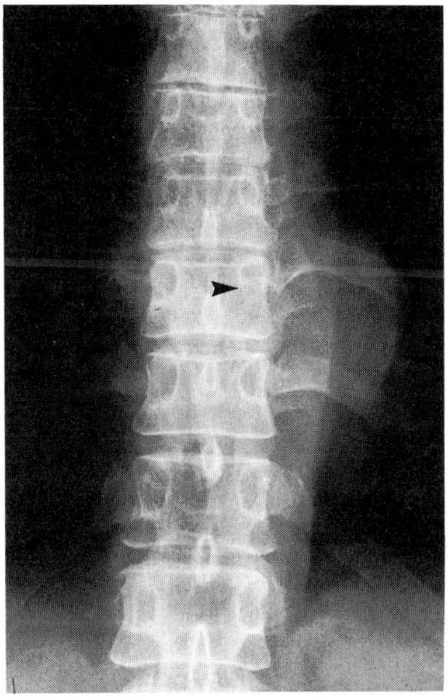

Figure 8.6 Portion of a dorsal spine radiograph showing a paravertebral shadow on the left side due to a neurofibroma which has eroded the inferior portion of the left pedicle of T10 (arrowhead). This radiograph is from a patient with segmental NF who presented with pain in the T10 myotome and café au lait patches in the T10 and T11 dermatomes on the left. There were no other features of neurofibromatosis and no family history. (Radiograph provided by Dr H. Saxton, Department of Radiology, Guy's Hospital, and reproduced with his permission.)

infarction, which would cause irreversible damage. Spinal neurofibromas may enlarge during pregnancy. Spinal neurofibromas are best diagnosed by MRI, but plain radiographs may show widening of the intervertebral foramina (Figure 8.6); if MRI (Figure 8.7) is not available, myelography and CT provide an alternative method. These neurofibromas may arise at any level from C1 (Ferner, Honavar and Gullan, 1989) to the cauda equina (Figure 8.8c,d). Bucci *et al.* (1990) reported the successful removal of five such tumours at the C1–2 level from the anterior aspect of the cord via a posterolateral approach. In a remarkable case, multiple neurofibromas at the craniocervical junction had caused atlantoaxial subluxation that was associated with, and may have caused, bilateral arteriovenous fistulas (Hasegawa *et al.*, 1989).

8.12 SPINAL MENINGOCELES

Meningoceles are herniae of the spinal theca. In neurofibromatosis they are usually lateral herniations of the theca in the thoracic region, although

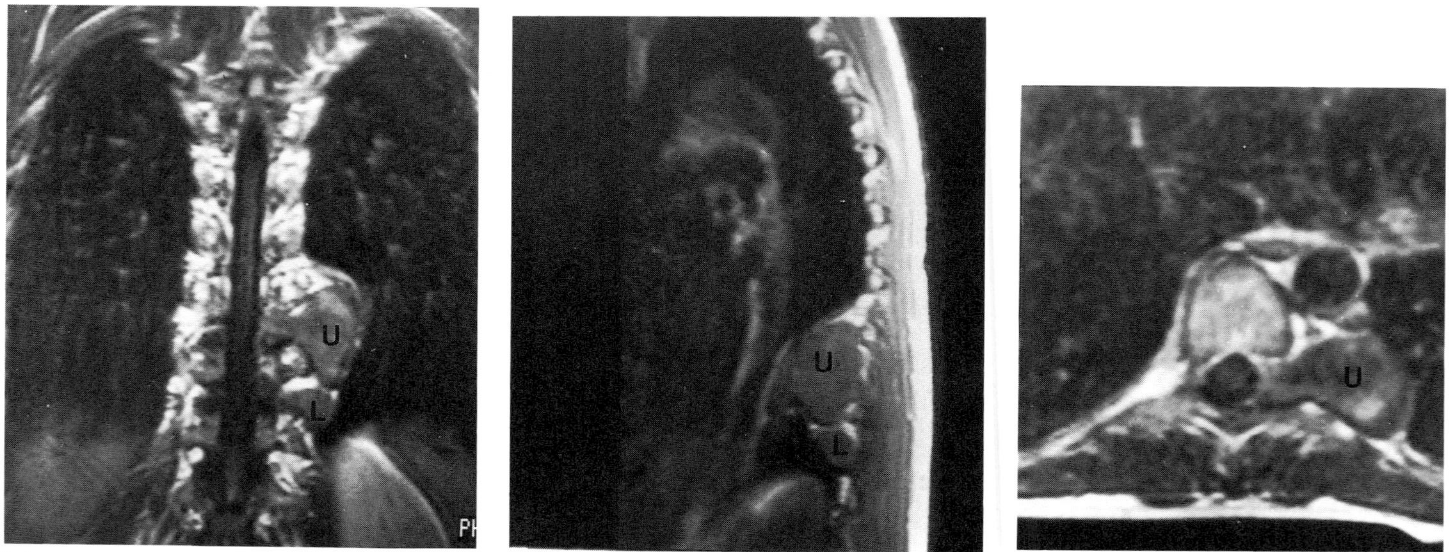

(a) (b) (c)

Figure 8.7 (a) T2-weighted coronal MRI scan (SE TR 415/TE 20); (b) sagittal scan (TR SE 685/TE 20); and (c) T2-weighted axial scan (TR SE 500/TE 20) from the same patient as in Figure 8.6 showing two neurofibromas. The upper (U) lies on the T10 root and extends into the intervertebral foramen but not the spinal canal (a). The lower (L) extends up to, but not into, the intervertebral foramen. (Scans provided by Dr J. Bingham and Dr T. Cox, Philip Harris Nuclear Magnetic Resonance Unit, UMDS, Guy's Hospital, and reproduced with their permission.)

they sometimes occur in the cervical region (So and Li, 1989). In a review of the 88 reports of thoracic meningocele in the world literature, 85% were in patients with NF1 (Erkulvrawatr *et al.*, 1979). In most cases the meningocele was an incidental finding revealed by plain radiographs taken for other reasons. Meningoceles cause paravertebral masses with scalloping of the vertebrae, which can be difficult to distinguish from that produced by dumb-bell neurofibromas on plain radiographs. Their true nature can be revealed by contrast myelography or, more simply, by CT or MRI. Although thoracic meningoceles are usually asymptomatic, paraparesis has been reported in 9% of cases and minor symptoms in another 8%. Headache has been a feature in 3% of cases and has been speculatively attributed to low cerebrospinal fluid (CSF) pressure such as occurs after lumbar puncture (Erkulvrawatr *et al.*, 1979).

8.13 INTRAMEDULLARY SPINAL CORD TUMOURS

Although earlier series included cases of NF2 in which intramedullary tumours are very common, there have been cases reported of intramedullary gliomas in NF1, and their frequency probably exceeds that in the general population (Ilgren, Kinnier-Wilson and Stiller, 1985). They usually present with a progressive paraparesis with sensory impairment below the level of the lesion and impairment of sphincter control at a fairly early stage. MRI is the best method of imaging these lesions, and myelography backed up by CT is now an inferior alternative. It is usual to confirm the diagnosis by neurosurgical biopsy and to give the patient radiotherapy.

8.14 NEUROFIBROMATOSIS AND PERONEAL MUSCULAR ATROPHY

Rare examples of progressive sensorimotor peripheral neuropathy have been reported in association with neurofibromatosis. This diagnosis must be made with care because the accumulation of multiple root lesions can produce a clinical picture resembling peroneal muscular atrophy (Figure 8.8). Electrophysiological examination of the lower limbs alone in our case could have been interpreted as due to the axonal type of hereditary motor and sensory neuropathy (type 2), but the normal electrophysiological findings in the upper limbs refuted that diagnosis. The neurological deficit was due to multiple neurofibromata on the cauda equina roots which were demonstrated by myelography (Figure 8.8).

However, in some cases of NF1, peroneal muscular atrophy has been due to neuropathy, which has been called neurofibromatous neuropathy (Thomas *et al.*, 1990). Thomas and Eames (1971) reported a man with multiple café au lait patches and axillary freckling (fulfilling diagnostic

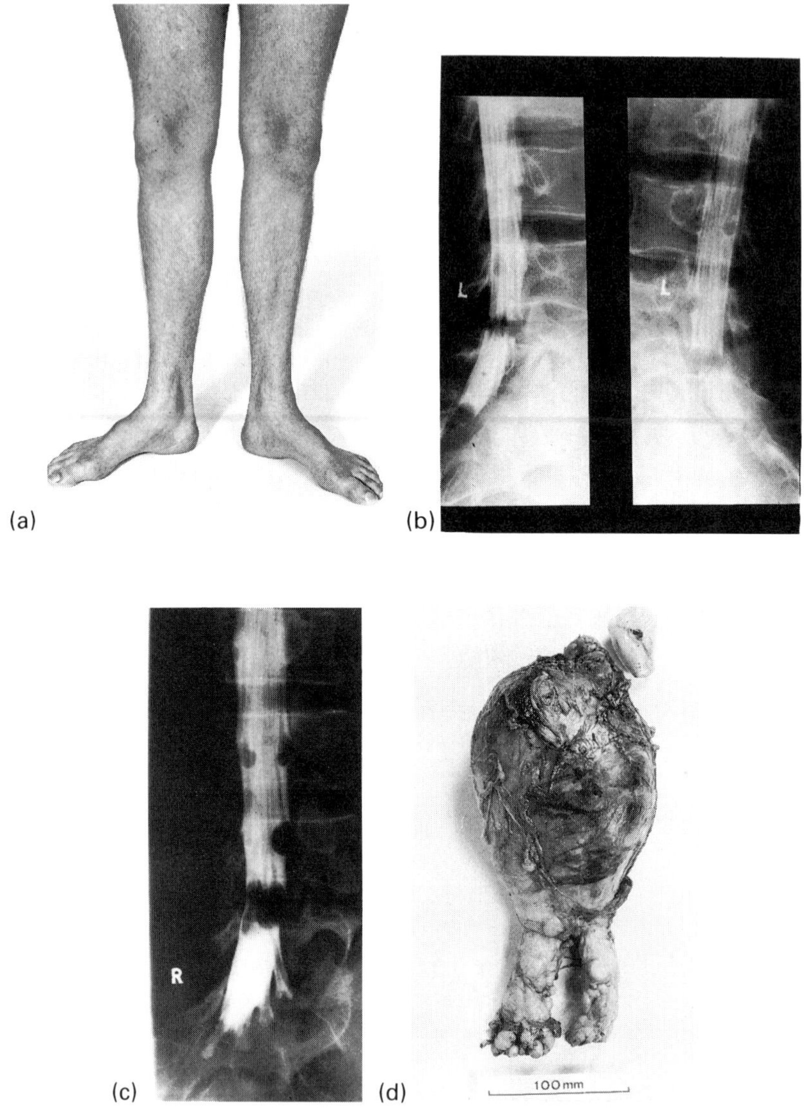
(a)
(b)
L
L
(c)
R
(d)
100 mm

(e)
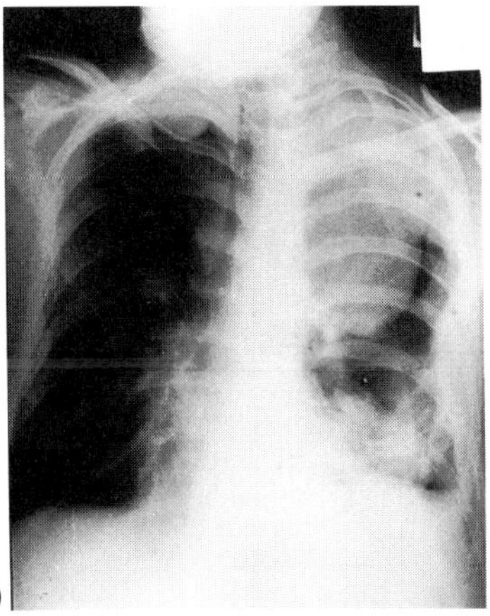

Figure 8.8 (a) The legs of a man aged 27 years with NF1 who had had bilateral progressive weakness and numbness of his legs for 18 months, producing peroneal muscular atrophy. The leg muscles showed evidence of denervation on electromyography and the sural nerve action potentials were markedly reduced. However, the upper limb sensory and motor nerve conduction were normal. (b) The neurological deficit was attributed to multiple neurofibromas on the cauda equina nerve roots. (Myelogram provided by Dr R.D. Hoare and reproduced with his permission.) (c) Seven years later the neurofibromas had enlarged, but there was no evidence of a generalized neuropathy. (Myelogram provided by Dr T. Cox and reproduced with his permission.) (d) One year later a malignant Schwannoma was excised from the left sciatic nerve. (Photograph provided by Professor Lord McColl.) (e) He had multiple metastases including these in the lung, and died soon afterwards despite treatment with adriamycin.

criteria for NF1) who had clinical and electrophysiological features of the axonal form of peroneal muscular atrophy. There was no family history except of foot drop and subcutaneous lumps in one leg reported in a brother, and the family was not available for genetic studies. The patient had no dermal neurofibromas but the nerves exhibited irregular thickenings along their course. A superficial peroneal nerve biopsy showed neurofibroma-like tissue in a subperineurial sleeve surrounding a central core of more normal endoneurial tissue (Figure 8.9). In a subsequent report the authors discuss whether this case may represent a different disease rather than a rare variant of NF1 (Thomas *et al.*, 1990). They also presented another similar case of peroneal muscular atrophy associated with NF1-like features in which the nerve biopsy findings were identical to those in Figure 8.9. This man's father had NF1-like features but without peroneal muscular atrophy. Four cases of peroneal muscular atrophy associated with NF1 were reported in abstract by Murphy, Bosch and Cancilla (1980). Three cases were all in the same family and one was

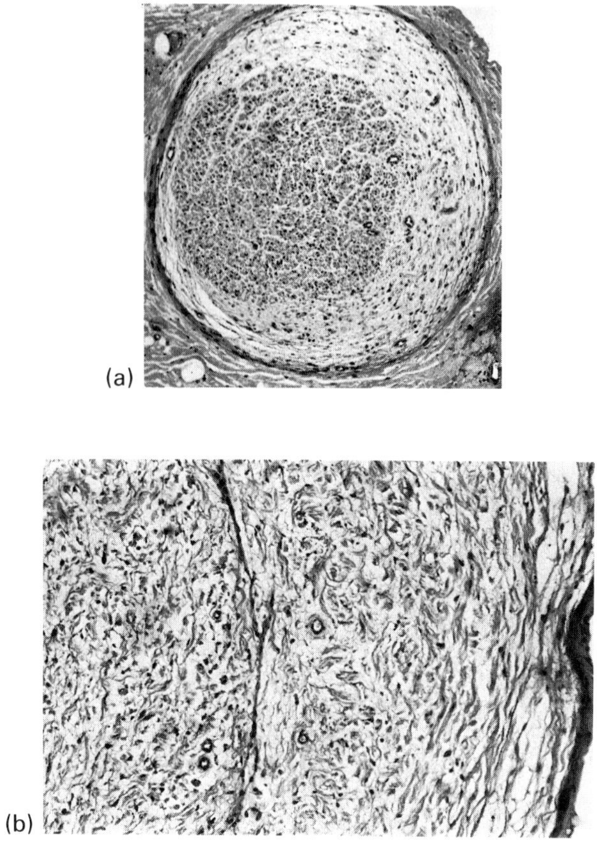

Figure 8.9 (a) Transverse section through a fascicle from the superficial peroneal nerve biopsy of a patient with NF1 and peroneal muscular atrophy showing a central area of compact tissue surrounded by a loose subperineurial zone. Haematoxylin and eosin stain, × 100. (b) Higher power view of the subperineurial region showing interlacing bundles of collagen fibrils within which blood vessels and nuclei of fibroblasts and blood vessels are visible. × 350. (Reproduced from Thomas *et al*. (1990) with permission.)

sporadic. Although the nerve conduction studies only showed moderate reduction of nerve conduction velocity (suggesting the axonal form of hereditary motor and sensory neuropathy), nerve biopsies in two showed onion bulb formation. Bradley, Richardson and Frew (1974) described a woman with NF1 and a progressive sensorimotor axonal neuropathy causing peroneal muscular atrophy; she also had complete bilateral deafness with a progressive onset in childhood. Her two daughters had mild subclinical neurophysiological evidence of axonal neuropathy and one also had multiple café au lait patches but no other features of NF1; they also had partial albinism, infantile deafness and a dominantly inherited abnormality of the iris in which strands are attached to the posterior of the periphery of the cornea, called Axenfeld's defect. The postmortem examination of another patient with NF1 disclosed diffuse thickening of the peripheral nerves with degeneration of nerve fibres, proliferation of fibroblasts and an increase of mucoid interstitial material, but the clinical findings were not reported (Lambers and Ortiz de Zarate, 1952).

A few patients have been reported with NF2 and peroneal muscular atrophy associated with neurofibromatous changes in the peripheral nerves consisting of lamellated processes probably derived from perineurial cells (Ohnishi and Nada, 1972; Thomas *et al.*, 1990).

8.15 PERIPHERAL NERVE NEUROFIBROMAS

Although the commonest neurofibromas in NF1 are those that arise in the dermis and produce the characteristic multiple sessile or pedunculated lumps (dermal neurofibromas), it is also common for more deeply situated tumours to arise along the course of nerves (nodular neurofibromas). Those within the spinal canal have already been discussed, but tumours may arise at any site from the proximal roots to the most peripheral nerve branches. Benign neurofibromas usually produce little in the way of neurological deficit and few symptoms and simply present as lumps, which may become very large (Figure 8.10). The occurrence of pain and progressive neurological deficit can occur with benign tumours compressing the nerve from which they originate. However, such symptoms give rise to concern about the possibility of malignant change.

8.16 MALIGNANT PERIPHERAL NERVE TUMOURS

Malignant change in neurofibromas is rare, but does occur and accounts for the greater incidence of malignant peripheral nerve tumours in NF1 than the general population. In the Baylor neurofibromatosis programme, 24 (3.5%) of 693 patients had neurofibrosarcoma and nine of these cases developed after enrolment into the programme for other reasons (Riccardi and Powell, 1989). From a Japanese autopsy series of 122 cases of NF1, 19.7% died of malignant Schwannoma, 13% of neurofibrosarcoma and 10% of glioma (Okada and Shozawa, 1984). Although these percentages are biased estimates from hospital-based series, a few cases of malignant peripheral nerve tumours are regularly reported, even in population studies of NF1. Two of 138 cases had malignant peripheral nerve tumours in the southeast Wales population study (Huson, Harper and Compston, 1988). In a study of 30 malignant Schwannomas collected in a Danish centre serving 1.5 million people

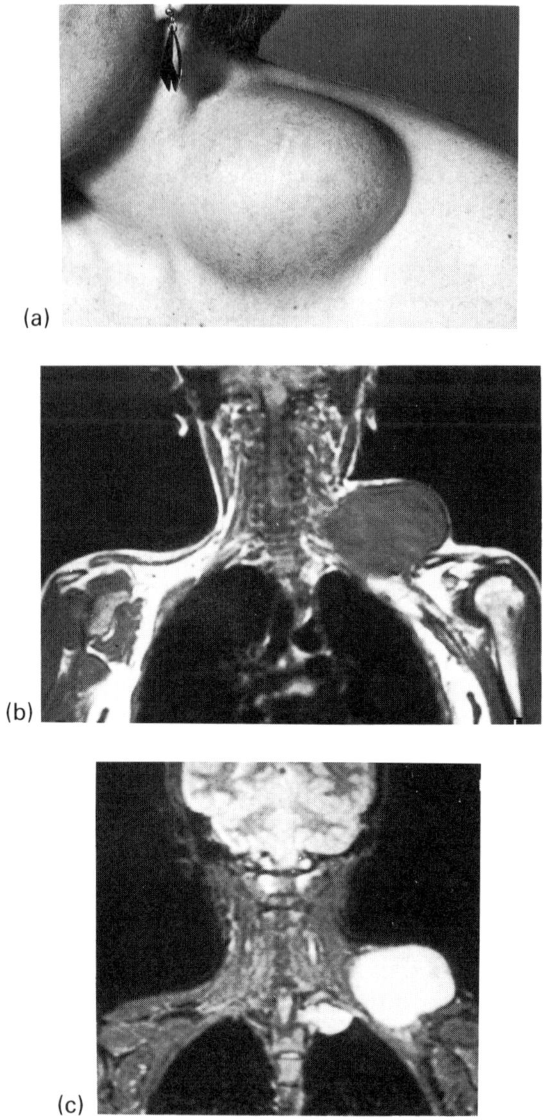

Figure 8.10 (a) Large painless neurofibroma arising from the left brachial plexus. There was no associated neurological deficit. (b) T1-weighted coronal image (SE TR 595/TE 20). A large nodular plexiform neurofibroma is seen to be arising from the left brachial plexus. (c) T1-weighted coronal image (IR TR 1800/TE 30) following intravenous injection of gadolinium-DTPA causing enhancement of the neurofibroma arising from the brachial plexus. In addition a separate neurofibroma on the left T2 root is shown lying in the intervertebral foramen. These neurofibromas were not causing pain or neurological deficit. The larger one was removed without producing any deficit.

over about 18 years, eight occurred in patients with NF1 (Bojsen-Mller and Myhre-Jensen, 1984). Malignant peripheral nerve tumours include neurofibrosarcomas, malignant Schwannomas, angiosarcomas and malignant Schwannomas with rhabdomyoblastic differentiation termed malignant 'Triton' tumours (Bojsen-Mller and Myhre-Jensen, 1984; Brooks, Freeman and Enterline, 1985; Konishi *et al.*, 1986; Brown, Tornos and Evans, 1992). Their pathology is described in Chapter 6.

Malignant tumours may occur at any site in the peripheral nervous system, but are said to arise most commonly from plexiform neurofibromas. Posterior mediastinal tumours are not uncommon and, while usually benign, may undergo malignant change (Ardissone *et al.*, 1986). A recent report has indicated that neurofibrosarcomas may also, albeit rarely, arise from the dermis (Dabski, Reiman and Muller, 1990). Tumours sometimes arise in the field of irradiation for another neoplasm (Ducatman *et al.*, 1986; Dabski, Reiman and Muller, 1990), raising the possibility that they are radiation-induced. They usually present as progressively enlarging masses without pain or other symptoms, as in two-thirds of a recent series of 31 cases (Nambisan *et al.*, 1984). However, the occurrence of pain and sensory or motor deficit in the territory of the nerve involved should also give rise to concern about malignant change since such symptoms are uncommon in benign neurofibromas, even the large benign plexiform neurofibromas associated with NF1. They are extremely malignant and difficult to treat.

Malignant Schwannomas in patients with NF1 have an even worse prognosis than in those without, and occur at a younger age (Nambisan *et al.*, 1984). Of eight patients with malignant Schwannomas and NF1, only 38% survived 5 years compared with 64% of 11 patients with malignant Schwannomas not associated with NF1 (Bojsen-Mller and Myhre-Jensen, 1984).

In a series of patients with dermal neurofibrosarcoma, two of three with NF1 died within 2 years, while only one of 10 patients with dermal neurofibrosarcoma without NF1 died of their neoplasm (Dabski, Reiman and Muller, 1990). In a series of malignant nerve sheath tumours, 13 cases associated with NF1 had a worse 5-year survival rate (26.5%) than 18 cases without NF1 (50.9%, $p < 0.05$) (Nambisan *et al.*, 1984).

The only favourable prognostic factor for malignant peripheral nerve tumours has been a tumour site compatible with wide excision. One woman was still alive 14 years after excision and immediate amputation for a malignant Schwannoma in the upper arm (Bojsen-Mller and Myhre-Jensen, 1984). Of 11 patients with malignant Schwannoma and NF1 in a pathological series (Daimaru, Hashimoto and Enjoji, 1985), only two (18%) survived 5 years, one still being alive 5.8 years after simple excision of a tumour from the back and one having died 11.5 years after wide excision and irradiation of a 'huge' tumour of the ulnar nerve.

Surgical excision with a wide margin is the recommended primary treatment (Nambisan *et al.*, 1984). Where wide excision is not possible, adjuvant radiotherapy may be appropriate, but chemotherapy has not so far been found beneficial. Recurrences or metastases after initial treatment carry a very poor prognosis. Treatment with radiotherapy or chemotherapy is often attempted (Figure 8.8), but successful results have not been reported.

8.17 PSYCHIATRIC CONSEQUENCES

Patients with NF1 may have learning difficulties in childhood and their average IQ is lower than that of the general population. Some have to cope with the serious complications that the disease may cause, including the possibility of disfigurement. There is a danger that ignorance of the features of the disorder by both medical personnel and patients will exaggerate the risks and lead to a form of 'neurofibromatosis neurosis' which affects anxiety-prone patients who have been misdiagnosed as having NF1. We have seen patients with such a neurosis who actually had multiple lipomas, Klippel–Trenaunay syndrome, non-specific skin rashes or even pityriasis rosea or urticaria pigmentosa.

Suggestions that patients with NF1 suffer from psychiatric disease more than the rest of the population have to be evaluated with care. Samuelsson (1981) and Samuelsson and Riccardi (1989) found that a third of the 74 patients in a quasi-population study in Gothenburg, Sweden had psychiatric conditions. The affected patients had a wide range of disorders, including six with alcoholism and others with incompletely investigated problems such as dementia with blindness and deafness. However, there were seven patients with depression and six with anxiety. Riccardi and Eichner (1986) report that there were no instances of psychosis or dementia in their series of 238 patients attending the Baylor neurofibromatosis clinic, but admit that many complained of symptoms of anxiety and depression. Neither of these reports included a control group. Ferner and Hughes (unpublished data) found that diagnosed psychiatric illness was no more common in 103 patients with NF1 than in age- and sex-matched controls. Furthermore, the scores of the patients on a formal test of depression and anxiety were no different from those of the controls. Reports of anxiety and depression in series of patients with NF1 may therefore merely reflect the background prevalence of these common disorders in the community. Although patients with NF1 may have somatic symptoms that cause them concern, most seem able to cope with these symptoms as well as the rest of the community. The exceptions are those who have coincidental mental retardation.

REFERENCES

Afifi, A.K., Dolan, K.D., Van Gilder, J.C. and Fincham, R.W. (1988) Ventriculomegaly in neurofibromatosis-1. Association with Chiari type I malformation. *Neurofibromatosis*, **1**, 299–305.

Alvord, E.C. and Lofton, S. (1988) Gliomas of the optic nerve or chiasm. *J. Neurosurg.*, **68**, 85–98.

Ardissone, F., Andrion, A., D'Alessandro, L. *et al.* (1986) Neurogenic intrathoracic tumors. A clinicopathological review of 92 cases. *Thorac. Cardiovasc. Surg.*, **34**, 260–4.

Blau, J.N. (1987) The epidemiology of migraine headache, in *Migraine* (ed. J.N. Blau), Chapman & Hall, London, pp. 451–77.

Bojsen-Mller, M. and Myhre-Jensen, O. (1984) A consecutive series of 30 malignant schwannomas. Survival in relation to clinico-pathological parameters and treatment. *Acta Pathol. Microbiol. Immunol. Scand. [A].*, **92**, 147–55.

Bradley, W.G., Richardson, J. and Frew, I.J.C. (1974) The familial association of neurofibromatosis, peroneal muscular atrophy, congenital deafness, partial albinism, and Axenfeld's defect. *Brain*, **97**, 521–32.

Brasfield, R.D. and Das Gupta, T.K. (1972) Von Recklinghausen's disease: a clinicopathological study. *Ann. Surg.*, **175**, 86–104.

Brooks, J.S., Freeman, M. and Enterline, H.T. (1985) Malignant 'Triton' tumors. Natural history and immunohistochemistry of nine new cases with literature review. *Cancer*, **55**, 2543–9.

Brown, R.W., Tornos, C. and Evans, H.L. (1992) Angiosarcoma arising from malignant schwannoma in a patient with neurofibromatosis. *Cancer*, **70**, 1141–4.

Bucci, M.N., McGillicuddy, J.E., Taren, J.A. and Hoff, J.T. (1990) Management of anteriorly located C1–C2 neurofibromata. *Surg. Neurol.*, **33**, 15–18.

Canale, D.J. and Bebin, J. (1972) Von Recklinghausen disease of the nervous system. In *Handbook of Clinical Neurology, Vol. 14, The Phakomatoses* (eds P.J. Vinken and G.W. Bruyn), North Holland Publishing, Amsterdam, pp. 132–62.

Chono, Y., Ueno, K., Nunomura, M. *et al.* (1985) Von Recklinghausen's disease associated with occlusion of bilateral middle cerebral artery, moyamoya phenomenon, and anterior communicating artery aneurysm. Report of an autopsy case. *Neurol. Med. Chir. (Tokyo)*, **25**, 209–14.

Dabski, C., Reiman, H.M., Jr and Muller, S.A. (1990) Neurofibrosarcoma of skin and subcutaneous tissues. *Mayo. Clin. Proc.*, **65**, 164–72.

Daimaru, Y., Hashimoto, H. and Enjoji, M. (1985) Malignant peripheral nerve-sheath tumors (malignant schwannomas). An immunohistochemical study of 29 cases. *Am. J. Surg. Pathol.*, **9**, 434–44.

Deans, W.R., Bloch, S., Leibrock, L. *et al.* (1982) Arteriovenous fistula in patients with neurofibromatosis. *Radiology*, **144**, 103–7.

Ducatman, B.S., Scheithauer, B.W., Piepgras, D.G. *et al.* (1986) Malignant peripheral nerve sheath tumors. A clinicopathologic study of 120 cases. *Cancer*, **57**, 2006–21.

Duquenne, M., Denet, S., Weryha, G. *et al.* (1990) Steinert's disease associated with neurofibromatosis. *Presse Medicale*, **19**, 1636.

Editorial (1990) Epilepsy and disorders of neuronal migration. *Lancet*, **336**, 1035–6.

Eljamel, M.S. and Foy, P.M. (1989) Multiple meningiomas and their relation to neurofibromatosis. Review of the literature and report of seven cases. *Surg. Neurol.*, **32**, 131–6.

Erkulvrawatr, S., Gammal, T.E., Hawkins, J. *et al.* (1979) Intrathoracic meningoceles and neurofibromatosis. *Arch. Neurol.*, **36**, 557–9.

Ferner, R.E., Honavar, M. and Gullan, R.W. (1989) Spinal neurofibroma presenting as atlanto-axial subluxation in von Recklinghausen neurofibromatosis. *Neurofibromatosis,* **2**, 43–6.

Ferner, R.E., Chaudhuri, R., Bingham, J. *et al.* (1993) Magnetic resonance imaging in neurofibromatosis 1. The nature and evolution of increased intensity T2 weighted lesions and their relationship to intellectual impairment. *J. Neurol. Neurosurg. Psychiatr.*, **56**, 492–5.

Frank, E., Brown, B.M. and Wilson, D.F. (1989) Asymptomatic fusiform aneurysm of the petrous carotid artery in a patient with von Recklinghausen's neurofibromatosis. *Surg. Neurol.*, **32**, 75–8.

Hasegawa, H., Bitoh, S., Katoh, A. and Tamura, K. (1989) Bilateral vertebral arteriovenous fistulas and atlantoaxial dislocation associated with neurofibromatosis – case report. *Neurol. Med. Chir. (Tokyo),* **29**, 55–9.

Hilal, S.K., Solomon, G.E., Gold, A.P. and Carter, S. (1971) Primary arterial occlusive disease in children, parts I and II. *Radiology*, **99**, 71–94.

Hochstrasser, H., Boltshauser, E. and Valavanis, A. (1988) Brain tumors in children with von Recklinghausen neurofibromatosis. *Neurofibromatosis,* **1**, 233–9.

Holt, J.F. and Kuhns, L.R. (1976) Macrocranium and macrencephaly in neurofibromatosis. *Skeletal Radiol.*, **1**, 25–8.

Horie, A., Shigemi, U., Fukushima, T. and Tamaka, K. (1974) Neurofibromatosis complicated by intracranial brain tumours. *Acta Pathol. Jpn.*, **24**, 705.

Hornstein, L. and Borchers, D. (1989) Stroke in an infant prior to the development of manifestations of neurofibromatosis. *Neurofibromatosis,* **2**, 116–20.

Horwich, A., Riccardi, V.M. and Francke, U. (1983) Brief clinical report: aqueductal stenosis leading to hydrocephalus – an unusual manifestation of neurofibromatosis. *Am. J. Med. Genet.*, **14**, 577–81.

Hosoda, K., Kanazawa, Y., Tanaka, J. *et al.* (1986) Neurofibromatosis presenting with aqueductal stenosis due to a tumor of the aqueduct: case report. *Neurosurgery,* **19**, 1035–7.

Huson, S.M., Harper, P.S. and Compston, D.A.S. (1988) Von Recklinghausen neurofibromatosis. *Brain,* **111**, 1355–81.

Ilgren, E.B., Kinnier-Wilson, L.M. and Stiller, C.A. (1985) Gliomas in neurofibromatosis: a series of 89 cases with evidence for enhanced malignancy in associated cerebellar astrocytomas. *Pathol. Annu.*, **20** (Pt 1), 331–58.

Konishi, N., Hiasa, Y., Shimoyama, T. *et al.* (1986) Malignant 'triton' tumor with metastatic hemangiopericytoma in a patient associated with von Recklinghausen's disease. *Acta Pathol. Jpn.*, **36**, 459–69.

Lambers, K. and Ortiz de Zarate, J.C. (1952) Zentrale und periphere Neurofibromatose unter besonderer Berücksichtigung ihrer Beziehungen zür hypertrophischen Neuritis. *Dtsch. Z. Nervenheil.*, **169**, 289–307.

Laue, L., Comite, F., Hench, K. *et al.* (1985) Precocious puberty associated with neurofibromatosis and optic gliomas. Treatment with luteinizing hormone releasing hormone analogue. *Am. J. Dis. Child.*, **139**, 1097–1100.

Levisohn, P.M., Mikhael, M.A. and Rothman, S.M. (1978) Cerebrovascular changes in neurofibromatosis. *Dev. Med. Child. Neurol.*, **20**, 789–93.

Lewis, R.A. and Riccardi, V.M. (1981) Von Recklinghausen neurofibromatosis. Incidence of iris hamartomata. *Ophthalmology*, **88**, 348–54.

McKennan, K.X. (1991) Neurofibromatosis type 1 – A rare case resulting in conductive hearing loss. *Otolaryngol. Head Neck Surg.*, **104**, 868–72.

Milstein, J.M., Geyer, J.R., Berger, M.S. and Bleyer, W.A. (1989) Favorable prognosis for brainstem gliomas in neurofibromatosis. *J. Neurooncol.*, **7**, 367–71.

Mitsuhashi, T., Hashimoto, R., Nagahama, S. and Nagata, Y. (1991) Intrasellar cavernous angioma in neurofibromatosis. *Hum. Pathol.*, **22**, 623–4.

Mulvihill, J.J., Parry, D.M., Sherman, J.L. *et al.* (1990) Neurofibromatosis 1 (Recklinghausen disease) and neurofibromatosis 2 (bilateral acoustic neurofibromatosis). *Ann. Intern. Med.*, **113**, 39–52.

Murphy, M.J., Bosch, E.P. and Cancilla, P. (1980) Neurofibromatosis and peroneal muscular atrophy. *Neurology*, **30**, 404–5.

Nambisan, R.N., Rao, U., Moore, R. and Karakousis, C.P. (1984) Malignant soft tissue tumors of nerve sheath origin. *J. Surg. Oncol.*, **25**, 268–72.

North American Study Group for Optic Glioma (1989) Tumor spread in unilateral optic glioma. Study report No. 2. *Neurofibromatosis*, **2**, 195–203.

Office of Population Censuses and Surveys (1987) *Mortality Statistics. Cause.* Series DH2 no. 14 (HMSO, London).

Ohnishi, A. and Nada, O. (1972) Ultrastructure of the onion bulb-like lamellated structure observed in the sural nerve in a case of von Recklinghausen's disease. *Acta Neuropath. (Berl.)*, **20**, 258–63.

Okada, E. and Shozawa, T. (1984) Von Recklinghausen's disease (neurofibromatosis) associated with malignant pheochromocytoma. *Acta Pathol. Jpn.*, **34**, 425–34.

Pellock, J.M., Kleinman, P.K., McDonald, B.M. and Wixson, D. (1980) Childhood hypertensive stroke with neurofibromatosis. *Neurology*, **30**, 656–9.

Pikus, A. (1990) In (ed. J.J. Mulvihill) Neurofibromatosis 1 (Recklinghausen disease) and neurofibromatosis 2 (bilateral acoustic neurofibromatosis): an update. *Ann. Intern. Med.*, **113**, 39–52.

Riccardi, V.M. (1981) Von Recklinghausen's neurofibromatosis. *N. Engl. J. Med.*, **305**, 1617–1627.

Riccardi, V.M. and Eichner, J.E. (1986) *Neurofibromatosis: Phenotype, Natural History and Pathogenesis*, Johns Hopkins University Press, Baltimore, pp. 1–305.

Riccardi, V.M. and Powell, P.P. (1989) Neurofibrosarcoma as a complication of von Recklinghausen neurofibromatosis. *Neurofibromatosis*, **2**, 152–65.

Riviello, J.J., Jr., Marks, H.G., Lee, M.S. and Mandell, G.A. (1988) Aqueductal stenosis in neurofibromatosis. *Neurofibromatosis*, **1**, 312–17.

Rosman, N.P. and Pearce, J. (1967) The brain in multiple neurofibromatosis (von Recklinghausen's disease): a suggested neuropathology basis for the associated mental defect. *Brain*, **90**, 829–37.

Rubenstein, A.E. (1986) Neurofibromatosis. A review of the clinical problem. *Ann. N.Y. Acad. Sci.*, **486**, 1–13.

Rubenstein, A.E., Mytilineoau, C., Yahr, M.D. and Revoltella, P. (1981) Neurological aspects of neurofibromatosis, in *Advances in Neurology. Neurofibromatosis (von Recklinghausen Disease)* (eds V.M. Riccardi and J.J. Mulvihill), Raven Press, New York, pp. 11–21.

Rubinstein, L.J. (1986) The malformative central nervous system lesions in the central and peripheral forms of neurofibromatosis. A neuropathological study of 22 cases. *Ann. N.Y. Acad. Sci.*, **486**, 14–29.

Samuelsson, B. (1981) Neurofibromatosis (von Recklinghausen's Disease). A clinical-psychiatric and genetic study. Goteborg Univ. Thesis.

Samuelsson, B. and Riccardi, V.M. (1989) Neurofibromatosis in Gothenburg, Sweden. III. Psychiatric and social aspects. *Neurofibromatosis*, **2**, 84–106.

Sasaki, O., Ishii, R., Koike, T. and Tanaka, R. (1984) Multiple cerebrovascular occlusive disease associated with neurofibromatosis. *No. To. Shinkei.*, **36**, 159–66.

Scharenberg, K. (1971) Neurofibromatosis (von Recklinghausen's disease), in *Pathology of the Nervous System* (ed. J. Minckler), McGraw-Hill, New York, pp. 1906–11.

Senveli, E., Altinors, N., Kars, Z. *et al.* (1989) Association of von Recklinghausen's neurofibromatosis and aqueduct stenosis. *Neurosurgery*, **24**, 99–101.

Shorvon, C.D. (1990) Epidemiology, classification, natural history, and genetics of epilepsy. *Lancet*, **336**, 93–6.

So, C.B. and Li, D.K. (1989) Anterolateral cervical meningocele in association with neurofibromatosis: MR and CT studies. *J. Comput. Assist. Tomogr.*, **13**, 692–5.

Sobata, E., Ohkuma, H. and Suzuki, S. (1988) Cerebrovascular disorders associated with von Recklinghausen's neurofibromatosis: a case report. *Neurosurgery*, **22**, 544–9.

Taboada, D., Alonso, A., Moreno, J. *et al.* (1979) Occlusion of the cerebral arteries in Recklinghausen's disease. *Neuroradiology*, **18**, 281–4.

Tada, T., Shigeta, H., Kobayashi, H. *et al.* (1988) Trochlear nerve meningioma in von Recklinghausen's disease. *Neurochirurgia (Stuttg.)*, **31**, 226–7.

Thomas, P.K. and Eames, R.A. (1971) Neurofibromatous neuropathy, in *Actualités de Pathologie Neuromusculaire: Advances in Neuromuscular Diseases* (eds G. Serratrice and H. Roux), Riker, Paris, p. 612.

Thomas, P.K., King, R.H., Chiang, T.R. *et al.* (1990) Neurofibromatous neuropathy. *Muscle Nerve*, **13**, 93–101.

Weichert, K.A., Dine, M.S., Benton, C. and Silverman, F.N. (1973) Macrocranium and neurofibromatosis. *Pediatr. Radiol.*, **107**, 163–6.

Wertheimer, T., Dechaume, J., Lecuire, J. and Moulin, J. (1957) Reflexions sur la coexistence de neurinomes multiples, de meningiomes et gliomes encephalique dans la maladie nerveuse de Recklinghausen (à propos des chitoneuromas). *Neurochirurgie*, **3**, 145.

Wolf, P.A., Kannel, W.B., Cupples, L.A. and D'Agostino, R.B. (1987) Risk factor intervention in cardiovascular and cerebrovascular disease, in *The Heart and Stroke* (ed. A.J. Furlan), Springer-Verlag, Heidelberg, pp. 331–55.

9

Intellect in neurofibromatosis 1

R.E. Ferner

9.1 INTRODUCTION

Intellectual impairment in neurofibromatosis 1 has been recognized since the beginning of the century (Preiser and Davenport, 1918). Findings were often based on school performance using examination results, number of years of education and personal assessment of academic success, rather than on objective intelligence tests or behavioural measures. Recent research has established that patients with NF1 may have a low intellectual quotient (IQ), specific learning difficulties, behavioural problems or a combination of these (Riccardi and Eichner, 1986; Eliason, 1988; Ferner and Hughes, unpublished data). However, severe intellectual handicap is rare. Psychologists have long debated whether a general intelligence factor exists that can be measured by IQ or whether intellectual ability is multifaceted. Studies on NF1 have included both measurement of IQ and tests of information processing.

9.2 INTELLECTUAL QUOTIENT

9.2.1 Full-scale IQ

Although some patients with NF1 display superior academic ability, the majority have an IQ in the low average range and about 8–10% are mentally retarded (IQ less than 70). Borberg (1951) found that 48 out of 71 patients tested had an IQ between 70 and 90, 16 had scores above 90 and 7 had an IQ less than 70. Riccardi and Eichner (1986) found that 8.4% of 203 patients tested were mentally retarded compared with about 3% of the general population. Mental retardation varied according to age so that

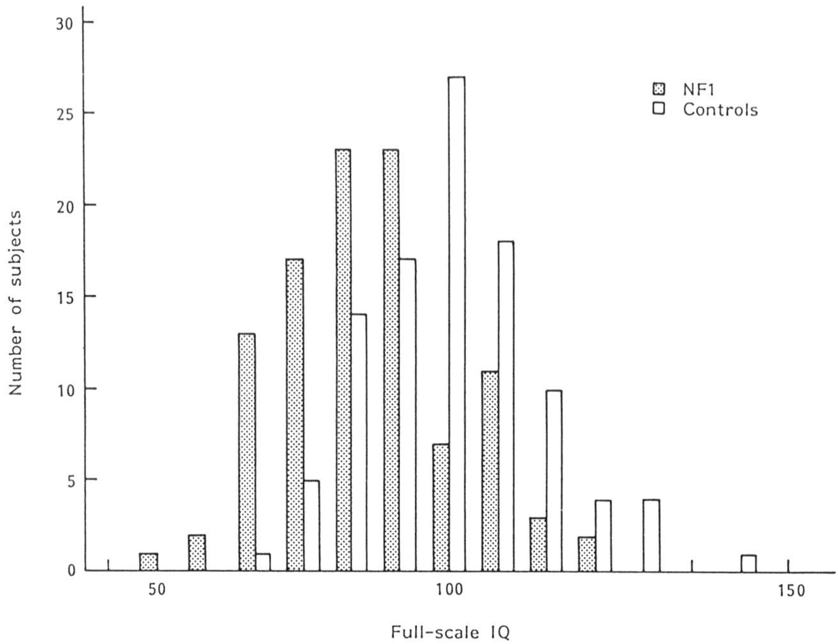

Figure 9.1 The distributions of full-scale IQ in 103 NF1 patients and 105 control subjects (Ferner and Hughes, unpublished data).

11.4% of preschool children had IQ scores below 70, whilst 7% of school children and only 3.4% of adult patients were mentally retarded. The reason for this age discrepancy has not been clarified and longitudinal studies are required to unravel its significance.

In an unpublished study, Ferner and Hughes used the Wechsler Intelligence Scales for children and adults (WISC-R and WAIS-R; Wechsler, 1976, 1981) to test 103 patients with NF1 between the ages of 6 and 75 years in southeast London. The patients were compared with 105 control subjects matched for age, sex and socioeconomic status. The IQ distributions of patients and controls were approximately normal (Figure 9.1). There was a highly significant difference in the means of the full-scale, verbal and performance scores between the NF1 and control groups. The mean full-scale IQ score of the patients was 88.5 (range 51–129), with a mean verbal IQ of 90.5 and a performance IQ of 88.1. The mean full-scale IQ of the control subjects was 101.8 (range 74–146), with a mean verbal IQ of 102.4 and a performance IQ of 101.5. In this study, 8% of patients and none of the controls were mentally retarded. In the highest range of ability, only 10% of patients had full-scale IQ scores above 110 compared with 21% of controls.

9.2.2 Differences between verbal and performance IQ

Eliason (1986) selected a group of 23 children with NF1 aged between 6 and 13 years who were known to have learning problems. She assessed them using the WISC-R and found a mean full-scale IQ of 93 (range 62–114), a verbal IQ of 100 and a performance IQ of 87. One child was mentally retarded with a full-scale IQ score of 62. Eliason noted that in 48% of the sample the verbal IQ scores were greater than performance scores by at least 15 points, and only two children had the opposite pattern of performance scores significantly higher than verbal scores. These results differ from findings in the general population where verbal–performance differences of more than 15 points (in either direction) occur in only 25% of children. In a further study, Eliason (1988) compared 32 children with NF1 and school learning problems with a matched group of children with learning difficulties that were not attributable to a specific medical cause. The NF1 children had higher verbal than performance IQs, whereas the comparison group attained higher scores on performance than verbal tests. Varnhagen *et al.* (1988) tested 16 children with NF1 and compared them with nine unaffected sibling controls. They divided the patients into a mild group with café au lait patches and neurofibromas and a severe group with complications such as scoliosis and seizures. The IQ scores for patients and controls were in the average range, but were lower in the severely affected group than the unaffected siblings. The patients in the severe group had a significantly higher verbal than performance IQ, and this discrepancy was not seen in the other groups. Wadsby, Lindehammar and Eeg-Olofsson (1989) noted that the majority of 27 children with NF1 functioned in the average range of intelligence. However, out of 22 subjects tested on the WISC-R, 12 had significantly higher verbal than performance scores, whilst five gained better results on performance tests than verbal tests. Five children showed no significant difference between their verbal and performance abilities. However, in our larger study of 103 NFI patients, there was no discrepancy between verbal and performance IQ.

9.3 SPECIFIC LEARNING DIFFICULTIES

A child who has a specific learning difficulty will fail to achieve his or her full academic potential regardless of cultural or socioeconomic background and in the absence of overt neurological, genetic or general medical problems. The disorder may be evident despite a normal or, more rarely, above-average intelligence. About 6–9% of school children in the general population have some form of learning difficulty (Aron *et al.*, 1990). Learning difficulties in NF1 are estimated to be much more common and about 40–60% of patients are affected (Riccardi, 1984; Eliason, 1988; Wadsby, Lindehammar and Eeg-Olofsson, 1989; Aron *et al.*, 1990; Ferner and Hughes, unpublished data). Although learning difficulties are more common in males in the general population, in NF1 they are equally common in both sexes. Characteristically, patients with learning difficulties experience problems with visuo-spatial tasks, memory, sustained attention, coordination, language and behaviour, which may cause underachievement in reading, writing and mathematics.

9.3.1 Visuo-spatial problems

Eliason (1988) found that children with NF1 had significant problems with visual perception. They performed badly on five separate visuo-spatial tasks, the Bender Visual Motor Gestalt Test (Koppitz, 1963), Benton Visual Retention Test–Multiple Choice Form (Benton and Stone, 1970) and Judgement of Line Orientation (Benton, Varney and Hamsher, 1976). In the Bender Visual Motor Gestalt Test, visual perception and spatial concepts are tested by asking the child to copy nine geometric designs, which are judged on form, shape and pattern. This test also requires fine motor coordination and memory skills. The Benton Visual Retention Test–Multiple Choice Form assesses perceptual matching ability and is applicable to children in the age range 6–8 years. The child is shown a geometric figure and selects a matching figure from a choice of four designs. The Judgement of Line Orientation is used for children over 8 years and requires subjects to predict the angle that would be produced if two separate lines were to intersect. Eliason showed that 56% of the NF1 group had isolated visual–perceptual problems detected by these tests compared with only 6% of the other learning difficulty group.

Varnhagen *et al.* (1988) tested spatial memory in seven mildly affected NF1 patients, five severely affected NF1 patients and five NF1 siblings. They noted that NF1 children were less adept at tasks of spatial memory than their unaffected siblings and that children with severe NF1 showed more deficits than those with mild disease.

Wadsby, Lindehammar and Eeg-Olofsson (1989) performed the Frostig development test of visual perception (Frostig, Maslow and Welty Lefever, 1963) on 11 children. They obtained measures of hand–eye coordination, figure–ground discrimination (focusing on a specific letter, number or figure in a text), and determination of constancy of shape, position in space and spatial relationships. They found that four of the children were impaired on one or more of these measures.

We have examined visuo-spatial ability, divided attention and speed of reaction in 103 NF1 patients and 105 matched controls (Ferner and Hughes, unpublished data) using the computerized Salford Tracking

Task (Willumeit, Ott and Neubert, 1983). The subjects used a 'mouse' to track a target moving randomly on the computer screen in a horizontal axis. Simultaneously the subjects were required to press a response button when they detected peripheral visual stimuli appearing at irregular intervals. The response measure, the root mean square deviation of the distance from the target during a 1 min trial, was significantly greater in the NF1 patients than the controls. The mean reaction time to 10 peripheral stimuli per trial was also recorded and was significantly slower in the NF1 subjects than the controls. Forty-one patients showed poor awareness of spatial relationships and impaired hand–eye coordination compared with four controls, irrespective of age. Many patients had difficulty in moving the 'mouse' smoothly across the table and tended to hold it upside down. They were unaware of the position of the 'mouse' on the table without looking directly at it.

The Wechsler block design subtest comprises a series of cards with designs of increasing complexity in red and white, and a set of blocks whose sides are painted in combinations of red and white. The subject is shown one design at a time from the cards and is required to reproduce it by choosing and assembling the appropriate blocks within a time limit. We detected poor constructional and perceptual skills in the patient group compared with the controls (Ferner and Hughes, unpublished data).

9.3.2 Organization and planning

Poor planning and organizational ability have been shown in some NF1 patients with visuo-spatial impairment (Varnhagen *et al.*, 1988; Bellerman, 1989). Sixteen NF1 children demonstrated significantly impaired planning skills on a trail making task (Armitage, 1946) compared with their nine unaffected siblings (Varnhagen *et al.*, 1988). Bellerman (1989) observed that children with NF1 tend to be unable to integrate and organize new information and do not manage their time efficiently, resulting in untidy, unstructured classwork.

9.3.3 Memory

Three studies suggest that patients with NF1 have impairment of short-term memory, although long-term memory is normal. Varnhagen *et al.* (1988) measured auditory serial recall in 16 children with NF1 and nine controls. The patients recalled significantly fewer words in the correct order than their unaffected sibling controls. Eliason (1988) found that 60% of non-NF1 children with learning difficulties had language or memory deficits without visuo-spatial problems compared with 4% of NF1 children. Although NF1 subjects were more likely to present with visuo-spatial problems in isolation, 30% of them also had memory deficits on the Rey Auditory Verbal Learning Test (Lezak, 1983) in addition to visuo-perceptual problems.

In our southeast London study on adults and children (Ferner and Hughes, unpublished data), we tested short-term and delayed verbal memory recall. The NF1 patients recalled significantly fewer words immediately and after a delay of 20 min compared with the control group. Preliminary results from testing with the computerized Sternberg Memory Task suggest that NF1 patients have impaired scanning ability and difficulty with short-term memory retrieval compared with their controls. This task assesses high-speed scanning ability and retrieval from short-term memory (Sternberg, 1975).

9.3.4 Attention deficit

> He was certainly slow over his books – but more from a constitutional inability to fix his attention on his tasks than from want of capacity to understand them. His temperament it could not be denied was heedless to the last degree: he acted recklessly on his first impulses, and rushed blindfold at all his conclusions.

This portrayal of the character Armadale by Wilkie Collins (1864) reflects the predicament of patients with a short attention span. They fail to maintain alertness, are unable to select one source of information rather than another, and cannot process two tasks simultaneously.

Eliason (1988) showed that NF1 children responded slowly to a computerized Continuous Performance Test (Lindgren and Lyon, 1983), in which they were asked to press a space bar every time a target sequence of letters appeared. Although their responses were slower and less accurate than those of normal children, they were comparable to those of children with learning difficulties from other causes.

In our southeast London study (Ferner and Hughes, unpublished data), we administered an automated continuous attention task in which the subjects monitored a series of 200 consecutive digits and pressed the response button when three odd or three even numbers appeared in a row (Wesnes and Warburton, 1983). Fifty-eight per cent of patients compared with 22% of controls were unable to attempt the task. Such failure might be due to impaired attention, slow information processing or a combination of both. Of those who completed the test, the patients had significantly fewer correct responses and more false positive responses than the controls.

9.3.5 Coordination

NF1 patients may have considerable impairment of gross and fine motor coordination in the absence of detectable neurological lesions (Riccardi and

Eichner, 1986; Aron *et al.*, 1990; Ferner and Hughes, unpublished data). Their problems are similar to those described in children with motor learning difficulties from other causes (McKinlay, 1987) and are not related to IQ results. Clumsiness may prevent them from riding a bicycle, tying shoelaces, participating in sports, holding a pen correctly or using scissors. Poor manual dexterity results in ill-formed handwriting and immature drawing. Dunn and Roos (1989) noted that eight out of 28 children had incoordination that could not be explained by tumour or hydrocephalus. We found that 43% of 103 patients had coordination problems of this nature (Ferner and Hughes, unpublished data).

9.3.6 Language disorders

The American Education for all Handicapped Children Act (Public Law, 1975) referred to learning problems in language as 'disorders of one or more of the basic psychological processes involved in comprehending or using language, either spoken or written, which result in difficulty listening, thinking, speaking, reading, writing or doing mathematical calculations'.

Language disorders may accompany other learning problems in patients with NF1 (Eliason, 1988; Ferner and Hughes, unpublished data). Solot *et al.* (1990) evaluated language problems in 23 children with NF1 and 10 normal sibling controls. The sex ratio of language problems in the NF1 patients was equal. The NF1 patients had delayed language development and slow acquisition of vocabulary. They made significant syntactic, semantic and phonological errors. Their problems also included motor dyspraxia resulting in mispronunciations, incorrect sequencing of sounds and abnormal prosody. Preliminary results from the study revealed that 11 patients and two sibling controls suffered from articulation disorders. Twelve patients and no controls had voice disorders including hypernasality, hoarseness and vocal nodules. Nine patients and one sibling control had a language learning problem, but none of the NF1 patients or controls had impaired hearing.

Fourteen of our 103 patients exhibited hypernasal speech, two had speech delay and one patient was dysarthric owing to a brain stem glioma. In contrast, two control subjects had delayed language development and none had hypernasal speech (Ferner and Hughes, unpublished data).

9.3.7 Behaviour

Patients with NF1 may suffer from a particular pattern of behaviour disturbance (Riccardi and Eichner, 1986; Bellerman, 1989; Ferner and Hughes, unpublished data). They may be impulsive, uruly and socially imperceptive. Their misjudgement of non-verbal communication such as gestures and facial expression may lead them to behave in an inappropriate and intrusive fashion. Wadsby, Lindehammar and Eeg-Olofsson (1989) interviewed the parents and teachers of 27 children with NF1 and asked them to describe the child's character and behaviour. Nine children displayed sleep disturbance, impaired concentration and hyperactivity.

Varnhagen *et al.* (1988) administered the Pre-Adolescent Mood Scale to children under 14 years (McNair, Lorr and Droppleman, 1971) and the Profile of Mood States (Schokman-Gates, 1983) to older children. They noted that children with NF1 displayed aggressive tendencies compared with their unaffected siblings and felt that this was indicative of their hyperactive behaviour. In our study, two out of 42 children required special education despite above average intelligence, because of disruptive behaviour (Ferner and Hughes, unpublished data).

9.3.8 Reading, writing, mathematics

Each of the learning problems mentioned above may contribute to the patient's inability to read, write, spell and copy from the blackboard. For instance visuo-spatial difficulties may cause letters and numbers to be reversed, omitted or rotated. Inability to distinguish 'figure–ground' (section 9.3.1) may cause poor tracking from left to right and from line to line. Numbers may be placed in an incorrect column resulting in mathematical errors (Bellerman, 1989).

Wadsby, Lindehammar and Eeg-Olofsson (1989) found that seven out of 27 children with NF1 had difficulties with reading and writing based on teachers' reports. In our study, we assessed reading ability with the Schonell Graded Word Reading Test (Schonell and Schonell, 1956) and National Adult Reading Test (Nelson, 1982). Twenty-six per cent of patients compared with 5% of controls had impaired reading skills; 41% of patients reported that they were below average in mathematics at school; and 60% had clumsy writing and made frequent spelling errors (Ferner and Hughes, unpublished data).

A psychologist's appraisal of an 8-year-old child with a severe learning difficulty encapsulates the problems faced by many children with NF1.

> X was friendly, lively and co-operative during the assessment; he found it hard to sit still for long. He is a boy of exceptionally high intelligence (full scale IQ 139) but his visuo-spatial skills are comparatively weak. He has impairment of visual short term memory and very poor motor skills; he has experienced related severe difficulties with spelling, drawing, copying, free writing and written arithmetic. More specifically his spelling is at least 2 years below the level usually attained by a boy of his age and intelligence. He makes both visual and phonological errors and is ignorant of

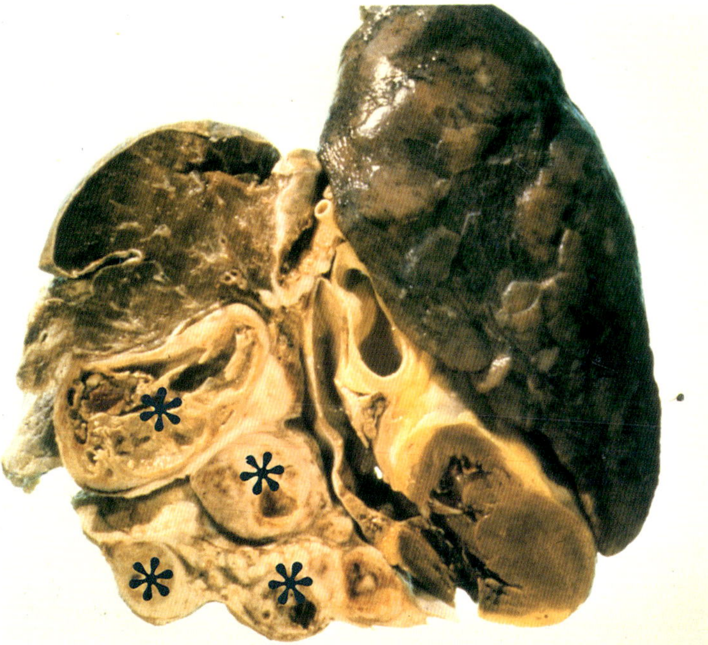

Plate 1 Mediastinal neurofibrosarcoma. Marked compression and displacement of the right lung and the heart by four tumour nodules (asterisks).

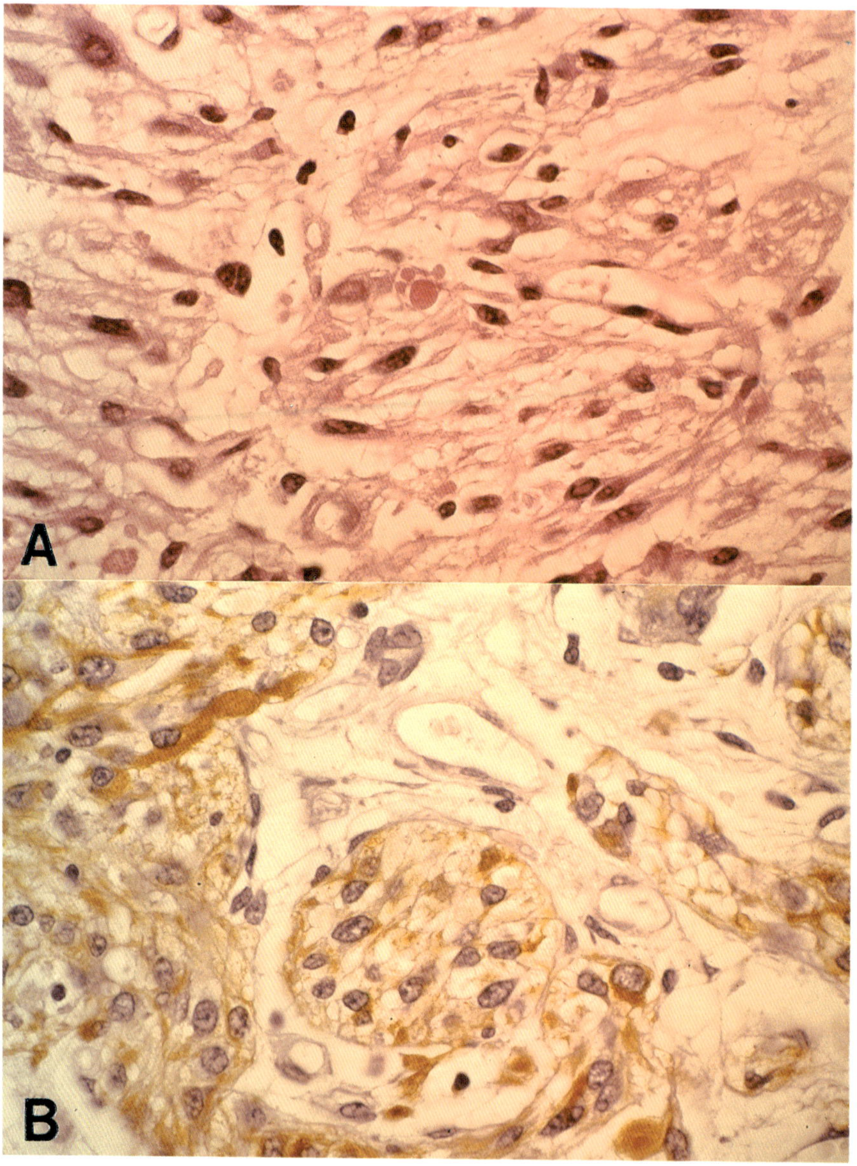

Plate 2 Optic pathway glioma. (A) Glial tumour with features of a pilocytic astrocytoma including bipolar tumour cells and protein droplets. H & E, × 400. (B) Immunocytochemical demonstration of glial fibrillary acidic protein (GFAP) which confirms the astrocytic nature of the tumour. Note the pseudofascicular growth pattern. GFAP immunohistochemical reaction, × 400.

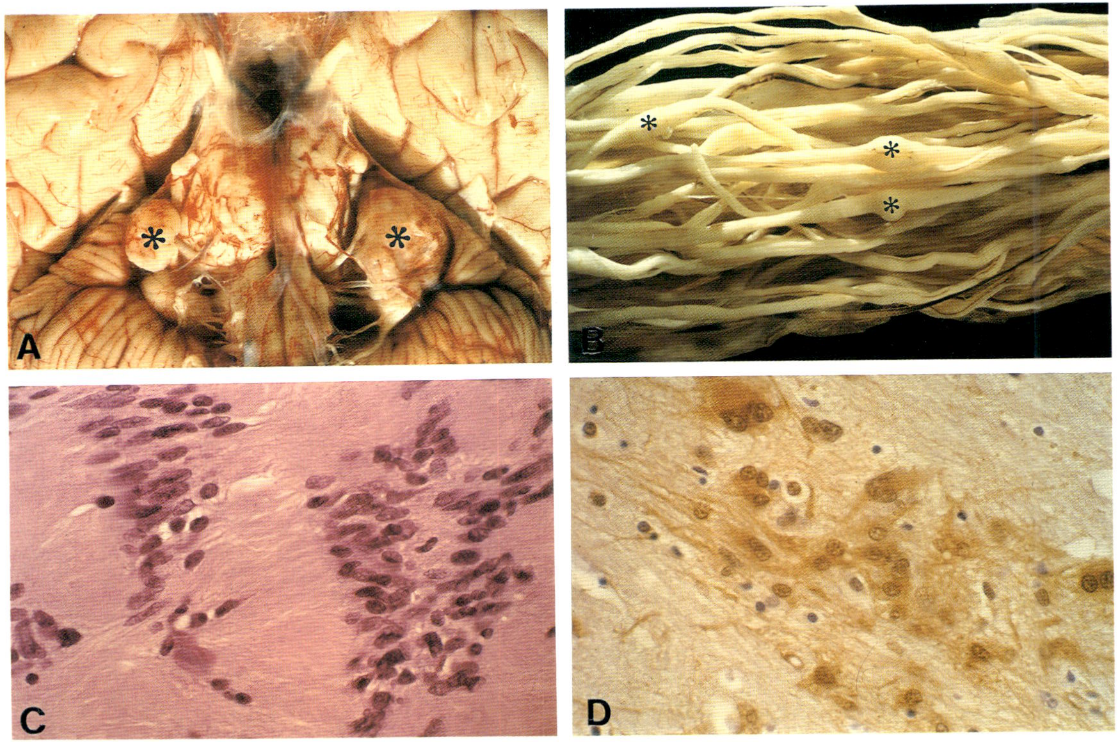

Plate 3 Characteristic neuropathological manifestations of NF2. (A) Bilateral Schwannomas originating from the eighth cranial nerve (asterisks). (B) Multiple Schwannomas in nerve roots of the cauda equina. Some of the tumours are labelled by asterisks. (C) Microscopic appearance of a Schwannoma with nuclear palisading (Antoni type A architecture). H & E, × 400. (D) Glial microhamartoma of the cerebral cortex. Moderately polymorphic cell population with strong immunoreactivity for S100 protein. S100 immunohistochemical reaction, × 400.

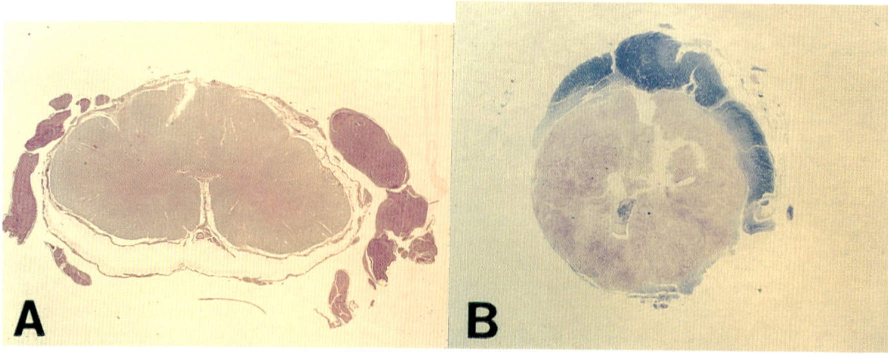

Plate 4 Multiple Schwannomas of spinal nerve roots (A) and pilocytic astrocytoma of the cervical spinal cord (B) in a patient with NF2. The spinal tumour in (B) has caused striking compression and displacement of the adjacent cord, which is reduced to the rim of the blue-stained tissue above. (A) H & E; (B) Luxol–Nissl stain.

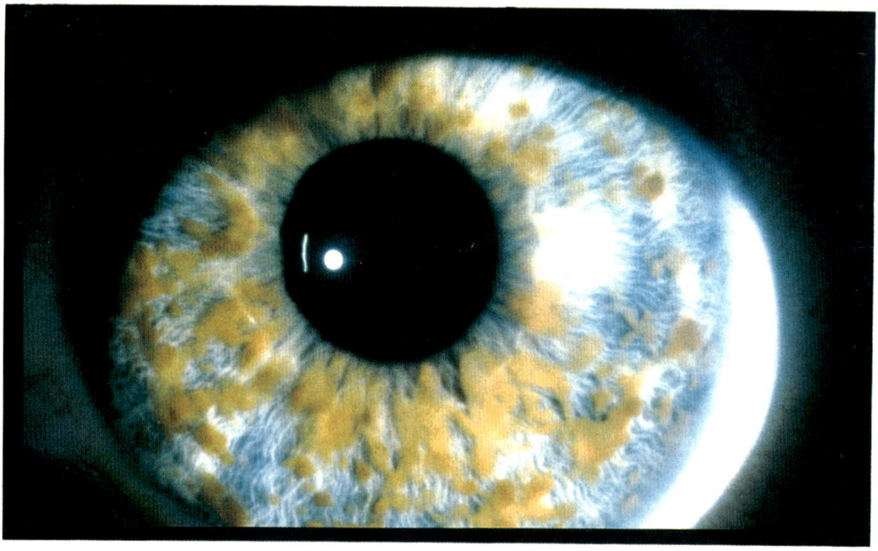

Plate 5 Iris nodules in a patient with NF1. (Photograph courtesy of W. Church.)

spelling rules. His continuous writing is fluent, imaginative and logical, but is marred by poor spelling and punctuation and by untidy handwriting. He finds writing a physical effort. His written arithmetic is below average: he understands calculation procedures but finds written sums visually confusing. In conclusion X is an intellectually gifted child with a specific learning difficulty. He needs to be given appropriate help with spelling and writing if he is to fulfil his potential and avoid becoming unhappy and frustrated at school.

(personal communication, Sylvia Moody, 1989)

9.4 SPECIAL SCHOOL ATTENDANCE AND REMEDIAL TEACHING

The British Education Act of 1981 declares that a child has special educational needs if 'he has a significantly greater difficulty in learning than the majority of children of his age; or if he has a disability which either prevents or hinders him from making use of educational facilities of a kind generally provided in schools . . . for children of his age'.

In their southeast Wales population study, Huson, Harper and Compston (1988) used a retrospective assessment of education to give an approximate measure of intellectual impairment in NF1. They reported that 10% of 124 NF1 patients attended special school, and 17% required remedial teaching. By contrast, 95% of healthy individuals with affected parents attended an ordinary school and only 5% attended remedial classes. The education attainments of the patients differed from those of the controls. Ninety-five of the 124 NF1 patients had completed their education; of these, four gained GCE 'O' level passes and only one the higher GCE 'A' level educational qualification. Twenty-two of the 45 unaffected siblings had completed their education; of these, one gained 'O' level qualifications, four obtained 'A' level qualifications and three took university courses.

We found that 34% of patients attended special school or remedial classes compared with only 4% of a matched control group (Ferner and Hughes, unpublished data).

In Sweden, Samuelsson (1981) classified 71 patients retrospectively on school performance as normal, remedial class level or special school level. She noted that 45% exhibited 'mild mental retardation', and in general did not acquire any vocational skills. In a later Swedish study on 27 children with NF1 aged between 2 and 15 years, Wadsby, Lindehammar and Eeg-Olofsson (1989) asked teachers to categorize each child as clearly above normal; above normal; normal; below normal; clearly below normal. The teachers felt that eight out of the 17 school children performed below average and thought that three of this group were functioning below their intellectual capabilities.

9.5 AETIOLOGY OF INTELLECTUAL IMPAIRMENT IN NF1

The aetiology of intellectual impairment on NF1 has not been determined, but the following possible influences on intelligence will be examined:

- migrational disorders
- age and sex
- socio-economic factors
- macrocephaly
- short stature
- disease severity
- neurological disorders
- psychiatric problems
- physical appearance.

9.5.1 Migrational abnormalities in the brain

(a) Postmortem findings

The anatomical basis of intellectual impairment in NF1 has not been studied systematically and only one pathological study has addressed the problem. Rosman and Pearce (1967) examined the histology of the brains of 10 patients with NF1 and five control cases. An assessment of intellectual performance was based on IQ testing in two cases and on clinical, social and occupational history in the other cases. Five patients had intellectual impairment and the remaining five cases were in the average range of ability. The brains of intellectually impaired patients showed disorders of cerebral architecture with random orientation of neurons and disarray of normal cortical lamination. In addition, heterotopias in the subcortical white matter were found in all of these cases. Neuronal heterotopias, single, paired or in small groups, were present in the deep white matter in three brains. Glial nodules were detected in the cerebral cortex of one patient. Less severe changes were noted in the brains of those with average intelligence and there was no gross disorder of cerebral development. In three of these cases the cortical architecture was disordered with misdirection of neurons, poor demarcation of the cortical layers and ectopic neurons in the subpial molecular layer. Heterotopic neurons were present in the subcortical white matter, but none were present in the deep cerebral white matter. These changes were absent in the brains of five control subjects. Rosman and Pearce (1967) suggested that intellectual impairment in NF1 is due to migrational abnormalities in the developing fetus.

In our southeast London study (Ferner and Hughes, unpublished data), postmortem examinations were performed on two patients: one was mentally retarded and the other was a lawyer with above-average intellectual ability. One patient had been diagnosed during life as having multiple cerebral infarcts and the other as having multiple sclerosis. Both diagnoses were confirmed by the neuropathological examination. There was no evidence of heterotopias, hamartomas or neoplasia in either patient. A postmortem examination was also performed on a 73-year-old man with NF1 who was not part of the southeast London study. He had not had a formal intellectual assessment, but had completed secondary school education and had worked as a builder. He died from postoperative complications following surgery for atlanto-axial subluxation caused by a neurofibroma on the odontoid peg (Ferner, Honavar and Gullen, 1989). He was found to have a small island of ectopic grey matter in the deep cerebellar white matter, but no cerebral heterotopias.

(b) Magnetic resonance imaging studies

On the basis of Rosman and Pearce's findings, Duffner and her colleagues (1989) assessed school performance and carried out magnetic resonance imaging (MRI) of the brain in 30 school children. They found that intellectual problems did not correlate with migrational abnormalities in the brain, and they did not detect any grey matter heterotopias. However, they noted increased-intensity lesions on T2-weighted images in about 60% of children. The nature of the lesions was uncertain, but they occurred predominantly in the basal ganglia, thalamus, brain stem and cerebellum. Duffner *et al.* (1989) postulated that these lesions were slow-growing gliomas or hamartomas.

Dunn and Roos (1989) attempted to correlate abnormalities on brain MRI with learning difficulties in 31 children with NF1. Learning difficulties were detected in 23 children, including eight children with incoordination. Sixteen children had increased-signal lesions on T2-weighted images, predominantly in the basal ganglia, cerebellum and brain stem. However, only 11 of these children had learning problems and five were asymptomatic. Of the 15 children who had no increased-signal lesions on MRI, 12 had intellectual problems and three did not. There was no association between learning difficulties and the presence of these T2-weighted abnormalities on MRI.

Ferner *et al.* (1993) drew similar conclusions when they performed brain MRI scans on 38 patients with an age range of 3–63 years, including 14 children (Table 9.1). The subjects underwent neurological examination and assessments of IQ and information processing. Seven patients did

Table 9.1 Abnormalities on MRI head scans in 38 patients with NF1

Abnormalities	*n*
Known associations	
Increased-intensity T2-weighted lesions	13
Optic nerve glioma	6
Parenchymal glioma	3
Dilated ventricles	4
Increased-intensity T1-weighted lesions	1
Total no. of patients affected	24
Other associations	
Multiple sclerosis	2
Vascular disease	2
Cerebral atrophy	2
Chromophobe adenoma	1
Posterior fossa arachnoid cyst	1
Meningeal dysplasia	1
Venous malformation arising from corpus striatum vessels	1
Total no. of patients affected	10
Total no. of patients with:	
abnormal scans	28
normal scans	10

Some patients had more than one abnormality.
Source: Ferner *et al.* (1993).

not undergo formal psychological testing and their intellectual ability was evaluated on school performance and occupation.

Six of the 38 patients were mentally retarded, with a full scale IQ ranging between 51 and 67. One of these patients had a normal scan. Three cases had abnormalities on scan which were thought to be unrelated to their NF1, these were multiple sclerosis, confirmed by CSF examination, cerebral atrophy (with microcephaly) and multiple vascular lesions, verified at postmortem and not the kind associated with NF1. One patient had an optic nerve glioma and meningeal dysplasia due to shunt infection (Table 9.1). Only one patient had a single increased-intensity T2-weighted lesion in the deep white matter adjacent to the right insular cortex (Table 9.2).

Nineteen patients had an IQ in the range 70–89; seven of these patients had normal scans. General abnormalities included multiple vascular lesions; pituitary adenoma; optic nerve glioma (two cases); parenchymal glioma (three cases); and dilated ventricles of unknown aetiology (two

Table 9.2 Sites of increased-intensity lesions on T2-weighted scans in 13/38 patients with NF1

Sites	*Number of patients*
Basal ganglia	11
Cerebellum	4
Brain stem	3
Lateral ventricle wall	2
Cerebral peduncle	2
Corpus callosum	2
Frontal lobe	1
Parietal lobe	1
Internal capsule	1
Optic tract	1
Insular cortex	1

Source: Ferner *et al.* (1993).

cases). Increased-intensity lesions on T2-weighted images were seen in eight patients and were found predominantly in the basal ganglia, cerebellum and brain stem.

Thirteen patients had an IQ in the range 91–112; two patients had normal scans. General abnormalities included optic nerve glioma (three cases); venous malformation in the right thalamus; multiple sclerosis confirmed at postmortem (see section 9.5.1a); posterior fossa arachnoid cyst; plexiform neurofibroma extending into the left temporal fossa; dilated ventricles; and right frontal lobe atrophy of unknown aetiology. Four of this group had increased-intensity T2-weighted lesions in the basal ganglia (Figure 9.2), cerebellum, cerebral peduncle and optic tract.

Overall, 13 patients had increased-intensity lesions on T2-weighted images of the type described by Duffner *et al.* (1989) and Dunn and Roos (1989). However, only one of these patients had an IQ less than 70 and there was no demonstrable relationship between intellectual impairment and the presence of these abnormalities on MRI.

Current studies have, therefore, shown no correlation between intellectual impairment and the presence of increased-intensity lesions on T2-weighted images (Duffner *et al.* 1989; Dunn and Roos, 1989; Ferner *et al.* 1993). This finding is surprising in the light of Rosman and Pearce's neuropathological study, which demonstrated a clear relationship between intellectual impairment and migrational abnormalities in the brain. It is possible that MRI has failed to detect abnormalities in the cerebral architecture. Further radiological studies with positron emission tomography and neuropathological investigation are necessary to elucidate the problem.

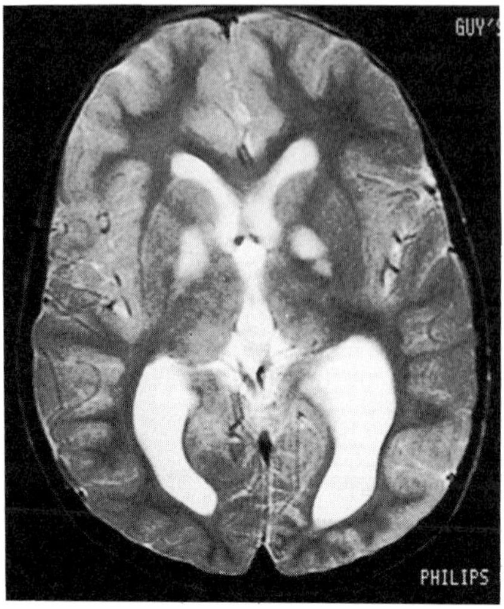

Figure 9.2 T2-weighted axial image (TR SE 1920/TE 80) in an asymptomatic patient with NF1. There are increased-intensity lesions in the globus pallidus on both sides and the lateral and third ventricles are dilated. (MRI scan provided by Dr J. Bingham and Dr T. Cox, Department of Radiological Science, UMDS, Guy's Hospital, and reproduced with their permission.)

9.5.2 Age and sex

Age has an obvious effect on performance in IQ tests. This factor could not account for the observed differences between the NF1 and control subjects since the Wechsler IQ battery is standardized for age. In our southeast London study (Ferner and Hughes, unpublished data), we found that sex did not influence performance on the Wechsler IQ tests in NF1 patients or controls. However, females in both control and patient groups performed slightly worse than the males on the Salford Tracker Task of visuo-spatial ability.

9.5.3 Socio-economic group

Socio-economic group is known to be correlated with IQ in the population as a whole and this correlation was confirmed in our southeast London study (Figure 9.3). The mean IQ of patients in the highest socio-economic groups (1 and 2) was higher than that of groups 3 and 4, which was in turn higher than that of group 5. The IQ differences between the NF1 group and the controls were significant irrespective of socio-economic status. We also assessed the socio-economic group of the subject taking part in the study and of the parent who was the wage-earner (Ferner and

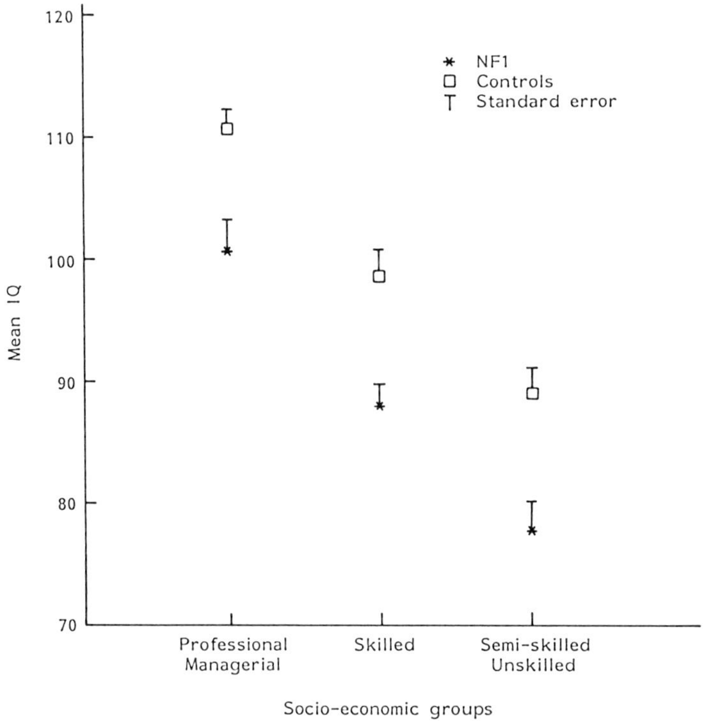

Figure 9.3 Full-scale IQ in patients and controls according to socio-economic group (means and SE).

Hughes, unpublished data). The NF1 patients showed a tendency to drift down in social class compared with their parent, a tendency that was not observed in the control subjects.

9.5.4 Macrocephaly

Huson, Harper and Compston (1988) reported that 45% of 115 NF1 patients had head circumferences above the 97th centile compared with 15% of 40 controls, but found no relationship between the occurrence of macrocephaly and intellectual impairment. We found that 56.9% of 103 patients had a head circumference above the 98th centile compared with 30% of 105 controls (Ferner and Hughes, unpublished data). However, the mean full-scale IQ of the patients with macrocephaly was 89, which was not significantly different from those with a normal head circumference (full-scale IQ 87). The high number of controls with large heads may be explained by the fact that heads have increased in size over the last 40 years (personal communication from Locks, the oldest hatmakers in

England). Locks sold a hat to Lord Nelson before he left for the Battle of Trafalgar, and his head circumference was only 57 cm. Today the most common head circumference for the hats sold by this firm is 59 cm!

9.5.5 Short stature

In the general population, short stature has been associated with a poor educational level and low IQ (Teasdale, Sorensen and Owen, 1989). About a third of patients with NF1 are shorter in height than the third centile (Huson, Harper and Compston, 1989; Ferner and Hughes, unpublished data), but no association between short stature and intellectual impairment has been established.

9.5.6 Disease severity

Varnhagen *et al.* (1988) noted that children with 'severe' NF1 (with complications such as seizures and scoliosis) performed worse on tasks of visuo-spatial ability than children with mild NF1. However, the numbers in the study were very small. We assessed the general medical and neurological complications in both patients and controls in our southeast London study (Ferner and Hughes, unpublished data). The patients with disease complications had a mean IQ of 88 (SD 14), which was not significantly different from the mean IQ of 90 (SD 15.4) of those without complications.

9.5.7 Psychiatric complications

In a retrospective study of 69 patients in Sweden, Samuelsson and Riccardi (1989) noted mental illness in 33% of subjects. Problems included depression, anxiety and sleep disturbance. They found a significant relationship between mental illness and intellectual impairment, but did not perform IQ testing. Our patients did not suffer from more psychiatric illness than their controls (Ferner and Hughes, unpublished data). There was no significant difference in the anxiety and depression scores between the two groups on the Spielberger Anxiety Trait Inventory for Children (Spielberger, Gorsuch and Lushene, 1970) or The Hospital Anxiety and Depression Scale (Zigmond and Snaith, 1983). Two patients and two control subjects had depression severe enough to require treatment. One patient and two controls suffered from alcoholism. In addition, one patient had been treated for a psychotic illness and one had been diagnosed as suffering from anorexia nervosa. Psychiatric problems did not adversely affect intellectual performance in our study. The mean

IQ of patients with psychiatric problems was 87 and the mean IQ for those without psychiatric illness was 88.

9.5.8 Physical appearance

Hett, Mather and Dewar (1989) reported the case of a sailor with NF1 who was ostracized by his Royal Navy shipmates because of his unsightly facial neurofibromas. Society is often prejudiced against those with an atypical facial appearance, and a person with a facial disfigurement may experience a severe social handicap (Bull, 1990). We noted that 33% of patients had experienced hostile reactions from strangers because of unsightly neurofibromas. However, these patients did not have more intellectual difficulties than the rest of the patients. In addition, they had a similar rate of marriage to the control group despite their cosmetic problems (Ferner and Hughes, unpublished data).

9.6 TREATMENT

The intellectual problems in NF1 are not thought to be progressive (Riccardi and Eichner, 1986; Samuelsson and Samuelsson, 1989), but longitudinal studies are needed to confirm this impression. It is imperative to diagnose intellectual impairment as early as possible so that educational assistance may be given to the child. The child's teacher, physician and educational psychologist should be requested to perform a full assessment of his or her capabilities and potential. This will allow an educational programme to be drawn up that is tailored to the child's individual needs. Severe intellectual impairment in NF1 is so unusual that other NF1-related (tumour, hydrocephalus) or unrelated causes should be considered (e.g. fragile X syndrome).

A child with learning problems benefits from a structured environment with one-to-one teaching when possible. Visuo-spatial problems may be tackled by using colour-coded cues to mark the beginning and end of words and lines, giving verbal instructions when possible, and providing large-print books, tape recorders and typewriters. Crossword puzzles enrich vocabulary and improve spelling and writing. Exercises emphasizing the position of the body in space, finger painting and clay modelling increase the child's confidence (Bellerman, 1989). Clearly marked files, timetables and a diary will aid memory and facilitate organization of work.

A child with attention deficit and behavioural problems requires a framework of consistent rules, reinforcement of social skills and minimal distraction. The acquisition of computer skills may improve concentration. A small number of carefully selected children respond to the judicious use of stimulant drugs such as methylphenidate (Aron *et al.*, 1990).

Intellectual problems are a major complication of NF1, but their aetiology has not been determined. Further psychometric, radiological and pathological studies are needed to unravel the causes. If learning difficulties are not diagnosed in early childhood, they engender frustration and underachievement and may result in social isolation in adult life.

REFERENCES

Armitage, S.G. (1946) An analysis of certain psychological tests for the evaluation of brain damage. *Psychol. Monogr.*, **60** (277).

Aron, A.M., Rubenstein, A.E., Wallace, S.A. and Halperin, J.C. (1990) Learning disabilities in neurofibromatosis, in *Neurofibromatosis: A Handbook for Patients, Families, and Healthcare Professionals* (eds A.E. Rubenstein and B.R. Korf), Thieme, New York, Ch. 5, pp. 55–8.

Bellerman, P. (1989) What is it like to have a learning disability?, in *Achieving in spite of . . .* National Neurofibromatosis Inc., Florida, pp. 4–13.

Benton, A. and Stone, F.B. (1970) *Visual Retention Test – Multiple Choice Form*, Department of Neurology, University of Iowa, Iowa City.

Benton, A., Varney, N. and Hamsher, K. (1976) *Judgement of Line Orientation*, Department of Neurology, University of Iowa, Iowa City.

Borberg, A. (1951) Clinical and genetic investigations into tuberous sclerosis and Recklinghausen's neurofibromatosis. *Acta Psychiatr. Neurol. Scand. [Suppl.]*, **71**, 1–239.

Bull, R. (1990) Society's reactions to facial disfigurement. *Br. Psychol. Soc. Newsletter*, **7**, 10–12.

Duffner, P.K., Cohen, M.E., Seidel, F.G. and Shucard, D.W. (1989) The significance of MRI abnormalities in children with neurofibromatosis. *Neurology*, **39**, 373–8.

Dunn, D.W. and Roos, K.L. (1989) Magnetic resonance imaging evaluation of learning difficulties in neurofibromatosis. *Neurofibromatosis*, **2**, 1–5.

Education Act (1981) Her Majesty's Stationery Office, London, Ch. 60, pp. 1–21.

Eliason, M.J. (1986) Neurofibromatosis: implications for learning and behaviour. *J. Dev. Behav. Pediatr.*, **7**, 175–9.

Eliason, M.J. (1988) Neuropsychological patterns: neurofibromatosis compared to developmental learning disorders. *Neurofibromatosis*, **1**, 17–25.

Ferner, R.E., Honavar, M. and Gullen, R.W. (1989) Spinal neurofibroma presenting as atlanto-axial subluxation in von Recklinghausen neurofibromatosis. *Neurofibromatosis*, **2**, 43–6.

Ferner, R.E., Chaudhuri, R., Bingham, J. *et al.* (1993) Magnetic resonance imaging in neurofibromatosis 1. The nature and evolution of increased intensity T2 weighted lesions and their relationship to intellectual impairment. *J. Neurol. Neurosurg. Psychiatr.*, in press.

Frostig, M., Maslow, P. and Welty Lefever, D. (1963) *The Marianne Frostig Developmental Test of Visual Perception Standardization*, Consulting Psychologists Press, Palo Alto.

Hett, D.A., Mather, S. and Dewar, E.P. (1989) Von Recklinghausens' disease of the nerves: a modern day social response. *J. R. Nav. Med. Serv.*, **75**, 139–41.

Huson, S.M., Harper, P.S. and Compston, D.A.S. (1988) Von Recklinghausen neurofibromatosis: a clinical and population study in South East Wales. *Brain*, **111**, 1355–81.

Koppitz, E. (1963) *The Bender Gestalt Test with Young Children*, Grune and Stratton, New York.

Lezak, M. (1983) *Neuropsychological Assessment*, Oxford University Press, New York.

Lindgren, S.D. and Lyon, D. (1983) *PACE: Pediatric Assessment of Cognitive Efficiency*, Department of Paediatrics, University of Iowa, Iowa City.

McKinlay, I. (1987) Children with motor learning difficulties: not so much a syndrome – more a way of life. *Physiotherapy*, **11**, 635–8.

McNair, D.M., Lorr, M. and Droppleman, L.F. (1971) *Profile of Mood States*, Education and Industrial Testing Service, San Diego, CA.

Nelson, H.E. (1982) *National Adult Reading Test (NART) Test Manual*, NFER-Nelson, Windsor, Berkshire.

Preiser, S.A. and Davenport, C.B. (1918) Multiple neurofibromatosis (von Recklinghausen's disease) and its inheritance. *Am. J. Med. Sci.*, **156**, 507–41.

Public Law (1975) *Education for all Handicapped Children Act*, Federal Register, Washington, D.C.

Riccardi, V.M. (1984) Neurofibromatosis as a model for investigating hereditary vs environmental factors in learning disabilities. In *The Developing Brain and its Disorders* (eds M. Arima, Y. Suzuki and H. Yabuuchi), University of Tokyo Press, Tokyo.

Riccardi, V.M. and Eichner, J.E. (1986) Psychosocial aspects, in *Neurofibromatosis: Phenotype, Natural History and Pathogenesis*, Johns Hopkins University Press, Baltimore, Ch. 11, pp. 150–61.

Rosman, N.P. and Pearce, J. (1967) The brain in multiple neurofibromatosis (von Recklinghausen's disease): a suggested neuropathological basis for the associated mental defect. *Brain*, **90**, 829–38.

Samuelsson, B. (1981) Neurofibromatosis (von Recklinghausen's disease): a clinical-psychiatric and genetic study. University of Gothenburg. Thesis.

Samuelsson, B. and Riccardi, V.M. (1989) Neurofibromatosis in Gothenburg, Sweden. III. Psychiatric and social aspects. *Neurofibromatosis*, **2**, 84–106.

Samuelsson, B. and Samuelsson, S. (1989) Neurofibromatosis in Gothenburg, Sweden. Background, study design and epidemiology. *Neurofibromatosis*, **2**, 6–22.

Schokman-Gates, K. (1983) The development and investigation of the Pre-Adolescent Mood Scale. Presented at the Psychologist's Association of Alberta Annual Conference, Edmonton, Alberta, Canada.

Schonell, F.J. and Schonell, F.E. (1956) *Diagnostic and Attainment Testing Including a Manual of Tests, their Nature and Use, Recording and Interpretation*, Oliver and Boyd, Edinburgh.

Solot, C.B., Zackai, E.H., Obringer, A.C. *et al.* (1990) Communication disorders in children with neurofibromatosis type 1, in *Neurofibromatosis: a Handbook for Patients, Families, and Heathcare Professionals* (eds A.E. Rubenstein and B.R. Korf), Thieme, New York, Ch. 6, pp. 59–70.

Spielberger, C.D., Gorsuch, R.L. and Lushene, R.E. (1970) *Manual for the State-Trait Anxiety Inventory (Self-evaluation Questionnaire)*, Consulting Psychologists Press, Palo Alto, CA.

Sternberg, S. (1975) Memory scanning: new findings and current controversies. *Q. J. Exp. Psychol.*, **27**, 1–32.

Teasdale, T.W., Sorensen, T.I.A. and Owen, D.R. (1989) Fall in association of height with intelligence and educational level. *Br. Med. J.*, **298**, 1290–1.

Varnhagen, C.K., Lewin, S., Das, J.P. *et al.* (1988) Neurofibromatosis and psychological processes. *J. Dev. Behav. Pediatr.*, **5**, 257–65.

Wadsby, M., Lindehammar, H. and Eeg-Olofsson, O. (1989) Neurofibromatosis in childhood: neuropsychological aspects. *Neurofibromatosis*, **2**, 251–60.

Wechsler, D. (1976) *Wechsler Intelligence Scale for Children-Revised*, The Psychological Corporation, New York.

Wechsler, D. (1981) *Wechsler Adult Intelligence Scale-Revised,* The Psychological Corporation, New York.

Wesnes, K. and Warburton, D.M. (1983) Effects of smoking on rapid information processing performance. *Neuropsychobiology*, **9**, 223–9.

Willumeit, H.P., Ott, H. and Neubert, W. (1983) Simulated car driving as a useful technique for the determination of residual effects and alcohol interaction after short- and long-acting benzodiazepines. *Psychopharmacology [Suppl.]*, **1**, 182–92.

Zigmond, A.S. and Snaith, R.P. (1983) The Hospital Anxiety and Depression Scale. *Acta Psychiatr. Scand.*, **67**, 361–7.

10

Ophthalmological manifestations of neurofibromatosis 1 and 2

V.A. Purvin and D.W. Dunn

10.1 INTRODUCTION

Ophthalmological manifestations of neurofibromatosis are of interest in several respects. Individuals with neurofibromatosis may come to medical attention first because of eye problems. The presence of an orbital neurofibroma or Schwannoma, an optic nerve glioma or meningioma or congenital glaucoma should prompt a search for additional signs of neurofibromatosis. Second, some lesions, such as iris nodules, are seen so often in NF1 that a thorough eye examination may be useful in confirming a suspected diagnosis. In addition, the eye and orbit are commonly affected by the complications of neurofibromatosis 1 (NF1).

The exact frequency of ophthalmological complications of neurofibromatosis is difficult to determine. Many of the older studies are flawed by lack of attention to diagnostic criteria for neurofibromatosis and most do not separate NF1 from the less common neurofibromatosis 2 (NF2). The incidence of eye involvement has probably been underestimated by physicians who have not performed a detailed ophthalmological examination and who may have overlooked iris nodules and choroidal hamartomas. Two recent studies have given some indication of the incidence of ophthalmological manifestations. Lewis and Riccardi (1981) studied 77 individuals with NF1, combining both a careful examination for neurofibromatosis and a complete ophthalmological survey. They found that 77% of their patients had Lisch nodules and 51% had choroidal hamartomas. In their series, 25% of patients had neurofibromas or café au lait spots involving the eyelid, 25% had prominent corneal nerves or posterior embryotoxon (maldevelopment of the posterior corneal layers), 12% had possible optic nerve glioma, 10% strabismus, 9% retinal lesions and 5% neurofibroma of the conjunctiva. Huson, Jones and Beck (1987) reviewed ophthalmological manifestations of neurofibromatosis as part

Table 10.1 Ophthalmological manifestations of neurofibromatosis

NF1
Eyelids
eyelid cutaneous neurofibroma
eyelid plexiform neurofibroma
eyelid café au lait spots
congenital ptosis
Orbit
orbital neurofibroma
congenital aplasia of greater wing of sphenoid
congenitally small orbit
Anterior segment
Lisch nodules
prominent corneal nerves
Glaucoma
congenital
acquired
Retina
choroidal hamartomas
Optic nerve
optic nerve glioma
NF2
Anterior segment
posterior subcapsular cataracts
Retina
combined pigment epithelial and retinal hamartoma
Optic nerve
meningioma

of a prevalence study in southeast Wales. They found that 95% of individuals with neurofibromatosis had iris nodules. In a group of 53 patients who had a complete ophthalmological examination, Huson, Jones and Beck were able to identify choroidal hamartomas in 35%, neurofibromas on the eyelids in 16%, prominent corneal nerves in 6%, presumed conjunctival neurofibromas in one patient and bilateral optic atrophy due to optic nerve glioma in one patient.

In this chapter we will discuss the specific ophthalmological manifestations of neurofibromatosis; these are summarized in Table 10.1. Our emphasis will be on recognition of lesions that may prompt an evaluation for, or confirm a diagnosis of, neurofibromatosis, and on potential complications that should be sought on follow-up examinations.

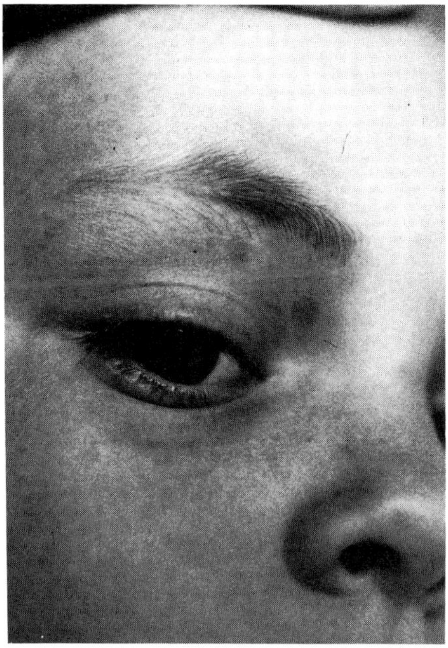

Figure 10.1 Two café au lait spots on the right upper lid of a child with NF1.

10.2 LIDS

Eyelid involvement in neurofibromatosis ranges from small, asymptomatic lesions to massive, severely disfiguring tumours with orbital extension. Café au lait spots, one of the defining features for NF1, were found on the eyelids in two of 77 patients reported by Lewis and Riccardi (1981). These sharply demarcated, hyperpigmented macules are identical to those found on other body surfaces, and do not require any specific treatment (Figure 10.1).

Congenital ptosis, unassociated with lid or orbital tumour, was found in approximately 9% of NF1 patients in one series (Hall, 1986). In our series of 81 children with NF1, three exhibited this type of ptosis (Dunn, 1987). Unilateral involvement is as common as bilateral (Hall, 1986). The basis for this congenital anomaly is unclear.

Dermal neurofibromas, sometimes termed fibroma molluscum in the older literature, are a characteristic feature of NF1. These dome-shaped or pedunculated lesions are common on the eyelid, occurring in 16% of patients with neurofibromatosis in one series (Huson, Jones and Beck, 1987). They usually become evident at puberty when their growth rate increases in association with hormonal changes. Similar growth may occur during pregnancy. These tumours are benign and rarely represent a problem to the patient.

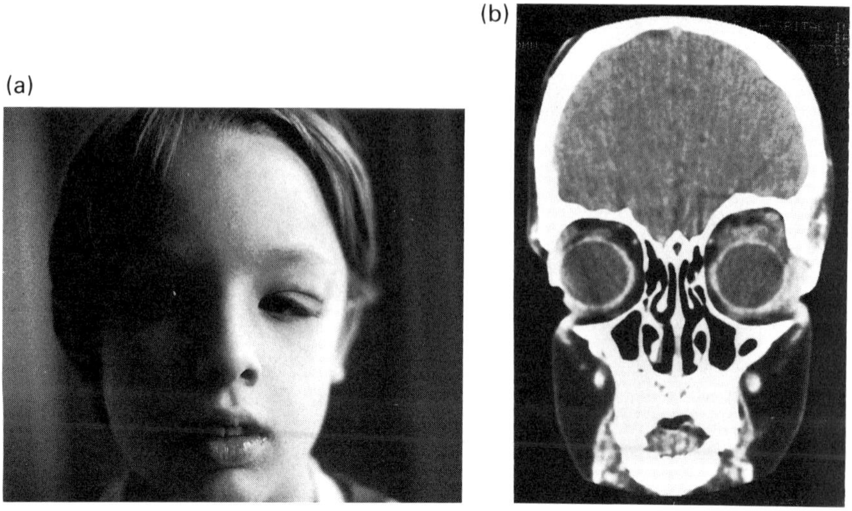

Figure 10.2 (a) Characteristic 'sigmoid' ptosis due to plexiform neurofibroma arising in the lateral portion of the left upper lid. (b) Coronal CT scan of the same patient demonstrating abnormal soft tissue superior and lateral to the left globe. Enlargement of the involved orbit is also seen. (Reproduced from Dunn, 1987.)

Plexiform neurofibromas involve the eyelid less often than dermal neurofibromas, occurring in less than 5% of individuals with NF1. However, they pose much more of a threat to vision and appearance and are often extremely difficult to treat. These tumours usually arise in the lateral portion of the upper lid causing a characteristic 'sigmoid' ptosis (Figure 10.2). Although they are congenital tumours, patients usually present between the ages of 2 and 5 years (Francois, 1972). Initially there is fullness of the lid; over time, progressive growth causes a nodular thickening sometimes termed 'a bag of worms' appearance. Overlying skin changes range from mild thickening to severe overgrowth with hyperpigmentation (elephantiasis neuromatosa). Involvement is nearly always unilateral. Pathologically, these tumours are composed of interwoven bundles of Schwann cells, peripheral nerve axons and endoneurial fibroblasts, usually with widespread invasion of soft tissue. A well-demarcated cellular perineurial sheath defining individual tumour cords is a distinctive feature (Jakobiec and Jones, 1979).

Plexiform neurofibromas affect surrounding tissues in a variety of ways. Francois (1972) has described a syndrome of plexiform neurofibroma of the upper lid with unilateral facial hemihypertrophy involving both soft tissue and bone plus ipsilateral glaucoma with buphthalmos. Glaucoma occurs in about 50% of patients with eyelid plexiform neurofibroma (Walsh and Hoyt, 1969). Associated bony abnormalities are common, including enlargement of the orbit and defects in temporal, frontal and/or sphenoid bones. About 25% of these lid tumours extend to involve the orbit (Francois, 1972) (see below).

These tumours exhibit relentless growth in most cases. Because of interdigitation with normal tissue, complete excision is rarely feasible. Many patients are treated with repeated surgical procedures aimed at debulking the tumour with variable results. In rare instances these tumours may undergo malignant (sarcomatous) transformation (Schatz, 1971; Jakobiec, Font and Zimmerman, 1985).

10.3 ORBIT

Neurofibromatosis can affect the orbit in a variety of ways. Exophthalmos may be caused by a mass lesion (most commonly an optic nerve glioma or neurofibroma), a congenitally small orbit, buphthalmos secondary to congenital glaucoma, or bony defects of the orbital floor or roof. Defects of orbital bones may occur as a congenital anomaly or may be acquired secondary to progressive tumour growth causing remoulding of adjacent bone (Figure 10.3). Aplasia or hypoplasia of the greater wing of the sphenoid allows forward displacement of the temporal lobe with communication of normal brain pulsations to the orbit, causing pulsatile exophthalmos (Binet *et al.*, 1969) (Figure 10.4). This condition can be distinguished from a carotid-cavernous fistula by absence of an orbital or cranial bruit and by absence of arterialized conjunctival and episcleral veins (Bullock and Bartley, 1986). Rarely, defects of orbital bones may cause enophthalmos rather than proptosis. In such cases, ocular pulsations may also be observed (Dabezies and Walsh, 1961; Savino, Glaser and Luxenburg, 1977). Anomalous development of orbital and facial bones may also cause hypertelorism, found in eight out of 34 patients in one series (Wolters *et al.*, 1986).

Orbital neurofibromas may be divided into three types: primary, plexiform and diffuse. Primary neurofibroma is an unusual type of orbital mass lesion, accounting for only 1% of biopsied orbital tumours. These tumours are less commonly associated with neurofibromatosis than are the plexiform type. Only 12% of patients reported by Francois (1972) and one of nine reported by Krohel *et al.* (1985) had neurofibromatosis. Onset is usually between the third and fifth decade. Initial symptoms are typically pain and double vision. Common signs include proptosis, downward deviation of the globe and limitation of eye movements usually affecting supraduction. Additional findings may include disc oedema or pallor secondary to optic nerve compression, choroidal folds and acquired hypermetropia as a result of pressure on the posterior globe and occasionally anaesthesia in the distribution of the frontal nerve. Primary neurofibromas usually exhibit slowly progressive growth

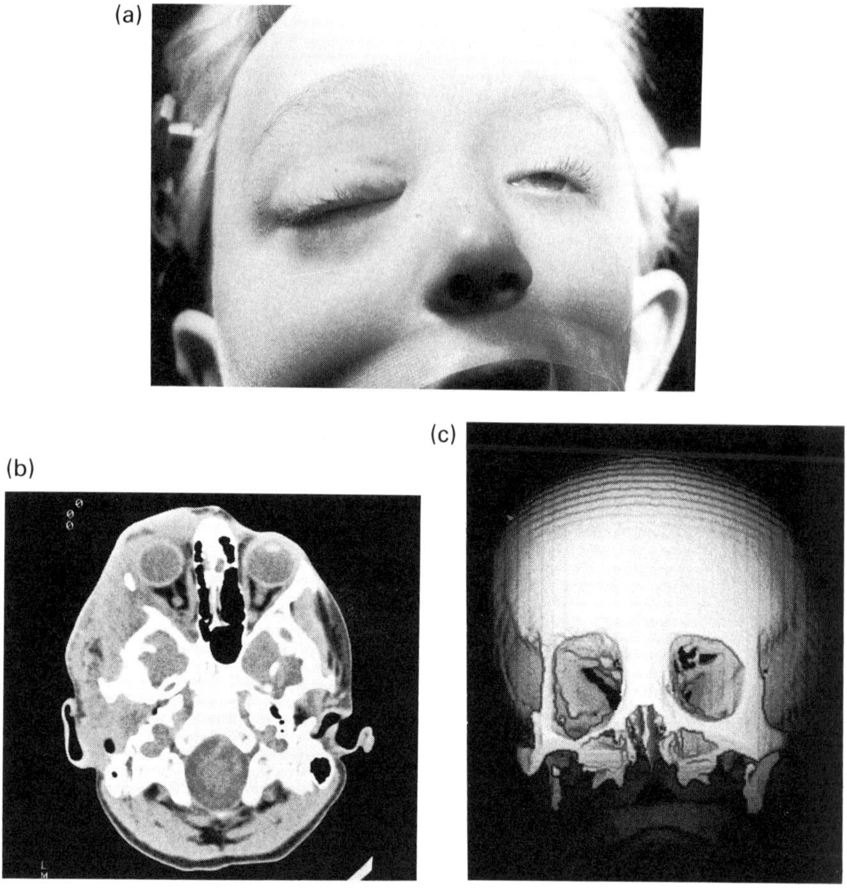

Figure 10.3 (a) Seven-year-old boy with NF1 and a plexiform neurofibroma involving the right orbit. (b) Axial CT scan of this patient reveals extensive tumour involving the orbit and temporal fossa with associated bony erosion of the lateral orbital wall. (c) Three-dimensional reconstructed CT scan shows marked enlargement of the right orbit with widening of the superior orbital fissure. (Photograph and scans courtesy of Dr Ronald Martin.)

causing increasing proptosis. These tumours are thought to originate from branches of the ophthalmic division of the fifth cranial nerve. They are usually well encapsulated and are less vascular than the plexiform type. Thus they can usually be dissected free from adjacent orbital tissues, and if removed in entirety they do not recur. Primary orbital neurofibromas may occasionally be multiple with or without associated neurofibromatosis (Krohel *et al.*, 1985; Shields *et al.*, 1990).

(a) (b)

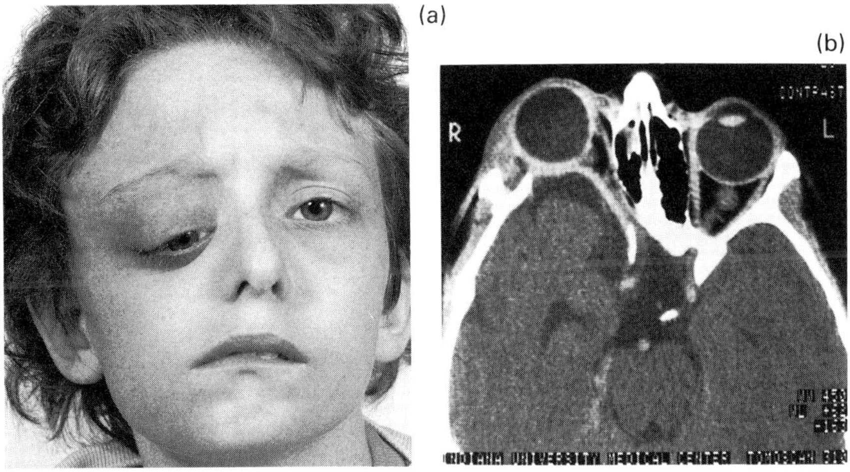

Figure 10.4 (a) Twelve-year-old girl with NF1 and right-sided proptosis. There is also downward displacement of the right orbit and mild thickening of the upper lid. (b) Axial CT scan reveals absence of the greater wing of the sphenoid on the right with forward herniation of the temporal lobe into the orbit. There is mild thickening of soft tissue lateral to the globe.

Orbital plexiform neurofibromas are thought to arise in the lid and extend posteriorly to involve orbital structures (see above). These lesions can best be defined by computed tomography (CT) (Zimmerman *et al.*, 1983; Reed *et al.*, 1986). CT scans typically show a contrast-enhancing, irregular soft-tissue mass with orbital deformity (Figure 10.3). Thickening of lids and periorbital soft tissue is the most constant finding, lending support to the idea of a more superficial origin for this tumour (Reed *et al.*, 1986). Other observations have included thickening of the extraocular muscles, irregular nodularity and enhancement of the optic nerve sheath (presumed to result from involvement of posterior ciliary nerves) and increased density of intraconal fat. Thickening and enhancement of the uvea/sclera has been found in patients with associated buphthalmos due to congenital glaucoma. Bony abnormalities are also well delineated by CT. Changes include orbital enlargement, often with thinning of orbital bones, dysplasia of the greater or lesser wings of the sphenoid, downward tilting or box-like enlargement of the sella and deformity of the posterior lateral ethmoid bones (Francois, 1972).

Diffuse neurofibroma is distinguished from the plexiform type by absence of a distinct perineurial sheath. This tumour is not invariably associated with neurofibromatosis (Jakobiec and Jones, 1979).

Because of their tendency to grow in and around normal structures, treatment of the plexiform and diffuse types of neurofibroma is difficult.

Tenzel *et al.* (1977) have suggested removal of these lesions with *en bloc* resection. If the tumour remains lateral, resection can often be accomplished with preservation of good levator function. For larger lesions, other authors have recommended either selective and repeated resections (Krueger *et al.*, 1979) or more radical excision (orbital exenteration) in patients with no useful vision (Jackson, Laws and Martin, 1983).

10.4 ANTERIOR SEGMENT

Several abnormalities of the anterior segment are particularly notable in patients with neurofibromatosis. Iris nodules are a defining feature of NF1. These lesions have been called Lisch nodules, although similar findings were described by Waardenburg in 1918, and by Goldstein and Wexler in 1930, before the report by Lisch in 1937. They are pigmented hamartomas consisting of large fusiform melanocytes (Perry and Font, 1979). These nodules cause no symptoms. They can occasionally be detected on a general examination as yellow-brown lesions in an individual with neurofibromatosis and lightly coloured irides. They are much more readily seen using biomicroscopy. Iris nodules are smooth, dome-shaped lesions of up to 2 mm in diameter. They vary from clear to lightly pigmented and usually have very distinct borders. Their elevation and soft translucency distinguish them from the more common flat iris naevus (Plate 5).

The number of iris nodules increases progressively with age. Lewis and Riccardi (1981) found iris nodules in three of 16 children under 5 years of age and in 92% of individuals aged 6 years or more. In the series of Flueler, Boltshauser and Kilchhufer (1986), 33% of the children under 6 years of age, 87% of those 6–12 years of age and 100% of those over 12 years of age had iris nodules. Similarly, Zehavi, Romano and Goodman (1986) found nodules in 40% of children under 10 years of age and in 18 of 20 individuals aged 11 years or more.

Iris nodules are occasionally unilateral, especially in children. Their presence and number do not correlate with severity of disease (Lewis and Riccardi, 1981). In one series their number correlated with skin manifestations (Zehavi, Romano and Goodman, 1986), but this was probably due to both lesions becoming more prevalent over time. When correction was made for age, no such correlation was found (Lewis and Riccardi, 1981).

Iris nodules rarely occur in individuals who do not have neurofibromatosis. Greene and Gordon (unpublished data) were able to identify one patient with iris nodules who did not have neurofibromatosis and Huson, Jones and Beck (1987) found that one of their 150 controls had two iris nodules and no additional evidence of neurofibromatosis. Though not pathognomonic for neurofibromatosis, iris nodules occur predominantly

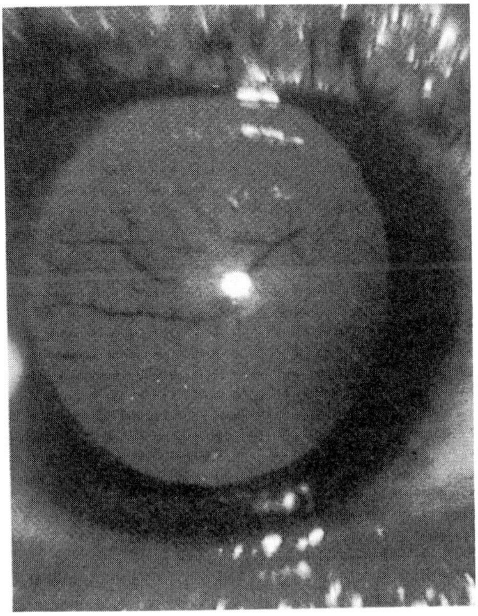

Figure 10.5 Enlarged corneal nerves in a patient with multiple endocrine neoplasia. (Reproduced from Grayson, 1983, with permission of C.V. Mosby.)

in individuals with NF1. Thus the presence or absence of iris nodules may help confirm or exclude a diagnosis of NF1. Since iris nodules occur in 90–100% of adults with neurofibromatosis, if a child of an individual with neurofibromatosis reaches 12 years of age without developing café au lait spots or iris nodules, the diagnosis of neurofibromatosis can be ruled out with reasonable assurance. If an individual presents with one manifestation of neurofibromatosis, e.g. café au lait spots or cutaneous neurofibromas, the finding of iris nodules confirms the diagnosis of NF1.

Other abnormalities of the iris occur rarely. Individuals with large numbers of iris nodules may develop ectropion uveae, a distortion of the iris in which the posterior pigment epithelium is displaced anteriorly (Greenwald and Weiss, 1984). Malignant melanoma of the iris is a rare complication of neurofibromatosis (Goldstein and Wexler, 1930; Woog *et al.*, 1982).

The cornea is occasionally involved in patients with neurofibromatosis. Enlarged corneal nerves were found in three of 53 neurofibromatosis patients examined by Huson, Jones and Beck (1987) and in 17 of the 77 individuals with neurofibromatosis reported by Lewis and Riccardi (1981) (Figure 10.5). Both diffuse enlargement and nodular thickening have been described in neurofibromatosis. Diffuse enlargement is in no way pathognomonic for neurofibromatosis, and it is sometimes seen in normal individuals, especially in the elderly (Grayson, 1983). Other conditions associated with increased visibility of corneal nerves include keratoconus, Refsum's disease, leprosy, ichthyosis, congenital glaucoma and Fuch's dystrophy (Grayson, 1983). Marked nodularity is more distinctively abnormal than diffuse thickening and should prompt a search for one of the above conditions. Enlargement of corneal nerves has also been noted in association with multiple endocrine neoplasia type 3 characterized by mucosal neuromas, phaeochromocytoma and medullary thyroid carcinoma (Font and Ferry, 1972). Corneal enlargement and clouding is a typical finding in congenital glaucoma sometimes associated with NF1. Corneal anaesthesia with secondary neurotropic keratitis may occur in NF2 secondary to involvement of the fifth cranial nerve in the cerebello-pontine angle by vestibular Schwannoma. Unilateral keratoconus in a patient with neurofibromatosis has also been described (Walsh and Hoyt, 1969).

Involvement of the conjunctiva, episclera and sclera by neurofibroma or Schwannoma has been described, but is quite unusual (Dabezies and Penner, 1961). Melanocytosis of these structures has also been observed (Goldstein and Wexler, 1930).

The lens is not involved in individuals with NF1; however, lens involvement has been reported in individuals with NF2 (Pearson-Webb, Kaiser-Kupfer and Eldridge, 1986; Kaiser-Kupfer *et al.*, 1989). Kaiser-Kupfer *et al.* (1989) examined 47 patients from 11 families with NF2 and found that none of these individuals had iris nodules. Of 20 patients with vestibular Schwannoma, 17 had bilateral posterior subcapsular cataracts. Only two of 24 patients without vestibular Schwannoma had similar lens opacities. The youngest patient with such a cataract in this series was 19 years. The lens abnormalities may be seen prior to the onset of symptoms from vestibular Schwannomas and thus routine eye examination in individuals at risk for developing NF2 may help predict those individuals destined to develop vestibular Schwannomas and thus allow early removal of the tumours.

10.5 GLAUCOMA

Glaucoma has been associated with plexiform neurofibromas of the orbit and with involvement of uveal structures by neurofibromas. The glaucoma may be congenital or acquired. When congenital, it presents with an enlarged globe (buphthalmos) and cloudy cornea (Satran, Letson and Seljeskog, 1980). Both the congenital and acquired forms are nearly always unilateral.

Grant and Walton (1968) proposed four possible mechanisms for glaucoma associated with neurofibromatosis. First, there may be infiltration of the angle with neurofibroma visible on gonioscopy. Second, there may be closure of the angle by thickening of the ciliary body or choroid. Third, there can be late onset of glaucoma following development of secondary fibrovascular tissue in the angle. Finally, glaucoma may reflect an associated failure of angle structure development. These authors felt that the first three explanations were more likely.

Medical treatment of this congenital form of glaucoma has been almost uniformly unsuccessful. Surgical options include goniotomy, filtering procedures and cyclocryotherapy. Despite aggressive treatment, visual outcome in this condition is often very poor.

10.6 RETINA AND CHOROID

Lesions of the choroid are second only to iris nodules in frequency. In Lewis and Riccardi's series (1981), 51% of individuals had lesions involving the choroid, and in the series of Huson, Jones and Beck (1987) 35% had such lesions. These lesions may be difficult to visualize with direct ophthalmoscopy. They are small, flat or minimally elevated, yellow-white to brown, avascular lesions (Figure 10.6). Though visible with indirect ophthalmoscopy, they are more readily seen as hypofluorescent lesions on fluorescein angiography, although occasionally there may be areas of hyperfluorescence due to atrophy of the overlying retinal pigment epithelium. These choroidal lesions have been variously termed pigmented hamartomas, naevi or café au lait spots of the fundus (Cotlier, 1977; Savino, Glaser and Luxenburg, 1977; Huson, Jones and Beck, 1987), probably all terms for the same lesion (Archer and Nevin,

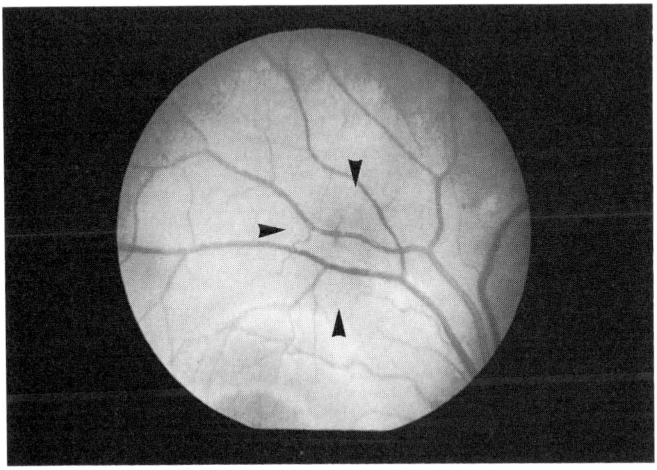

Figure 10.6 Fundus photograph of a large, pigmented choroidal naevus (arrowheads). (Courtesy of Dr John Minturn.)

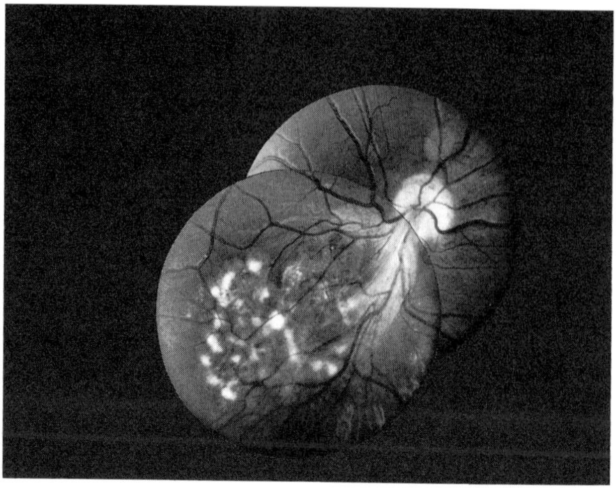

Figure 10.7 Combined hamartoma of the retina and retinal pigment epithelium in a patient with NF2. (Courtesy of Dr W.F. Hoyt.)

1977). In most cases there is no histological confirmation. Choroidal involvement may occasionally take the form of diffuse neurofibroma. This occurs in eyes extensively damaged by associated congenital glaucoma (Brownstein and Little, 1957).

In contrast to choroidal hamartomas, retinal lesions are relatively uncommon in neurofibromatosis. Glial hamartomas identical to those seen in tuberous sclerosis have been described. These nodular masses originate in the nerve fibre layer separate from the optic disc (Archer and Nevin, 1977). Persistent myelination of the nerve fibre layer may also occur with increased frequency in patients with neurofibromatosis.

Another unusual manifestation of neurofibromatosis is combined pigment epithelial and retinal hamartoma. These lesions are slightly elevated with dilatation and tortuosity of retinal vessels overlying an area of diffuse hyperpigmentation of the retinal pigment epithelium (Figure 10.7). Fluorescein angiography usually shows tortuosity and leakage from vessels within the lesion (Schachat *et al.*, 1984). This rare hamartoma usually occurs in isolation and is thought to be congenital. Its association with neurofibromatosis was first described by Cotlier (1977) in a patient with NF2. An additional patient with NF2 and a combined retinal pigment epithelial and retinal hamartoma was recently described by Landau *et al.* (1990). Three other patients described by Gass (1987) had this type of retinal lesion associated with café au lait spots in two cases and with a diagnosis of neurofibromatosis without further description in the third case.

10.7 OPTIC NERVES AND CHIASM

Mass lesions of the anterior visual pathways are a relatively common complication of NF1. These lesions may be hyperplastic nerves, hamartomas or gliomas. Meningiomas may occur in NF2. Of this group, the vast majority are low-grade gliomas, probably accounting for more than 90% of masses of the anterior visual pathway in neurofibromatosis. In contrast, the proportion of neurofibromatosis in series of gliomas of the anterior visual pathway has ranged from 10 to 65%, with an average of 25% (Chutorian *et al.*, 1965; Hoyt and Baghdassarian, 1969; Wong and Lutow, 1972; Miller, Iliff and Green, 1974; Oxenhandler and Sayers, 1978; DeSousa *et al.*, 1979; Stern, DiGiacinto and Houspian, 1979; Wright, McDonald and Call, 1980; Borit and Richardson, 1982; Rush *et al.*, 1982; Tenny *et al.*, 1982; Gould, Hilal and Chutorian, 1987).

The frequency of optic pathway gliomas in NF1 has ranged from 1.5 to 15%. Huson, Jones and Beck (1987) found a 1.5% prevalence of symptomatic optic pathway tumours, but did not use neuroimaging to reveal asymptomatic lesions. The radiographic studies of Lewis *et al.* (1984) and Listernick *et al.* (1989), which included both asymptomatic and symptomatic lesions, demonstrated a 15% prevalence of optic pathway tumour in patients with NF1. However, only one-third of Lewis *et al.*'s patients and one-fifth of Listernick *et al.*'s patients had clinical evidence of these lesions.

Examination of patients with optic pathway gliomas shows varying degrees of visual loss and proptosis. Visual field changes are non-specific. The optic disc may be oedematous, pale or may appear normal. Optociliary shunt vessels, a characteristic finding in optic nerve sheath meningiomas, occur rarely with optic nerve gliomas. The rare occurrence of a glioma confined to the optic nerve head has been associated with NF2 (Dossetor, Landau and Hoyt, 1989).

The pathology and natural history of these lesions has been a long-standing area of controversy. Optic nerve gliomas were initially considered neoplasms meriting aggressive surgical and/or radiation therapy. However, in 1969 Hoyt and Baghdassarian suggested a very different natural history. They noted that three-quarters of their patients with optic pathway gliomas who received no treatment had unchanged or actually improved visual acuity over long periods of follow-up. They thus concluded that these tumours are 'congenital, non-neoplastic and self-limited'. In contrast, Chutorian *et al.* (1965) maintained that these lesions are low-grade astrocytic tumours capable of neoplastic growth and responsive to radiation therapy. In an actuarial analysis, Alvord and Lofton (1988) found markedly variable growth rates in histologically similar optic pathway gliomas. At the present time the consensus seems

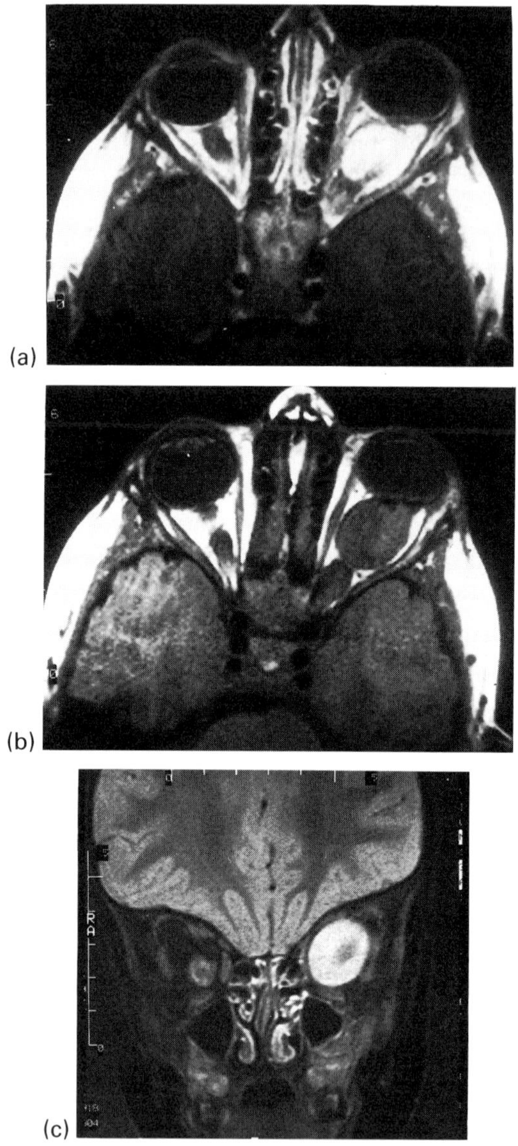

Figure 10.8 (a) T1-weighted axial MRI scan (TR 600, TE 20) showing a large fusiform optic nerve glioma with kinking on the left and mild optic nerve enlargement on the right in a patient with NF1. (b) Gadolinium-enhanced T1-weighted axial MRI scan reveals difference in signal intensity between optic nerve and surrounding tumour. (c) Proton-density coronal MRI scan (TR 2000, TE 30) again demonstrating optic nerve encased in tumour. This perineurial pattern of glial proliferation is thought to be characteristic of optic nerve glioma associated with NF1.

to be that these optic pathway gliomas represent a heterogeneous group of tumours.

This variable growth potential is of particular concern in the case of an optic nerve glioma confined to a single intraorbital optic nerve. If the natural history of this lesion includes progressive intracranial spread with eventual involvement of the contralateral optic nerve, then aggressive surgery is warranted. McDonnell and Miller (1983) reported a single case of posterior growth of a glioma confirmed histologically and followed radiologically. Alvord and Lofton (1988) found that 5% of unilateral optic nerve gliomas subsequently extended into the chiasm and the North American Study Group for Optic Glioma (1989) found chiasmal invasion in four of 106 cases of unilateral optic nerve glioma.

The optic pathway gliomas that occur in patients with NF1 may have a different natural history from those in unaffected individuals, but there are conflicting data regarding this issue. Rush *et al.* (1982) noted longer survivals in individuals with chiasmal gliomas and NF1. Similarly, Wright, McNabb and McDonald (1989) found more aggressive tumour behaviour in patients with optic gliomas without neurofibromatosis. Alvord and Lofton (1988) in contrast found that patients with neurofibromatosis had more frequent recurrence of intraorbital gliomas following surgical excision. Imes and Hoyt (1986) in their study of optic chiasmal gliomas found no overall difference in tumour behaviour in neurofibromatosis versus non-neurofibromatosis patients. These authors noted that neurofibromatosis patients were more likely to die of other tumours than from the effect of their chiasmal gliomas.

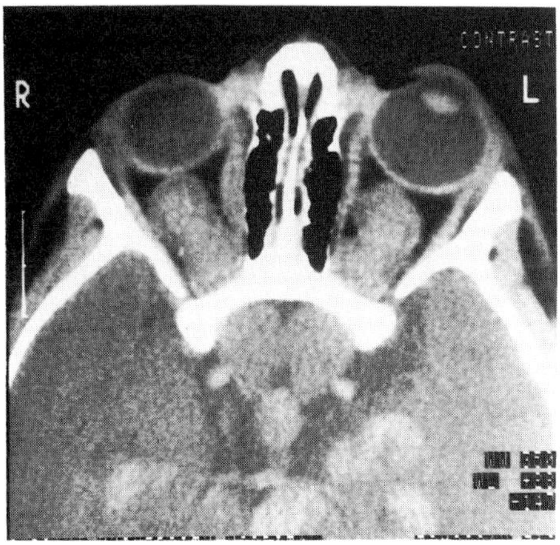

Figure 10.9 Contrast-enhanced CT scan showing bilateral optic nerve and chiasmal glioma. This pattern of diffuse bilateral tubular expansion is considered pathognomonic for NF1.

In addition to possible differences in tumour behaviour, there may be characteristic radiographic changes in optic pathway gliomas that are associated with neurofibromatosis. Seiff *et al.* (1987) described an optic nerve glioma with a compact core seen on an MRI scan as low signal intensity on T2-weighted images with a higher-intensity circumferential component, a finding they felt was distinctive for neurofibromatosis (Figure 10.8). This appearance correlates nicely with the pathological study of optic nerve gliomas by Stern, Jakobiec and Houspian (1980), in which they found a pattern of perineurial astrocytic proliferation to be characteristic of neurofibromatosis-associated tumours. Other patterns seen particularly in individuals with neurofibromatosis include bilateral tubular thickening of the optic nerves and diffuse enlargement of the chiasm plus optic nerves (Figure 10.9). Globular suprasellar mass lesions without optic nerve or tract involvement are more commonly seen in

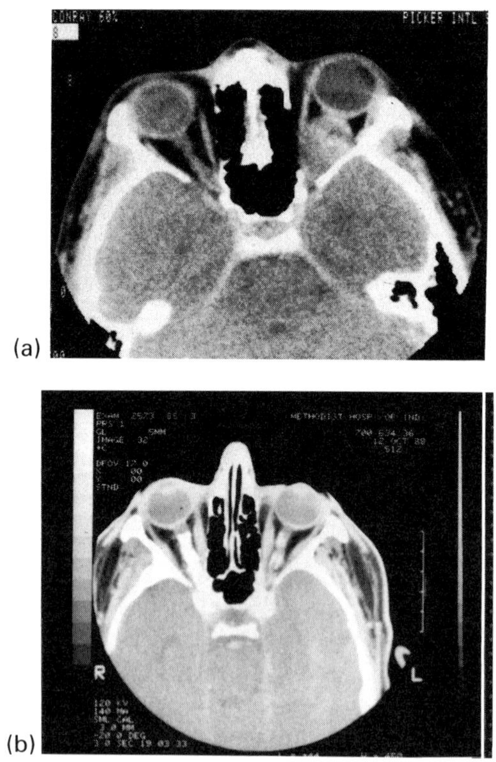

Figure 10.10 (a) CT scan of optic nerve glioma. There is fusiform enlargement of the entire intraorbital optic nerve. (b) CT scan of the orbit in a patient with bilateral optic nerve sheath meningiomas showing typical 'tram-track' calcification along mildly and diffusely enlarged optic nerves.

individuals with no evidence of neurofibromatosis (Fletcher, Imes and Hoyt, 1986).

Another issue regarding radiographic studies in optic pathway gliomas is the reliability of modern techniques in differentiating these tumours from other mass lesions. For intraorbital optic nerve lesions, Jakobiec *et al.* (1984) felt that they could distinguish meningiomas from gliomas based on radiographic features in at least 75% of cases. Gliomas are more often large fusiform masses with kinking and buckling, whereas meningiomas cause a diffusely enlarged nerve often with expansion behind the globe or at the orbital apex. The margins of a glioma are typically clear-cut; meningiomas usually have irregular excrescent margins with frequent calcification (Figure 10.10). With suprasellar lesions the differential diagnosis is usually less of a problem. Fletcher, Imes and Hoyt (1986) felt that only large globular masses require histological examination. They felt that in the individual with NF1 a confident diagnosis of glioma could be made without biopsy when there was tubular thickening of the optic nerve and chiasm or extension of the mass from the chiasm along the optic tract (Figure 10.11).

Decisions regarding treatment of optic pathway gliomas are hampered by our uncertainty concerning the natural history of these tumours and by the lack of randomized prospective trials comparing different treatment modalities. For intraorbital optic nerve gliomas, management

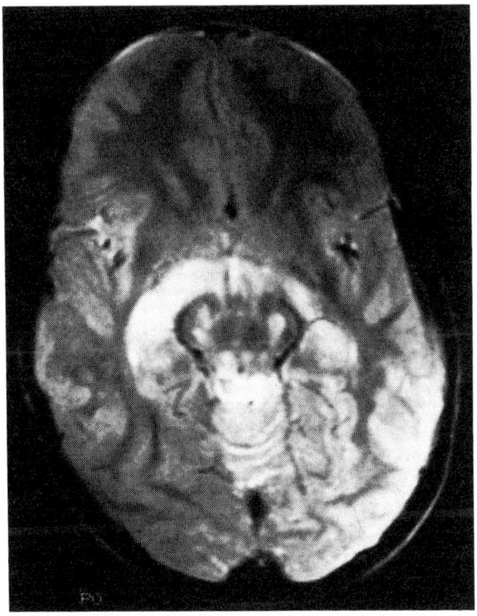

Figure 10.11 T2-weighted axial MRI scan showing bilateral optic tract extension from a chiasmal glioma in a patient with NF1.

options include observation, biopsy with or without resection and radiation. Biopsy is indicated for those cases in which radiographic differentiation between optic nerve glioma and meningioma cannot be made with confidence (Jakobiec *et al.*, 1984). In the individual with unilateral optic nerve glioma and neurofibromatosis, surgical resection should be undertaken when there is severe proptosis, marked visual loss or radiographic evidence of progression with associated reduction in vision. At the present time, the infrequency of posterior extension of unilateral optic nerve gliomas and the tendency for multifocal tumour growth in patients with neurofibromatosis suggest careful clinical and radiographic follow-up of patients without surgery when there is retained vision and only mild or moderate proptosis. Although radiation may slow the growth of optic nerve gliomas, surgical resection is preferred when therapy is indicated.

Surgical resection is rarely appropriate for chiasmal gliomas. For globular suprasellar tumours, partial resection of an exophytic component may occasionally be indicated (Bynke, Kagstrom and Tjernstrom, 1977). In the majority of optic chiasmal gliomas, attempts at debulking do not improve vision and in fact may cause further impairment of optic nerve function and neuroendocrine status. Asymptomatic lesions, which constitute the majority of chiasmal gliomas in neurofibromatosis patients, do not require treatment. If there is clinical or radiographic evidence of progression, treatment options include radiation and chemotherapy. The appropriate choice may depend on the age of the patient. Packer *et al.* (1988) have used a combination of actinomycin D and vincristine without radiotherapy in children 5 years of age or less. This approach allows delay in institution of radiation therapy and thus avoids the deleterious effects of radiation therapy on cognitive and neuroendocrine function seen most commonly in younger children. Cranial radiation with doses above 4500 cGy may be effective, the reported response ranging from 46 to 91% (Packer *et al.*, 1982; Gould, Hilal and Chutorian, 1987; Easle *et al.*, 1988; Edwards, 1990; Tarbell, 1990). Radiotherapy may shrink the tumour and delay tumour growth, but less often causes improvement in visual or endocrine function. Long-term beneficial effects on prognosis remain difficult to prove (Imes and Hoyt, 1986; Easle *et al.*, 1988). Complications of radiation therapy seen in 43% of cases include cognitive delay, endocrine dysfunction, vascular occlusion and the occurrence of second tumours.

For the individual with neurofibromatosis a number of questions still remain. The NIH consensus group on neurofibromatosis recommended neuroimaging studies only for symptomatic patients, a position not widely accepted by neurologists or neurosurgeons in the USA. If one accepts the proposition that only symptomatic lesions should be treated, then neuroimaging in asymptomatic patients may not be warranted. If one decides to image asymptomatic individuals with neurofibromatosis, then there are few data to suggest when such studies should be carried out or how often they should be repeated. If a mass lesion is found in an asymptomatic individual there are again no data to suggest how often neuroimaging studies should be repeated. Good prospective studies are sorely needed for defining the natural history of these tumours. The heterogeneity of these tumours is now recognized. Developments in molecular genetics may define factors important in tumour growth and give us a means of predicting which of the tumours will grow and become symptomatic and thus merit aggressive therapy.

REFERENCES

Alvord, E.C. and Lofton, S. (1988) Gliomas of the optic nerve or chiasm. *J. Neurosurg.*, **68**, 85–98.

Archer, D.B. and Nevin, N.C. (1977) Neurofibromatosis-von Recklinghausen's disease, in *Hereditary Retinal and Choroidal Diseases*, Vol. II (ed. A.E. Krill), Harper & Row, Hagerstown, pp. 1193–218.

Binet, E.F. *et al.* (1969) Orbital dysplasia in neurofibromatosis. *Radiology*, **93**, 829–33.

Borit, A. and Richardson, E.P., Jr (1982) The biological and clinical behavior of pilocytic astrocytomas of the optic pathways. *Brain*, **105**, 161–87.

Brownstein, S. and Little, J.M. (1957) Ocular neurofibromatosis. *Ophthalmology*, **90**, 1595–9.

Bullock, J.D. and Bartley, G.B. (1986) Dynamic proptosis. *Am. J. Ophthalmol.*, **102**, 104–10.

Bynke, H., Kagstrom, E. and Tjernstrom, K. (1977) Aspects of the treatment of gliomas of the anterior visual pathway. *Acta Ophthalmol.*, **55**, 269–80.

Chutorian, A.M. *et al.* (1965) Optic gliomas in children. *Neurology*, **14**, 83–95.

Cotlier, E. (1977) Café-au-lait spots of the fundus in neurofibromatosis. *Arch. Ophthalmol.*, **95**, 1990–3.

Dabezies, O.H., Jr and Penner, R. (1961) Neurofibroma or neurilemmoma of the bulbar conjunctiva. *Arch. Ophthalmol.*, **66**, 73.

Dabezies, O.H., Jr and Walsh, F.B. (1961) Pulsating enophthalmos in association with neurofibromas of the eyelid. *Trans. Am. Acad. Ophthalmol. Otolaryngol.*, **65**, 885–94.

DeSousa, A.L. *et al.* (1979) Optic chiasmatic glioma in children. *Am. J. Ophthalmol.*, **87**, 376–81.

Dossetor, F., Landau, K. and Hoyt, W.F. (1989) Optic disk glioma in neurofibromatosis type 2. *Am. J. Ophthalmol.*, **108**, 602–3.

Dunn, D.W. (1987) Neurofibromatosis in childhood. *Curr. Probl. Pediatr.*, **17**, 445–597.

Easle, J.D. *et al.* (1988) Controversy in the management of optic pathway gliomas – 29 patients treated with radiation therapy at Baylor College of Medicine from 1967 through 1987. *Neurofibromatosis*, **1**, 248–51.

Edwards, M.S.B. (1990) Management and treatment of chiasmatic gliomas, in *Optic Gliomas in Neurofibromatosis*, National Neurofibromatosis Foundation, New York, pp. 123–6.

Fletcher, W.A., Imes, R.K. and Hoyt, W.F. (1986) Chiasmal gliomas: appearance and long-term changes demonstrated by computerized tomography. *J. Neurosurg.*, **65**, 154–9.

Flueler, U., Boltshauser, E. and Kilchhufer, A. (1986) Iris hamartoma as diagnostic criterion in neurofibromatosis. *Neuropediatrics*, **17**, 183–5.

Font, R.L. and Ferry, A.P. (1972) The phakomatoses. *Int. Ophthalmol. Clin.*, **12**, 1–50.

Francois, J. (1972) Ocular aspects of the phakomatoses, in *Handbook of Clinical Neurology*, Vol. 14 (eds P.J. Vinken *et al.*), Elsevier, New York, pp. 619–67.

Gass, J.D.M. (1987) Combined pigment epithelial and retinal hamartoma, in *Stereoscopic Atlas of Macular Diseases: Diagnosis and Treatment* (ed. E.A. Kelin), C.V. Mosby, St Louis, pp. 620–5.

Goldstein, I. and Wexler, D. (1930) Melanosis uveae and melanoma of the iris in neurofibromatosis. *Arch. Ophthalmol.*, **3**, 288.

Gould, R.D., Hilal, S.K. and Chutorian, A.M. (1987) Efficacy of radiotherapy in optic gliomas. *Pediatr. Neurol.*, **3**, 29–32.

Grant, W.M. and Walton, D.S. (1968) Distinctive gonioscopic findings in glaucoma due to neurofibromatosis. *Arch. Ophthalmol.*, **79**, 127–34.

Grayson, M. (1983) *Diseases of the Cornea*, 2nd edn, C.V. Mosby, St Louis.

Greenwald, M.J. and Weiss, A. (1984) Ocular manifestations of the neurocutaneous syndromes. *Pediatr. Dermatol.*, **2**, 98–117.

Hall, B.D. (1986) Congenital lid ptosis associated with neurofibromatosis. *Am. J. Med. Genet.*, **25**, 595–7.

Hoyt, W.F. and Baghdassarian, S.A. (1969) Optic glioma of childhood: natural history and rationale for conservative management. *Br. J. Ophthalmol.*, **53**, 793–8.

Huson, S., Jones, D. and Beck, L. (1987) Ophthalmic manifestations of neurofibromatosis. *Br. J. Ophthalmol.*, **71**, 235–8.

Imes, R.D. and Hoyt, W.F. (1986) Childhood chiasmal gliomas: update on the fate of patients in the 1969 San Francisco study. *Br. J. Ophthalmol.*, **70**, 179–82.

Jackson, I.T., Laws, E.R. and Martin, R.D. (1983) The surgical management of orbital neurofibromatosis. *Plast. Reconstr. Surg.*, **71**, 751–8.

Jakobiec, F.A. and Jones, I.S. (1979) Neurogenic tumors, in *Diseases of the Orbit* (eds I.S. Ones and F.A. Jakobiec), Harper & Row, Hagerstown, pp. 371–84.

Jakobiec, F.A. *et al.* (1984) Combined clinical and computed tomographic diagnosis of orbital glioma and meningioma. *Ophthalmology*, **91**, 137–55.

Jakobiec, F.A., Font, R.L. and Zimmerman, L.E. (1985) Malignant peripheral nerve sheath tumors of the orbit: a clinico-pathologic study of eight cases. *Trans. Am. Ophthalmol. Soc.*, **83**, 332–66.

Kaiser-Kupfer, M. *et al.* (1989) The association of posterior capsular lens opacities with bilateral acoustic neuromas in patients with neurofibromatosis type 2. *Arch. Ophthalmol.*, **107**, 541–4.

Krohel, G.B. *et al.* (1985) Localized orbital neurofibromas. *Am. J. Ophthalmol.*, **100**, 458–64.

Krueger, W. *et al.* (1979) Plexiform neurofibroma of the head and neck. *Am. J. Surg.*, **138**, 517–20.

Landau, K. *et al.* (1990) Retinal hamartoma in neurofibromatosis 2. *Arch. Ophthalmol.*, **108**, 328–9.

Lewis, R.A. and Riccardi, V.M. (1981) Von Recklinghausen neurofibromatosis: prevalence of iris hamartoma. *Ophthalmology*, **88**, 348–54.

Lewis, R.A. *et al.* (1984) Von Recklinghausen neurofibromatosis: II. Incidence of optic nerve gliomata. *Ophthalmology*, **91**, 929–35.

Lisch, K. (1937) Ueber Beteiligung der Augen, insbesondere das Vorkommen von Irisknotchen bei der Neurofibromatose (Recklinghausen). *Z. Augenheilkde*, **93**, 137–43.

Listernick, R. *et al.* (1989) Optic gliomas in children with neurofibromatosis type 1. *J. Pediatr.*, **114**, 788–92.

McDonnell, P. and Miller, N. (1983) Chiasmatic and hypothalamic extension of optic nerve glioma. *Arch. Ophthalmol.*, **101**, 1412–15.

Miller, N.R., Iliff, W.J. and Green, W.R. (1974) Evaluation and management of gliomas of the anterior visual pathways. *Brain*, **97**, 743–54.

North American Study Group for Optic Glioma (1989) Tumor spread in unilateral optic glioma. Study report No. 2. *Neurofibromatosis*, **2**, 195–203.

Oxenhandler, D.C. and Sayers, M.P. (1978) The dilemma of childhood optic gliomas. *J. Neurosurg.*, **48**, 34–41.

Packer, R.J. *et al.* (1982) Optic glioma. Long-term follow-up of 85 histopathologically verified cases. *Ophthalmology*, **89**, 1213–19.

Packer, R.J. *et al.* (1988) Treatment of chiasmatic/hypothalamic gliomas of childhood with chemotherapy: an update. *Ann. Neurol.*, **23**, 79–85.

Pearson-Webb, M.A., Kaiser-Kupfer, M.I. and Eldridge, R. (1986) Eye findings in bilateral acoustic (central) neurofibromatosis: association with presenile lens opacities and cataracts but absence of Lisch nodules. *N. Engl. J. Med.*, **315**, 1553–4.

Perry, H.D. and Font, R.L. (1979) Iris nodules in neurofibromatosis: electron microscopic findings. *Invest. Ophthalmol. Vis. Sci. [Suppl.]*, **18**, 204.

Reed, D. *et al.* (1986) Plexiform neurofibromatosis of the orbit: CT evaluation. *AJNR*, **7**, 259–63.

Rush, J.A. *et al.* (1982) Optic glioma: long term follow-up of 85 histopathologically verified cases. *Ophthalmology*, **89**, 1213–19.

Satran, L., Letson, R.D. and Seljeskog, E.L. (1980) Neurofibromatosis with congenital glaucoma and buphthalmos in a newborn. *Am. J. Dis. Child.*, **134**, 182–3.

Savino, P.J., Glaser, J.S. and Luxenburg, M.N. (1977) Pulsating enophthalmos and choroidal hamartomas: two rare stigmata of neurofibromatosis. *Br. J. Ophthalmol.*, **61**, 483–8.

Schachat, A.P. *et al.* (1984) Combined hamartomas of the retina and retinal pigment epithelium. Discussion by J.D.M. Gass. *Ophthalmology*, **91**, 1609–15.

Schatz, H. (1971) Benign orbital neurilemmoma sarcomatous transformation in von Recklinghausen's disease. *Arch. Ophthalmol.*, **86**, 268–73.

Seiff, S.R. *et al.* (1987) Orbital optic glioma in neurofibromatosis. Magnetic resonance diagnosis of perineural arachnoidal gliomatosis. *Arch. Ophthalmol.*, **105**, 1689–92.

Shields, J. *et al.* (1990) Multiple orbital neurofibromas unassociated with von Recklinghausen's disease. *Arch. Ophthalmol.*, **108**, 80–3.

Stern, J., DiGiacinto, G.V. and Houspian, E.M. (1979) Neurofibromatosis and optic glioma: clinical and morphological correlations. *Neurosurgery*, **4**, 524–8.

Stern, J., Jakobiec, F.A. and Houspian, E.M. (1980) The architecture of optic nerve gliomas with and without neurofibromatosis. *Arch. Ophthalmol.*, **98**, 505–11.

Tarbell, N.J. (1990) Radiation therapy in the management of patients with optic chiasm gliomas, in *Optic Gliomas in Neurofibromatosis*, National Neurofibromatosis Foundation, New York, pp. 149–58.

Tenny, R.T. *et al.* (1982) The neurosurgical management of optic glioma: results in 104 patients. *J. Neurosurg.*, **57**, 452–8.

Tenzel, R.R. *et al.* (1977) Surgical treatment of eyelid neurofibromas. *Arch. Ophthalmol.*, **95**, 479–83.

Waardenburg, P.J. (1918) Heterochramie en melanosis. *Ned. Tijdschr. Geneeskd.*, **2**, 1453–5.

Walsh, F.B. and Hoyt, W.F. (1969) *Clinical Neuro-ophthalmology*, 3rd edn, Vol. 3, Williams & Wilkins, Baltimore, pp. 1942–57.

Wolters, E. *et al.* (1986) Hypertelorism in neurofibromatosis. *Neuropediatrics*, **17**, 175–7.

Wong, I.G. and Lubow, M. (1972) Management of optic glioma of childhood: a review of 42 cases, in *Neuro-ophthalmology*, C.V. Mosby, St Louis, pp. 51–60.

Woog, J.J. *et al.* (1982) Neurofibromatosis of the eyelid and orbit. *Int. Ophthalmol. Clin.*, **22**, 157–87.

Wright, J.E., McDonald, W.I. and Call, N.B. (1980) Management of optic nerve gliomas. *Br. J. Ophthalmol.*, **64**, 545–52.

Wright, J.E., McNabb, A.A. and McDonald, W.I. (1989) Optic nerve glioma and the management of optic nerve tumors in the young. *Br. J. Ophthalmol.*, **73**, 967–74.

Zehavi, C., Romano, A. and Goodman, R.M. (1986) Iris (Lisch) nodules in neurofibromatosis. *Clin. Genet.*, **29**, 51–5.

Zimmerman, R.A. *et al.* (1983) Computed tomography of orbital-facial neurofibromatosis. *Radiology*, **146**, 113–16.

11

Orthopaedic manifestations of neurofibromatosis

J. Fairbank

11.1 INTRODUCTION

A number of the protean manifestations of neurofibromatosis require surgical treatment. This chapter is concerned with aspects of neurofibromatosis that affect the musculoskeletal system, including the spine and cranium. The important conditions discussed include spinal deformity, neurofibromas and other tumours affecting the spinal cord and peripheral nerves, pseudoarthrosis of long bones, especially the tibia, limb gigantism associated with plexiform neurofibromas, and less common problems, such as pectus excavatum. The radiological manifestations of neurofibromatosis frequently cause diagnostic difficulties, giving neurofibromatosis the reputation, like syphilis, of being a mimic of many other conditions. This chapter does not include pathological information, which is described in Chapter 6. Most of the published data relate to neurofibromatosis 1 (NF1), but because most reports pre-date the clear distinction of NF1 from NF2, it is not always possible to distinguish the two conditions in the orthopaedic and neurosurgical literature. Where the distinction is not possible, the term NF has been used in this chapter.

Many of the orthopaedic and spinal problems of NF1 are age-related, and when these conditions are present in very young children the diagnosis of NF1 may easily be missed. About 10% of children with NF1 have serious cosmetic or functional involvement of the musculoskeletal system (Cole and Myers, 1978; Huson, Harper and Compston, 1988). The diagnosis should be considered whenever the clinician is confronted by:

- serious scoliosis;
- pseudoarthrosis of a long bone;
- hypertrophy of a part;
- an unusual radiographic lesion of bone.

The skeletal manifestations of the disease may precede the appearance of neurofibromas by many years. It is important to seek a family history of NF1 and to look for café au lait spots.

11.2 SURGICAL TREATMENT: GENERAL CONSIDERATIONS

If a patient requires an anaesthetic, it is important to remember that NF1 may be complicated by phaeochromocytoma. Phaeochromocytoma, which has inexplicably escaped the attention of orthopaedic textbook authors, has caused the unexpected death of at least one patient in my experience, when the diagnosis had eluded physicians for several years (Kalff, Shapiro and Lloyd, 1982). The diagnosis and management of phaeochromocytoma are discussed in Chapter 13. Reviews of phaeochromocytoma and other anaesthetic complications of NF1 have been published by Fisher (1975), Yamashita, Matsuki and Oyama (1977) and Van Aken, Scherer and Lawin (1982). The most recent, and valuable, by Hull (1986) considers the anaesthetic management of phaeochromocytoma.

All surgery involving bone in NF1 is blighted by the high risk of pseudoarthrosis. Special efforts have to be made in all patients to avoid this complication. The multisystem nature of NF1 frequently faces surgeons with cases that present formidable difficulties in their management. A number of surgical disciplines may be required to manage an individual patient.

11.3 RADIOLOGY

The radiological manifestations of NF1 are notorious for presenting diagnostic difficulties (Klatte, Fraken and Smith, 1976), especially in children (Crawford and Bagamery, 1986). They include a high frequency of skeletal involvement, with bone deformities arising directly from the destruction by neurofibromatous tissue or from aberrations of skeletal growth and development of body parts or systems (Binet and Markarian, 1974). A variety of malignant bone tumours have been described with NF1, including fibrosarcoma, malignant fibrous histiocytoma, chordoma and osteosarcoma (Ducatman, Scheithauer and Dahlin, 1983; Sharif and Tucker, 1985; Wamer *et al.*, 1985; Sørensen, Mulvihill and Nielsen, 1986), although these are very rare (Voutsinas and Wynne-Davies, 1983). These cases are sporadic, and may even be coincidental. The main radiological manifestations of NF are as follows.

(a) Focal gigantism

This is the result of hypertrophy of a bone, digit or entire limb. An example is shown in Figures 11.1 and 11.2. Unusual lengthening or shortening of a bone is a feature of NF (Gupta *et al.*, 1985).

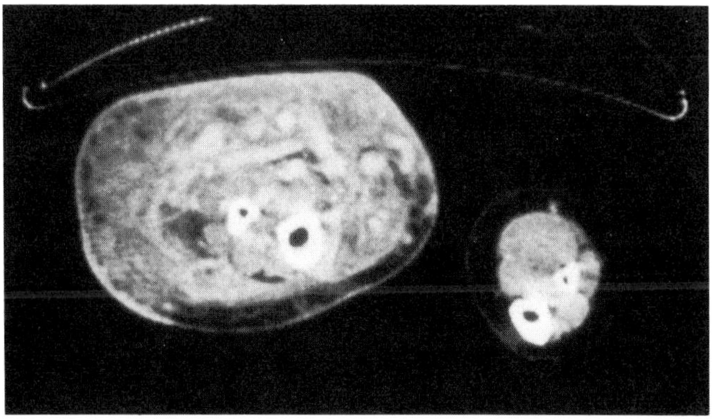

Figure 11.1 Axial CT scan of the calves of a young adult female with NF1 and gigantism. The gigantic left lower limb is much larger than the right.

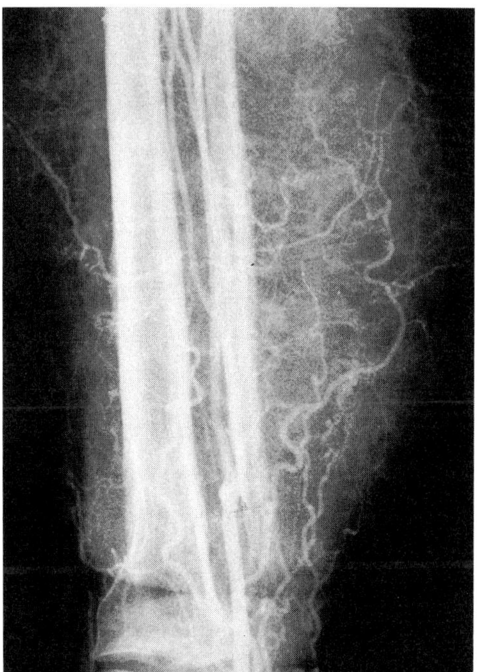

Figure 11.2 Angiogram of the gigantic left lower limb shown in Figure 11.1.

(b) Cortical bone defects

These are usually caused by NF tissue irritating the periosteum (Pitt, Mosher and Edeiken, 1972).

(c) Bone cyst formation

Cyst-like rarefactions occur as a result of proliferation of tissue within the medullary cavity (Schwartz and Ramos, 1980; Faure *et al.*, 1986; Gross *et al.*, 1989).

(d) Bowing of long bones

Bowing of long bones is a common feature of NF1, and may pre-date pseudoarthrosis formation (Figure 11.3).

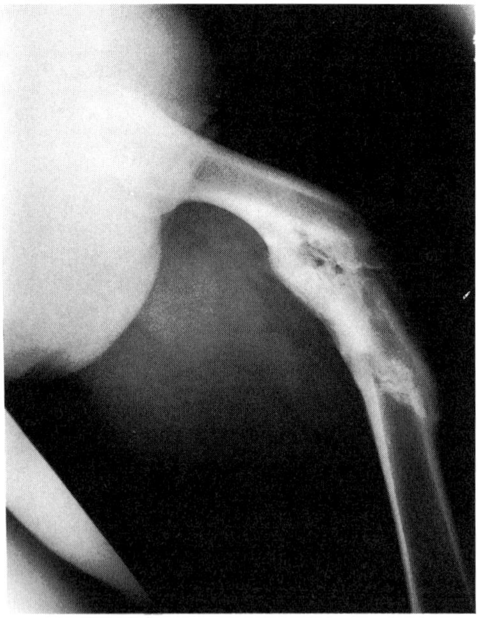

Figure 11.3 Radiograph of the femur of a patient with NF1, showing bowing secondary to pseudoarthrosis.

(e) Pseudoarthrosis of long bone

This is a common feature of NF1 (*vide infra*). Pseudoarthrosis is either the development of a false joint in a long bone or the failure of a fracture or osteotomy to unite with bone in, say, 6 months (opinions vary as to the time scale and to differences from the related definitions of non-union).

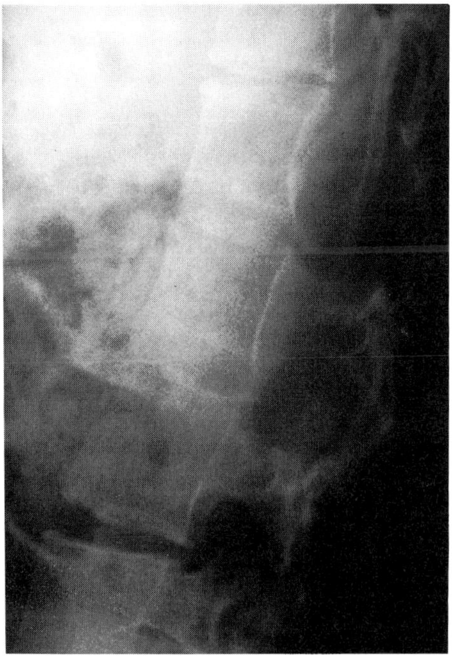

Figure 11.4 Lateral radiograph of the lumbar spine of an adolescent with NF1, showing vertebral scalloping and foraminal enlargement by neurofibromas.

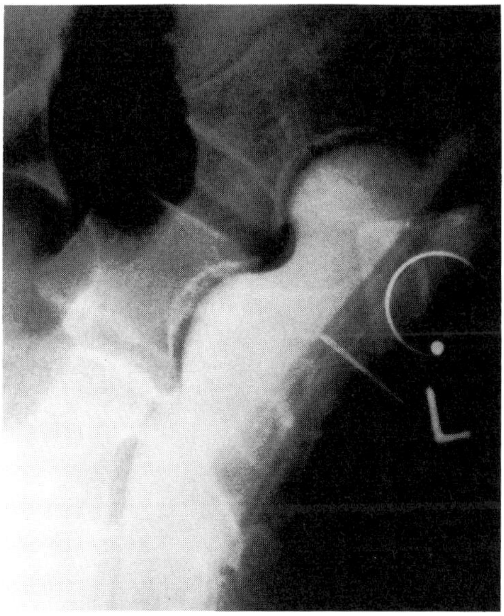

Figure 11.5 Myelogram of the upper lumbar spine of the same patient as in Figure 11.4, showing that vertebral scalloping is related to dural expansion.

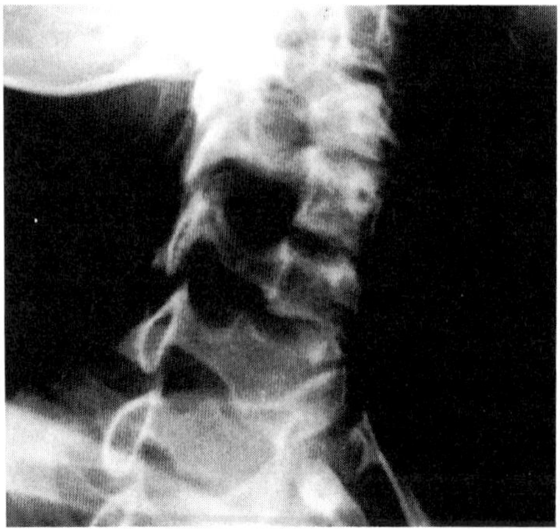

Figure 11.6 Lateral radiograph of the cervical spine showing marked enlargement of the intervertebral foramina between C4 and C5, and C5 and C6, as a result of neurofibromas on the C5 and C6 spinal nerve roots.

(f) Spine

The spine may be affected in NF1 by scalloping of the posterior margin of vertebral bodies (Casselman and Mandell, 1979), enlargement of the intervertebral foramina, defective pedicles or dysplasia of the vertebral bodies causing some types of spinal deformity (Figures 11.4, 11.5 and 11.6). These changes can occur when the spinal contents are normal, and may be a developmental anomaly (Heard and Payne, 1962). They can also indicate a dumb-bell tumour, saccular dilatation of the dura (dural ectasia) or the abnormally extensive protusion of the dura out of the intervertebral foramen (Figure 11.7) (Sammons and Thomas, 1959). The formation of a lateral meningocele with loss of the pedicles may be associated with loss of spinal stability (O'Neill, Whatmore and Booth, 1983). This ranges from minor subluxations to major single level dislocations, which may occur at any level in the spine (Curtis *et al.*, 1969; Mandell, 1978; Hvorslev and Reiter, 1979; Yong-Hing, Kalamchi and MacEwen, 1979; Winter and Edwards, 1981; Rockower, McKay and Nason, 1982; Isu *et al.*, 1983). Thoracic meningoceles have been reported in association with NF1, but are rare (see also Chapter 8). Pohl (1933) was the first to report thoracic meningoceles in association with NF. They present as a large soft-tissue or cystic masses protruding from the mediastinum. They may be accompanied by structural defects in the pedicle, enlargement of the intervertebral foramina and vertebral body anomalies (Erkulvrawatr *et al.*, 1979; Crawford, 1989). In a review of 70 cases of thoracic meningocele, of which 85% had NF, Miles, Pennybacker

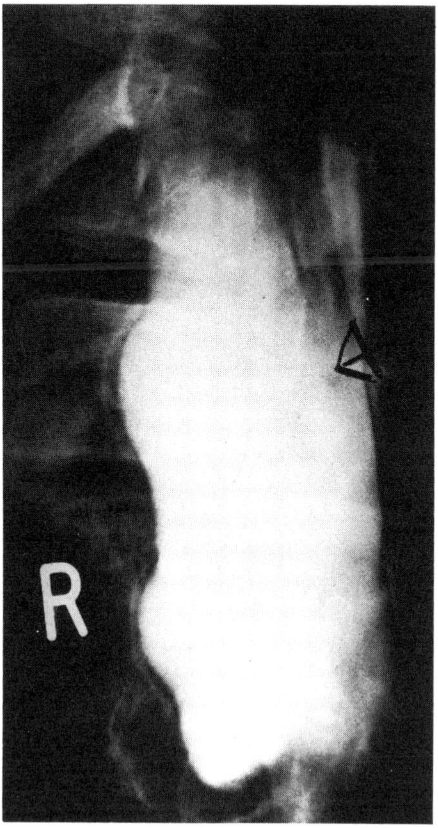

Figure 11.7 A thoracic meningocele demonstrated by myelography.

and Sheldon (1969) reported severe paraplegia in only six cases, and minor neurological impairment in seven. Nearly a quarter had significant pain.

(g) Intra-articular neurofibromas

Intra-articular neurofibromas or other tumours may disrupt joint mechanics (Baker, Tchang and Greenspan, 1982; Lachiewicz *et al.*, 1983).

(h) Skull

Macrocranium and macrocephaly are recognized features of NF1. In one study, 44% of 52 patients had cranial capacities above the 95th centile, and this finding was unrelated to intracranial tumours (Holt and Kuhn, 1976). Sphenoid dysplasia is a rare, but classic feature of NF (Chapter 7).

This was first described by Le Wald (1933), and may present with pulsatile exophthalmos (Binet *et al.*, 1969). The frequency of sphenoid dysplasia in NF is said to be 33% (Burrows, 1963). The value of modern imaging techniques in its diagnosis has been reviewed by Harkens and Dolan (1990). Other skull and facial anomalies that occur in NF1 include mandibular enlargement, osseous dysplasia of the lambdoid suture and foraminal enlargement. In one study, these and other abnormalities were found in 92% of 38 patients with NF (D'Ambrosio, Langlais and Y, 1988).

11.4 SPINAL TUMOURS

Schwannomas are common on the spinal nerve roots in NF2 and tumours sometimes occur on the spinal nerve roots in NF1. Fortunately, many of these spinal tumours present with radicular pain, and can be identified clinically at an early stage (McAlheny and Netsky, 1955). Conventionally the pain is continuous, and worse at night (Austin, 1959). There may be focal fasciculation, which is often asymmetrical. Cord compression will cause spasticity and weakness, especially on the side of the tumour, with pain and temperature loss on the opposite side (Chapter 8).

Plain radiographs may be normal or show evidence of symmetrical enlargement of a single intervertebral foramen. Imaging may include computed tomography (CT) in combination with myelography, or magnetic resonance imaging (MRI). Either technique will indicate the site of the tumour, although the precise pathology can only be determined by biopsy. Lumbar puncture and neurophysiological investigations are not usually needed. Angiography is only helpful if a haemangioma or arteriovenous malformation is suspected (Holt and Wright, 1948; Bull, 1952).

It is usually best to attempt excision of symptomatic neurofibromas only (Love and Dodge, 1952). Attempted excision of a neurofibroma in association with a kyphosis has long been recognized to have a catastrophic effect on spinal cord function (Cobb, 1948). Curtis *et al.* (1969) described paraplegia in association with spinal angulation or tumour, or both. Lonstein *et al.* (1980) and Winter, Lonstein and Anderson (1988) placed NF second only to congenital deformity as a cause of neurological deficit in association with spinal deformity. Miller (1936) found that paraplegia was due to a kyphotic angulation in more than half of his 20 paraplegic patients with NF. The series of Winter, Lonstein and Anderson (1988) included some formidable deformities, with a mean kyphosis of 132° in 33 patients, of whom six were paraplegic and six had respiratory distress. In the 27 who had surgery, laminectomy was worse than useless. They confirmed the value of combined anterior and posterior surgery, with prolonged rigid immobilization. These authors found that the severity of the deformity often prevented the use of instrumentation.

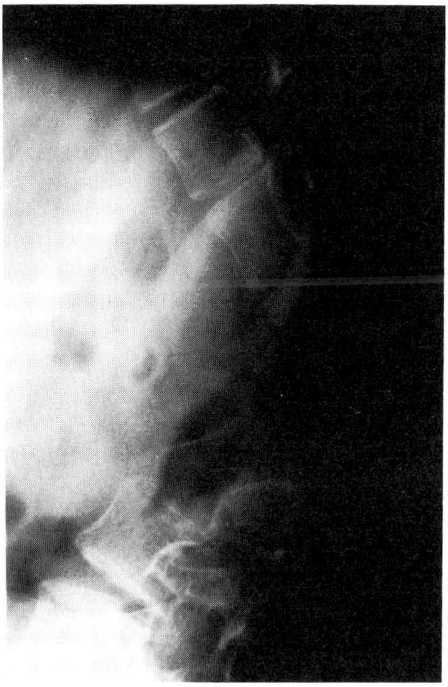

Figure 11.8 Lateral radiograph of the thoracolumbar spine of an adolescent with NF1 showing a thoracolumbar kyphosis.

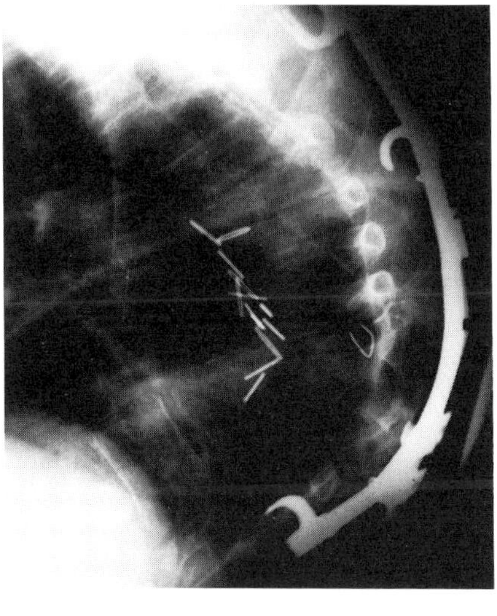

Figure 11.9 The spine shown in Figure 11.10, fused front and back with posterior compression and distraction Harrington rods.

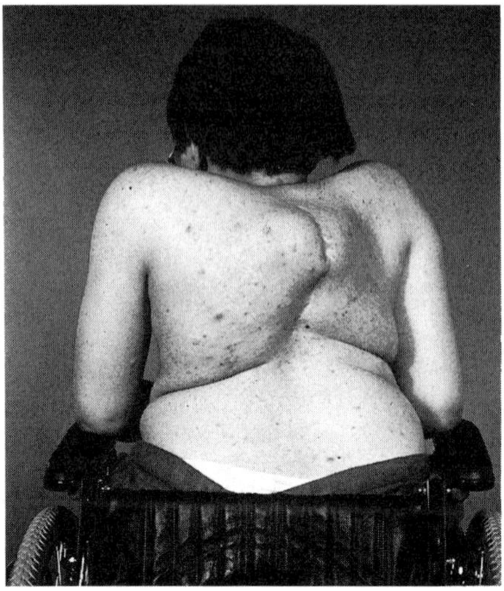

Figure 11.10 Rear view of the patient shown in Figures 11.8 and 11.9.

In this very complex group of patients, halo traction and halo cast may be of considerable value in correcting and stabilizing the deformity (Figures 11.8, 11.9 and 11.10).

11.5 SPINAL DEFORMITY

11.5.1 Introduction

Spinal curvatures are common in NF1, and may be the presenting feature. The incidence of deformity is dependent on the source of clinical material. A recent study in a multidisciplinary NF clinic found scoliosis in 23 of 220 patients with NF1 (10.5%) (Akbarnia *et al.*, 1992). The classic description is of two main varieties of curve, the dystrophic (Figures 11.11 and 11.12) and the idiopathic, with widely varying prognoses (Cobb, 1950).

The proportion of these two patterns of curve depends on the source of the data. Crawford (1987, 1989) estimated that there is a 7:1 ratio of idiopathic to dystrophic curves. Chaglassian, Riseborough and Hall (1976) reviewed 141 cases of NF, and found 37 with spinal deformity, of whom 16 had dystrophic-type curves and 20 idiopathic-type curves. Other series are reviews of cases presenting with spinal deformity, and are therefore likely to be biased in favour of the short dysplastic curves (Lawson, Moe and Pedras, 1973; Calvert, Edgar and Webb, 1989; Sirois and Drennan, 1990).

Leatherman and Dickson (1988) do not recognize a kyphoscoliotic pattern but recognize four main types of spinal deformity in NF. These

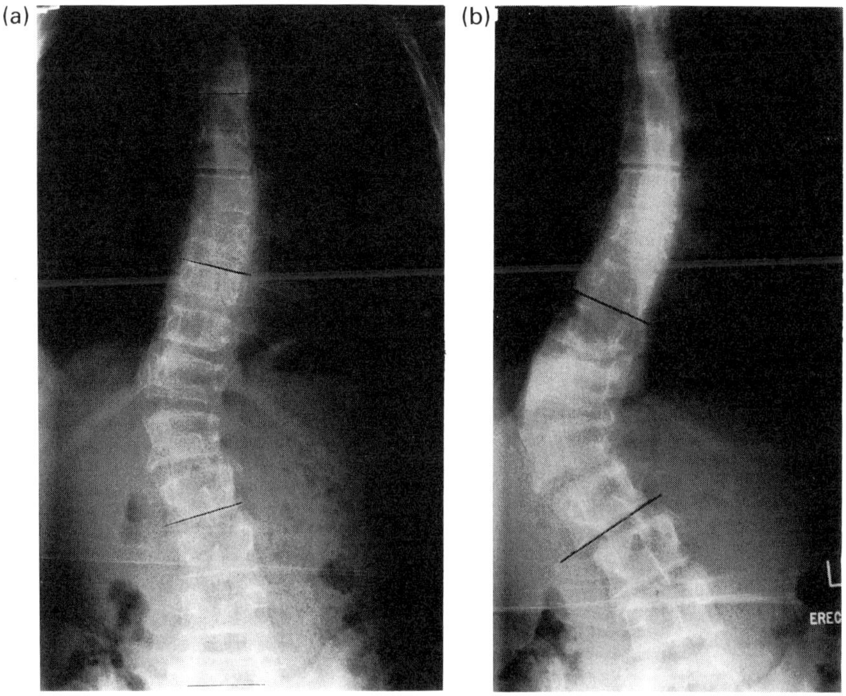

Figure 11.11 (a) A short dysplastic thoracolumbar scoliosis in an adolescent with NF. (b) The same curve 12 months later.

authors have strongly promoted a hypothesis that all scolioses, regardless of aetiology, have a lordotic element that is vital in their production. The types that they recognize are as follows.

- An inconsequential non-structural lumbar curve consequent on unequal leg lengths caused by local hypertrophy.
- The idiopathic-type long lordoscoliosis.
- The dystrophic, short angular lordoscoliosis.
- An angular thoracic or cervical kyphosis, which can occur alone or more usually above a compensatory lordosis that has rotated to the side.

Most authors agree that the dystrophic curve is short and sharp, involves four to six segments, and causes distortions of the vertebral bodies and ribs. There is severe wedging and rotation, with wide neural foramina, rib thinning and scalloping. These may be mistaken for congenital curves, until inspection of earlier films demonstrates the evolution of the deformity from normal-shaped curves. These curves appear early in childhood, and are relentlessly progressive, even when

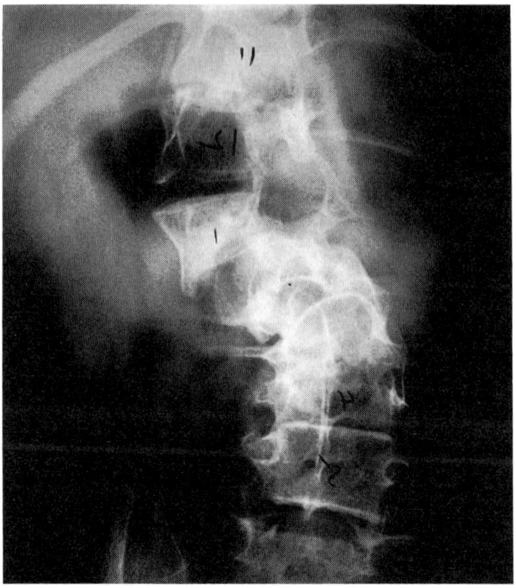

Figure 11.12 Another dysplastic curve in an adult with NF1.

growth is finished (Crawford, 1989). They cannot be controlled by bracing, and require early fusion. Some of these are associated with kyphosis, and correction of these complex deformities carries a high risk both of paraplegia and pseudoarthrosis, as well as loss of correction even after what seems a comprehensive anterior and posterior fusion.

It is essential that before corrective surgery is attempted, the contents of the spinal canal are investigated for neurofibromas by MRI or myelography. If a laminectomy is performed to remove a tumour, it should be accompanied by a spinal fusion. In most authors' estimation, this sort of surgery is sometimes followed by a severe dystrophic lordoscoliosis (Winter, 1984), but in Leatherman and Dickson's view (1988) this is the norm. Surgery attempted after paraplegia has occurred is often unrewarding.

The 'idiopathic' pattern of scoliosis may be convex to the left or to the right, and can be managed in the same way as conventional idiopathic scoliosis by an instrumented posterior fusion. Even in this group, there is a high incidence of pseudoarthrosis in those treated surgically (13%, according to Crawford (1989)). If there is any element of a dystrophic pattern, the curve may take on all the difficulties encountered in the dystrophic type (*vide infra*) (Scott, 1965; Chaglassian, Riseborough and Hall, 1976; Savini and Vicenzi, 1976; Winter *et al.*, 1979; Lonstein *et al.*, 1980; Crawford, 1981; Savini *et al.*, 1983; Hsu, Lee and Leong, 1984; Akbarnia, 1985). Spontaneous dislocation of one vertebra has been reported in NF in association with dural ectasia. All the skills of the spinal surgeon are required to correct and fuse this rare deformity, which is usually associated with progressive paraplegia (Curtis *et al.*, 1969; Rockower, McKay and Nason, 1982; Stone *et al.*, 1987; Winter, 1991).

11.5.2 Cervical spine

The cervical spine is prone to multilevel malalignments and kyphotic deformity, especially in association with a dystrophic-type curve in the thoracic spine. Of 102 patients with spinal deformity and NF1 referred to a recognized scoliosis centre (Twin Cities), only four involved the cervical spine (Winter *et al.*, 1979), whereas a centre with an interest in the cervical spine found 17 of 56 patients referred with NF (Yong-Hing, Kalamchi and MacEwen, 1979). Curtis *et al.* (1969) found that the neck was involved in four out of eight patients with NF and paraplegia. Verbiest (1989) found one example with an atlanto-axial subluxation among seven cases of cervical neurofibromas. In three cases these were associated with an anterior subluxation of a vertebra. The cervical spine showed a significant or severe kyphosis resulting from deformation of the vertebral bodies. Other recent case reports of dislocation of the dens (Crawford, 1989) and atlanto-axial dislocation (Hasegawa *et al.*, 1989) contain reviews of the literature of NF and the cervical spine. In the most recent series of eight cases, Craig and Govender (1992) draw attention to massive spondylophyte formation and dural ectasia, each in a single case. These authors once again stress that combined anterior and posterior surgery is required to stabilize the necks of these patients.

11.6 PSEUDOARTHROSIS OF LONG BONES

11.6.1 Introduction

Pseudoarthrosis appearing in any long bone in infancy usually turns out to be associated with NF. Much the most frequent site is the tibia, but pseudoarthrosis has been observed in all of the other long bones. Even so, affection of the tibia is rare. The incidence of congenital pseudoarthrosis of the tibia is 1 in 250 000 live births. NF has been implicated in between 50 and 90% of cases of congenital pseudoarthrosis of the tibia (Wellwood, Bulmer and Graff, 1971; Andersen, 1976b; Crawford, 1981; Morrissey, Riseborough and Hall, 1981; Boyd, 1982; Morrissey, 1982; Murrat and Lovell, 1982).

11.6.2 Boyd classification

The Boyd classification has been used to subclassify congenital pseudoarthrosis of the tibia. It is not clear from the literature whether use of this classification system influences management, as few, if any, series have sufficient patients to answer this question (Andersen, 1973). No controlled trial of treatment modalities have been attempted. However, there may be some value in the system for defining prognosis. To my knowledge, no attempt has been made to validate this classification system.

- **Type I**. There is anterior bowing and a defect in the tibia at birth. Other congenital deformities may also be present (Figure 11.13).

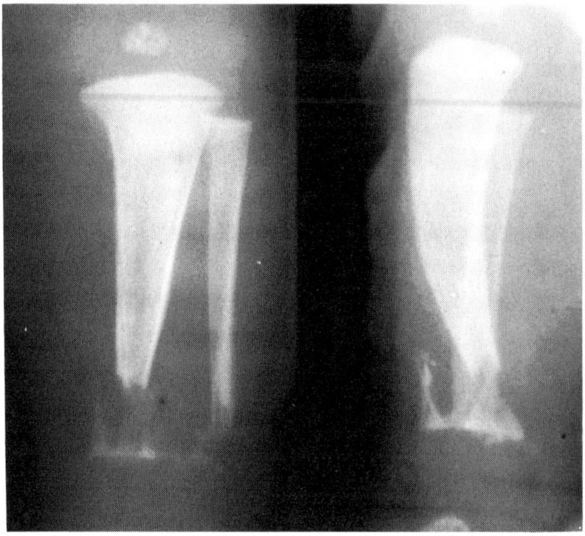

Figure 11.13 Neonatal pseudoarthrosis of the tibia and fibula (type I).

- **Type II**. There is anterior bowing and an hourglass constriction of the tibia present at birth. Spontaneous fracture or fracture following minor trauma often occurs before the age of 2 years. The tibia is tapered rounded and sclerotic, with obliteration of the medullary canal (Figure 11.14). This is the most common type, and that most usually associated with NF. Prognosis is poor. Recurrent fractures occur but their incidence decreases with age until skeletal maturity, when the problem stops.
- **Type III**. This develops in a congenital cyst, usually at the junction of the middle and distal thirds of the tibia. Anterior bowing may precede or follow the development of a fracture (Figure 11.15). The prognosis after treatment is more benign, and good results have been maintained into adult life.

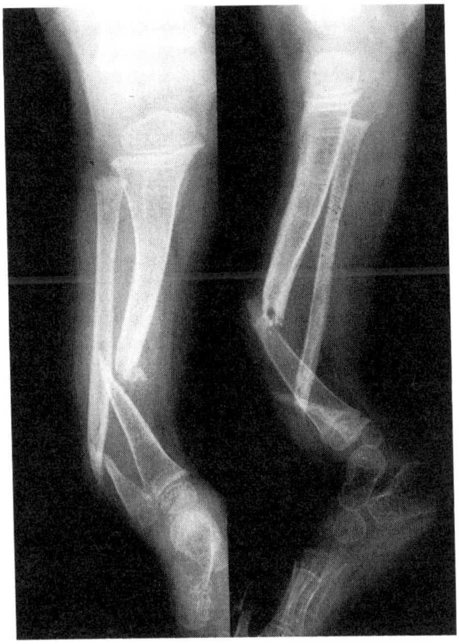

Figure 11.14 Pseudoarthrosis of the tibia and fibula (type II).

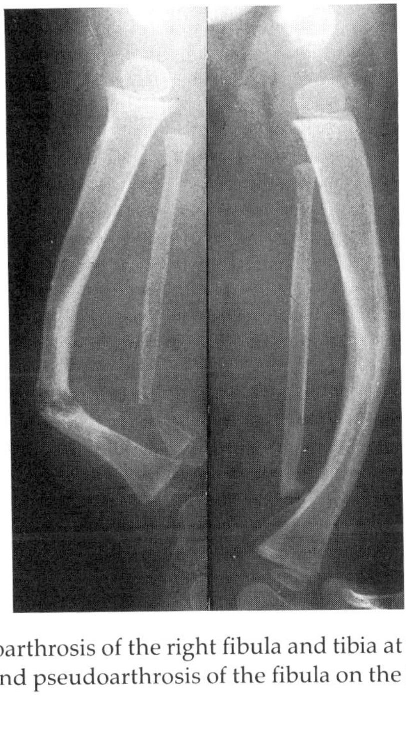

Figure 11.15 Pseudoarthrosis of the right fibula and tibia at the site of a cyst, and bowing of the tibia and pseudoarthrosis of the fibula on the left (type III).

(a)

(b)

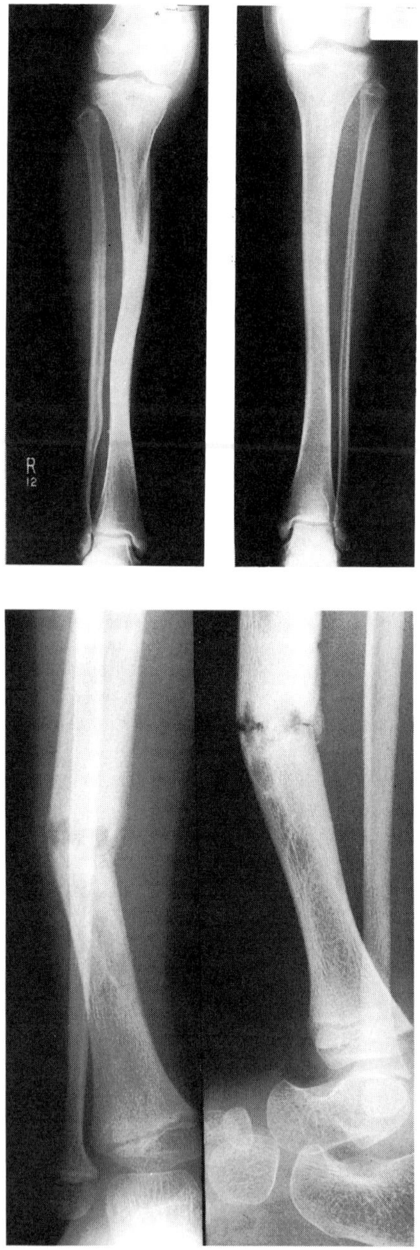

Figure 11.16 (a) Radiograph of the lower limb of a patient with NF1 showing an area of sclerosis of the right tibia at risk of becoming a pseudoarthrosis (type IV). (b) Stress fracture through an area of sclerosis in the tibia (type IV).

- **Type IV**. In this group, the pseudoarthrosis originates in a sclerotic segment of bone in the classic location, without narrowing of the tibia. The medullary canal is more or less completely obliterated. A stress fracture gradually develops in the cortex, which may develop into a full-blown pseudoarthrosis. The prognosis of this pattern is good, especially if it is caught early (Figure 11.16).
- **Type V**. This consists of a dysplastic tibia in conjunction with a dysplastic fibula. If a pseudoarthrosis occurs, the prognosis is better if only one bone is affected. If both bones fracture, then the prognosis is as Type II (Figure 11.17).

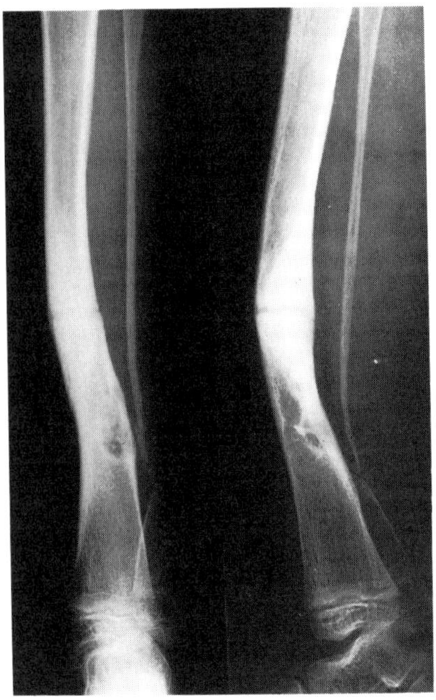

Figure 11.17 Radiograph of the lower limb of a child with NF1 showing a tibial pseudoarthrosis through a dysplastic tibia in combination with severe dysplasia of the fibula (type V).

- **Type VI**. Pseudoarthrosis occurs in the site of an intramedullary neurofibroma or Schwannoma. This pattern is very rare.

An anterolateral bow is the typical pattern in pseudoarthrosis of the tibia, whilst the rare posterior medial bow is said to carry a more benign prognosis.

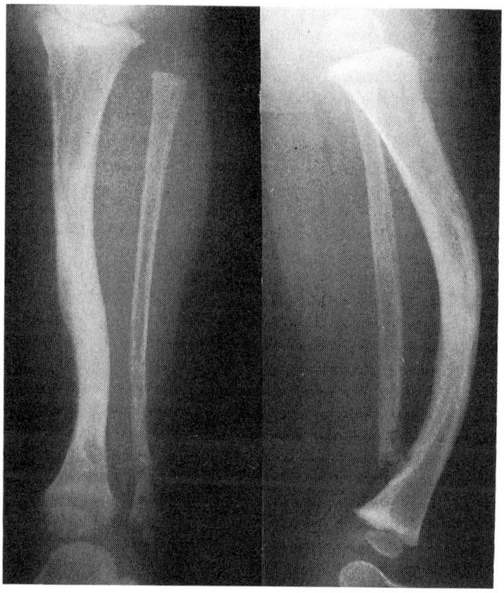

Figure 11.18 Pseudoarthrosis of the fibula, combined with bowing of the tibia.

11.6.3 Fibula

Pseudoarthrosis of the fibula often precedes or accompanies pseudoarthrosis of the tibia. Grades of severity proceed from bowing without pseudoarthrosis, through fibular pseudoarthrosis with or without ankle deformity, to a pseudoarthrosis combined with ankle deformity (Figure 11.18). The worst is when a pseudoarthrosis of the fibula is combined with latent pseudoarthrosis of tibia. It can even occur after apparently successful management of a tibial pseudoarthrosis.

Management is by brace treatment (with an outside iron and inside T-strap). At maturity the fibular deformity is managed by supramalleolar osteotomy through 'normal' bone. An alternative is the creation of a synostosis between the fibular stump and the tibia.

11.6.4 Other long bones

The ulna can be the site of a congenital or acquired pseudoarthrosis. Management is currently by any of the three modern techniques described in section 11.7 (Cobb, 1968; Shertzer, Bickel and Stubbins, 1969; Allieu *et al.*, 1981; Ali and Hooper, 1982; Bayne, 1985; Ostrowski, Eilert and Waldsten, 1985; Bell, 1989; Rajaratnam, Shanker and Varughese, 1989). An example of pseudoarthrosis of the ulna is shown in Figure 11.19.

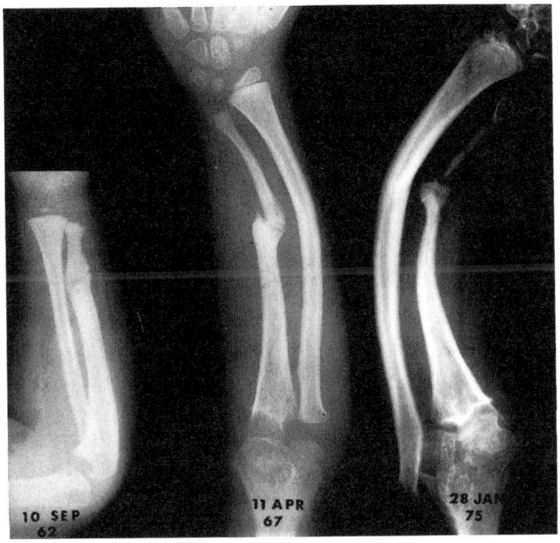

Figure 11.19 Pseudoarthrosis of the ulna in NF1.

The radius may develop a pseudoarthrosis either alone or in combination with the ulna (Sprague and Brown, 1974; Greenberg and Schwarz, 1975; Richen *et al.*, 1976; Masihuz-Zaman, 1977; Cleveland, Gilsanz and Wilkinson, 1978; Manske, 1979; Gregg *et al.*, 1982; Bayne, 1985; Herring and Roach, 1985; Bell, 1989; Kameyama and Oqawa, 1990). The femur is a very rare site for congenital pseudoarthrosis (Hunt and Pugh, 1961). The clavicle, a membrane bone, rarely develops a pseudoarthrosis in NF (Alldred, 1963). There are two case reports of humeral pseudoarthrosis (Crawford and Bagamery, 1986; Floyd and Percy-Lancaster, 1987).

11.7 MANAGEMENT OF PSEUDOARTHROSIS OF THE TIBIA AND OTHER LONG BONES

11.7.1 Introduction

Many different treatment modalities have been attempted for congenital pseudoarthrosis of the tibia. Boyd and Sage (1958) found that 23 different surgical procedures had been performed on 91 patients (167 operations) with only a 56% success rate. Newer techniques such as vascularized bone graft (Chen, Yu and Wang, 1979; Hagan and Bunke, 1982; Leung, 1983; Pho *et al.*, 1985), electrical stimulation (Bassett, Caulo and Kort, 1979, 1981; Sutcliffe and Goldberg, 1982; Paterson and Simonis, 1985) and bone transport (Ilizarov, 1971; Ilizarov and Gracheva, 1971) have all shown promising results, and are discussed in more detail in this section.

However, as is common in the surgery of rare diseases, no clinical trials have been performed. This is compounded by the difficulties in defining outcome measures and in agreeing an appropriate period of follow-up. Most would accept skeletal maturity as a suitable time, a view that is supported by at least one long-term review (Crossett *et al.*, 1989).

Many patients have been treated by amputation, either as a primary procedure (Andersen, 1976a,b), or more usually as a salvage procedure after multiple attempts to treat the pseudoarthrosis by other means (Aitken, 1959; Edvardsen, 1973; Masserman, Peterson and Bianco, 1974; McCarthy, 1982; Jacobsen *et al.*, 1983). Even in those cases where union is achieved, it may be in the presence of shortening, angular deformity and unsightly scarring, and at a price of multiple hospital admissions and surgical procedures (Hardinge, 1972; Sofield and Millar, 1959).

The surgical procedures traditionally available used to include osteotomy (Hallock, 1938), onlay grafts (Boyd, 1941; Boyd and Fox, 1948), bypass grafts (McFarland, 1951), pedicle grafts (Farmer, 1952) and intramedullary rods (Charnley, 1956). In most cases these methods have been superseded by three approaches that are currently in favour: electrical stimulation, vascularized bone grafting and bone transport. However, two recent publications have stressed the value of intramedullary nailing (Anderson *et al.*, 1992; Baker, Cain and Tullos, 1992). There is one recent abstract report of prophylactic bypass grafting in 10 cases culled from across North America with favourable results in seven (Wong, Strong and Gillespie, 1992).

11.7.2 Electrical stimulation

Electrical stimulation has a long history, but in modern times was popularized by Brighton *et al.* (1975), who used direct current stimulation to promote fusion. The scientific basis of this technique remains controversial. There is a bioelectric potential within normal bone, and the osteoblast, chondrocyte, fibroblast and other connective tissue cells are sensitive to an electric field. In a direct current environment there is a strong tendency to lay down new bone at the cathode and to resorb bone at the anode. The crystalline mineral component of bone (mainly calcium hydroxyapatite) exhibits piezoelectric effects under mechanical stress, and the small local currents created may be important for bone remodelling. Electromagnetic fields may create similar currents within the bone. Sutcliffe and Goldberg (1982) and Bassett, Caulo and Kort (1981) used surface coils to create a pulsed magnetic field to promote bone formation, and this method has been applied by these authors to congenital pseudoarthrosis of the tibia. Electrical stimulation has also been applied successfully to congenital pseudoarthrosis by Paterson and Simonis (1985).

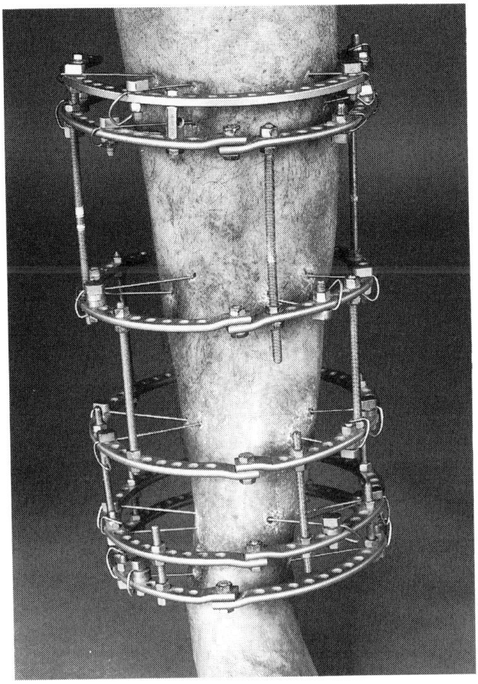

Figure 11.20 An Ilizarov frame applied to a tibia for bone transport to achieve leg lengthening and healing of a pseudoarthrosis.

11.7.3 Free vascularized bone grafts

Free vascularized bone grafts (usually from the fibula) have been used successfully over the last decade to fill a gap in the tibia and other long bones, especially in the forearm, after the pseudoarthrosis has been excised (Chen, Yu and Wang, 1979; Weiland and Daniel, 1980; Gilbert, 1982; Pho *et al.*, 1985; de Boer *et al.*, 1988). This technique is currently the method of choice in our institution.

11.7.4 Bone transport

Ilizarov, in Russia, developed a system of external fixation using steel rings attached to bone by fine wires in tension (Ilizarov, 1971, Ilizarov and Gracheva, 1971) (Figure 11.20). He has demonstrated the feasibility of transporting a healthy segment of diaphyseal bone into the defect left after the excision of the bone segment, which contained the pseudoarthrosis. Considerable preoperative planning is required. A scaffolding of steel rings is constructed with the aid of interconnecting bars. These bars are threaded. Nuts on the threaded bars can be adjusted progressively over the period of the bone transport (often several months) so that the rings attached to the transported bone can be carried from proximal to distal until its lower end contacts the distal stump of the tibia. The wires, which are sometimes especially flattened to reduce their profile, gradually cut through the skin like cheesewire. The segment to be transported is separated from the proximal diaphysis by a corticotomy (a division of the cortex of the bone leaving the medulla intact), and is gradually carried distally as new bone develops behind it (at a speed of 1–2 mm per day). If necessary, the transported segment and the distal fragment of bone can be transported together, lengthening the limb. In addition it is possible to correct angular or even rotatory deformities with this technique. The neurovascular structures appear to adapt to the gradual changes in the architecture of the limb, although careful neurological and vascular examination is mandatory throughout the procedure. Pain is a good guide to the occurrence of problems. This can be often treated by slowing down the rate of progress of the transported segment.

This technique has become widely adopted in the West in special centres, and a few reports in English of its use in congenital pseudoarthrosis of the tibia have begun to appear (Fabry *et al.*, 1988). It demands considerable skill to apply this technique successfully, and a cooperative patient and parents. It is normally carried out as an outpatient procedure, and the patient or parent performs the twice-daily adjustments to the frame and takes care of the pin track sites, a task to which both parties adapt surprisingly well.

11.7.5 Gigantism

This complication of NF1 may involve any part of the body from a whole limb to a single digit. There may be deformity, which ranges from mild anisomelia to a hypertrophied limb weighing more than the rest of the child (Praharaj *et al.*, 1969; Crawford, 1981, 1986; Pearn, Viljoen and Beighton, 1983). It is frequently found in association with a plexiform neurofibroma, but the precise relationship between these manifestations of NF remains unclear.

Overgrowth tends either to affect the skin and underlying soft tissue, producing abundant elephantine skin, or all musculoskeletal elements including bone and muscle. If the face or head is involved, there may be grotesque disfigurement, with impairment of vision and facial muscle function. Some unfortunate patients have repeated subperiosteal haemorrhage into the hypertrophied limb (Sane, Yunis and Greer, 1971; Kullmann and Wouters, 1972; Yaghmal and Tafazoll, 1977; Locht, Huebert and McFarland, 1981; Floyd and Percy-Lancaster, 1987). The management of these unpleasant deformities either requires plastic surgery (Littlewood, 1983), tolerance or amputation.

11.8 MISCELLANY

(a) Pectus excavatum

Pectus excavatum was present in 31% of 675 patients in one series (Riccardi, 1992), and has been described in a series of 704 patients whose deformity was corrected surgically (Shamberger and Welch, 1988). Four of these cases had NF, which may be seen as a chance association. However, Beals and Fraser (1976) have reported a family with NF showing this characteristic (see also Chapter 13).

(b) Spondylolisthesis

Spondylolisthesis has been reported in association with NF (McCarroll, 1950; Hunt and Pugh, 1961; Mandell, 1978; Winter *et al.*, 1979; Winter and Edwards, 1981). It may well be that this reflects the normal prevalence of spondylolisthesis in the population (2–5%). In one large series, 3.5% of skeletons from South Africa had spondylolysis, with no racial predilection (Eisenstein, 1978).

(c) Rib penetration

Major and Huizenga (1988) reported two cases of penetration of the spinal canal by ribs, sufficient to cause spinal cord compression, and other cases involving penetration of the intervertebral forameina have been described by Flood, Butt and Dickson (1986).

(d) Carpal tunnel syndrome

Carpal tunnel syndrome due to neurofibromas of the median nerve has been reported (Bowen and Bennett, 1984).

ACKNOWLEDGEMENTS

I am very grateful for the generous help of my orthopaedic, radiological and neurosurgical colleagues in Birmingham and Oxford for supplying material from their collections to illustrate this chapter. I have received particular help from Dr Nick Evans, Dr Philip Anslow and Mr Peter Burge. A further important source of radiographs was the excellent radiology museum of the Institute of Orthopaedics, University College, London, who were most generous in their assistance. Professor John Kenwright kindly provided the illustration of the Ilizarov frame.

REFERENCES

Aitken, T. (1959) Amputation as a treatment for certain lower-extremity congenital abnormalities. *J. Bone Joint Surg. [Am.]*, **41-A**, 1267–85.

Akbarnia, B.A. (1985) Spinal deformity in neurofibromatosis, in *The Pediatric Spine*, (eds D.S. Bradford and R.M. Hensinger), Thieme, New York, pp. 350–67.

Akbarnia, B.A., Gabriel, K.R., Beckman, E. and Chalk, D. (1992) Prevalence of scoliosis in neurofibromatosis. *Spine*, **17**, S244–8.

Ali, M.S. and Hooper, G. (1982) Congenital pseudoarthrosis of the ulna due to neurofibromatosis. *J. Bone Joint Surg. [Br.]*, **64-B**, 600–2.

Alldred, A.J. (1963) Congenital pseudoarthrosis of the clavicle. *J. Bone Joint Surg. [Br.]*, **45-B**, 312–19.

Allieu, Y., Gomis, R., Yoshimura, M. *et al.* (1981) Congenital pseudoarthrosis of the forearm. Two cases treated by free vascularized fibular graft. *J. Hand Surg.*, **6**, 475–81.

Andersen, K.S. (1973) Radiological classification of congenital pseudoarthrosis of the tibia. *Acta Orthop. Scand.*, **44**, 719.

Andersen, K.S. (1976a) Congenital pseudoarthrosis of the leg. Late results. *J. Bone Joint Surg. [Am.]*, **58-A**, 657–62.

Andersen, K.S. (1976b) Congenital pseudoarthrosis of the tibia and neurofibromatosis. *Acta Orthop. Scand.*, **47**, 108–11.

Anderson, D., Schoenecker, P., Sheridan, J. *et al.* (1992) Use of an intramedullary rod for the treatment of congenital pseudoarthrosis of the tibia. *J. Bone Joint Surg. [Am.]*, **74-A**, 161–8.

Austin, G. (1959) The significance and nature of pain in tumours of the spinal cord. *Surg. Forum*, **10**, 782.

Baker, J., Cain, T. and Tullos, H. (1992) Intramedullary fixation for congenital pseudoarthrosis of the tibia. *J. Bone Joint Surg. [Am.]*, **74-A**, 169–78.

Baker, N.D., Tchang, F.K. and Greenspan, A. (1982) Liposarcoma complicating neurofibromatosis. Report of two cases. *Bull. Hosp. Jt. Dis. Orthop. Inst.*, **42**, 172–86.

Bassett, C., Caulo, N. and Kort, J. (1981) Congenital 'pseudarthroses' of the tibia: treatment with pulsing electromagnetic fields. *Clin. Orthop.*, **154**, 136–49.

Bayne, L.G. (1985) Congenital pseudoarthrosis of the forearm. *Hand Clinics*, **1**, 457–65.

Beals, R.K. and Fraser, W. (1976) Familial congenital bowing of the tibia with pseudoarthrosis and pectus excavatum: report of a kindred. *J. Bone Joint Surg. [Am.]*, **58-A**, 545.

Bell, D. (1989) Congenital forearm pseudoarthrosis: report of six cases and review of the literature. *J. Pediatr. Orthop.*, **9**, 438–43.

Binet, E.F. and Markarian, B. (1974) Osseous lesions in adolescence with known neurofibromatosis. *N.Y. State J. Med.*, **74**, 2401–4.

Binet, E., Kieffer, S., Martin, S. *et al.* (1969) Orbital dysplasia in neurofibromatosis. *Radiology*, **93**, 829–33.

Bowen, J. and Bennett, J. (1984) An unusual case of carpal tunnel syndrome. *Del. Med. J.*, **56**, 227–30.

Boyd, H. (1941) Congenital pseudoarthrosis: treatment by dual bone grafts. *J. Bone Joint Surg.*, **23**, 497–515.

Boyd, H.B. (1982) Pathology and natural history of congenital pseudoarthrosis of the tibia. *Clin. Orthop.*, **166**, 5–13.

Boyd, H. and Fox, K. (1948) Congenital pseudoarthrosis: follow-up study after massive bone-grafting. *J. Bone Joint Surg. [Am.]*, **30-A**, 274–83.

Boyd, H.B. and Sage, F.P. (1958) Congenital pseudoarthrosis of the tibia. *J. Bone Joint Surg. [Am.]*, **40-A**, 1245.

Brighton, C.T., Freidenberg, Z.A., Zemsky, L.M. *et al.* (1975) Direct current stimulation of nonunion and congenital pseudarthrosis. *J. Bone Joint Surg. [Am.]*, **57-A**, 368.

Bull, J. (1952) Spinal meningiomas and neurofibromas. *Acta Radiol.*, **40**, 283.

Burrows, E. (1963) Bone changes in orbital neurofibromatosis. *Br. J. Radiol.*, **36**, 549–61.

Calvert, P., Edgar, M. and Webb, P. (1989) Scoliosis in neurofibromatosis. The natural history with and without operation. *J. Bone Joint Surg. [Br.]*, **71**, 246–51.

Casselman, E.S. and Mandell, G.A. (1979) Vertebral scalloping in neurofibromatosis. *Radiology*, **131**, 89–94.

Chaglassian, J.H., Riseborough, E.J. and Hall, J.E. (1976) Neurofibromatosis scoliosis. Natural history and results of treatment in thirty-seven cases. *J. Bone Joint Surg. [Am.]*, **58-A**, 695–702.

Charnley, J. (1956) Congenital pseudarthrosis of the tibia treated by intramedullary nail. *J. Bone Joint Surg. [Am.]*, **38–A**, 283–90.

Chen, C., Yu, Z. and Wang, Y. (1979) A new method of treatment of congenital tibial pseudarthrosis using free vascularised fibular graft: a preliminary report. *Ann. Acad. Med. Singapore*, **8**, 465–73.

Cleveland, R.H., Gilsanz, V. and Wilkinson, R.H. (1978) Congenital pseudarthrosis of the radius. *AJR*, **30**, 955–7.

Cobb, J. (1948) Outline for the study of scoliosis, in *Instructional Course Lectures*, J.W. Edwards, Ann Arbor, pp. 261–75.

Cobb, J. (1950) Discussion. *J. Bone Joint Surg. [Am.]*, **58–A**, 695–702.

Cobb, N. (1968) Neurofibromatosis and pseudarthrosis of the ulna. A case report. *J. Bone Joint Surg. [Br.]*, **50-B**, 146–9.

Cole, W.G. and Myers, N.A. (1978) Neurofibromatosis in childhood. *Aust. N.Z. J. Surg.*, **48**, 360–5.

Craig, J. and Govender, S. (1992) Neurofibromatosis of the cervical spine. A report of eight cases. *J. Bone Joint Surg. [Br.]*, **74–B**, 575–8.

Crawford, A.H. (1981) Neurofibromatosis in childhood. *AAOS Instr. Course Lect.*, **30**, 56–74.

Crawford, A. (1986) Neurofibromatosis in children. *Acta Orthop. Scand. [Suppl.]*, **218**, 1–60.

Crawford, A. (1987) Neurofibromatosis in childhood. *Instruct. Course Lect.*, **30**, 56.

Crawford, A. (1989) Pitfalls of spinal deformities associated with neurofibromatosis in children. *Clin. Orthop.*, **245**, 29–42.

Crawford, A.H., Jr and Bagamery, N. (1986) Osseous manifestations of neurofibromatosis in childhood. *J. Pediatr. Orthop.*, **6**, 72–88.

Crossett, L., Beatty, J., Betz, R. *et al.* (1989) Congenital pseudarthrosis of the tibia. Long-term follow-up study. *Clin. Orthop.*, **245**, 16–18.

Curtis, B.H., Fisher, R.L., Butterfield, W.L. *et al.* (1969) Neurofibromatosis with paraplegia. Report of eight cases. *J. Bone Joint Surg. [Am.]*, **51-A**, 843–61.

D'Ambrosio, J., Langlais, R. and Y.R.S., (1988) Jaw and skull changes in neurofibromatosis. *Oral Surg. Oral Med. Oral Pathol.*, **66**, 391–6.

de Boer, H., Verbout, A., Nielsen, H. *et al.* (1988) Free vascularised fibular graft for tibial pseudarthrosis. *Acta Orthop. Scand.*, **59**, 425–9.

Ducatman, B.S., Scheithauer, B.W. and Dahlin, D.C. (1983) Malignant bone tumors associated with neurofibromatosis. *Mayo Clin. Proc.*, **58**, 578–82.

Edvardsen, P. (1973) Resection osteosynthesis and Boyd amputation of congenital pseudoarthrosis of the tibia. *J. Bone Joint Surg. [Br.]*, **55-B**, 179–82.

Eisenstein, S. (1978) Spondylolysis. A skeletal investigation of two population groups. *J. Bone Joint Surg. [Br.]*, **60-B**, 488–94.

Erkulvrawatr, S., El Gammal, T., Hawkins, J. *et al.* (1979) Intrathoracic meningoceles and neurofibromatosis. *Arch. Neurol.*, **36**, 557–9.

Fabry, G., Lammens, J., Melkebeek, J. *et al.* (1988) Treatment of congenital pseudarthrosis with the Ilizarov technique. *J. Pediatr. Orthop.*, **8**, 67–70.

Farmer, A. (1952) The use of composite pedicle graft for pseudarthrosis of the tibia. *J. Bone Joint Surg. [Br.]*, **34-B**, 591–600.

Faure, C., Laurent, J., Schmit, P. *et al.* (1986) Multiple and large non-ossifying fibromas in children with neurofibromatosis. *Ann. Radiol. (Paris)*, **29**, 369–73.

Fisher, M.M. (1975) Anaesthetic difficulties in neurofibromatosis. *Anaesthesia*, **30**, 648–50.

Flood, B., Butt, W. and Dickson, R. (1986) Rib penetration of the intervertebral foraminae in neurofibromatosis. *Spine*, **11**, 172–4.

Floyd, A. and Percy-Lancaster, R. (1987) The elephant woman: neurofibromatosis associated with pseudarthrosis of the humerus. *J. Bone Joint Surg. [Br.]*, **69-B**, 121–3.

Gilbert, A. (1982) Les transfer osseux libres vascularisés dans le traitement de la pseudarthrose congenitale, in *Conferance Enseignment SO.F.C.O.T.*, Expansion Scientifique Française, Paris, pp. 30–1.

Greenberg, L. and Schwarz, A. (1975) Congenital pseudarthrosis of the distal radius. *South Med. J.*, **68**, 1053–4.

Gregg, P.J., Price, B.A., Ellis, H.A. *et al.* (1982) Pseudarthrosis of the radius associated with neurofibromatosis. A case report. *Clin. Orthop.*, **171**, 175–9.

Gross, M., Soberman, N., Dorfman, H. *et al.* (1989) Case report 556: Multiple non-ossifying fibromas of long bones in a patient with neurofibromatosis. *Skel. Radiol.*, **18**, 389–91.

Gupta, S., Tuli, S., Srivastava, T. *et al.* (1985) Skeletal overgrowth with modelling error in neurofibromatosis. *Clin. Radiol.*, **36**, 643–5.

Hagan, K. and Bunke, H. (1982) Treatment of congenital pseudarthrosis of the tibia with free vascularised bone graft. *Clin. Orthop.*, **166**, 34.

Hallock, H. (1938) The use of multiple small bone transplants in the treatment of pseudarthrosis of tibia of congenital origin or following osteotomy for correction of congenital deformity. *J. Bone Joint Surg.*, **20**, 648–60.

Hardinge, K. (1972) Congenital anterior bowing of tibia: the significance of different types in relationship to pseudarthrosis. *Ann. R. Coll. Surg. Engl.*, **51**, 17–30.

Harkens, K. and Dolan, K. (1990) Correlative imaging of sphenoid dysplasia accompanying neurofibromatosis. *Ann. Otol. Rhinol. Laryngol.*, **99**, 137–41.

Hasegawa, H., Bitoh, S., Katoh, A. *et al.* (1989) Bilateral vertebral arteriovenous fistulas and atlantoaxial dislocation associated with neurofibromatosis – case report. *Neurol. Med. Chir. (Tokyo)*, **29**, 55–9.

Heard, G. and Payne, E. (1962) Scalloping of the vertebral bodies in von Recklinghausen's disease of the nervous system (neurofibromatosis). *J. Neurol. Neurosurg. Psychiatr.*, **25**, 345–51.

Herring, J. and Roach, J. (1985) Congenital pseudarthrosis of the radius: clinical conference. *J. Pediatr. Orthop.*, **5**, 367–9.

Holt, J. and Kuhn, L. (1976) Macrocranium and macrencephaly in neurofibromatosis. *Skeletal Radiol.*, **1**, 25–8.

Holt, J. and Wright, G. (1948) The radiological features of neurofibromatosis. *Radiology*, **51**, 647.

Hsu, L.C.S., Lee, P.C. and Leong, J.C.Y. (1984) Dystrophic spinal deformities in neurofibromatosis. Treatment by anterior and posterior fusion. *J. Bone Joint Surg. [Br.]*, **66-B**, 495–9.

Hull, C. (1986) Phaeochromocytomas: diagnosis, preoperative preparation and anaesthetic management. *Br. J. Anaesth.*, **58**, 1453–68.

Hunt, J.C. and Pugh, D.C. (1961) Skeletal lesions in neurofibromatosis. *Radiology*, **76**, 1–20.

Huson, S.M., Harper, P.S. and Compston, D.A.S. (1988) Von Recklinghausen neurofibromatosis: a clinical and population study in southeast Wales. *Brain*, **111**, 1355–81.

Hvorslev, V. and Reiter, S. (1979) A case of neurofibromatosis with severe osseous disease of the thoracic spine. *Pediatr. Radiol.*, **8**, 1–253.

Ilizarov, G. (1971) Basic principles of transosseous compression and distraction osteosynthesis. *Ortop. Traumatol. Protez.*, **32**, 7–15.

Ilizarov, G. and Gracheva, V. (1971) Bloodless treatment of congenital pseudarthrosis of the crus with simultaneous elimination of shortening using dosed distraction. *Ortop. Traumatol. Protez.*, **32**, 42–6.

Isu, T., Miyasaka, K., Abe, H. *et al.* (1983) Atlantoaxial dislocation associated with neurofibromatosis. Report of three cases. *J. Neurosurg.*, **58**, 451–3.

Jacobsen, S., Crawford, A., Millar, E. *et al.* (1983) The Syme amputation in patients with congenital pseudarthrosis of the tibia. *J. Bone Joint Surg. [Am.]*, **65-A**, 533–7.

Kalff, V., Shapiro, B. and Lloyd, R.E.A. (1982) The spectrum of phaeochromocytoma in hypertensive patients with neurofibromatosis. *Arch. Intern. Med.*, **142**, 2092–8.

Kameyama, O. and Oqawa, R. (1990) Pseudarthrosis of the radius associated with neurofibromatosis: report of a case and review of the literature. *J. Pediatr. Orthop.*, **10**, 128–31.

Klatte, E.C., Fraken, E.A. and Smith, J.A. (1976) The radiographic spectrum in neurofibromatosis. *Semin. Roentgenol.*, **11**, 17–33.

Kullmann, L. and Wouters, H.W. (1972) Neurofibromatosis, gigantism and subperiosteal haematoma. Report of two children with extensive subperiosteal bone formation. *J. Bone Joint Surg. [Br.]*, **54-B**, 130–8.

Lachiewicz, P.F., Salvati, E.A., Hely, D. *et al.* (1983) Pathological dislocation of the hip in neurofibromatosis. A case report. *J. Bone Joint Surg. [Am.]*, **65-A**, 414–15.

Lawson, E., Moe, J. and Pedras, C. (1973) Spinal deformity and neurofibromatosis – natural history, classification, and treatment. *J. Bone Joint Surg. [Am.]*, **55-A**, 1321–2.

Leatherman, K. and Dickson, R. (1988) Deformities associated with neurofibromatosis, in *The Management of Spinal Deformities*, John Wright, London, pp. 235–51.

Leung, P. (1983) Congenital pseudarthrosis of the tibia: three cases treated by free vascularised iliac crest graft. *Clin. Orthop.*, **175**, 45.

Le Wald, L. (1933) Congenital absence of the superior orbital wall associated with pulsating exopthalmos. A report of four cases. *Am. J. Radiol.*, **30**, 756–64.

Littlewood, A. (1983) The vascular features of plexiform neurofibroma with some observations on the importance of preoperative angiography and the value of preoperative intra-arterial embolisation. *Br. J. Plast. Surg.*, **36**, 501–6.

Locht, R.C., Huebert, H.T. and McFarland, D.F. (1981) Subperiosteal hemorrhage and cyst formation in neurofibromatosis: a case report. *Clin. Orthop.*, **155**, 141–6.

Lonstein, J.E., Winter, R.B., Moe, J.H. *et al.* (1980) Neurologic deficits secondary to spinal deformity. *Spine*, **5**, 331–55.

Love, J. and Dodge, H. (1952) Dumbbell (hourglass) neurofibromas affecting the spinal cord. *Surg. Gynecol. Obstet.*, **94**, 1961.

Major, M. and Huizenga, B. (1988) Spinal cord compression by displaced ribs in neurofibromatosis. A report of three cases. *J. Bone Joint Surg. [Am.]*, **70-A**, 1100.

Mandell, G.A. (1978) The pedicle in neurofibromatosis. *Am. J. Radiol.*, **130**, 675–8.

Manske, P.R. (1979) Forearm pseudarthrosis–neurofibromatosis: case report. *Clin. Orthop.*, **139**, 125–7.

Masihuz-Zaman (1977) Pseudarthrosis of the radius associated with neurofibromatosis. A case report. *J. Bone Joint Surg. [Am.]*, **59-A**, 977–8.

Masserman, R., Peterson, H. and Bianco, A. (1974) Congenital pseudarthrosis of the tibia: a review of the literature and 52 cases from the Mayo Clinic. *Clin. Orthop.*, **99**, 140–5.

McAlheny, H. and Netsky, M. (1955) Compression of the spinal cord by extramedullary neoplasms. *J. Neuropathol. Exp. Neurol.*, **14**, 276.

McCarroll, H. (1950) Clinical manifestations of congenital neurofibromatosis. *J. Bone Joint Surg. [Am.]*, **32-A**, 601.

McCarthy, R.E. (1982) Amputation for congenital pseudarthrosis of the tibia. Indication and techniques. *Clin. Orthop.*, **166**, 21.

McFarland, B. (1951) Pseudarthrosis of the tibia in childhood. *J. Bone Joint Surg. [Br.]*, **33-B**, 36–46.

Miles, J., Pennybacker, J. and Sheldon, P. (1969) Intrathoracic meningocele: its development and association with neurofibromatosis. *J. Neurol. Neurosurg. Psychiatr.*, **32**, 99–110.

Miller, A. (1936) Neurofibromatosis with reference to skeletal changes, compression myelitis and malignant degeneration. *Arch. Surg.*, **32**, 109.

Morrissey, R.T. (1982) Congenital pseudoarthrosis of the tibia. A long-term follow-up study. *Clin. Orthop.*, **166**, 14–20.

Morrissey, R.T., Riseborough, E.J. and Hall, J.E. (1981) Congenital pseudoarthrosis of the tibia. *J. Bone Joint Surg. [Br.]*, **63-B**, 367–75.

Murrat, H.H. and Lovell, W.W. (1982) Congenital pseudarthrosis of the tibia: a long-term follow-up study. *Clin. Orthop.*, **166**, 14.

O'Neill, P., Whatmore, W.J. and Booth, A.E. (1983) Spinal meningoceles in association with neurofibromatosis. *Neurosurgery*, **13**, 82–4.

Ostrowski, D.M., Eilert, R.E. and Waldsten, G. (1985) Congenital pseudarthrosis of the ulna: a report of two cases and a review of the literature. *J. Pediatr. Orthop.*, **5**, 463–7.

Paterson, D. and Simonis, R. (1985) Electrical stimulation in the treatment of congenital pseudarthrosis of the tibia. *J. Bone Joint Surg. [Br.]*, **67-B**, 454.

Pearn, J., Viljoen, C. and Beighton, P. (1983) Limb overgrowth – clinical observations and nosological considerations. *S. Afr. Med. J.*, **64**, 905–8.

Pho, R., Levack, B., Satku, K. *et al.* (1985) Free vascularised fibular graft in the treatment of congenital pseudarthrosis of the tibia. *J. Bone Joint Surg. [Br.]*, **67-B**, 64–70.

Pitt, M., Mosher, J. and Edeiken, J. (1972) Abnormal periosteum and bone in neurofibromatosis. *Radiology*, **103**, 143–6.

Pohl, R. (1933) Meningocele im Baustraum unter dem Bilde cine intrathorakalen Rundschattens. *Röntgenpraxis*, **5**, 749.

Praharaj, K.C., Mohanta, K.D., Nanda, B.K. *et al.* (1969) Congenital hemihypertrophy with neurofibromatosis. *Indian J. Med. Sci.*, **23**, 146–50.

Rajaratnam, K., Shanker, J. and Varughese, S. (1989) Pseudarthrosis of the ulna due to neurofibromatosis: a case report. *Injury*, **20**, 239–40.

Riccardi, V.M. (1992) *Neurofibromatosis. Phenotype, Natural History and Pathogenesis*, 2nd edn, Johns Hopkins University Press, Baltimore, p. 385.

Richen, P., Kranik, A., VanHerpe, L. *et al.* (1976) Congenital pseudarthrosis of both bones of the forearm. *J. Bone Joint Surg. [Am.]*, **58-A**, 1032–3.

Rockower, S., McKay, D. and Nason, S. (1982) Dislocation of the spine in neurofibromatosis. A report of two cases. *J. Bone Joint Surg. [Am.]*, **64-A**, 1240–2.

Sammons, B. and Thomas, D. (1959) Extensive lumbar meningocele associated with neurofibromatosis. *Am. J. Radiol.*, **81**, 1021.

Sane, S., Yunis, E. and Greer, R. (1971) Subperiosteal or cortical cyst and intramedullary neurofibromatosis – uncommon manifestations of neurofibromatosis. A case report. *J. Bone Joint Surg. [Am.]*, **53-A**, 1194–200.

Savini, R. and Vicenzi, G. (1976) Deformities of the spine in neurofibromatosis. Clinical and radiographic study of 46 cases. *Ital. J. Orthop. Traumatol.*, **9**, 13–24.

Savini, R., Parisini, P., Cervellati, S. *et al.* (1983) Surgical treatment of vertebral deformities in neurofibromatosis. *Ital. J. Orthop. Traumatol.*, **9**, 13–24.

Schwartz, A. and Ramos, R. (1980) Neurofibromatosis and multiple nonossifying fibromas. *Am. J. Radiol.*, **135**, 617–19.

Scott, J.C. (1965) Scoliosis and neurofibromatosis. *J. Bone Joint Surg. [Br.]*, **47-B**, 240–6.

Shamberger, R. and Welch, K. (1988) Surgical repair of pectus excavatum. *J. Pediatr. Surg.*, **23**, 615–22.

Sharif, H. and Tucker, A. (1985) Rare skeletal manifestations in neurofibromatosis complicated with sarcoma. *Br. J. Radiol.*, **58**, 371–4.

Shertzer, J., Bickel, W. and Stubbins, S. (1969) Congenital pseudarthrosis of the ulna. *Minn. Med.*, **52**, 1061–6.

Sirois, J. and Drennan, J. (1990) Dystrophic spinal deformity in neurofibromatosis. *J. Pediatr. Orthop.*, **10**, 522–6.

Sofield, H. and Millar, A. (1959) Fragmentation, realignment, and intramedullary rod fixation of deformities of the long bones in children. A ten year appraisal. *J. Bone Joint Surg. [Am.]*, **41-A**, 1371–91.

Sorensen, S.A., Mulvihill, J.J. and Nielsen, A.N. (1986) Long-term follow-up of von Recklinghausen neurofibromatosis. Survival and malignant neoplasms. *N. Engl. J. Med.*, **314**, 1010–15.

Sprague, D. and Brown, G. (1974) Congenital pseudarthrosis of the radius. *J. Bone Joint Surg. [Am.]*, **56-A**, 191–4.

Stone, J., Bridwell, K., Shackelford, G. *et al.* (1987) Dural ectasia associated with spontaneous dislocation of the upper part of the thoracic spine in neurofibromatosis. A case report and review of the literature. *J. Bone Joint Surg. [Am.]*, **64-A**, 1079–83.

Sutcliffe, M. and Goldberg, A. (1982) The treatment of congenital pseudarthroses of the tibia with pulsing magnetic fields: a survey of 52 cases. *Clin. Orthop.*, **166**, 45.

Van Aken, H., Scherer, R. and Lawin, P. (1982) A rare intraoperative complication in a child with von Recklinghausen's neurofibromatosis. *Anaesthesia*, **37**, 827–9.

Verbiest, H. (1989) Benign spinal tumors: clinical experience, in *The Cervical Spine*, J.B. Lippincott, Philadelphia, pp. 723–5, 732–8.

Voutsinas, S. and Wynne-Davies, R. (1983) The infrequency of malignant disease in diaphyseal aclasis and neurofibromatosis. *J. Med. Genet.*, **20**, 345–9.

Wamer, R.P., Kini, K.R., Raju, U. *et al.* (1985) Neurofibromatosis and malignancy. *Clin. Pediatr.*, **24**, 584–5.

Weiland, A. and Daniel, R. (1980) Congenital pseudarthrosis of the tibia: treatment with vascularised autogenous fibular grafts. A preliminary report. *Johns Hopkins Med. J.*, **147**, 89–95.

Wellwood, J.M., Bulmer, J.H. and Graff, D.J.C. (1971) Congenital defects of the tibia in siblings with neurofibromatosis. *J. Bone Joint Surg. [Br.]*, **53-B**, 314–19.

Winter, R.B. (1984) Thoracic lordoscoliosis in neurofibromatosis: treatment by a Harrington rod with sublaminar wiring. Report of two cases. *J. Bone Joint Surg. [Am.]*, **66-A**, 1102–6.

Winter, R. (1991) Spontaneous dislocation of a vertebra in a patient who had neurofibromatosis. Report of a case with dural ectasia. *J. Bone Joint Surg. [Am.]*, **73-A**, 1402–4.

Winter, R.B. and Edwards, W.C. (1981) Case report: Neurofibromatosis with lumbosacral spondylolisthesis. *J. Pediatr. Orthop.*, **1**, 91–6.

Winter, R.B., Moe, J.H., Bradford, D.S. *et al.* (1979) Spine deformity in neurofibromatosis. A review of one hundred and two patients. *J. Bone Joint Surg. [Am.]*, **61-A**, 677–94.

Winter, R., Lonstein, J. and Anderson, M. (1988) Neurofibromatosis hyperkyphosis: a review of 33 patients with kyphosis of 80 or greater. *J. Spine Disorders*, **1**, 39.

Wong, J., Strong, M.L. and Gillespie, R. (1992) Prophylactic bypass grafting of the pre-pseudarthrotic tibia in neurofibromatosis. *J. Bone Joint Surg. [Br.]*, **74-B**, Suppl. II, 137–8.

Yaghmal, I. and Tafazoll, M. (1977) Massive subperiosteal hemorrhage in neurofibromatosis. *Radiology*, **122**, 439–41.

Yamashita, M., Matsuki, A. and Oyama, T. (1977) Anaesthetic considerations on von Recklinghausen's disease (multiple neurofibromatosis). Abnormal response to muscle relaxants. *Anaesthetist*, **26**, 317–18.

Yong-Hing, K., Kalamchi, A. and MacEwen, G.D. (1979) Cervical spine abnormalities in neurofibromatosis. *J. Bone Joint Surg. [Am.]*, **61-A**, 695–9.

12

Malignancy: epidemiologically associated cancers

J.J. Mulvihill

12.1 INTRODUCTION

Cancer is a frequently cited and much feared complication of neurofibromatosis. In fact, it only occurs slightly more frequently in neurofibromatosis patients than in the general population.

In reviewing the epidemiological evidence for malignant neoplasms in neurofibromatosis 1 (NF1), the following summary conclusion was reached by me and my co-author (Hope and Mulvihill, 1981):

> Although . . . malignancy is, beyond question, part of NF, reliable estimates of the frequency of malignancies are unavailable owing to a lack of formal epidemiologic studies. Nonetheless, even biased collections of cases of neoplasms complicating NF show such peculiarities in age at tumor diagnosis, tumor type, and multiplicity of tumors that certain associations seem valid. The associations are informative from a pathogenetic viewpoint, presenting two areas of uncertainty concerning the origin of the disease. First, tumors derived from the neural crest tend to support the thesis that NF is a neurocristopathy. The excesses of sarcomatous neural degeneration, pheochromocytoma, and possibilities of neural beginnings of rhabdomyosarcoma strengthen this argument. The multiple mucosal neuroma syndrome (multiple endocrine neoplasia, type III) strikingly resembles NF, except for the important absence of neurofibromas. On the other hand, the appearance of Wilms' tumor and leukemia with NF (as well as the bone dysplasias) suggests that the disease is not confined to the neural crest, but is due to a genetic defect, present in all cells, that affects cells outside of the neural crest. Furthermore, some tumors surely of neural crest origins are not seen to excess, like cutaneous melanoma and tumors of the argentaffin,

> chromaffin, and APUD (amine-precursor, uptake, and decarboxylation) cell types, including pancreatic islet cells, thyroid C cells, and the endocrine cells of the gastric and intestinal mucosa. Also, some malignancies expected in any large patient population (lung, breast, gastrointestinal, and prostate) are infrequent in the literature.
>
> It may be surprising that the literature, as we view it, so poorly supports some prevalent notions about malignancy in NF. In turn, the inconsistencies provide questions deserving study. By determining the relationship between various malignancies and NF, the pathogenesis and etiology of both pathologic processes may be better understood than they are now. Future reports should include information on age at diagnosis, family history, and precise location and histology of the associated malignancies.

This chapter is an update of that prior review. It summarizes the basis for those conclusions that still seem valid and gives details about areas that have emerged or have been clarified by intervening studies. The present review excludes neurofibromatosis 2 (NF2), all benign tumours (except central nervous system (CNS) tumours) and the molecular genetic epidemiology of cancer in NF1.

The principal questions are: What cancers occur to a statistically significant excess in persons with NF1? For any associated cancers, what is the magnitude of the excess? And, what are the clinical implications? In the intervening 13 years, two substantial case series (Huson, Harper and Compston, 1988; Riccardi, 1992) and one retrospective cohort study have been carried out. The firm association of adenocarcinoma of the duodenum and ampulla of Vater with NF1 has been made by case reports.

12.2 IS THERE A SIGNIFICANT EXCESS?

An ideal investigation would count the number of people in a defined population with cancer, with neurofibromatosis and with both disorders. Such an ideal study has not been conducted and evidence of a significant association comes from three imperfect approaches.

- The least vigorous, but most often used method is the collection of patients with both disorders, often reported simply as case reports, with little sense of a denominator that would permit quantification of the risk. Such reports generate hypotheses for testing for valid qualitative associations and for launching definitive studies.
- Consecutive patients with one disorder could be studied for the other disorder as a cross-sectional study. Some estimate of the expected frequencies of cases can be derived by knowing the frequency of the separate traits. The frequency of NF1 is 1 in 3000–4000, but the frequency of cancer must be calculated from the age-, year, sex- and

race-specific rates for the same geographic area. Since one out of four people gets cancer in a lifetime, 25% would be the expected frequency if a group of NF1 patients were followed from birth until death.

- The final approach would follow a well-ascertained cohort of NF1 patients for the occurrence of cancer. This could be done retrospectively or, ideally, prospectively. Large cross-sectional studies of NF1 have been conducted in Denmark, Michigan, southeast Wales and at the Baylor College of Medicine (Texas) (Table 12.1); only the Danish population has been followed up for a long time.

12.2.1 The cross-sectional studies

Each cross-sectional study defined and ascertained cases of malignancy in different ways. Borberg (1951) visited virtually all Danish hospitals, except a few specialty hospitals outside Copenhagen, and reviewed charts dated from 1924 through 1943, ending 1 January 1944. From the 84 probands, he made family visits and identified 128 additional patients through physical examination and family history. Crowe, Schull and Neel (1956) started with the University of Michigan hospital records and reviewed charts for 16 years from 1934 through 1950. The review identified 161 definite and 66 dubious cases. After a cycle of patient contacts, new records from 1951 through 1953 at the University Hospital were reviewed, leading to another 32 cases. A few cases were specifically referred to the study, and four state institutions (three for the mentally deficient and one for epileptics) were likewise surveyed. On the occasion of family studies, 86 additional cases were identified giving a total of 223 cases. The prevalence survey in southeast Wales (Huson, Harper and Compston, 1988) used seven sources: direct contact with general practitioners and selected consultants; hospital records from 1969 through 1986, coded with neurofibromatosis and related complications; charts coded as scoliosis or pseudoarthrosis from 1954 through 1986, at an orthopaedic hospital; a neuropathology registry, a dermatology histological register (for neurofibroma) and medical genetics records, all at the University Hospital of Wales, 1972 through 1986; and a newspaper story eliciting participation. This strategy led to finding 119 cases, of which 93 were acceptable. Family study added 51 cases living in the area, giving a total prevalence as of 1 June 1985 of 135 cases. Finally, the Neurofibromatosis Institute Clinical Research Programme of the Baylor College of Medicine (Riccardi, 1992) was a referral clinic that emerged from a general clinical genetics service. Although Riccardi (1992), a champion in the field, insists his series is 'reasonably instructive about the general character and natural history of NF', case ascertainment was clearly passive and not a systematic search of all cases in a geographic region, as attempted in the other series.

Table 12.1 Malignant and central nervous system tumours in neurofibromatosis cohorts

	Denmark 44	*Denmark 83*	*Michigan 50*	*Wales 85*	*Baylor 91*[a]	*Total*[b]
Neurofibromatosis patients (*n*)	172	212	223	135	579	1149
Number with malignancy (%)	26 (15)	70 (33)	23 (10)	6 (4)	115 (20)	151 (13)
Number with two or more tumours (% of these with any malignancy)	2 (8)	15 (21)	4 (17)	1 (17)	?	>20 (>13)[a]
Optic pathway glioma	5	6	2	2	50	60
Brain (other) and spinal cord	6	16	6	0	22	44
Vestibular Schwannoma	1	1	4	0	0	5
Sarcoma	3	11	6	0	39	56
Phaeochromocytoma	0	3	1	1	2	7
Lung	0	2	0	0	–[a,c]	2
Breast	4	7	0	1	–[a,c]	8
Colorectum	1	5	2	0	–[a,c]	7
Ovary	0	4	0	0	0	4
Leukaemia/lymphoma	0	4	2	0	1	7
Other						
Carcinoid	0	0	0	2	1	3
Penis	0	0	0	1	0	1
Oesophagus	1	0	0	0	0	0
Stomach	6	12	1	0	0	13
Other	1	14	3	0	11[a,c]	28

For ease of reference the columns are headed by the site of study and the year case accrual ended: Denmark 44 is Borberg (1951) with case accrual ending in 1944; Denmark 83 is Sørensen, Mulvihill and Nielsen (1986a,b); Michigan 50 is Crowe, Schull and Neel (1956); Wales 85 is Huson, Harper and Compston (1988); and Baylor 91 is Riccardi (1992).

[a] Baylor 91 excludes optic pathway gliomas and other brain tumours from the definition of malignancy.

[b] Total excludes Denmark 44, which is included in Denmark 83.

[c] The 11 other cancers include lung, breast and bowel cancers.

In the four cross-sectional studies (i.e. excluding the retrospective cohort study of Sørensen, Mulvihill and Nielsen, 1986a,b), the frequency of malignancy including CNS tumours, was 4–20%, the highest being in Baylor (Riccardi, 1992), where modern imaging techniques and ascertainment bias could contribute to a high figure. The frequency of patients with malignancy who had a second malignancy was 8% or 17% in the cross-sectional studies. Comparison of the tumour types with the general pattern of common cancers in the general population, even of children, points to a clear excess of certain cancers that are otherwise exceedingly rare: optic pathway glioma, other brain and spinal cord tumours, and sarcomas.

12.2.2 The retrospective cohort study

As pointed out elsewhere (Mulvihill, 1986), the Danish study (Sørensen, Mulvihill and Nielsen, 1986a,b) is the only retrospective cohort study of NF1. Although the initial ascertainment by Borberg (1951) had the usual hospital ascertainment bias, once the cohort was closed in 1944, Borberg had no substantial involvement with members of the cohort. Hence, the groups represents a true picture of the natural (as opposed to the clinical) history of NF1 in a nearly nationwide survey.

The follow-up study ended on 1 June 1983, by which time 70 patients (33%) of the original 212 probands and affected relatives had developed a malignancy (once again, defined here as a malignant neoplasm or benign CNS tumour; deep or cutaneous neurofibromas were not considered as malignancies). With the excellent records of the Danish cancer registry, thorough follow-up and the record linkage systems in Denmark, the mortality and cancer status of all but two of the 212 patients in the original cohort were determined. (These two had migrated to the USA and could not be found.) The numbers of expected cancers for those who were alive on 1 January 1944 were calculated by applying the age-, year- and sex-specific incidence of total cancer to the corresponding numbers of years-at-risk in the cohort, namely 1694 person-years of follow-up for probands and 2145 person-years for relatives.

In the total cohort, the point estimate of the relative risk for malignancy was 2.5 (53 cases observed versus 20.8 expected) with confidence intervals that excluded 1.0 and reached statistical significance (Table 12.2). The excess was largely in probands whose relative risk total was 4.0 (confidence interval (CI), 2.8–5.6) and was significant in each sex. The point estimate was always higher in females than in males and was statistically significant even for female relatives (relative risk of 1.9; CI, 1.1–3.1). The true relative risk probably lies between 4.0 (the risk of the probands, biased toward severe cases) and 1.5 (the risk of incidentally diagnosed relatives, biased toward mild cases).

Table 12.2 Occurrence of new malignant tumours in patients with NF1 according to sex, proband status and vital status

Group	*Male patients*		*Female patients*		*Total*	
	n	*Relative risk (CI)*	*n*	*Relative risk (CI)*	*n*	*Relative risk (CI)*
Probands (alive 1 January 1944)						
Observed	14	3.5	20	4.4	34	4.0
Expected	4.0	(1.9–5.9)	4.5	(2.7–6.8)	8.5	(2.8–5.6)
Relatives (alive 1 January 1944)						
Observed	4	0.9	15	1.9	19	1.5
Expected	4.4	(0.3–2.3)	7.9	(1.1–3.1)	12.3	(0.9–2.4)
Total cohort (alive 1 January 1944)						
Observed	18	2.1	35	2.8	53	2.5
Expected	8.4	(1.3–3.4)	12.4	(2.0–3.9)	20.8	(1.9–3.3)

CI denotes 95% confidence interval for relative risk.
Modified from Sørenson, Mulvihill and Nielsen (1986a,b).

Owing to the potentially large number of separate tumour types, expected numbers of cancers were not calculated for specific tumour types. In the general population, the lung, prostate and colon-rectum in men and breast, colon-rectum and uterus in women account for over half of all tumour sites. In contrast, in the Danish NF1 cohort, nervous system tumours accounted for 47% of all malignant conditions (Table 12.1). Finally, in the general population, a second cancer develops in 4% of persons with a first cancer (Storm *et al.*, 1985), whereas 15 of 70 neurofibromatosis patients (21%) with a first malignancy developed a second malignancy.

12.3 TUMOUR-SPECIFIC ASSOCIATIONS

Despite the lack of quantitative estimates, the cross-sectional and retrospective cohort studies give credible evidence for the validity of the association of NF1 with some CNS tumours (especially glioma of the optic pathway), phaeochromocytoma and neurofibrosarcoma. The common adult cancers do not seem to be associated with NF1, nor does Wilms' tumour, which was considered a candidate association before (Hope and Mulvihill, 1981).

With a decade of additional experience, the arguments seem strengthened that certain leukaemias and adenocarcinoma of the ampulla of Vater (not previously suspected) are validly associated tumours. The predominant leukaemias seem to be non-lymphocytic leukaemias of childhood, in particular xantholeukaemia (Bader and Miller, 1978; Laroche *et al.*, 1985; Goerg *et al.*, 1989; Kaneko *et al.*, 1989). Duodenal tumours with neurohumoral secretions seem to occur to excess and include periampullary tumours and carcinoids that produce somatostatin (Garcia *et al.*, 1978; Klein, Clemens and Cameron, 1989; Ohtsuki *et al.*, 1989; Burke *et al.*, 1990; Colarian *et al.*, 1990).

With passage of time, the cross-sectional studies could be revisited to yield much more quantitative information about tumour-specific risks than is now available.

12.4 CANCER IN CHILDREN WITH NF1

Retrospective studies are lacking and cross-sectional studies are usually based on a review of patients' records at a paediatric hospital. A prior review (Hope and Mulvihill, 1981) totalled 362 patients from the literature, of which 32 had optic nerve glioma, nine other gliomas, seven neurofibrosarcomas and seven other malignancies, totalling 15% of the entire series. Additional series (Lefkowitz *et al.*, 1990) emphasized the occurrence of multiple primary cancers in children with neurofibromatosis, as well as the possible excess of rhabdomyosarcoma. Results of the Children's Hospital of Philadelphia series suggested an excess of optic glioma patients when the *NF1* gene was inherited from a father (Schneider *et al.*, 1986). Furthermore, there seemed to be a concordance of histological tumour types when malignancies affected multiple family members (Hartley *et al.*, 1990). Some epidemiological rigour was added to the suspected excess of brain tumours in children with NF1: the New York state tumour registry series detected a relative risk of at least 6.2 for a prior history of neurofibromatosis in a case-control study of brain tumours (Baptiste *et al.*, 1989). Likewise in Italy, a 2.9 excess over expected numbers of children with cancer and neurofibromatosis was seen in a survey of 11 institutions belonging to the Italian Society of Pediatric Hematology and Oncology (Mosso *et al.*, 1987). Five of the seven Italian children with cancer and neurofibromatosis inherited the *NF1* gene from their mothers. An estimated 1% of all childhood cancer is attributed to NF1 (Bader, Kantor and Rubenstein, 1981; Bader, 1986).

With regard to the controversial issue of optic pathway gliomas (Aylsworth, 1990), estimates range between 0.9 and 15%, the higher being in patients screened by sensitive neuroimaging techniques. A typical series (Listernick *et al.*, 1989) scanned 65 children with no visual abnormalities and detected optic gliomas in 15%, especially in those with plexiform neurofibromas of the eyelid and glaucoma. Because of dilemmas in effective therapy, it is not clear whether detecting such tumours in asymptomatic children is beneficial. Hence, nothing has emerged, in my opinion, to challenge the NIH Consensus Development Conference recommendation that routine radiographic screening by computed tomography or magnetic resonance imaging be performed only in NF1 patients with symptoms (Stumpf, 1988).

12.5 CLINICAL IMPLICATIONS

12.5.1 Counselling

In describing the prognosis of a newborn or individual newly diagnosed with NF1, it is appropriate to anticipate the issue of risk for malignancy because some other counsellor or reading material will otherwise raise the issue. Although Riccardi (1992) criticizes our prior review as an 'attempt to play down the major excessive malignancies in NF1', I see nothing in the intervening literature that would lead me to advise routine diagnostic screening for cancer in everyone with the *NF1* gene. The physician or counsellor should increase the patient and family's awareness that any pain, tumour or unusual growth be rapidly brought to medical attention.

At the same time, there is support for reassurance that the absolute risk for cancer in NF1 is on average not so different from the general population (namely, a relative risk of 1.5–4.0). For certain rare tumours, optic pathway glioma and neurofibrosarcoma, there is an enormous but unquantified relative risk. However, a role for screening NF1 persons with no signs or symptoms is tenuous. Therapy for optic pathway tumours is based on symptoms and not just the presence of tumour. As for neurofibrosarcomas, absolute risk is so minute that they all do not meet criteria for a condition that should be screened for. Apart from the rare child who has already had one malignancy, there is no useful marker of which NF1 patients are more predisposed to malignancy than others.

12.5.2 Therapy and prognosis

If a person with NF1 does develop cancer, there is no evidence that the prognosis is any different from individuals with the same tumour and stage but without NF1 (Bader, 1986). Hence, there is no reason to modify therapy just because the patient has NF1.

12.6 CONCLUSION

A modification of our original conclusion, given 12 years of additional prospective, would read:

> Without doubt cancer is part of NF1. Confirmed estimates of the frequency of malignancies seen to excess are unavailable, owing to a lack of formal epidemiologic studies beyond the Danish retrospective cohort. In contrast, the types of cancers associated with NF1 are well known because even biased collections of cases of tumors complicating NF1 show peculiarities in the age of tumor diagnosis and of tumor type, as well as a multiplicity of tumors in the same person. The relative risk of neurofibrosarcoma, pheochromocytoma, and optic pathway glioma are surely high, but the absolute risk is low.
>
> The associations are important in clinical management and they further shed light on the pathogenesis of tumors in general and NF1 in particular. Some tumor types seem to support the hypothesis that neurofibromatosis is a neurocristopathy, whereas others do not. A new but rare tumor association is that of neurohumoral secreting tumors in the duodenum and the ampulla of Vater.

REFERENCES

Aylsworth, A. (ed.) (1990) *Neurofibromatosis: Optic Gliomas in Neurofibromatosis*, Conference Series Vol. 2, The National Neurofibromatosis Foundation, New York.

Bader, J.L. (1986) Neurofibromatosis and cancer. *Ann. N.Y. Acad. Sci.*, **486**, 57–65.

Bader, J.L. and Miller, R.W. (1978) Neurofibromatosis and childhood leukemia. *J. Pediatr.*, **92**, 925–9.

Bader, J.L. *et al.* (1980) Neurofibromatosis (NF) and other genetic defects associated with childhood cancer. *Am. J. Hum. Genet.*, **32**, 97A.

Bader, J.L., Kantor, A.F. and Rubenstein, A.E. (1981) Increased risk of cancer with neurofibromatosis. *Proc. Am. Soc. Clin. Oncol.*, **20**, 339.

Baptiste, M. *et al.* (1989) Neurofibromatosis and other disorders among children with CNS tumors and their families. *Neurology*, **39**, 487–92.

Borberg, A. (1951) Clinical and genetic investigations into tuberous sclerosis and Recklinghausen's neurofibromatosis: contribution to elucidation of interrelationship and eugenics of the syndromes. *Acta Psychiatr. Neurol. [Suppl.]*, **71**, 1–239.

Burke, A.P. *et al.* (1990) Somatostatin-producing duodenal carcinoids in patients with von Recklinghausen's neurofibromatosis: a predilection for black patients. *Cancer*, **7**, 1591–5.

Colarian, J., Pietruck, T., LaFave, L. and Calzada, R. (1990) Adenocarcinoma of the ampulla of Vater associated with neurofibromatosis. *J. Clin. Gastroenterol.*, **12**, 118–19.

Crowe, F.W., Schull, W.J. and Neel, J.V. (1956) *A Clinical, Pathological and Genetic Study of Multiple Neurofibromatosis*, Charles C. Thomas, Springfield, Illinois.

Garcia, J.C. *et al.* (1978) Ellison syndrome and neurofibromatosis in a 13-year-old boy. *J. Paediatr.*, **93**, 982–4.

Goerg, C. *et al.* (1989) Neurofibromatosis and acute monocytic leukemia in adults. *Cancer*, **64**, 1717–19.

Hartley, A.L. *et al.* (1990) Sarcomas in three generations of a family with neurofibromatosis. *Cancer Genet. Cytogenet.*, **45**, 245–8.

Hope, D.G. and Mulvihill, J.J. (1981) Malignancy in neurofibromatosis, in *Neurofibromatosis (von Recklinghausen Disease): Genetics, Cell Biology and Biochemistry. Advances in Neurology*, Vol. 29 (eds V.M. Riccardi and J.J. Mulvihill), Raven Press, New York, pp. 33–56.

Huson, S.M., Harper, P.S. and Compston, D.A.S. (1988) Von Recklinghausen neurofibromatosis: a clinical and population study in South-East Wales. *Brain*, **111**, 1355–81.

Kaneko, Y. *et al.* (1989) Chromosome pattern in juvenile chronic myelogenous leukemia, myelodysplastic syndrome and acute leukemia associated with neurofibromatosis. *Leukemia*, **3**, 36–41.

Klein, A., Clemens, J. and Cameron, J. (1989) Periampullary neoplasms in von Recklinghausen's disease. *Surgery*, **106**, 815–19.

Laroche, L. *et al.* (1985) Xantholeucèmie associée a une neurofibromatose de von Recklinghausen (NFR). *Ann. Dermatol. Venereol.*, **112**, 731–2.

Lefkowitz, I.B. *et al.* (1990) Neurofibromatosis and cancer: incidence and management, in *Neurofibromatosis: A Handbook for Patients, Families and Healthcare Professionals*, (eds A.E. Rubenstein and B.R. Korf), Thieme, New York, pp. 99–110.

Listernick, R. *et al.* (1989) Optic gliomas in children with neurofibromatosis type 1. *J. Pediatr.*, **114**, 788–92.

Mosso, M.L. *et al.* (1987) Neurofibromatosis and malignant childhood cancers: a survey in Italy, 1970–83. *Tumori*, **73**, 209–12.

Mulvihill, J.J. (1986) Neurofibromatosis: a genetic epidemiologist's point of view. *Ann. N.Y. Acad. Sci.*, **486**, 38–44.

Ohtsuki, Y. *et al.* (1989) Duodenal carcinoid (somatostatinoma) combined with von Recklinghausen's disease: a case report and review of the literature. *Acta Pathol. Jpn.*, **39**, 141–6.

Riccardi, V.M. (1992) *Neurofibromatosis: Phenotype, Natural History and Pathogenesis*, 2nd edn, The Johns Hopkins University Press, Baltimore.

Schneider, M. *et al.* (1986) Childhood neurofibromatosis: risk factors for malignant disease. *Cancer Genet. Cytogenet.*, **21**, 347–54.

Sørensen, S.A., Mulvihill, J.J. and Nielsen, A. (1986a) Long-term follow-up of von Recklinghausen neurofibromatosis: survival and malignant neoplasms. *N. Engl. J. Med.*, **314**, 1010–15.

Sørensen, S.A., Mulvihill, J.J. and Nielsen, A. (1986b) On the natural history of von Recklinghausen neurofibromatosis. *Ann. N.Y. Acad. Sci.*, **486**, 30–7.

Storm, H.H. *et al.* (1985) Summary: multiple primary cancers in Denmark, 1943–80. *Nat. Cancer Inst. Mongr.*, **68**, 411–30.

Stumpf, D. (1988) Concensus development conference on neurofibromatosis. *Arch. Neurol.*, **45**, 575–8.

13

Medical complications of neurofibromatosis 1

R.E. Ferner

13.1 INTRODUCTION

Neurofibromatosis 1 (NF1) is a systemic disorder affecting ectodermal and mesodermal tissues, and its medical complications display marked heterogeneity. Hypertension is the commonest associated general medical disorder, but some of the reported associations are rare and I have tried to indicate which may be merely due to coincidence.

13.2 HYPERTENSION

The most important general medical disorder to occur in NF1 is hypertension, which affects about 6% of patients (Riccardi and Eichner, 1986). The hypertension may have no apparent cause, i.e. it may be due to essential hypertension. However, there is an increased incidence of phaeochromocytoma (section 13.3), coarctation of the aorta and renovascular hypertension.

Renovascular hypertension occurs in about 2% of patients (Huson, 1989; Ferner and Hughes, unpublished data). The renal arterial lesion may be major or small vessel stenosis, aneurysm formation or extrinsic compression by an adjacent tumour. Four variants of renal artery stenosis have been described in NF1: a pure intimal form; advanced intimal; intimal and aneurysmal; and nodular (Reubi, 1945; Salyer and Salyer, 1974). Renal artery stenosis is not usually discovered until the patient presents with hypertension, which may be in the perinatal period, childhood or adult life. In a review of 16 published cases of renovascular hypertension, the diagnosis was made before the age of 20 years in all but one patient, and the renal artery stenosis was bilateral in four (Bourke and Gatenby, 1971). Riccardi and Eichner (1986) undertook digital subtraction angiography in 50 patients and found no renovascular abnormalities in the absence of systemic hypertension. Five of their nine patients with hypertension had renal artery abnormalities, including fusiform arterial narrowing, aneurysms and secondary revascularization. It is possible that the true frequency of renovascular hypertension is greater since subtle intrarenal lesions may not be demonstrated even with digital subtraction angiography (Pollard *et al.*, 1989).

Unfortunately, operation on renovascular lesions has an unpredictable outcome. Even surgery for a main renal artery stenosis may not produce a permanent cure because of the presence of intrarenal lesions and re-stenosis of reimplanted arteries (Pollard *et al.*, 1989).

Because of the increased incidence of hypertension, and especially potentially curable causes of hypertension, it is important that NF1 patients have their blood pressure monitored regularly. In children and young adults this is particularly important and should be carried out at least annually.

13.3 PHAEOCHROMOCYTOMA

Phaeochromocytomas are uncommon tumours that secrete catecholamines and occasionally vasoactive polypeptides, serotonin and substance P. They occur in about 1 in 1000 hypertensive patients in the general population and 6% are familial (Cryer, 1985). Between 5 and 25% of patients with a phaeochromocytoma have NF1, but the frequency of these tumours among all NF1 patients is less than 1%. Phaeochromocytomas also occur with increased frequency in other neurocutaneous disorders, including tuberous sclerosis, Sturge-Weber syndrome, von Hippel-Lindau syndrome and multiple endocrine neoplasia syndromes (section 13.4). Although phaeochromocytomas are uncommon in NF1, prompt diagnosis is essential as they may cause severe hypertension and cardiovascular compromise, which are potentially lethal. A phaeochromocytoma is particularly hazardous during anaesthesia and in pregnancy. However, surgical resection of a phaeochromocytoma offers a good chance of cure from the hypertension and the tumour.

The commonest situation for a phaeochromocytoma is the adrenal medulla, but 10% are outside the adrenal, wherever nests of primitive neural crest cells have survived, anywhere from the base of the skull to the epididymis. The commonest ectopic site is the organ of Zuckerkandl – a cluster of neural crest cells on the sympathetic chain, situated close to the abdominal aorta and near the origin of the inferior mesenteric artery (Chan and Wang, 1989). About 12% of phaeochromocytomas are malignant, and those that are malignant are usually extra-adrenal (Ross and Griffith, 1989). Metastases occur in the liver, nervous system, lungs, lymph nodes and skeleton.

Headache is the commonest symptom of phaeochromocytoma, occurring in about 60% of patients. The headache is of sudden onset, lasts for about 15 min and may be frontal or occipital. Some patients have concomitant nausea, vomiting and neckache, and the symptoms are reported to be more severe in patients with paroxysmal hypertension. Blurring of vision, homonymous hemianopia and scotomata scintillating in time with the heart beat are found in 10% of cases. There is a risk of cerebral ischaemia, fits and transient loss of consciousness. A third of patients experience anxiety, tremor and a feeling of impending doom. Palpitations due to cardiac arrhythmias and chest pain due to myocardial ischaemia occur, and catecholamine cardiomyopathy is the cause of death in 58% of cases (Ross and Griffith, 1989). Other vascular manifestations include claudication and gangrene of the limbs. Prominent sweating, either constant or nocturnal, occurs in 50% of cases and may be confined to the upper half of the body. Weight loss has been found in 7% of patients, and less common symptoms include abdominal pain, nausea and constipation (Ross and Griffith, 1989). Tumours in extra-adrenal sites may give rise to unusual symptoms such as terminal haematuria in bladder phaeochromocytomas.

The key clinical finding is either sustained or paroxysmal hypertension and is found in nearly all patients with an actively secreting tumour. The presence of a phaeochromocytoma should be suspected in patients with persistent hypertension that is difficult to treat, where the pulse pressure is narrow and when hypertension is made worse by beta-blocker drugs (Ross and Griffith, 1989).

It is not cost-effective to screen all patients with NF1 for phaeochromocytoma, but patients should be carefully assessed and monitored for hypertension and suggestive symptoms. Biochemical diagnosis can be made by measuring 24 h urinary or plasma concentrations of catecholamines, vanillylmandelic acid and other metabolites (adrenaline and noradrenaline), but false positive results can occur. Most tumours are in the abdomen and can be detected by computed tomographic scanning from the level of the diaphragm to the aortic bodies. The method is less sensitive for tumours smaller than 2 cm, and for ectopic and recurrent tumours. Alternative techniques include ultrasonography, arteriography, venous sampling with measurement of catecholamine concentrations at different sites, adrenal scintigraphy with meta-iodobenzylguanidine, and magnetic resonance imaging, which may become the method of choice, especially for localizing extra-adrenal tumours (Chan and Wang, 1989).

If possible, the tumour should be removed. Special precautions should be taken to produce complete alpha and beta blockade beforehand to prevent catastrophic fluctuations in blood pressure and dysrhythmias during surgery. In some pateints with multiple or malignant tumours, surgery is not feasible and long-term alpha and beta blockade should be used (Drury, 1989).

13.4 MULTIPLE ENDOCRINE NEOPLASIA SYNDROMES

The multiple endocrine neoplasia (MEN) syndromes comprise three distinct autosomal dominant conditions each having almost complete penetrance by the age of 70 years. They are considered here because their features overlap with NF1, and many of their associated tumours have a neural crest origin (Knudson, 1981). Nevertheless, an association with NF1 has not been established (Hope and Mulvihill, 1981) and these conditions are described here as an aid towards differential diagnosis.

MEN 1 comprises diffuse hyperplasia or adenomas of the parathyroid glands, pituitary, pancreatic islets and sometimes the adrenal cortex (Schimke, 1986). Some patients have lipomas, thymomas or Schwannomas.

The most common form of MEN is type 2A, which is manifested by medullary carcinoma of the thyroid C cells, phaeochromocytoma and sometimes parathyroid adenoma or hyperplasia. Medullary carcinoma of the thyroid is the first manifestation and usually causes death from metastatic disease by the fifth decade. Hyperplasia of the thyroid C cells (which have a neural crest origin) occurs before the development of carcinoma. Prospective screening by detecting a rise in calcitonin levels after stimulation with an infusion of pentagastrin or calcium helps diagnosis and improves prognosis (Gagel *et al.*, 1988). Thyroidectomy for C cell hyperplasia is curative and substantially increases life expectancy. Genetic linkage studies have shown that the gene for MEN 2A is located on chromosome 10 and genetic prediction using inherited DNA markers can be undertaken in families with two or more affected members (Ponder, 1990) (see Note, p. 328).

MEN 2B embraces phaeochromocytoma, medullary carcinoma of the thyroid and multiple mucosal neuromas. Patients have a Marfanoid apearance and may develop ganglioneuromatosis (Schimke, 1986). It has been postulated that patients with MEN 2B have mutations at the same locus on chromosome 10 as MEN 2A patients (Jackson *et al.*, 1988).

In the MEN syndromes, phaeochromocytomas are more often bilateral, ectopic, multifocal and malignant than in sporadic cases (Chan and Wang, 1989). Prospective screening for relatives of affected families is recommended yearly between the ages of 5 and 35 years and at increasing intervals after this age. Early detection of phaeochromocytoma may be carried out using computed tomography and radioisotope scans, but there is a cumulative risk of radiation. Biochemical screening has been used, but is associated with poor compliance when 24 h urinary catecholamines are assayed. Plasma catecholamines measured after exercise combined with plasma levels of chromogranin, a protein secreted with catecholamines, has been advocated as a reliable method for detecting early disease (Gagel *et al.*, 1988).

13.5 NEUROBLASTOMA

Although neuroblastomas have been reported with NF1 (Knudson, 1981; Schorry *et al.*, 1989), Hope and Mulvihill (1981) doubted whether these reports represent more than a chance association. None were discovered in two recent population studies (Huson, Harper and Compston, 1988; Ferner and Hughes, unpublished data). Because of their possible association with NF1 and their undoubted origin from neural crest cells, a brief account of neuroblastomas is appropriate. Neuroblastomas may arise either from the adrenal medulla or anywhere in the sympathetic nervous system. The tumour is the commonest neoplasm of early childhood and occurs in the first 4 years of life with a peak incidence of 2 years. Patients usually present with an abdominal mass, by which time metastases have often already occurred. Neuroblastomas cause increased urinary excretion of catecholamines and vanillylmandelic acid. Patients with localized disease, young babies under 1 year of age and those with a small primary tumour and distant metastases confined to the liver, skin and bone marrow have a good prognosis (Evans, 1980). Occasionally the malignant neuroblast cells differentiate into mature ganglion cells to produce a benign ganglioneuroma. Multidrug regimens may produce remissions and autologous bone transplantation with high dose melphalan may prolong survival (Nesbit, 1990).

13.6 CARDIOVASCULAR SYSTEM

The occurrence of renal artery stenosis causing hypertension is the commonest and most important example of vascular involvement in NF1, and has been discussed at the beginning of this chapter. Despite several reports of stenosis or occlusion of intracranial arteries in NF1, it is doubtful whether the occurrence of stroke from this cause is greater than in the non-NF1 population (Chapter 8). Vascular abnormalities may affect the gastrointestinal tract in NF1, but their frequency is unknown as some lesions may be clinically silent. The most common site is the origin of major vessels, and severe compromise of the gastrointestinal vasculature may cause bowel infarction (Riccardi and Eichner, 1986).

Cardiovascular involvement resulting from coarctation and aneurysm of the aorta and from extrinsic compression by neurofibromas in the mediastinum and thorax have been reported in NF1 (Riccardi and Eichner, 1986). There is no clear evidence that congenital heart defects occur with increased frequency in NF1. Lin and Garver (1988) reviewed the literature over the last 30 years and found that there were five structural defects and one conduction defect in the largest series of 78 patients (Neiman *et al.*, 1974). They were of the opinion that two of these patients with pulmonary stenosis and juxtaductal aortic coarctation had Noonan's syndrome rather than NF1.

There have been anecdotal case reports of hypertrophic obstructive cardiomyopathy in association with NF1 (Fitzpatrick and Emanuel, 1988) and I have seen one example. When the cause has been compression by neurofibromas impinging on the outflow tracts, the association with NF1 is undoubtedly real (Pung and Hirsch, 1955). In cases of idiopathic hypertrophic obstructive cardiomyopathy, the question still arises whether the association is coincidental. The patients present with chest pain on exertion and a systolic murmur. Electrocardiography demonstrates left ventricular hypertrophy and the diagnosis is made using cross-sectional and M-mode echocardiography, cardiac catheterization and angiography. It has been hypothesized that the hypertrophy of the myocardium is due to a defect of neural crest cells, to stimulation of the myocardium by nerve growth factor or to abnormal metabolism of catecholamines (Fitzpatrick and Emanuel, 1988).

13.7 RESPIRATORY SYSTEM

Neurogenic tumours are among the rarest neoplasms arising from the lung parenchyma (Roviaro *et al.* 1983). Benign intrapulmonary neurofibromas are found infrequently in NF1 and are associated with a good prognosis. They are usually asymptomatic and are diagnosed on routine chest radiography, but very large tumours may cause cough or dyspnoea. Malignant Schwannomas occur rarely and cause death by widespread metastases. Excision of intrapulmonary neurogenic tumours in NF1 is advocated because they carry a greater risk of malignancy than isolated intrapulmonary tumours (Spiro, 1990).

Mediastinal tumours in NF1 are usually neurofibromas and they originate in the posterior mediastinum or spread from the retroperitoneal space, the cervical paraspinal areas and other parts of the thorax. Posterior mediastinal masses may also be ganglioneuromas, neural crest tumours, Schwannomas, malignant tumours of nerve sheath origin (Heimberger, Battersby and Velios, 1963) and meningoceles. Ardissone *et al.* (1986) reviewed 92 cases of intrathoracic neurogenic tumours and found that 93.5% were benign and included ganglioneuromas, Schwannomas and neurofibromas. Among 13 patients with neurofibromas, four had NF1. Malignant neoplasms were found in 6.5% and were diagnosed as neurofibrosarcomas and ganglioneuroblastomas.

Neurofibromas and Schwannomas may produce scalloping and erosion of adjacent vertebral bodies and ribs, and in about 5% of cases they extend into the spinal canal. The tumours are frequently asymptomatic, but pain along the course of the nerve is encountered. Intraspinal extension may be clinically silent or produce pyramidal signs. Malignancy is uncommon but can only be excluded by surgical excision, and individual lesions should be monitored and removed if they enlarge progressively or cause symptoms (Goldstraw, 1990).

Scoliosis is a lateral curvature of the spine that is usually associated with rotation, but significant kyphosis is uncommon. The occurrence and management of scoliosis in NF1 are discussed in Chapter 11. The rotation of the spine produces a reduction in lung volume and impaired mechanical function in severe cases, which may result in respiratory and cardiac failure. Cardiorespiratory problems are encountered more frequently if the scoliosis is in the upper part of the spine and is not eliminated by forward flexion (Ogilvie, 1990). Respiratory failure resulting from severe scoliosis caused the death of one patient in my series of 103 patients.

Deformities of the sternum, including pectus excavatum and pectus carinatum, have been reported in as many as 30% of patients with NF1 (Riccardi and Eichner, 1986). However, this association may have been overemphasized since I have found a significant degree of pectus excavatum in only 2% of cases. These chest deformities do not cause respiratory problems, but pectus carinatum may itself be the result of airflow obstruction in childhood.

The coincidental occurrence of bilateral upper lobe pulmonary fibrosis with secondary cyst formation and vascular changes and NF1 was reported by Davis and Kaplan (1978). Both sexes are said to be affected and the symptoms start in adult life. Patients complain of a non-productive cough and dyspnoea on exertion, but there are no abnormal physical signs. Chest radiography reveals bilateral reticulonodular shadowing in the upper zones and there is a restrictive ventilatory defect with reduced transfer factor. The condition is slowly progressive and death occurs from respiratory failure (Stack and Thomas, 1990). However, the association of idiopathic pulmonary fibrosis is certainly rare, and may be only coincidental since no examples were identified in 238 patients by Riccardi and Eichner (1986), 135 patients by Huson, Harper and Compston (1988) or my own 103 patients.

13.8 GASTROINTESTINAL TRACT

13.8.1 Carcinoid tumours

Carcinoid tumours have been reported in association with NF1 and were found in two of 135 patients in the south Wales population study (Huson,

Harper and Compston, 1988). Carcinoid tumours are slow-growing neoplasms of the enterochromaffin cells usually in the gut. The tumours usually arise in the ileum, but may occur anywhere in the small intestine. They are also found in organs that are derived from the embryonic foregut, i.e. bronchi, stomach, pancreas and thyroid. Obendorfer introduced the term 'carcinoid' in 1907 to emphasize the comparatively benign behaviour of the tumour (Hough *et al.*, 1983). Histologically the ileal carcinoid tumour exhibits dense clusters of cells that histochemically show an argentaffin reaction (Oates, 1980). It has been postulated that the neurofibromas in NF1 and carcinoid tumours have a common neuroendocrine origin (Fernandez *et al.*, 1988) and in one case report an intestinal neurofibroma showed evidence of transition into a carcinoid tumour (Arnesjo *et al.*, 1983).

The carcinoid syndrome is almost always produced by tumours derived from enterochromaffin cells and the principal mediators are serotonin with tachykinins and histamine. Rarely, the syndrome is produced from ovarian or testicular teratomas. The syndrome consists of cutaneous flushing, diarrhoea, right-sided heart valve lesions, facial telangiectasia and bronchoconstriction. The liver is able to inactivate hormones released into the portal circulation, so that the syndrome manifests only after carcinoid tumours have metastasized to the liver.

The carcinoid syndrome can be diagnosed by finding raised levels of the serotonin metabolite, 5-hydroxyindoleacetic acid, in the urine. Surgical resection of the primary tumour results in cure if it has not metastasized, and patients may experience prolonged symptomatic relief if the liver metastases can be removed. Somatostatin and its analogue SMS201–995 improve diarrhoea, flushing and bronchoconstriction (Kvols *et al.*, 1986).

A striking feature of carcinoid tumours in NF1 is their tendency to occur in the duodenum and especially in the region of the ampulla of Vater. In a recent series, nine out of 16 carcinoid tumours located in the duodenum occurred in patients with NF1 (Dayal *et al.*, 1986). In contrast only 0.2–0.3% of these tumours are located on the ampulla of Vater in the general population (Hough *et al.*, 1983). Duodenal carcinoid tumours present in adult life. When associated with NF1 they are more common in black people (Burke *et al.*, 1990). Patients with duodenal carcinoid tumours may be asymptomatic, but eventually present with jaundice, upper intestinal bleeding or intestinal obstruction. Tumours larger than 2 cm have almost invariably metastasized when diagnosed. They may be treated by local excision with biliary diversion (Johnson and Weaver, 1981). Since carcinoid tumours and phaeochromocytomas may occur in the same patient with NF1, and carcinoid tumours may be asymptomatic, the duodenum should be examined in any patient undergoing surgery for phaeochromocytoma (Wheeler, Curley and Williams, 1986).

In addition to the association with NF1, patients with carcinoid tumours have been reported to have an increased risk of developing second tumours, notably gliomas and meningiomas (Hough *et al.*, 1983).

13.8.2 Gastrointestinal neurofibromas

In addition to carcinoid tumours, neurofibromas and other tumours of the gastrointestinal tract have been reported in NF1. Gastrointestinal tumours have been recognized in NF1 since von Recklinghausen described a patient in whom neurofibromas in the stomach and jejunum underwent malignant change (von Recklinghausen, 1882). Davis and Berk (1973) estimated that gastrointestinal neurofibromas develop in about 25% of NF1 patients, but conversely only 15% of patients with gastrointestinal neurofibromas have NF1. In a recent population study, Huson, Harper and Compston (1988) reported gastrointestinal neurofibromas in 2.1% of patients. In addition to neurofibromas, leiomyomas, ganglioneuromas and sarcomas have been identified. The most common location of neurofibromas is the jejunum followed by the stomach, but multiple sites of involvement have been reported. The tumours are usually situated in the serosa and some cases have hyperplasia of Auerbach's plexus, suggesting a disturbance of neuronal proliferation (Hochberg *et al.*, 1974).

The tumours occur in both sexes and symptoms usually occur in adulthood. They range from pain, dyspepsia and constipation to haematemesis and melaena. The tumours may also cause obstruction or perforation. Because of difficulties in identifying these tumours, the average time from symptom onset to diagnosis has been as long as 3 years (Hochberg *et al.*, 1974).

13.8.3 Gangliocytic paraganglioma

Gangliocytic paraganglioma is a duodenal tumour consisting of both neural and epithelial elements and there is some dispute as to whether it constitutes a hamartoma arising from maldevelopment of the pancreas or a relatively benign neoplasm (Stephens *et al.*, 1987). Of 50 cases reported, two were associated with NF1. The tumours usually occur in middle-aged males and present with epigastric pain and gastrointestinal haemorrhage, which can be cured by resection of the tumour. The two cases with NF1 were women. One presented with epigastric pain, nausea and vomiting with concomitant rise in alkaline phosphatase and the symptoms resolved after operation (Kheir and Halpern, 1984). The other patient was asymptomatic but undergoing surgery for bilateral phaeochromocytomas when she was discovered to have a carcinoid tumour and a duodenal gangliocytic paraganglioma. The patient died of myocardial infarction several months later and a postmortem examination showed no evidence that the tumour had spread beyond the duodenum (Stephens *et al.*, 1987).

13.8.4 Ganglioneuromatosis

Ganglioneuromatosis is a rare complication of NF1. It consists of dysplastic proliferation of the myenteric plexuses and ganglion cells in the small and large bowel, stomach and the oesophagus (Phat *et al.*, 1980). Patients present with abdominal discomfort and constipation.

13.9 UROGENITAL TRACT

Although Wilms' tumour, a highly malignant renal sarcoma occurring in children, has been reported in association with NF1, the association is extremely rare and probably coincidental (Chapter 12).

Neurofibromas in the retroperitoneal space may compress the urinary pelvis and calyces and cause hydronephrosis. Neurofibromas in the pelvis may compress or involve the bladder and urethra causing difficulty in micturition (Clark *et al.*, 1977; Batta, Gundian and Myers, 1989).

An uncommon but important issue is the occurrence of neurofibromas affecting the genitalia. Tumours at this site have obvious psychosexual consequences. Plexiform neurofibromas can cause hypertrophy of the perineal tissues and lead to misdiagnosis of an intersex state (Kaneti *et al.*, 1988). In one report an 11-year-old girl with NF1 had progressive enlargement of the clitoris and labium majus from early childhood. A biopsy revealed that the abnormal genital growth was due to a neurofibroma and she was treated with clitorectomy and clitoroplasty (Nogita *et al.*, 1990).

13.10 GROWTH DISTURBANCE

The most common general medical disturbance in NF1 is an abnormally short stature, which occurs in about a third of patients with NF1 (Huson, Harper and Compston, 1988; Ferner and Hughes, unpublished data). The cause of this short stature is not clear: in most cases there is no tumour, growth hormone deficiency or hypothyroidism, and an alteration of growth control related to the *NF1* gene is likely. In rare cases, short stature is associated with a chiasmal glioma and may be due to a hypothalamic disturbance (Schimke, 1990).

13.11 DISTURBANCES OF PUBERTY

Although precocious and delayed puberty have been reported in NF1, both are rare. Normally the onset of puberty is marked by increased growth of the genitalia and skeleton, development of secondary sexual characteristics and the capacity to produce children. These changes develop over a period of 4 years owing to the combined effects of sex steroids and growth hormone. Puberty is triggered by increased secretion of the pituitary gonadotrophins, follicle-stimulating hormone (FSH) and luteinizing hormone (LH), which are under the control of the hypothalamic gonadotrophin-releasing hormone, luteinizing hormone releasing hormone (LHRH). The age of onset of puberty varies widely around the world. In Britain the mean age is 11.5 years for boys and 10.5 years for girls.

When precocious puberty occurs in NF1, it is usually associated with an optic pathway glioma that has extended into the hypothalamus. For instance, Laue *et al.* (1985) reported three children with NF1 who all had optic gliomas, precocious puberty and high serum concentrations of sex steroids and gonadotrophins. Conventional treatment with surgery and radiotherapy is usually needed. In addition, the long-acting LHRH analogue, D-Trp6-Pro9-NEt-LHRH, can be used to reduce gonadotrophin and sex steroid levels. After treatment, secondary sexual characteristics may remain unchanged or regress. Reductions in growth rate and bone age maturation have been documented (Laue *et al.*, 1985).

Patients with NF1 should be distinguished from those with the McCune–Albright's syndrome, which comprises precocious puberty, irregular skin pigmentation and polyostotic fibrous dysplasia.

Delayed puberty has been reported in NF1, but is uncommon, affecting only 1.5% of the patients in the series of Huson, Harper and Compston (1988). Only two of 669 NF1 patients reported by Riccardi and Eichner (1986) had delayed puberty, and in one of these the delay was associated with, and possibly due to, hydrocephalus.

Since disturbances of sexual maturation are rare in NF1, and when present are often due to a structural lesion, their cause should always be carefully investigated. There are many other causes of delayed puberty, including constitutional and emotional factors, hypothalamic tumours, craniopharyngiomas, pituitary tumours, gonadal dysgenesis, chronic systemic disease, cranial irradiation and chemotherapy. If necessary, puberty may be induced in boys by regular intramuscular testosterone oenanthate and in girls by administering oral ethinyloestradiol (Wu, 1989).

13.12 PREGNANCY

There is no clear indication that NF1 leads to infertility, but patients may experience complications during pregnancy as a consequence of neurofibromatosis. In theory, uterine neurofibromas may cause difficulty in implantation of the fetus and vaginal neurofibromas may impede delivery, but in practice neurofibromas cause little difficulty. Jarvis and Crompton (1978) found no significant obstetric problems in 10 NF1 patients with 27 pregnancies. I have a patient who had a normal pregnancy and delivery despite a large vaginal neurofibroma.

Swapp and Main (1973) reported that 10 of 11 patients with NF1 developed hypertension during pregnancy. They hypothesized that the vascular changes of NF1 are triggered by pregnancy and that damaged arterioles could not expand to meet the rise in plasma volume and red cell mass, leading to relative stenosis to the organs supplied. It is particularly important to monitor blood pressure closely during and after pregnancy in women with NF1 because of the possibility that renal artery stenosis or phaeochromocytoma become evident at this time.

Pregnancy may cause an increase in the size and number of dermal neurofibromas, but according to Swapp and Main (1973) they often regress after delivery.

Renal artery stenosis and phaeochromocytoma may both be present during pregnancy. Phaeochromocytomas carry a high risk of mortality and morbidity for both mother and fetus. Careful monitoring of the blood pressure is particularly important in women planning conception and throughout pregnancy.

NOTE

The MEN 2A gene has recently been cloned making direct mutation analysis an approach for DNA analysis applicable to all families (Mulligan *et al.*, 1993).

REFERENCES

Ardissone, F., Andrion, A., D'Alessandro, L. *et al.* (1986) Neurogenic intrathoracic tumours, a clinicopathological review of 92 cases. *Thorac. Cardiovasc. Surg.*, **34**, 260–4.

Arnesjo, B., Idvall, I., Ihse, I. *et al.* (1983) Concomitant occurrence of neurofibromatosis and carcinoid of the intestine. *Scand. J. Gastroenterol.*, **8**, 637–43.

Batta, A.G., Gundian, J.C. and Myers, R.P. (1989) Neurofibromatosis presenting as perineal pain and urethral burning. *Urology*, **33**, 138–40.

Bourke, E. and Gatenby, P.B.B. (1971) Renal artery dysplasia with hypertension in neurofibromatosis. *Br. Med. J.*, **2**, 681–2.

Burke, A.P., Usaf, M.C., Sobin, L.H. *et al.* (1990) Somatostatin-producing duodenal carcinoids in patients with von Recklinghausen's neurofibromatosis. A predilection for black patients. *Cancer*, **65**, 1591–5.

Chan, F.L. and Wang, C. (1989) Imaging for adrenal tumours. *Clin. Endocrinol. Metab.*, **3**(1), 153–89.

Clark, W.C., Marlett, M.M., Prudencio, R.F. and Das Gupta, T.K. (1977) Neurofibromatosis of the bladder in children: case report and literature review. *J. Urol.*, **118**, 654–6.

Cryer, P.E. (1985) Phaeochromocytoma. *Clin. Endocrinol. Metab.*, **14**(1), 203–20.

D'Angio, G.J., Beckwith, J.B., Breslow, N.E. *et al.* (1978) Neurofibromatosis and interstitial lung disease. *Arch. Dermatol.*, **114**, 1368–9.

Davis, G.B. and Berk, R.N. (1973) Intestinal neurofibromas in von Recklinghausen's disease. *Am. J. Gastroenterol.*, **60**, 410–14.

Dayal, Y., Talberg, K.A., Nunnemacher, G. *et al.* (1986) Duodenal carcinoids in patients with and without neurofibromatosis. *Am. J. Surg. Pathol.*, **10**(5), 348–57.

Drury, P. (1989) Endocrine hypertension. *Med. Int.*, **64**, 2664–9.

Evans, A.E. (1980) Staging and treatment of neuroblastoma. *Cancer*, **45**, 1799–802.

Fernandez, M.T., Puig, L., Capella, G. *et al.* (1988) Von Recklinghausen neurofibromatosis with carcinoid tumor and submucous leiomyomas of the duodenum. *Neurofibromatosis*, **1**, 294–8.

Fitzpatrick, A.P. and Emanuel, R.W. (1988) Familial neurofibromatosis and hypertrophic cardiomyopathy. *Br. Heart J.*, **60**, 247–51.

Gagel, R.F., Armen, H., Tashjian, A.H., Jr *et al.* (1988) The clinical outcome of prospective screening for multiple endocrine neoplasia type 2a. *N. Engl. J. Med.*, **318**, 478–83.

Goldstraw, P. (1990) Mediastinal disorders, in *Respiratory Medicine* (eds R.A.L. Brewis, G.J. Gibson and D.M. Geddes), Baillière Tindall, London, Ch. 45, p. 1445.

Heimberger, I., Battersby, J.S. and Velios, F. (1963) Primary neoplasms of the mediastinum: a fifteen year experience. *Arch. Surg.*, **86**, 978–84.

Hochberg, F.H., Dasilva, A.B., Galdabini, J. and Richardson, E.P. (1974) Gastrointestinal involvement in von Recklinghausen's neurofibromatosis. *Neurology*, **24**, 1144–51.

Hope, D.G. and Mulvihill, J.J. (1981) Malignancy in neurofibromatosis. *Adv. Neurol.*, **29**, 33–56.

Hough, D.R., Usar, M.C., Chan, A. *et al.* (1983) Von Recklinghausen's disease associated with gastrointestinal carcinoid tumours. *Cancer*, **51**, 2206–8.

Huson, S.M. (1989) Recent developments in the diagnosis and management of neurofibromatosis. *Arch. Dis. Child.*, **64**, 745–9.

Huson, S.M., Harper, P.S. and Compston, D.A.S. (1988) Von Recklinghausen neurofibromatosis: a clinical and population study in southeast Wales. *Brain*, **111**, 1355–81.

Jackson, C.E., Norum, R.A., O'Neal, L.W. *et al.* (1988) Linkage between MEN 2B and chromosome 10 markers linked to MEN 2A. *Am. J. Hum. Genet.*, **43**, A147.

Jarvis, G.J. and Crompton, A.C. (1978) Neurofibromatosis and pregnancy. *Br. J. Obstet. Gynaecol.*, **85**, 844–6.

Johnson, L. and Weaver, M. (1981) Von Recklinghausen's disease and gastrointestinal carcinoids. *JAMA*, **245**, 2496.

Kaneti, J., Lieberman, E., Moshe, P. and Carmi, R. (1988) A case of ambiguous genitalia owing to neurofibromatosis – review of the literature. *J. Urol.*, **140**, 584–5.

Kheir, S.M. and Halpern, N.B. (1984) Paraganglioma of the duodenum in association with congenital neurofibromatosis. Possible relationship. *Cancer*, **53**, 2491–6.

Knudson, A.G., Jr (1981) A geneticist's view of neurofibromatosis. *Adv. Neurol.*, **29**, 237–42.

Kvols, L.K., Moertel, C.G., O'Connell, M.J. *et al.* (1986) Treatment of the malignant carcinoid syndrome: evaluation of a long-acting somatostatin analogue. *N. Engl. J. Med.*, **315**, 663–6.

Laue, L., Comite, F., Hench, K. *et al.* (1985) Precocious puberty associated with neurofibromatosis and optic gliomas. Treatment with luteinizing hormone releasing hormone analogue. *Am. J. Dis. Child.*, **139**, 1097–100.

Lin, A.E. and Garver, K.L. (1988) Cardiac abnormalities in neurofibromatosis. *Neurofibromatosis*, **1**, 146–51.

Mulligan, L.M., Kwok, J.B., Healey, C.S. *et al.* (1993) Germ-line mutations of the *RET* proto-oncogene in multiple endocrine neoplasia type 2A. *Nature*, **363**, 458–60.

Neiman, H.L., Holt, M.E., Stern, A.M. and Perry, B.L. (1974) Neurofibromatosis and congenital heart disease. *AJR*, **122**, 146–9.

Nesbit, M. (1990) Advances and management of solid tumours in children. *Cancer*, **65**, 696–702.

Nogita, T., Kawabata, Y., Tsuchida, T. *et al.* (1990) Clitoral and labial involvement of neurofibromatosis. *J. Am. Acad. Dermatol.*, **23**, 937–8.

Oates, J.A. (1980) Carcinoid syndrome, in *Harrison's Principles of Internal Medicine*, 9th edn (eds K.J. Isselbacher, R.D. Adams, E. Braunwald *et al.*), McGraw-Hill, New York, Ch. 91, pp. 476–9.

Oates, J.A. (1986) The carcinoid syndrome. *N. Engl. J. Med.*, **315**, 702–3.

Ogilvie, C.M. (1990) Symptoms and signs, in *Respiratory Medicine*, (eds R.A.L. Brewis, G.J. Gibson and D.M. Geddes), Baillière Tindall, London.

Phat, V.N., Sezeur, A., Danne, M. *et al.* (1980) Primary myenteric plexus alterations as a cause of megacolon in von Recklinghausen's disease. *Pathol. Biol.* (Paris), **28**, 585–8.

Pollard, S.G., Hornick, P., Macfarlane, R. and Calne, R.Y. (1989) Renovascular hypertension in neurofibromatosis. *Postgrad. Med. J.*, **65**, 31–3.

Ponder, B. (1990) Multiple endocrine neoplasia type 2. *Br. Med. J.*, **300**, 484–5.

Pung, S. and Hirsch, E.F. (1955) Plexiform neurofibromatosis of the heart and neck. *Arch. Pathol.*, **59**, 341–6.

Reubi, F. (1945) Neurofibromatose et lesions vasculaires. *Schweiz med. Wochenschrift*, **75**, 463–5.

Riccardi, V.M. and Eichner, J.E. (1986) *Neurofibromatosis: Phenotype, Natural History and Pathogenesis*, Johns Hopkins University Press, Baltimore.

Ross, E.J. and Griffith, D.N.W. (1989) The clinical presentation of phaeochromocytoma. *Q. J. Med.*, **71**, 485–96.

Roviaro, G., Montorsi, M., Varoli, F. *et al.* (1983) Primary pulmonary tumours of neurogenic origin. *Thorax*, **38**, 942.

Salyer, W.R. and Salyer, D.C. (1974) The vascular lesions of neurofibromatosis. *Angiology*, **25**, 510–18.

Schimke, R.N. (1986) Multiple endocrine neoplasia: search for the oncogenic trigger. *N. Engl. J. Med.*, **314**, 1315–16.

Schimke, R.N. (1990) The endocrine system in neurofibromatosis, in *Neurofibromatosis: a Handbook for Patients, Families, and Healthcare Professionals* (eds A.E. Rubenstein and B.R. Korf), Thieme, New York, Ch. 13, pp. 142–9.

Schorry, E.K., Stowens, D.W., Crawford, A.H. *et al.* (1989) Summary of patient data from a multidisciplinary neurofibromatosis clinic. *Neurofibromatosis*, **2**, 129–34.

Spiro, S.G. (1990) Lung tumours, in *Respiratory Medicine* (eds R.A.L. Brewis, G.J. Gibson and D.M. Geddes), Baillière Tindall, London, p. 874.

Stack, B.H.R. and Thomas, J. St. J. (1990) Pulmonary infiltrations, in *Respiratory Medicine* (eds R.A.L. Brewis, G.J. Gibson and D.M. Geddes), Baillière Tindall, London, p. 1188.

Stephens, M., Williams, G.T., Jasani, B. and Williams, E.D. (1987) Synchronous duodenal neuroendocrine tumours in von Recklinghausen disease. A case report of co-existing gangliocytic paraganglioma and somatostatin-rich glandular carcinoid. *Histopathology*, **11**, 1331–40.

Swapp, G.H. and Main, R.A. (1973) Neurofibromatosis in pregnancy. *Br. J. Dermatol.*, **80**, 431–5.

von Recklinghausen, K. (1882) *Uber die multiplen Fibrome der Haut und ihre Beziehung zu den multiplen Neuromen*, Hirschwald, Berlin.

Wheeler, M.H., Curley, I.R. and Williams, E.D. (1986) The association of neurofibromatosis, phaeochromocytoma and somatostatin-rich duodenal carcinoid tumour. *Surgery*, **100**, 1163–9.

Wu, F.C.W. (1989) Delayed puberty. *Med. Int.*, **64**, 2638–43.

14

Reconstructive surgery for neurofibromatosis

M.F. Angel, J.A. Persing and M.T. Edgerton

14.1 INTRODUCTION

The goals of reconstructive surgery in patients with neurofibromatosis are similar to those in patients with other conditions. The surgeon's first aim is to preserve function, both sensory (vision and hearing) and motor (deglutition, speech, respiration and muscle motion). Secondly, the surgeon aims to achieve an aesthetic appearance for the patient that is as normal as possible. The reconstructive considerations are different for the individual forms of neurofibromatosis. For example, in neurofibromatosis 1 (NF1), treatment for multiple skin and mass disorders predominates, while in neurofibromatosis 2 (NF2), facial nerve palsy treatment is the prime focus of attention for the reconstructive surgeon.

14.1.1 Factors affecting surgical interventions in NF1

(a) General factors

The reconstructive surgical effort is guided by a number of variables: the age of the patient, the type of NF1 involvement (plexiform neurofibroma, pigmented naevus, cutaneous pedunculated neurofibroma), site and growth rate of the neurofibromatosis tissue, and the associated functional and aesthetic deformities caused by the tissue overgrowth. Because of the multiplicity of factors involved, the ultimate treatment plan for a given patient is highly individualized. Individualized treatment plans notwithstanding, there are several guiding principles one can use in approaching a patient with NF1.

(b) Effect of type of NF1

Because NF1 is a progressive condition throughout childhood and early adulthood, it may be argued that the best chance for cure from the effects of this condition is total eradication of the involved tissues in early childhood. This is impractical, however, because the disease is diffuse and limits of the involvement are often unknown. Sacrifice of all the involved tissue would usually result in too great a functional loss or extraordinary disfigurement. The concept, therefore, of subtotal removal for this disease has been championed by several authors (Conley, 1972; Griffith *et al.*, 1972; Grabb *et al.*, 1980).

Before this view became predominant, however, several issues had to be resolved. In multiple series, the rate of malignant degeneration of neurofibromas has been between 2 and 16% (Hosoi, 1931; Preston, Walsh and Clarke, 1951; Feinman and Yakovac, 1970; Griffith *et al.*, 1972), with more recent studies giving a lower incidence of malignancy of approximately 2% (Griffith *et al.*, 1972; Knight, Murphy and Gottlieb, 1973; Maceri and Saxon, 1984). Total resection to remove a malignancy is therefore only indicated in a small number of cases (Aird, 1958; Feinman and Yakovac, 1970). Some have suggested that subtotal resection is harmful because it leads to malignant degeneration and is a stimulus for further tumour growth. However, this opinion has not been substantiated by the work of Griffith *et al.* (1972) and Maceri and Saxon (1984).

The type of NF1 aids the surgeon in his/her decision-making. There are three clinical presentations of NF1 that are of particular interest to plastic surgeons.

- A patient with **multiple dermal neurofibromas** presents with multiple nodules in the cutaneous tissue; during his or her lifetime, a patient may have hundreds of these lesions. Trying totally to eradicate all of these tumours is futile, so the goal of surgery therefore becomes removal of the cutaneous neurofibromas having the greatest effect on the patient's function and appearance.
- The **nodular plexiform neurofibroma** form is typified by a tortuous enlargement of peripheral nerves. This usually occurs deep within the tissue, involving major nerve trunks (often within the orbit, neck or trunk). Superficial excisions will therefore have only fleeting benefit.
- The **diffuse plexiform neurofibroma** form of NF1 is associated with massive enlargement of limbs and other bony structures. This regional gigantism may require not only removing soft tissue but also reducing bone bulk and decreasing limb growth.

(c) Effect of site of involvement

The site of involvement is a major factor in selecting the optimal reconstructive approach. Adkins and Ravitch (1977) found that masses in the head and neck area were the presenting complaint in 22% of patients, while soft-tissue masses in the extremities occurred in 16%. Bone disorders of the long bones (26%) and scoliosis (21%) were also important presenting complaints. Finally, central nervous system (CNS) involvement was noted in 8% of cases; some of these present at the skull base (Roland, Glasscock and Bojrab, 1986).

Reports by others (Davis, Edgerton and Hoffmeister, 1954; Mukherji, 1974; Grabb *et al.*, 1980; Bromley, Sherman and Goulian, 1981; Maceri and Saxon, 1984; Griffith, Lewis and McKinney, 1985; Shack, Reilley and Lynch, 1985; Spira and Riccardi, 1987) have likewise found a significant number of NF1 patients presenting with head and neck lesions. The recurrent theme, however, in all series of NF1 patients is the protean nature of the disease.

14.2 SURGICAL OPTIONS IN NF1

The extent of the tumour may prohibit complete resection without a total thickness removal of skin, subcutaneous tissue, motor and sensory

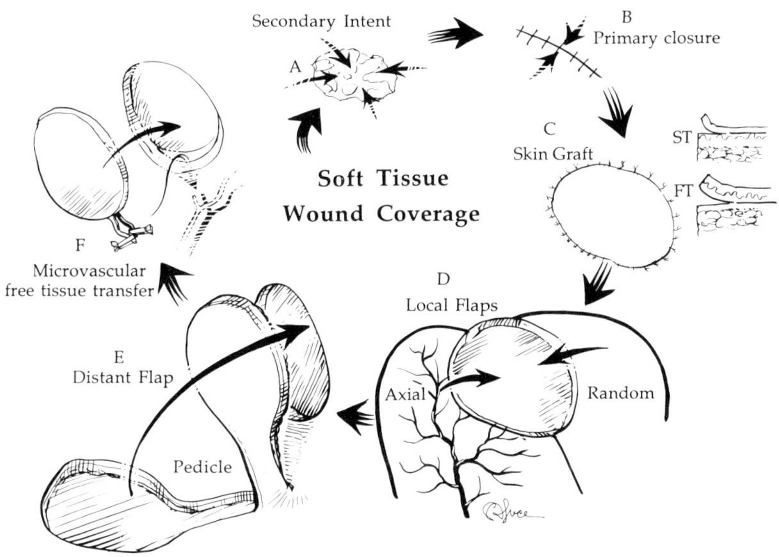

Figure 14.1 Hierarchy of wound closure. (a) Healing by secondary intention; this allows epithelialization and wound contraction leading to healing. (b) Direct closure. (c) Healing by skin grafts, which can be either split thickness (ST) or full thickness (FT). (d) Reconstruction by local flaps; these are based on transposition and rotation principles. (e) Reconstruction by distant flaps; tissue not in proximity to the wound is brought to it. (f) Reconstruction by free tissue transfer; tissue is isolated on its vascular pedicle, transferred to the wound and vascular continuity is re-established using microvascular technique.

nerves, eyelids and frontal bones (Davis, Edgerton and Hoffmeister, 1954; Crikelair and Cosman, 1968; Griffith *et al.*, 1972; Mukherji, 1974; Grabb *et al.*, 1980). Therefore, multiple subtotal resections over years is a prudent means of managing many of these large lesions (Grabb *et al.*, 1980). The soft-tissue defects thus produced can be approached by selection of either wound closure by secondary intention, direct closure, skin grafting or local or distant flaps (Figure 14.1).

14.2.1 Secondary intention

A hierarchy of wound management exists, and the first option to consider is allowing the wound to close secondarily (i.e. without further surgical intervention). The wound-healing phenomenon is primarily controlled by epithelialization and wound contraction. If a wound occurs over a stable bony surface, and is out of sight, secondary healing results in an unobtrusive contracture. However, if a wound in a mobile area is allowed to heal secondarily, this can lead to unwanted distortion of tissues, such as an ectropion of the lower eyelid or elbow contracture. Rarely is this treatment approach elected in healing with NF1 lesions.

14.2.2 Direct closure

The next approach is direct closure of the wound. A factor to be considered in decision-making is the orientation of the wound margins. Borges (1971, 1973) has commented on the importance of 'lines of least-tension' in the skin, and has mapped out patterns of these lines throughout the body (Figure 14.2). When planning an excision of skin anywhere on the body, and in particular on the face and around joints at the extremities, one should consider the orientation of these lines in order to place the long axis of the excision, if possible, parallel to them. This aids in wound closure and succeeds in reducing the amount and width of scarring postoperatively.

If a wound cannot be closed directly, one can either close the wound with a skin graft or use flaps.

14.2.3 Reconstruction by skin grafts

Skin grafts can be harvested from any part of the body. If the entire epidermis and dermis are transferred, this is a full-thickness graft. Thinner grafts incorporating only a portion of the dermis are known as split-thickness grafts (McGregor, 1980; Rudolph and Ballantyne, 1990). Skin thickness varies throughout the body, primarily due to height of the dermis, as the height of the epidermis remains relatively constant. Regions of increased thickness of the skin (legs, buttocks) are favoured

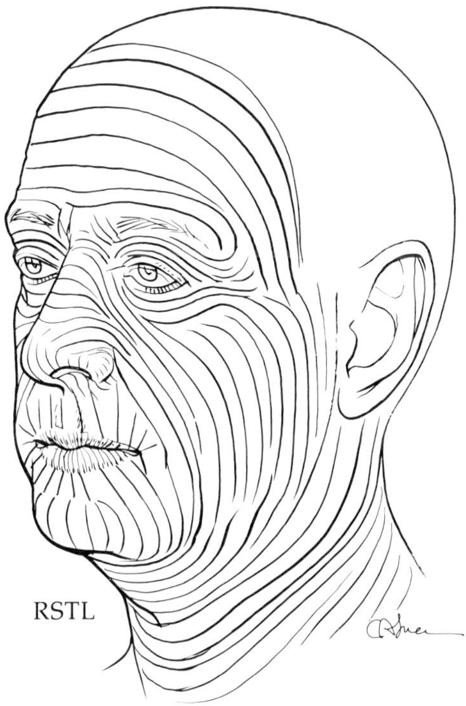

Figure 14.2 Resting skin tension lines (RSTL). Incisions placed parallel to them will heal with the best scar, while incisions perpendicular to them will heal with a less optimal scar owing to increased skin tension.

sites for split-thickness graft harvesting because of their ability to regenerate new skin readily from epithelium-producing elements deeper in the dermis, and their relatively hidden location on the body with normal garments.

When considering whether a graft is appropriate for a particular defect and what type, several factors are important. Colour match is a major consideration. In Caucasians the skin of the head and neck is 'pinker' than the rest of the body. Therefore, when one places a graft on the face, the graft should be harvested from the head and neck area to maintain this similarity. If a graft is taken from the leg or buttocks and placed on the face, it will appear sallow and yellow. In Black patients it may appear darker than the surrounding skin.

Full-thickness grafts retard wound contraction and distortion to a greater degree than split-thickness grafts, even if both types of graft are the same thickness by absolute measurement. This is an important observation, particularly when replacing skin defects about the eyelids,

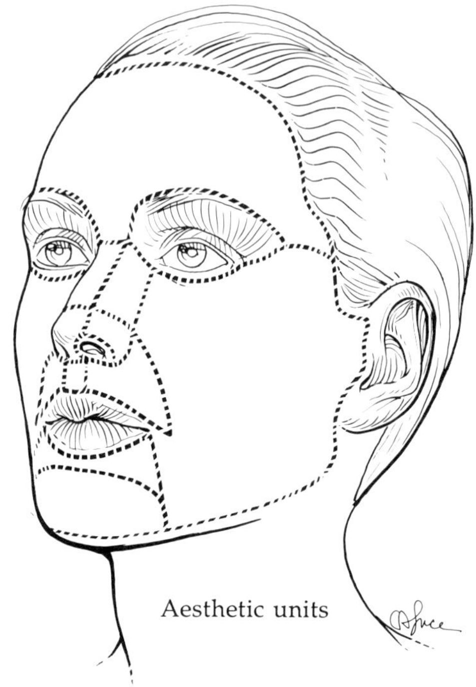

Figure 14.3 'Aesthetic units'. Skin grafts placed on the natural boundaries of the nose, chin, forehead and periorbital areas are less noticeable than those placed on only part of these units.

where wound contracture (even with thick split-thickness grafts) may lead to eyelid distortion and ectropion.

In grafting the face, the concept of 'aesthetic units' is also important (Figure 14.3). As noted by others (Menick, 1987), grafts placed on the natural boundaries of the nose, cheek, chin or forehead are less noticeable than those placed on only a part of these units. Preservation of the normal boundaries of an anatomical structure is more easily masked to the objective viewer (not as disfiguring), whereas interruption of these lines are readily recognized as abnormal.

The amount of trauma a given area will experience in everyday postoperative life also dictates the thickness of the chosen graft. One would want a thicker, more durable graft for the palms of the hand or soles of the feet than for the trunk, because of the more significant daily trauma to the hands and feet.

14.2.4 Reconstruction by local flaps

If the defect for reconstruction is too deep to be adequately reconstructed by skin grafts because the variation in height of the skin surface would be too noticeable, or if even minimal wound contracture is undesirable, skin flaps should be chosen as the best reconstruction alternative. There are an array of local flaps that can be used. Movement of these flaps is based on the principle of rotation or transposition (Figure 14.1), and is feasible because in most parts of the body there is some inherent laxity of skin. Rotation flaps are particularly useful for triangular-shaped defects, and transposition flaps are more suited to rectangular defects. Combinations of these flaps may be used for even the most complex geometric designs of wound defects.

Local flaps may be categorized (Daniel, 1975a,b; Daniel and Kerrigan, 1990) based on the pattern of blood supply to the skin, as random (nurtured by subdermal plexus of capillaries) or axial (a dominant blood vessel is identified extending to the subdermal plexus), or by whether the site of origin of the dominant blood vessel is through muscle (Ger, 1972; McGraw, 1986) or fascia (fasciocutaneous) (Ponten, 1981; Tolhurst, Haeseker and Zeeman, 1983).

In the head and neck region, nasolabial, cheek or glabellar local flaps are often used (Borges, 1973; Karapandzic, 1974; McGregor, 1980) because of local skin laxity. Skin laxity is also present in the torso, but to a lesser extent. In the scalp and four extremities, however, the skin is taut, which places limits on flap design. For these areas, musculocutaneous and fasciocutaneous flaps from other regions of the body are often used.

14.2.5 Tissue expanders

The use of tissue expanders has recently allowed the surgeon to increase the amount of local tissue that can be used for reconstruction, usually in local flaps. This technique was introduced by Radovan (1984) and involves the placement of an expandable receptacle under the desired quality soft tissue. Over the ensuing weeks, the expander is increased in size by the injection of saline through a subcutaneous port, and in so doing, increases the surface area of the overlying tissue by 60% or more.

While biophysical bases of this process are not yet entirely understood (Austad *et al.*, 1982; Manders *et al.*, 1984; Austad, Thomas and Pasyk, 1986), this technique has been used successfully in the scalp (Manders *et al.*, 1982), trunk (Argenta, 1984; Manders *et al.*, 1984) and extremities (Edgerton and Morgan, 1985; Van Beck and Adson, 1987). It also has a place in the management of defects in patients with NF1 (Figure 14.4).

14.2.6 Reconstruction with distant flaps

The next surgical option for NF1 reconstruction is closure by distant flaps, which are either of the pedicled or microvascular free tissue transfer type.

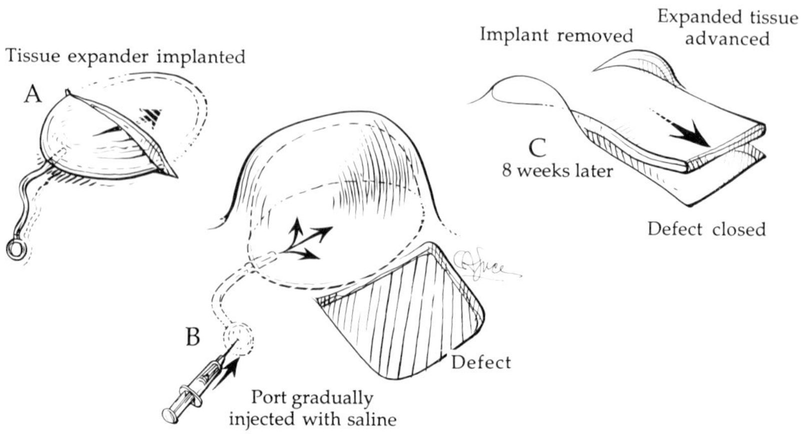

Figure 14.4 Tissue expansion. (A) The expander is first implanted; (B) after several weeks, expansion is commenced by injecting sterile saline percutaneously through the port; this is done as an outpatient and is well tolerated; (C) once expansion is complete, the expander is removed and flaps are transposed.

The pedicle of the flap is the bridge of tissue that provides circulation to the flap. Although successful in many cases, this technique often requires several lengthy steps before final closure of the wound is achieved. For this reason, their usefulness has been greatly decreased with the arrival of microsurgical techniques.

Using the operative microscope to transfer tissue from one region of the body to another, the design of the flap and its composition (skin only, skin plus muscle, etc.) can be fashioned to the particular requirements of the defect in question. Microvascular free tissue transfer has the additional advantage of avoiding the extreme body positioning needed for prolonged periods of time when the pedicle flap is used (Chicarilli and Davey, 1989). Microvascular transfer of flaps is now reliable, with overall success rates of approximately 95%, proving certain types of tissue transfer are now cost-effective (O'Brien and Morrison, 1987).

14.3 SPECIFIC RECONSTRUCTIONS

14.3.1 Scalp

The scalp (with its hairy skin) provides protection for the calvaria and ultimately the brain. It is often involved in NF1 lesions and is important in a patient's body image.

The scalp is highly vascular, being supplied by five paired arteries from the external (superficial temporal, postauricular and occipital) and internal (supraorbital and supratrochlear) carotid systems. There are rich

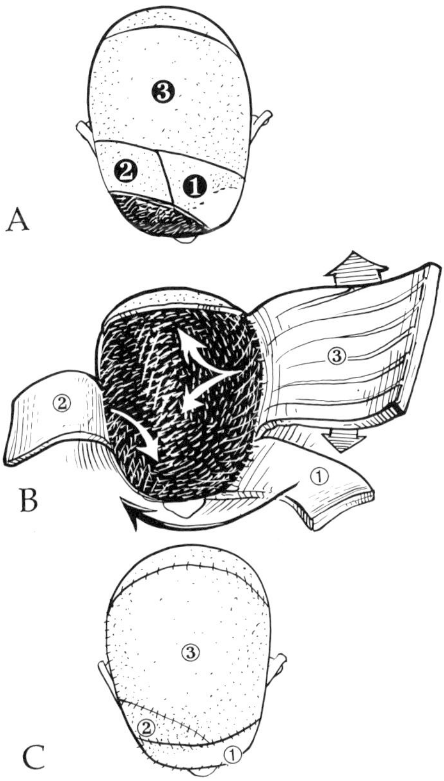

Figure 14.5 The three-flap procedure of Orticochea. (A) Flaps are initially outlined; (B) flaps are incised, elevated and galea is incised to allow further flap expansion (arrows); (C) flaps are rotated into new position.

anastomoses between these systems, which allow for significant variation in flap design to cover scalp defects. However, these anastomoses (Horowitz *et al.*, 1984) are variable and decrease with age. Pericranial flaps, which require support from an anastomotic network that crosses the midline of the skull in individuals older than 60 years, are particularly vulnerable to ischaemic flap loss. The scalp is also relatively inelastic compared with skin elsewhere owing to the fibrous nature of the galea aponeurosi. These features must all be taken into consideration when reconstructing the scalp.

Small wounds (2–4 cm) can often be closed primarily after undermining the skin edges and releasing skin tension from the galea. For larger lesions, local flaps can be used. For moderate-sized wounds (10–14 cm), the three-flap procedure of Orticochea (1967, 1971) (Figure 14.5) or tissue expansion (Manders *et al.*, 1982) may be used.

14.3.2 Forehead

The forehead, like the scalp, has rich blood supply, allowing many different flap designs. Unlike the scalp, however, the forehead is thinner and much more pliable, making reconstruction in this area easier.

Small to moderate defects in this area can be closed either primarily or by the use of local flaps as in other areas. The excision lines should be orientated transversely in the mid and upper forehead, and vertically near the glabella, so as to be parallel with the resting skin tension lines.

As defects increase in size, larger local flaps from the scalp or skin grafts are more desirable. The advantage of using local scalp tissue is that a large amount of well-vascularized tissue can be brought to the defect site. The major disadvantage is that the flap is a multiple-stage procedure. Alternatively, the major advantage of skin grafts is that they are easily performed with little donor site morbidity. Their use presupposes the presence of an adequately vascularized wound, e.g. when the pericranium on the skull is present. However, vascularization of the skin graft is only rarely successful if placed on bare bone. Vascularized tissue can be elevated as pericranial flaps to create a bed over the bare bone, which is suitable for grafting (Horowitz *et al.*, 1984; Terranova, 1990).

To get the best colour match for defects in the facial region, skin from the neck and supraclavicular area should be used. When a large area of the forehead needs to be skin grafted, consideration should be given to grafting the entire forehead (a single aesthetic unit). Clipper-shaving the scalp, followed by taking a large split-thickness graft from this site, has provided a large amount of excellent colour-matched tissue for this purpose with minimal donor site morbidity.

14.3.3 Eyelid and orbit

Eyelid and orbital involvement in NF1 (Munro and Martin, 1980; Van der Meulen *et al.*, 1982; Jackson, Laws and Martin, 1983; Marchac, 1984; Poole, 1989) is a relatively common presentation to the plastic surgeon. In Marchac's series (1984) of 21 patients presenting with NF1, 81% (17/21) had orbital/palpebral manifestation. The eyelids alone were involved in seven of these patients, with severe disease noted in the remaining 10.

Blepharoptosis (drooping eyelid) commonly occurs when NF1 involves the eyelid and orbital structures, severity depending on the location and the size of the tumour. Smith and English (1970) noted that the lid margin of the ptotic eyelid displays a 'peculiar sinuous configuration' because the tumour is located lateral to the levator muscle. As the tumour is often adjacent to the conjunctiva, in selected cases transconjunctival excision may be performed with no visible scars.

Exophthalmos (anterior displacement of the eye) and ptosis are

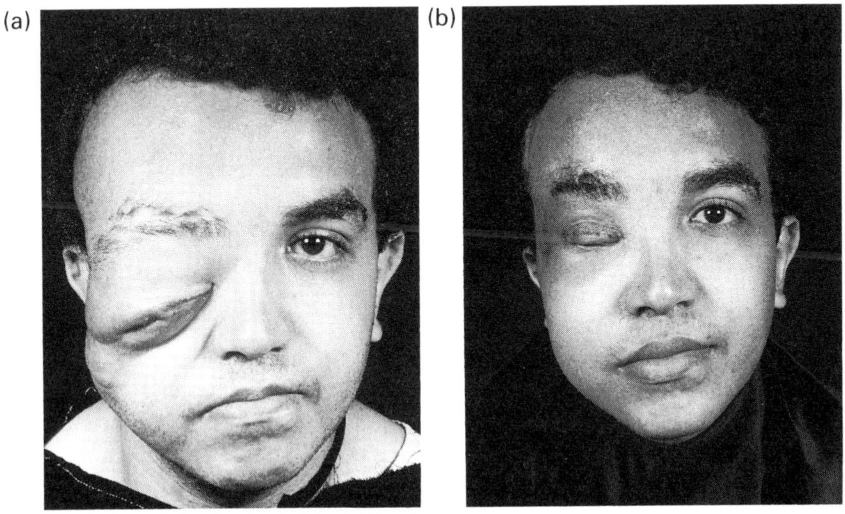

Figure 14.6 (A) Preoperative photograph of a young man with a long history of neurofibromatosis. The right eye was not functional at the time of initial consultation. (B) Early postoperative view. Although enucleation and prosthetic reconstruction was recommended, he declined the recommendation. He is quite content with permanent tarsorrhaphy.

common findings, and visual acuity is often decreased. Prior to any procedure, consultation with an ophthalmologist is important to assess extraocular muscle involvement and optic nerve function and to check for the presence of an optic nerve glioma.

Frequently, treatment of eyelid involvement in NF1 includes full-thickness resection of the eyelid with preservation on the lash border and levator muscle. However, enough lid tissue is left medially to close the wound, protect the globe and preserve lacrimal function (Figure 14.6).

For more involved cases, where the tumour has either (1) extended intracranially, (2) malpositioned the orbit or (3) produced massive exopthalmus while preserving visual function, a combined intra- and extracranial approach is necessary.

When vision is absent and the globe is massively proptotic, exenteration of the orbit may be useful. However, if it is elected to preserve the eye, either because of the patient's wishes or the presence of useable vision, excision and reconstruction requires a multidisciplinary approach involving plastic surgery, neurosurgery and ophthalmology services. The neurosurgical team first gains intracranial access to visualize the orbital roof, where herniation of the brain may be contributing to the exophthalmos (Figure 14.7). This is reduced, and the bony defect (usually in the sphenoid bone and posterior orbit) is reconstructed with bone grafts.

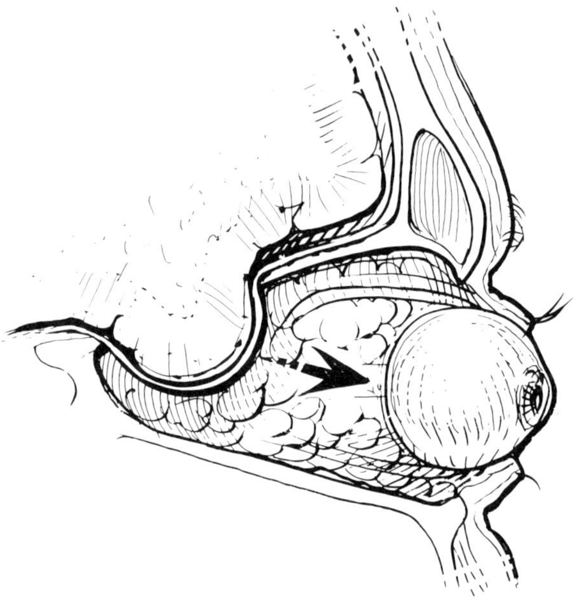

Figure 14.7 How brain herniation can be a cause of exophthalmus.

Attention is next directed to the questions of continued exophthalmos and dystopia. These entities require modification of the size and position of the orbit (Figure 14.8). This can be realized by placing platform grafts inferiorly while removing or elevating the orbital roof (Figure 14.9) (Edgerton, 1990).

Once these issues are dealt with, attention can be given to the canthal ligaments, lacrimal system and extraocular muscles. Canthal dystopia is treated by canthopexy (Figure 14.10), while lacrimal drainage obstruction is often treated by reconstruction of the system or diversion of tear flow by a dacryocystorhinostomy. Strabismus is dealt with by balancing of the extraocular muscles. In order to achieve a desirable result, a series of operations is often necessary.

14.3.4 Cheek and mid-face

NF1 involvement of the middle of the face is common. Fifty per cent of patients in the series of Griffiths, Lewis and McKinney (1985) had cheek involvement, while 15% had involvement of the parotid and 15% of the maxilla.

For small lesions, excision is easily performed and reconstructed. However, when lesions in this region are large, several difficult decisions arise. If there is extensive skin involvement that must be sacrificed, where

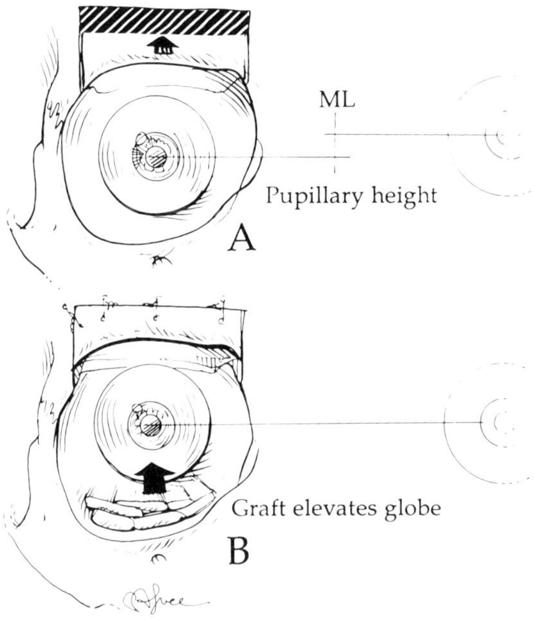

Figure 14.8 Vertical dystopia and its treatment. (a) Entire orbit has been lowered by the neurofibroma resulting in a decreased pupillary height. ML = midline. (b) This is treated by elevating the orbit and placing bone grafts on the orbital floor.

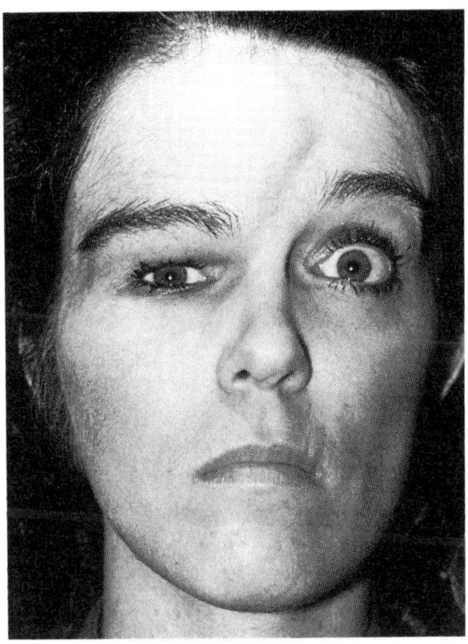

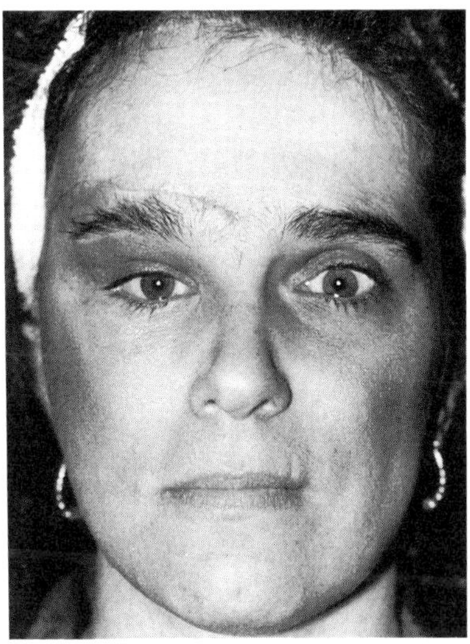

Figure 14.9 (a) Patient who previously had resection of neurofibromatosis tissue. Her major deficiencies at this time were orbital dystopia (right eye lower than left) and contour irregularity of the forehead. (b) After dystopia repair, as depicted in Figure 14.8, and forehead plasty.

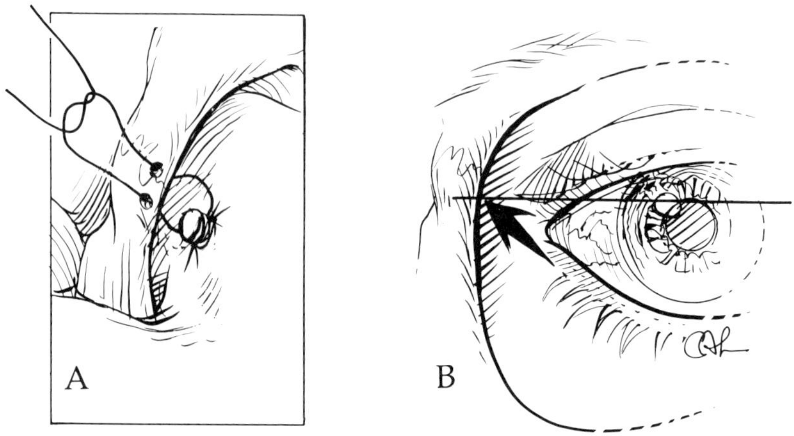

Lateral canthopexy

Figure 14.10 Technique of lateral canthopexy. Holes are made into the zygoma laterally and sutures are placed through these holes and through the lateral central tendon. This pulls the canthus laterally and posteriorly (A), resulting in a more normal fissural shape (B).

does one get the necessary amount of soft tissue? This may require local flaps from the neck or distant flaps. When the parotid gland region is involved, consideration has to be given to facial nerve function. Total resection of all involved tissue is often not possible without some damage to the facial nerve. In these situations a balance has to be made between disfigurement caused by tumour and the worry of loss of facial nerve function resulting from surgery.

(a) *Facial nerve issues*

A complete discussion of rehabilitation of facial nerve palsy will not be undertaken here, but the general principles of the care of the patient with facial nerve palsy are (1) to protect the function of the eye by preventing corneal exposure as a result of impaired eyelid function, (2) to allow facial movements and (3) to achieve facial symmetry. The first goal can be achieved by multiple measures such as tarsorrhaphy, placement of a gold weight in the upper lid and muscle transfers to effect closure of the eyelids, preventing drying of the cornea (May, 1986). When possible, grafting of the facial nerve can be carried out to improve facial symmetry (Conley, 1955; Conley and Baker, 1978). When not possible, static fascial slings may be used (Conley and Baker, 1978, 1979; May, 1986). Static fascial slings offer the advantages of simplicity and immediate benefit. However, the disadvantage of sling lengthening owing to gravity pull on the soft tissues of the face renders this option less acceptable for most younger patients in good health.

Nerve transfers (hypoglossal and accessory) likewise are relatively simple, and are effective in providing resting muscle tone, particularly in the lower two-thirds of the face. The disadvantages of this technique are: delayed onset of effect (neurite outgrowth of approximately 1 mm/day) of 6–8 months; donor site morbidity (tongue hemiatrophy with hypoglossal transfer; shoulder pain and noticeable muscle atrophy in some patients undergoing accessory nerve transfer); and lack of spontaneous and symmetrical movement.

To gain movement of the face and aid in symmetry, muscle slings such as the masseter and temporalis transfer may be used (Edgerton, Tuerk and Fisher, 1975; Rubin, 1977; Conley and Baker, 1978; May, 1986). Greater sophistication in dynamic muscle sling procedures, particularly in emphasizing individual variation in the type of normal smile and tailoring the operative procedure to reproduce individual muscle (zygomaticus, risoris, superior and inferior quadratus muscle) activity, has led to much improved results. However, although these muscle slings provide movement, it is not spontaneous or reflexive, and 'trick' movement must be learned to achieve balanced facial movement.

In NF2, when removal of vestibular Schwannoma has resulted in facial nerve palsy, with the facial nerve discontinuous with the brain stem, a different approach must be undertaken. Dynamic sling procedures may still be useful here, particularly in the elderly patient population, because of the rapid onset of benefit and often less concern about a perfectly symmetrical facial appearance, especially when it means a lengthy operative treatment plan (Edgerton, Tuerk and Fisher, 1975; Rubin, 1977; Conley and Baker, 1978; May, 1986).

In the younger patient, however, crossed facial nerve transfer may be an option (Anderl, 1977). In this situation, several nerve grafts are attached to the distal ends of the facial nerve on the unaffected side of the face, allowing a year for the nerve fibres to migrate into the graft on the affected side of the face. The nerve is then attached to the distal stump of the severed facial nerve on the affected side (Figure 14.11). The advantage of this technique is that symmetrical reflexive facial movement may be possible. The disadvantages of the crossed face nerve techniques include long periods of no spontaneous or induced facial movement (12–18 months), facial scarring (usually minimal), reduction in movement on the non-paralysed side of the face, and in NF2 patients the possibility of bilateral involvement of the vestibular (and therefore facial) nerves. Even though bilateral involvement of the vestibular nerves is very likely in these patients, surgical resection of the tumour does not lead inevitably to facial nerve paralysis, therefore this reconstructive approach still may be advocated in properly selected individuals.

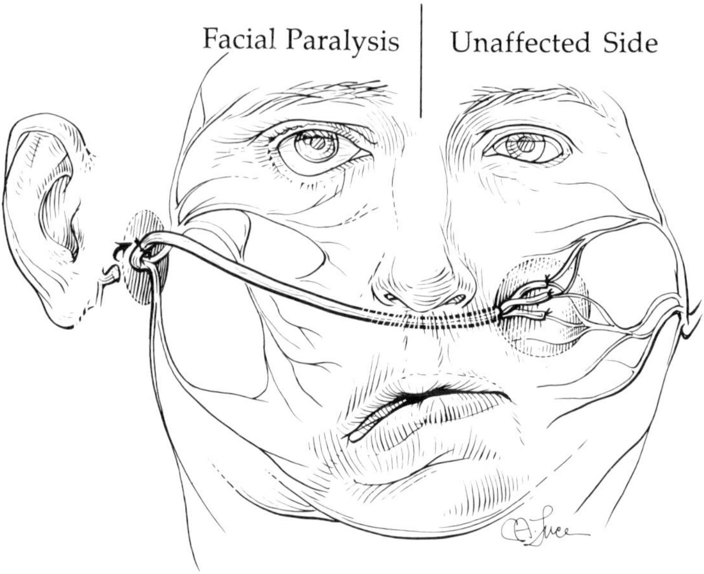

Figure 14.11 A crossed-nerve graft. A nerve graft is attached to the normal facial nerve on the patient's left and to the stump of the paralysed nerve on the patient's right.

In order to prevent atrophy of the facial musculature when the nerve is growing through the graft, a hypoglossal nerve transfer may provide support to the denervated muscles. The hypoglossal nerve may be reattached later to its normal distal end at the time of facial nerve grafting. However, if there has been a time lapse of greater than 2 years between the onset of facial nerve palsy and the proposed reinnervation, atrophy of the facial muscles may have already occurred, rendering this form of treatment less effective. Recent use of microvascular muscle transfer (such as the pectoralis minor, latissimus dorsi and gracilis muscles) attached to the crossed facial nerve graft may obviate this delay problem in the future (Hari, Ohmori and Torii, 1976; O'Brien, Franklin and Morrison, 1980; Manktelow and Zuker, 1984; Harrison, 1985; Terzis, 1987; O'Brien *et al.*, 1990).

The establishment of complete, spontaneous, symmetrical facial reanimation using nerve transfer or a combination of techniques is not entirely reliable as yet. However, further technical and biological improvements may allow this option to be more routinely successful and therefore more widely recommended.

(b) Nasal involvement

Bulk excess due to neurofibromatosis of the nose may be handled by standard closed (McDowell, Valone and Brown, 1952; Sheen and Sheen, 1987; Rees and Woodsmith, 1988) or open (Rethi, 1984) techniques. More extensive lesions may require degloving (Casson, Bonnato and Converse, 1974; Maniglia, 1986) or lateral rhinotomy (Bernard *et al.*, 1989). Bony reconstruction of the nose may require calvarial or rib grafts. Rib grafts incorporating segments of cartilage are optimal for dorsal nasal augmentation, owing to cartilage flexibility and resistance to resorption.

(c) Maxilla

When NF1 affects the maxilla, facial growth and occlusion may be disturbed. Orthognathic principles using Le Fort maxillary and mandibular osteotomies with orthodontic adjustment are often helpful (Figure 14.12). The basic principles in management are to correct dental malalignment when it appears to be a progressive abnormality, as soon as the deformity is judged to be of significant functional and cosmetic consequence, as long as the timing and type of surgery does not impair normal skeletal development and tooth eruption. However, bony asymmetry above may be acceptable, and even desirable, in non-occlusal regions in order to accommodate excesses in soft-tissue overgrowth.

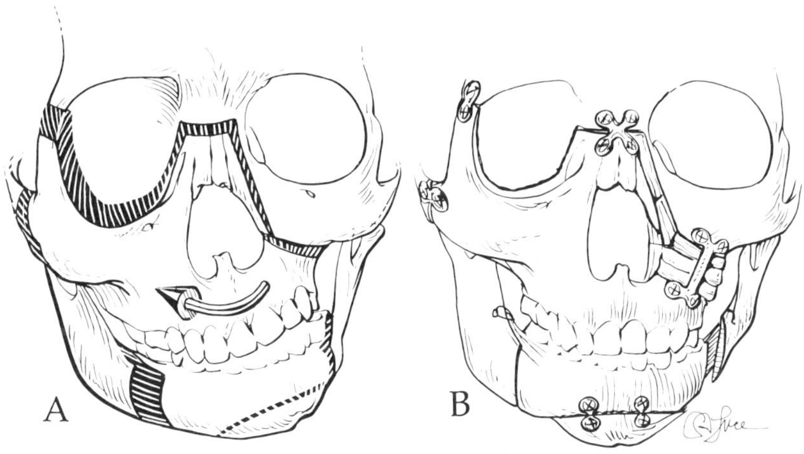

Figure 14.12 Reverse facial osteotomy of Munro. There is unequal growth of the facial skeleton because of neurofibromatosis. Osteotomies are outlined (A) and carried out, resulting in a more symmetrical structure (B).

14.3.5 Lower face and lip

The lips are complex structures serving many functions (speech, alimentation, expression, etc.). Their surfaces consist of skin as well as a dry vermillion and moist mucosal area. The major muscle of the lips (the orbicularis oris) primarily functions as a sphincter to maintain oral continence (prevent drooling) and to aid in speech. It works in concert with several pairs of elevating and depressing muscle groups. This complex interaction allows for the multiplicity of motions and emotions that can be communicated with the mouth (Zide, 1990).

NF1 may involve the lips, resulting in disfiguring enlargement. For small lesions (less than one-third of the lower lip or one-quarter of the upper), simple excision and closure is sufficient. For larger lesions, however, multiple procedures are often needed. Each procedure is aimed at correcting a particular lip defect (Figure 14.13). An example would be the Abbe flap (1898), which is the transfer of a full-thickness flap of either upper or lower lip to the other. The flap is pedicled by the labial vessels and is transposed into the lip defect. It is most useful for central defects, one-third to one-half the lip in size. For more lateral defects, the Estlander (1872) or fan flap (McGregor, 1980) are better reconstructive options.

Intraoral neurofibromatosis may involve mucosal structures. Batsakis' study (1979) found a 6.5% involvement. If oral/pharyngeal involvement is massive, tracheotomy may be required to maintain airway patency.

NF1 may lead to the development of macroglossia, which requires resection. There are several means of resecting the tongue, depending on the way the tongue is enlarged (Edgerton, 1960; Bjuggren, Jensen and Strombeck, 1968). Hemihypertrophy of the tongue may be best treated by asymmetrical resection of the tongue, including the lateral surface of the tongue. Diffuse macroglossia, however, may be best dealt with by a central resection of the tongue, leaving the lateral and anterior portions of the tongue intact (along with the laterally situated lingual nerves) in order to provide normal sensation of the tongue and avoid painful neuralgics.

It is important to deal with gingival involvement, because of its detrimental effect on tooth position and oral hygiene. Debulking of hypertrophic and hyperplastic tissue may be necessary to improve this situation.

14.3.6 Extremities

Multiple neurofibromas in NF1 may commonly occur in the extremities with great variance in size and number of lesions (Cohen, 1984). Treatment is therefore reserved for functional and cosmetic reasons. Asymmetrical, small nodules in hidden areas need not be removed. Occasionally, lesions at the belt/brassiere line should be removed because

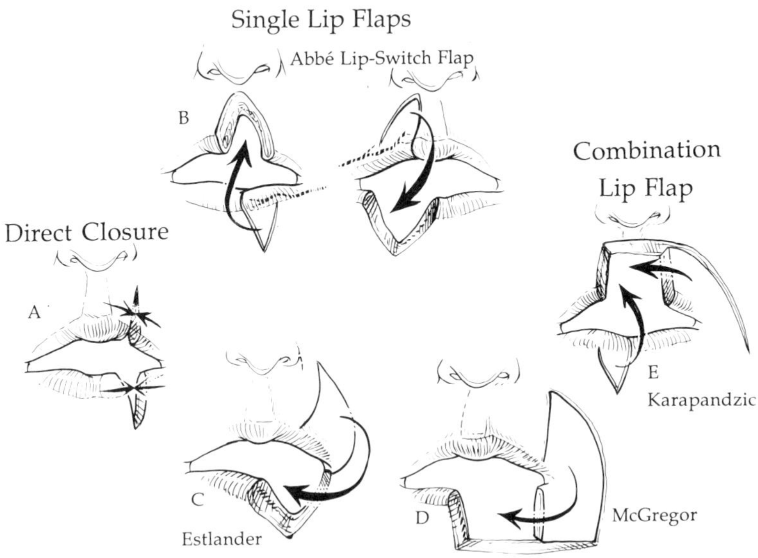

Figure 14.13 Techniques of lip reconstruction. (A) Direct closure can be undertaken for small defects. For larger defects there are many options; among the more common are lip flaps. (B) Abbe flap. (C) Estlander flap. (D) McGregor flap. (E) Karapandzic flap.

of interference with garment use. As in other areas, simple excision with closure is performed for smaller lesions. Large numbers of these small skin lesions may be removed expeditiously with diathermy alone, leaving the created defect to heal by wound contraction secondarily (Roberts and Crockett, 1985). Larger lesions may pose problems involving skin and soft-tissue reduction with or without bone removal. If the skin involvement is large, reconstruction of the defect as described earlier may involve local flaps, use of tissue expansion or distant flaps.

Growth of the nodular neurofibroma occurs by proliferating elements within the nerve sheath, resulting in a large mass or plexiform neurofibroma. In this case, resection of the nerve (whole or individual fascicles) with nerve grafting may be indicated if functional limitations due to compressive nerve palsy are appreciated. Malignant degeneration is uncommon, but should be suspected in patients with new-onset pain or rapid enlargement of the tumour size. If surgical excision is elected (ordinarily in the brachial and lumbar plexuses) the use of intraoperative nerve stimulation and recording is helpful to define non-functional elements within the neurofibroma (Figure 14.14). This electrophysiological technique defines optimal sites for resection and reconstruction better than any visual inspection method, and is most favourable for

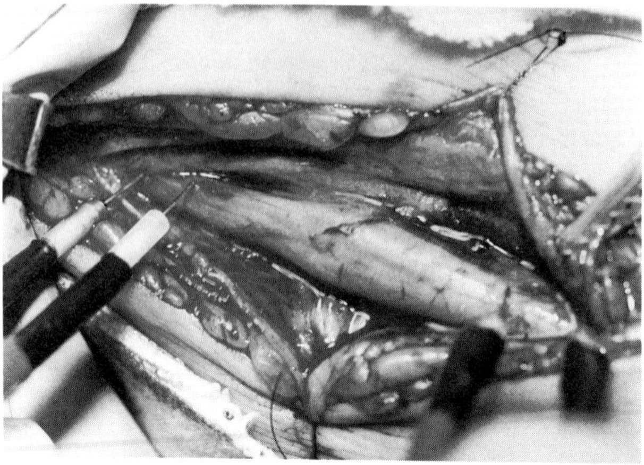

Figure 14.14 Intraoperative photograph of nerve stimulation to assess functional site of nerve in question. Action potential amplitude and conduction velocities can be assessed using this technique.

neural recovery. Nerve fascicles that are functioning but entrapped by the tumour may be spared using this approach.

Finally, the neurofibroma may lead to regional gigantism (Holt and Wright, 1948; Holt, 1978). Besides soft-tissue reduction, removal of some of the bone is needed. In some cases, epiphyseal stapling is performed to decrease the degree of subsequent bone growth.

14.3.7 Integument

(a) Café au lait spots

The skin hyperpigmentation, café au lait spots, may become a troublesome feature for those with NF1. Truncal and extremity involvement often may be covered with clothing and need not be addressed surgically. Blending skin make-up (e.g. Cover Mark) may be particularly useful in women to cover exposed areas of the face, hands and legs. When there is an accompanying overgrowth of tissue, hypertrichosis, or if a patient wishes to avoid repeated applications of cosmetics, skin excision may be the best option. Excision of these hyperpigmented areas with consideration given to lines of least tension, especially on the face, and reconstruction of the defect with grafts or flaps respecting aesthetic unit boundaries provide the most optimal results (Roberts and Crockett, 1985). Laser treatment of café au lait spots has not yet proven reliable enough to be recommended. Experimental work will further define its role in the treatment of these lesions in the future.

(b) Dermal neurofibromas

A common complaint of individuals with neurofibromatosis relates to their dermal neurofibromas. Because of the nature of the disease, cure cannot be achieved; however, as in other areas, one can treat specific symptomatic lesions. Surgical excision has been the mainstay of treatment (Preston, Walsh and Clarke, 1951; section 14.3.6). Others have tried other treatment modalities. Alt (1987) has reported favourable outcome in using dermabrasion for certain lesions. The more deeply the location of the lesions, however, the less likely this modality is of use. Likewise, laser therapy at present does not appear to offer any benefits over conventional surgery for these lesions.

14.4 CONCLUSION

There are many reconstructive options now available to those with neurofibromatosis. In order to achieve maximum benefit, individualized treatment plans that accurately define the needs of patients and costs of each option should be thoroughly assessed before any reconstructive step is elected. Technological advances continue to offer a wider and often more effective range of possibilities to consider.

REFERENCES

Abbe, R.A. (1898) A new plastic operation for the relief of deformity due to double harelip. *Med. Rec.*, **53**, 477.

Adkins, J.C. and Ravitch, M.M. (1977) The operative management of Von Recklinghausen's neurofibromatosis in children, with special reference to lesions of the head and neck. *Surgery*, **83**, 342.

Aird, I. (1958) *Companion in Surgical Studies*, E. & S. Livingstone, Edinburgh.

Alt, T.H. (1987) Therapeutic facial dermabrasion, in *Skin Surgery*, 6th edn (ed. E. Epstein), W.B. Saunders, Philadelphia, p. 327.

Anderl, H. (1977) Cross facial nerve grafting – up to 12 months of seventh nerve disruption, in *Reanimation of the Paralyzed Face* (ed. L.R. Robin), C.V. Mosby, St Louis, p. 263.

Argenta, L.C. (1984) Reconstruction of the breast by tissue expansion. *Clin. Plast. Surg.*, **11**, 257.

Austad, E.D. *et al.* (1982) Histomorphologic evaluation of guinea pig skin and soft tissue after controlled tissue expansion. *Plast. Reconstr. Surg.*, **70**, 704.

Austad, E.D., Thomas, S.B. and Pasyk, K.A. (1986) Tissue expansion: dividend or loan? *Plast. Reconstr. Surg.*, **70**, 63.

Batsakis, J.G. (ed.) (1979) *Tumors of the Head and Neck*, 2nd edn, Williams and Wilkins, Baltimore.

Bernard, P.J. *et al.* (1989) Complications following rhinotomy: review of 148 patients. *Ann. Otol. Rhinol. Laryngol.*, **98**, 684.

Bjuggren, G., Jensen, R. and Strombeck, J. (1968) Macroglossia and its surgical treatment. Indications and postoperative experiences from the orthodontic, phoniatric, and surgical points of view. *Scand. J. Plast. Surg.*, **2**, 116.

Borges, A.F. (1971) Historical review of the z and w plasty revisions of linear scars. *Intern. Surg.*, **56**, 182.

Borges, A.F. (1973) *Elective Incisions and Scar Revision*, Little, Brown and Co., Boston.

Bromley, G.S., Sherman, J.E. and Goulian, D. (1981) Neurofibromatosis – distribution and surgical treatment. *Ann. Plast. Surg.*, **8**, 272.

Casson, D.R., Bonnato, P.C. and Converse, J.M. (1974) The midface degloving procedure. *Plast. Reconstr. Surg.*, **53**, 102.

Chicarilli, A.N. and Davey, L.M.(1989) Rectus abdominis myocutaneous free flap reconstruction following a cranio-orbital-maxillary resection for neurofibrosarcoma. *Plast. Reconstr. Surg.*, **80**, 726.

Cohen, M.D. (1984) Neurofibromatosis manifested in the foot. *J. Am. Pediatr. Assoc.*, **74**, 1984.

Conley, J. (1955) Facial nerve grafting in treatment of parotid tumors. *Arch. Surg.*, **70**, 1955.

Conley, J. (1972) Neurogenic tumors of the head and neck. *J. Otol. Soc. Aust.*, **3**, 362.

Conley, J. and Baker, D.C. (1978) The surgical treatment of extratemporal facial paralysis: an overview. *Head Neck Surg.*, **1**, 12.

Conley, J. and Baker, D.C. (1979) Hypoglossal-facial nerve anastomosis for reinnervation of the paralyzed face. *Plast. Reconstr. Surg.*, **63**, 63.

Crikelair, G.F. and Cosman, B. (1968) Histologically benign, clinically malignant lesions of the head and neck. *Plast. Reconstr. Surg.*, **42**, 343.

Daniel, R.K. (1975a) The anatomical and hemodynamic characteristics of the cutaneous circulation and their influence on skin flap design, in *Skin Flaps* (eds W.C. Grabb and M.B. Myers), Little, Brown and Co., Boston, p. 111.

Daniel, R.K. (1975b) Toward an anatomical and hemodynamic classification of skin flaps. *Plast. Reconstr. Surg.*, **56**, 330.

Daniel, R.K. and Kerrigan, C.L. (1990) Principles and physiology of skin flap surgery, in *Plastic Surgery* (ed. J.C. McCarthy), W.B. Saunders, Philadelphia, p. 275.

Davis, W.B., Edgerton, M.T. and Hoffmeister, S.F. (1954) Neurofibromatosis of the head and neck. *Plast. Reconstr. Surg.*, **14**, 186.

Edgerton, M.T. (1960) The management of macroglossia when associated with prognathism. *Br. J. Plast. Surg.*, **3**, 117.

Edgerton, M.T. (1990) On impact of craniosynostosis and orbital development and its surgical treatment, in *Scientific Foundation and Surgical Treatment of Craniosynostosis* (ed. J. Persing), Williams & Wilkins, Baltimore.

Edgerton, M.T. and Morgan, R.F. (1985) Tissue expansion in reconstructive hand surgery: case report. *J. Hand Surg.*, **10A**, 754.

Edgerton, M.T., Tuerk, D.B. and Fisher, J.C. (1975) Surgical treatment of Moebius syndrome by platysma and temporalis transfers. *Plast. Reconstr. Surg.*, **55**, 305.

Estlander, J.A. (1872) En ny operation metod att aterstall fortord lapp ellekkind. *Finsak Lak-sall SK Hannal*, **14**, 1.

Feinman, N.L. and Yakovac, B.A. (1970) Neurofibromatosis in childhood. *J. Pediatr.*, **76**, 339.

Ger, R. (1972) Surgical treatment of the ulcerative lesions of the lower extremity. *Curr. Prob. Surg.*, **1**, 52.

Grabb, W.C. *et al.* (1980) Facial hamartomas in children: neurofibroma, lymphangioma and hemangioma. *Plast. Reconstr. Surg.*, **66**, 509.

Griffith, B.H. *et al.* (1972) Von Recklinghausen's disease in children. *Plast. Reconstr. Surg.*, **49**, 647.

Griffith, B.H., Lewis, V.L. and McKinney, P. (1985) Neurofibromas of the head and neck. *Surg. Gynecol. Obstet.* **160**, 534.

Hari, K., Ohmori, K. and Torii, S. (1976) Free gracilis muscle with microneurovascular anastomoses for treatment of facial paralysis. *Plast. Reconstr. Surg.*, **57**, 133.

Harrison, D.H. (1985) The pectoralis minor vascularized muscle graft for the treatment of unilateral facial palsy. *Plast. Reconstr. Surg.*, **95**, 206.

Holt, J.F. (1978) Neurofibromatosis in children. *AJR*, **130**, 615.

Holt, J.F. and Wright, E.M. (1948) The radiologic features of neurofibromatosis. *Radiology*, **51**, 647.

Horowitz, J.H. *et al.* (1984) Galeal-pericranial flaps in head and neck reconstruction, anatomy and application. *Am. J. Surg.*, **148**, 489.

Hosoi, K. (1931) Multiple neurofibromatosis: von Recklinghausen's disease. *Arch. Surg.*, **22**, 258.

Jackson, I., Laws, E.R. and Martin, R.D. (1983) The surgical management of orbital neurofibromatosis. *Plast. Reconstr. Surg.*, **71**, 751.

Karapandzic, M. (1974) Reconstruction of lip defects by local arterial flaps. *Br. J. Plast. Surg.*, **27**, 93.

Knight, W.A., Murphy, W.K. and Gottlieb, J.A. (1973) Neurofibromatosis associated with malignant neurofibroma. *Arch. Dermatol.*, **107**, 747.

Maceri, D.R. and Saxon, K.G. (1984) Neurofibromatosis of the head and neck. *Head Neck Surg.*, **6**, 842.

Manders, E.K. *et al.* (1982) Skin expansion to eliminate large scalp defects. *Ann. Plast. Surg.*, **9**, 131.

Manders, E.K. *et al.* (1984) Soft tissue expansion: concepts and complications. *Plast. Reconstr. Surg.*, **74**, 493.

Maniglia, A.J. (1986) Indications and techniques of midfacial degloving. *Arch. Otol. Head Neck Surg.*, **114**, 1588.

Manktelow, R.T. and Zuker, R.M. (1984) Muscle transplantation by fascicular paralysis territory. *Plast. Reconstr. Surg.*, **73**, 751.

Marchac, D. (1984) Intracranial enlargement of the orbital cavity and palpebral remodeling for orbitopalpebral neurofibromatosis. *Plast. Reconstr. Surg.*, **73**, 534.

May, M. (1986) *The Facial Nerve*, Thieme, New York.

McCraw, J.B. (1986) The recent history of myocutaneous flaps. *Clin. Plast. Surg.*, **7**, 13.

McDowell, F., Valone, J.A. and Brown, J.B. (1952) Bibliography and historical note on plastic surgery of the nose. *Plast. Reconstr. Surg.*, **10**, 149.

McGregor, I.A. (1980) *Fundamental Techniques of Plastic Surgery and Their Surgical Application*, 7th edn, Churchill Livingstone, Edinburgh.

Menick, F.J. (1987) Artistry in aesthetic surgery – aesthetic perception and the subunit principle. *Clin. Plast. Surg.*, **14**, 723.

Mukherji, M.M. (1974) Giant neurofibroma of the head and neck. *Plast. Reconstr. Surg.*, **53**, 184.

Munro, I.R. and Martin, P.D. (1980) The management of gigantic benign craniofacial tumors: the reverse facial osteotomy. *Plast. Reconstr. Surg.*, **65**, 777.

O'Brien, B. McC. and Morrison, W.A. (1987) *Reconstructive Microsurgery*, Churchill Livingstone, London.

O'Brien, B. McC., Franklin, J.D. and Morrison, W.A. (1980) Cross facial nerve grafts and microneurovascular free muscle transfer for long-established facial palsy. *Br. J. Plast. Surg.*, **33**, 202.

O'Brien, B. McC. *et al.* (1990) Results of management of facial palsy with microvascular free-muscle transfer. *Plast. Reconstr. Surg.*, **86**, 12.

Orticochea, M. (1967) Four flap scalp reconstruction technique. *Br. J. Plast. Surg.*, **20**, 159.

Orticochea, M. (1971) New three-flap reconstruction technique. *Br. J. Plast. Surg.*, **24**, 184.

Ponten, B. (1981) The fasciocutaneous flap: its use in soft tissue defects of the lower leg. *Br. J. Plast. Surg.*, **34**, 215.

Poole, M.D. (1989) Experiences in the surgical treatment of cranio-orbital neurofibromatosis. *Br. J. Plast. Surg.*, **42**, 155.

Preston, F.W., Walsh, W.S. and Clarke, T.H. (1951) Cutaneous neurofibromatosis: clinical manifestations and incidence of sarcoma in 61 male patients. *Arch. Surg.*, **64**, 813.

Radovan, C. (1984) Tissue expansion in soft-tissue reconstruction. *Plast. Reconstr. Surg.*, **74**, 482.

Rees, T.D. and Woodsmith, D. (1988) *Cosmetic Facial Surgery*, W.B. Saunders, Philadelphia.

Rethi, A. (1984) Reccourcissement du nez trop long. *Rev. Chir. Plast.*, **2**, 85.

Roberts, A.H.N. and Crockett, D.J. (1985) An operation for the treatment of cutaneous neurofibromatosis. *Br. J. Plast. Surg.*, **38**, 292.

Roland, P., Glasscock, M.E. and Bojrab, D.I. (1986) Neuromas of the skull base. *Otolaryngol. Head Neck Surg.*, **42**, 155.

Rubin, L.R. (1977) *Reanimation of the Paralyzed Face*, C.V. Mosby, St Louis.

Rudolph, R. and Ballantyne, D.L. (1990) Skin grafts, in *Plastic Surgery* (ed. J.G. McCarthy), W.B. Saunders, Philadelphia, p. 221.

Shack, B., Reilley, A.T. and Lynch, J.B. (1985) Neurofibromas of the head and neck. *South. Med. J.*, **78**, 801.

Sheen, J.H. and Sheen, A.P. (1987) *Aesthetic Rhinoplasty*, C.V. Mosby, St Louis.

Smith, B. and English, F.P. (1970) Classical eyelid border sign of neurofibromatosis. *Br. J. Ophthalmol.*, **54**, 134.

Spira, M. and Riccardi, V. (1987) Neurofibromatosis, *Clin. Plast. Surg.*, **14**, 315.

Terranova, W. (1990) The use of periosteal flaps in scalp and forehead reconstruction. *Ann. Plast. Surg.*, **25**, 450.

Terzis (1987) *Microreconstruction of Nerve Injuries*, W.B. Saunders, Philadelphia.

Tolhurst, D.E., Haeseker, B. and Zeeman, R.J. (1983) The development of the fasciocutaneous flap and its clinical applications. *Plast. Reconstr. Surg.*, **71**, 597.

Van Beck, A.L. and Adson, M.H. (1987) Tissue expansion in the upper extremity. *Clin. Plast. Surg.*, **14**, 535.

Van der Meulen, J.C. *et al.* (1982) The management of orbitofacial neurofibromatosis. *Ann. Plast. Surg.*, **8**, 213.

Zide, B.M. (1990) Deformities of the lips and cheeks, in *Plastic Surgery* (ed. J.G. McCarthy), W.B. Saunders, Philadelphia, p. 2009.

15

Neurofibromatosis 1: clinical management and genetic counselling

S.M. Huson and M. Upadhyaya

15.1 INTRODUCTION

Because of its extreme variability and large number of complications, neurofibromatosis 1 (NF1) is an extremely difficult disease to manage well. As so many different specialties may be involved, it is the coordination of medical care that presents the greatest challenge. Although neurofibromatosis 2 (NF2) has a much greater morbidity and mortality, it can be an easier disease to manage at an organizational level. The number of specialists involved in patient care is smaller and the variation in disease expression much less, particularly within families. For NF2, improved care may result from close follow-up with screening investigations such as brain stem auditory evoked responses and cranial imaging. For NF1 the best way of organizing patient follow-up and the use of screening investigations for specific complications (e.g. optic gliomas) are widely debated issues.

What is clear is that the patients and their families do want access to health professionals with experience of NF1. The British Neurofibromatosis Association, formerly called LINK (Let's Increase Neurofibromatosis Knowledge), was formed in 1981. The most frequent complaint of new members (C. Peperell, personal communication) is that they have been given inadequate information about the disease by their doctors and that no one person was prepared to coordinate their health care. A lot of the stimulus to health professionals to develop an interest in neurofibromatosis health care has resulted from the work of the lay associations. For NF1 patients, the health professional is continually performing a difficult 'balancing act', between providing adequate information and follow-up but not creating unnecessary anxiety. What makes this even more difficult is that very few large studies have formally evaluated the psychosocial experience of individuals with NF1, nor have different kinds of health care for NF1 patients been formally compared and evaluated.

15.2 STUDIES OF PATIENT CARE AND PSYCHOSOCIAL ISSUES

15.2.1 Patient care in the southeast Wales population study

In the southeast Wales study (Huson, Harper and Compston, 1988; Huson, 1989), we used a study questionnaire that included a section on patient's attitudes to the disease. In practice this was often not completed because it had already become obvious that the patient understood so little about NF1 that the answers would have been uninterpretable. Many patients regarded NF1 as 'just a skin complaint' and those with complications often had no idea that they were related to the disease. Those who had sought to inform themselves often had an exaggerated impression of their risk of malignancy or fear of becoming an 'elephant man'. We did discover by whom and at what age the diagnosis of NF1 had been made, the medical care received by the patients and the number who had received formal genetic counselling. All of these were taken as measures reflecting the level of health professional awareness of NF1 in the study area.

With regard to diagnosis, because café au lait spots are present by the age of 5 years, then the detection of six or more café au lait spots on any examination in childhood should raise the suspicion of NF1 and affected children should be diagnosed through the channels of routine child heath surveillance. 'Awareness' of the medical profession to the diagnosis of NF1 was indirectly assessed by studying by whom and at what age the diagnosis had been made in 135 individuals. The outcome is summarized in Table 15.1. Twenty of the 135 cases were diagnosed for the first time when assessed for the study. A further 10 individuals, all from one particularly large family, were aware of having the disease through discussion within the family, but, regarding it as 'just a skin complaint', never sought medical advice. The mean age of diagnosis in the remaining 105 cases was 17.7 years. The majority of these cases had not been diagnosed until early adulthood, when the appearance of neurofibromas had caused them to seek medical attention. In view of the improved child health surveillance in recent years, the data from those aged less than 18 years were analysed separately (Table 15.1). The findings are similar to those for the whole study population. Fifteen out of 41 children had not been diagnosed prior to the study and six of the remaining 26 presented because of a major disease complication. In a further four cases the diagnosis was only made during a hospital consultation for unrelated

Table 15.1 Age at diagnosis and specialty of assessing physician in the Welsh study population

Diagnosed by	*Number of cases*	*Number for whom age at diagnosis known*	*Mean age at diagnosis in years (range)*[a]
Total cohort (n = 135)			
Paediatrician	26	23	3.7 (0.3–15)
Dermatologist	21	18	23.0 (0.5–41)
Study[b]	20	20	22.1 (1–83)
General Practitioner	16	10	37.6 (4–67)
Neurologist	12	8	26.8 (12–46)
Family[b]	10	–	–
Orthopaedic Surgeon	9	9	12.8 (1–31)
General Physician	7	5	30.8 (18–54)
Plastic Surgeon	7	7	12.4 (1–24)
Ophthalmologist	3	3	4, 7, 35
Neurosurgeon	2	2	4, 33
Clinical Geneticist	1	1	4
General Surgeon	1	0	–
Individuals aged <18 years			
Paediatrician	20		2.7 (0.3–10)
Study	11		8.3 (1–15)
Family	4		–
Clinical Geneticist	1		4
Plastic Surgeon	1		1
Ophthalmologist	1		4
Orthopaedic Surgeon	1		11
Dermatologist	2		0.5, 15

[a] For numbers <5, age at diagnosis individually listed.
[b] See text for explanation.
Source: Huson (1989).

medical problems. Many parents said that they had pointed out the café au lait spots to various doctors, only to be told they were 'just birth marks'.

With regard to disease management, 94 of the 135 cases in the study population had had at least one hospital consultation for NF1 prior to their assessment for the study. Only 30 of the 135 were being regularly followed up in a hospital clinic and in half of these it was to monitor a specific disease complication (Table 15.2). None of the remaining 105 individuals were under regular review with their general practitioner for NF1. The medical histories of many of the patients demonstrated that

Table 15.2 Reason for hospital follow-up of 30 out of 135 NF1 patients in Welsh population study

Reason	*Number*
General overview of disease	15
Adults	5
Children (<18 years)	10
Because of disease complication	15
Neurological complications	5
Facial plexiform neurofibromas	3
Ophthalmological complications[a]	3
Orthopaedic complications	2
Endocrine complications	1
Follow-up after gastrointestinal surgery	1

[a] Including optic gliomas, as both individuals with this complication were followed only by an ophthalmologist.
Source: Huson (1989).

regular follow-up with more awareness of the disease would have avoided delay in diagnosis of complications and distress caused by uncertainty. There were three cases with hypertension, two due to renal artery stenosis and one due to phaeochromocytoma, which illustrated the value of regular follow-up. In all three of these cases the raised blood pressure had been a coincidental finding on examination when they had presented with another problem.

Only nine individuals from seven families had received formal genetic counselling and in four cases this was after they had completed their families. Although others had been informed of the mode of inheritance, the variation in disease severity and risks of complications had not been explained. Many parents with disease complications assumed that if they had children with NF1 they would have a similar disease presentation.

The study showed many areas for improvement in patient care for NF1. Although many of the disease complications are individually rare, their combined burden is significant. In the Welsh population, patients were not being diagnosed sufficiently early nor receiving appropriate follow-up and counselling.

15.2.2 Psychosocial burden of NF1

Given that there has been so little clinical and scientific research into NF1 until the last two decades, it is not surprising that even less attention has been paid to the psychosocial aspects of the disease. Fortunately this situation is now changing with such publications as those of Messner

(Messner, Gardner and Messner, 1985; Messner, Messner and Lewis, 1985; Messner and Smith, 1986); Ellis (1990); Ablon (1992, 1993) and Benjamin (Benjamin *et al.*, 1993). These studies highlight four main problems experienced by people with NF1. These are listed below, along with relevant quotations from some of the above studies.

- The unpredictable nature of NF1 makes it particularly difficult for the patient to cope with. One subject in the study of Ablon (1992) describes this in a far better way than we could:

  > Most diseases will unfold in a certain way – slower or faster. With NF, because the symptoms are so unpredictable and variable, you don't know whether there will be symptoms, what they might be, or if they will be serious. You never get your balance or equilibrium on how to deal with them. After one thing appears and you deal with it, here comes another. It is not just that there are big and little fires, there is always the worrying sign up that says 'Danger of Fire'. The psychological burden is always there, regardless of the extent of the physical problems. Even when the symptoms are minor you still know something is there. The internal stigmata make people carry themselves differently even though externally others can't see it.

- The potential cosmetic disfigurement associated with the disease is particularly difficult in a society where much value is placed on a person's appearance. In the study of Benjamin *et al.* (1993) 48% of 54 patients had had problems related to the cosmetic aspects of NF1. Teasing at school about the café au lait spots did not seem to be a concern, but teasing about other aspects of NF1 (e.g. clumsiness, learning difficulties and plexiform neurofibromas) had occurred. Many adults described changes in life-style to try to hide the cutaneous neurofibromas by changing mode of dress and avoiding activities like swimming. Those individuals who were undiagnosed at the time of first appearance of their cutaneous neurofibromas were particularly anxious about them.

  > As more neurofibromas have grown on my face I have had a much harder time finding work. Somehow I know it's what I look like . . .
  >
  > *Ablon (1992)*

- Schooling difficulties were also a major concern to the patients in the Benjamin study. Thirty-two per cent of affected individuals reported being unhappy at school and tended to have a small social circle ($n = 56$). Thirty per cent of affected individuals reported having truanted from school on more than one occasion and 60% of cases had had difficulties with school work in junior school. One of the patients had commented, 'I was unable to learn quickly, to grasp new things. I was then left alone and began to get further behind.' The children still in school at the time of the study seemed to be receiving more help with their learning difficulties than did the previous generation, with 30% of children being helped by an educational psychologist. Their parents, however, remained concerned about behaviour and teasing.

- The association of the Elephant Man with NF1 means that the media view of the disease is one causing severe deformity. Doctors often introduce NF1 as the 'Elephant Man's disease' even though the majority of the medical profession (including the present authors) now believe that the diagnosis in the Elephant Man was one of Proteus syndrome as discussed by Dr Clark in Chapter 17. Some NF1 families think that the link with the Elephant Man's story is helpful for raising public awareness of neurofibromatosis and as a lesson in human dignity. However, older patients, particularly those who were introduced to NF1 by a doctor as being the 'Elephant Man's disease', often find the association very painful.

> All through my teens from the time I was thirteen till I was twenty I thought I was going to eventually just look like the 'Elephant Man'. I believed that I was going to be 'the Elephant Lady'. That was why I didn't want to make any plans for the future, thinking, What if I end up like that? Now I really feel cheated because I know it was all a big mistake. It's no one's fault. I'm not blaming anyone. But that still is the stereotype now in people's minds.
>
> *Ablon (1993)*

- NF1 patients and their families are often highly critical of how the diagnosis of NF1 has been dealt with in their family. They also usually perceive their disease as more of a problem than their doctors. In the study of Benjamin *et al.* (1993) the patients were asked to indicate whether they were affected severely, moderately, mildly or minimally and this was then compared with a medically judged severity grading. There was no correlation between individual perception and medical classification of severity, with the majority of patients perceiving themselves more severely affected ($p < 0.0001$). Individuals who had been diagnosed later in life, had a child with NF1, or who were concerned about the cosmetic aspects of the disease perceived themselves more severely affected.

> When I was fifteen my mother took me to an internist who was, as I call it, 'a graduate of the Dachau school of medicine'. He said, 'You have neurofibromatosis. I think you should be sterilised, because you should not bring any more defective babies into the world'. And at that age with my emerging sexuality. It was horrible. It's

> just the worst story I have to tell about that hospital, despite how bad the other stories are!
>
> The doctor said, 'Your son may have neurofibromatosis. If he does, he'll probably develop a brain tumour. But we won't know whether he has neurofibromatosis for a year or more, so just don't worry about it. Bring him back next year'.
>
> *Ablon (1992)*

15.3 GENERAL MANAGEMENT

15.3.1 Overview

As the awareness for the need for one health professional to take an overview of the care of NF1 sufferers has increased, a number of different approaches to disease management have evolved. Riccardi, a pioneer in the field who established one of the first neurofibromatosis clinics, suggested the following protocol in a review article in 1981:

> . . . all persons with neurofibromatosis or at risk for it should routinely undergo an extensive evaluation aimed at confirming the diagnosis, identifying complications and monitoring progression. Evaluation should include the following procedures: intelligence quotient measurement and psychological testing; electroencephalography; audiography; slit-lamp ocular examination; radiological skeletal surveying with special attention to the skull, optic foramina and spine (and, in selected cases, internal auditory canals); cranial CT scanning with and without dye contrast, to include the orbits and optic chiasms; and measurement of 24 h urinary excretion levels of epinephrine and norepinephrine.

When we began our research in NF1 in 1983, no centre in the UK ran a specialist neurofibromatosis clinic. Discussions with colleagues in various disciplines suggested that some accepted the need to offer NF1 sufferers regular follow-up, but felt that screening investigations, such as those suggested by Riccardi, were unnecessary. Based on the experience of the Welsh study, we concluded that patients with NF1 should have regular clinical assessments, but none of the complications occur often enough to warrant biochemical or radiological screening (Huson, Harper and Compston, 1988, 1989). We recommended that because many of the complications develop early in life, children with the disease should be reviewed twice yearly. Particular attention should be paid to intellectual development so that the child can be channelled into appropriate schooling. In adults, unless a particular complication indicated more frequent review, annual clinical examination only was recommended. Having worked with this protocol for several years, it is now felt that even

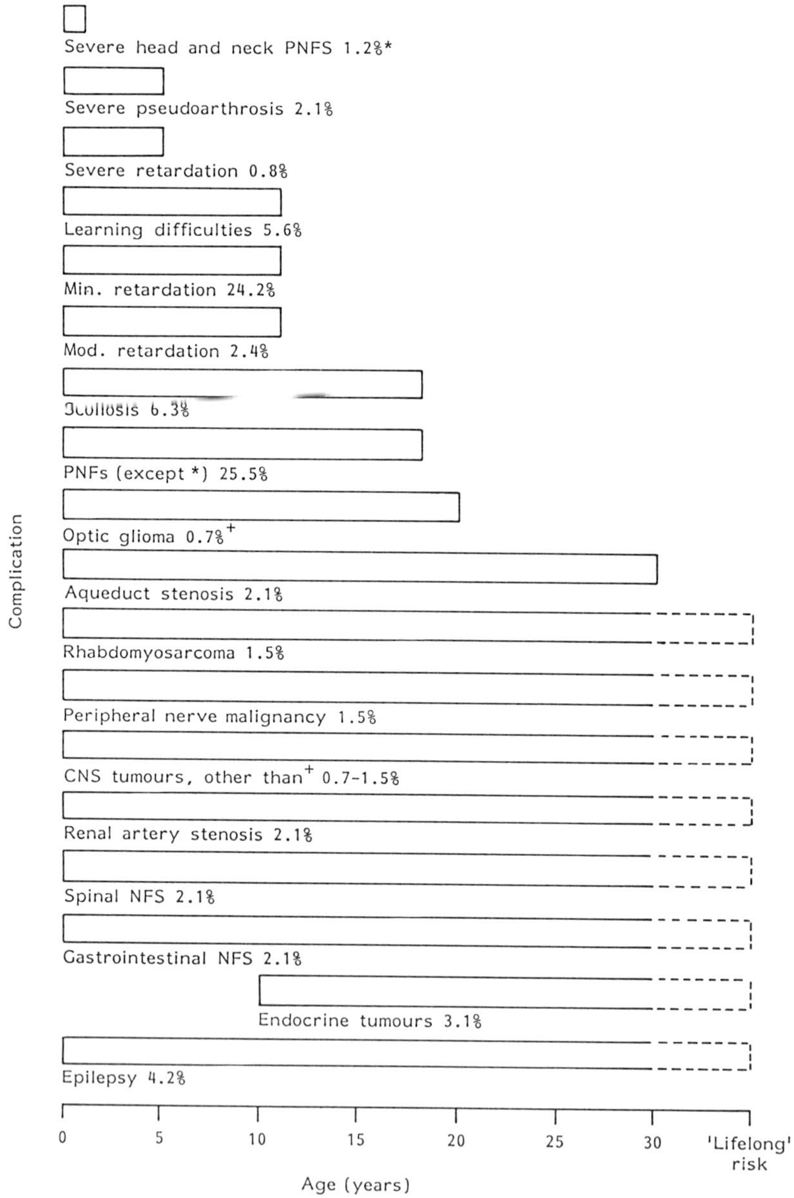

Figure 15.1 Age range at presentation and frequency of major NF1 complications. PNF plexiform neurofibroma; NFs neurofibromas. (Reproduced from Huson, Compston and Harper, 1989, with permission.)

for children twice-yearly review is too frequent. In the Oxford neurofibromatosis clinic we now review children only once a year unless a particular complication requires more frequent follow-up by a specific specialty. This is not a rigid approach. Often in the first year after the diagnosis of NF1 has been made in a child, the parents appreciate more frequent contact with the clinic as they gradually come to terms with information about NF1.

Each annual clinical assessment involves a general cutaneous examination to monitor the major disease features and then a general physical examination. At particular ages, particular complications should be sought. In Figure 15.1 the age ranges for presentation of the majority of NF1 complications are given. This can be used to assess what complications an individual of a given age is still at risk of developing; it can also be used for reassurance. For example, a young adult with no problems to date can be reassured that they now have no risk of certain complications, but monitored for those complications that might still occur. The age range during which a given feature may present was derived as follows, from review of previously published series: aqueduct stenosis (Horwich, Riccardi and Francke, 1983), endocrine tumours (Modlin *et al.*, 1979; Griffiths, Williams and Williams, 1987), CNS tumours (Lewis *et al.*, 1984; Ilgren, Kinnier-Wilson and Stiller, 1985), pseudoarthrosis (Morrissy, Riseborough and Hall, 1981), rhabdomyosarcoma (Hope and Mulvihill, 1981; Hartley *et al.*, 1988) and scoliosis (Chaglassian, Riseborough and Hall, 1976; Winter *et al.*, 1979); from the age of presentation in this study and that of Riccardi and Eichner (1986): plexiform neurofibroma. For intellectual handicap, it was assumed that severe developmental delay would have been identified by the age of 5 years and milder problems by the end of primary school education. The remaining complications have a 'life-long' risk of presentation because examples of each developing throughout life were found either in our series or the literature. Insufficient data are at present available to provide a more accurate age range. It is hoped that endeavours such as the National Neurofibromatosis Foundation (NNFF) clinical database may provide more specific data (Friedman, Birch and Greene, 1993). For some complications, there are peaks within the age range given. Rhabdomyosarcoma is an example: we have found these tumours to present most frequently in young children when they often arise in the pelvis (Huson, Harper and Compston, 1988; Hartley *et al.*, 1988). However, the risk is life-long because Hope and Mulvihill's review (1981) included a few adults with rhabdomyosarcoma elsewhere.

Although there is a low risk of the majority of these complications developing, it is important to draw attention to the high frequency of mild learning difficulties in children with NF1 as reviewed by Dr Ferner in Chapter 9. We have seen a considerable number of children who have been labelled as being lazy or uncooperative in the classroom setting, who on re-evaluation in the light of the diagnosis of NF1 have been found to have learning difficulties. Careful developmental monitoring is therefore essential in children with NF1, particularly in their early years at school, so that this kind of problem does not arise. If there is any doubt about the progress of a child with NF1, formal assessment by an educational psychologist can be extremely helpful.

15.3.2 The role of screening investigations

The general principles of screening (Cuckle and Wald, 1984) can be applied to the follow-up of patients with neurofibromatosis. The procedures used must be safe, simple and cheap. Whether costs should be a factor in designing screening protocols for specific complications of rare disease is a matter of debate. In our opinion, if the test is justified in the first place, then it makes sense to use the best possible technique (e.g. magnetic resonance imaging (MRI) rather than computed tomography (CT) for detection of vestibular Schwannomas in NF2). Screening protocols should have a high detection rate (a high proportion of affected individuals should yield a positive result) and a low false positive result (few unaffected individuals should yield a positive result). There should be a clear advantage in detecting the lesion in terms of treatment and natural history. Applying these principles to NF1, we do not believe that routine screening investigations for any disease complications are justified. All the complications that screening investigations would be necessary to detect (e.g. CNS tumours, phaeochromocytomas) are individually rare. In addition, no-one would actually treat some of the complications (e.g. optic gliomas) until they became symptomatic. Other complications are easily identified on routine clinical examination (e.g. hypertension due to renal artery stenosis or phaeochromocytoma, scoliosis). The 'non-screening' approach to managing NF1 patients was recommended by the NIH Consensus Conference Panel, who in their statement (1988) conclude that:

> . . . tests should be dictated by findings on clinical evaluation. Laboratory tests when aimed at asymptomatic patients are unlikely to be of value, particularly cranial computerised tomography, magnetic resonance imaging, electroencephalograms and evoked potentials.

Despite this statement some leading neurofibromatosis clinics still recommend routine cranial neuroimaging as part of the assessment in NF1. Listernick and Charrow (1990) recommend screening for optic gliomas because of the high proportion of asymptomatic cases only diagnosed because imaging studies are performed. In their series

(Listernick *et al.*, 1989) and that of Lewis *et al.* (1984), 15% of patients with NF1 had optic gliomas; however, only two out of 15 and 11 out of 33 of these lesions were clinically symptomatic in the respective studies. Riccardi (1992) is extremely dogmatic in his approach to routine neuroimaging in NF1:

> . . . in this day and age of concerns about the costs of health care, it is easy to understand a reluctance to adopt such an aggressive approach in the midst of apparent, even if declining, controversy. However it seems clear that until physicians who are immediately responsible for the health care of these children adopt a publicly stated, aggressive 'go get 'em' attitude, dozens, if not hundreds of children with NF1 will unnecessarily lose at least a portion of their sight each year.

We find this approach extremely difficult to accept because only a small proportion of asymptomatic optic gliomas will ever become symptomatic. In the southeast Wales population study, only two out of 135 (1.5%) of the population had symptomatic optic gliomas and none of the children have developed an optic glioma in the 6-year follow-up period to January 1992 (Cordeiro, Sampson and Huson, unpublished data).

Another problem with routine cranial imaging in NF1 is to know at what age the first scan should be performed and whether a negative scan at a given age means there is no further risk of optic glioma. A recent report by Listernick, Charrow and Greenwald (1992) throws some light on this question. They report on four children who all had initial normal cranial imaging studies between 3 and 11 months of age (three using CT and one MRI). A growth spurt in two children at 5 years 1 month and 5 years 9 months led to repeat scans and demonstration of chiasmal gliomas. A third child developed right proptosis at 20 months, secondary to an optic glioma with chiasmal extension. The fourth child was asymptomatic when a repeat scan showed extensive involvement of both optic nerves and the chiasm at 24 months of age; there has been no change in this tumour in 6 years of follow-up. These patients demonstrate that optic glioma in NF1 is an acquired lesion and that a negative early scan cannot be used for reassurance that no tumours will develop. As they have seen no children over the age of 6 years with negative neuroimaging who subsequently develop symptomatic tumours, Listernick, Charrow and Greenwald (1992) speculate that the period of greatest risk for the development of rapidly progressive tumours is during the first 5 years of life.

The other problem that emerges if MRI is used as the neuroimaging technique is the recognition of other CNS abnormalities. These are increased intensity lesions on T2-weighted images, which are seen in approximately 60% of children with NF1 (Duffner *et al.*, 1989; Chapter 9).

The nature of these lesions is as yet unclear, and although they appear to be benign, their recognition on a routine scan often causes parents unnecessary anxiety.

Although we do not agree with the routine use of screening investigations in NF1, their use in the clinical research setting is a different matter. For example, as a result of monitoring the outcome of his protocol investigations, Riccardi has ceased to do 24 h urine metadrenaline estimations because of the low frequency of phaeochromocytomas detected (Riccardi, 1992). With regard to the vexed issue of cranial neuroimaging, the only way the natural history of asymptomatic and symptomatic optic gliomas and the T2-weighted images seen on MRI scans can be be determined is by follow-up of cohorts of patients in a clinical research setting. The use of different body imaging techniques in the assessment and follow-up of plexiform neurofibromas is another important issue that this kind of study could address.

15.3.3 Management of specific disease features

(a) Neurofibromas

Of the major defining features, only neurofibromas cause the NF1 patient significant problems. Lisch nodules are never symptomatic. Café au lait spots do not cause actual symptoms, but sometimes children are embarrassed by them and teased at school. This is usually helped by the child beginning to understand about NF1 and having an easy explanation to give their friends about the café au lait spots. If patients are particularly distressed, treatment options are available as discussed by Drs Angel, Persing and Edgerton (section 14.3.7).

Dermal neurofibromas are associated with a number of problems. The principal one is their cosmetic appearance and the uncertainty as to how many will appear during a given individual's lifetime. In the Welsh study, 20% of the 94 patients (15 women, four men) were persistently distressed by their appearance (Huson, Harper and Compston, 1988). Unfortunately there is no treatment to prevent the development of neurofibromas. To offer patients the chance to have each neurofibroma removed as it develops is unrealistic. We encourage patients to come to terms with the variation in NF1 and its natural history, and through this to accept the appearance of their cutaneous neurofibromas. Patients are offered surgery for particularly large or unsightly lesions on exposed parts of the body or those that are a problem because of rubbing on clothing straps, etc. Patients are helped by having access to a plastic surgeon who is sympathetic to their problem and conscious of the importance of the cosmetic outcome of surgery (see Chapter 14 for review of the techniques available).

Dermal neurofibromas are rarely painful, but nodular lesions on large peripheral nerves and some plexiform neurofibromas can be painful and tender, particularly on palpation. Surgery for lesions involving the main nerve trunks must be carried out with great care by someone experienced in the field because of the risk of damage to the underlying nerve trunks (Chapter 14). The only actual physical symptom consistently reported in connection with dermal neurofibromas is pruritus. Some patients complain of general cutaneous pruritus, others find particular lesions itchy. This itchiness often occurs when neurofibromas are developing and resolves later. Twenty-one per cent of the patients in the Welsh study (Huson, Harper and Compston, 1988) reported pruritus of their neurofibromas and 18% (125 of 711) in the series of Riccardi (1992). Riccardi (1980, 1981) first reported pruritus associated with neurofibromas and the fact that patients often complain of itching in skin that has been exposed to blunt trauma where in turn a neurofibroma develops. Given the frequency of mast cells in neurofibromas, Riccardi (1980, 1981) proposed that the itching was caused by the release of chemicals such as histamine and that mast cells play a crucial part in control of neurofibroma growth. Riccardi has gone on to use the mast cell stabilizer, ketotifen, to treat pruritus and assess its effects on neurofibroma growth in the clinical setting. In 1987, he reported the outcome of a preliminary open label study in 15 patients. They received between 2 and 4 mg per day of ketotifen for between 30 and 43 months. Eleven patients noted improvement in neurofibroma-associated pruritus (or pain in association with subcutaneous or plexiform neurofibromas) and eight of the 11 patients had a general increase in well-being whilst on treatment. In addition there was a subjective decrease in neurofibroma size or slowing of tumour growth in most cases. In those who underwent surgery, there was a decrease in the amount of blood loss from the tumours noted at surgery. Blood loss is often profuse during operations on plexiform neurofibromas. Four of the 15 patients had no response to ketotifen administration, although one may have been non-compliant.

Given these encouraging results, Riccardi proceeded with a double-blind study involving 27 subjects (Riccardi, 1990, 1992) and found the effect on pruritus and pain was so marked that the patients could predict whether they were taking ketotifen or not. Riccardi concluded that the studies proved the value of ketotifen in five main areas: (1) itching, (2) pain and tenderness, (3) neurofibroma growth rate, (4) haemorrhage and (5) overall sense of patient well-being (Riccardi, 1992).

Although other centres have assessed the use of ketotifen, their results are less conclusive. Rubenstein (personal communication, 1992) embarked on a trial of its use in controlling pruritus, alternating drug or placebo for 2-month periods during an 8-month trial. From a clinic population of 400 NF1 patients, only 12 (3%) had persistent and generalized pruritus. In view of these small numbers, the trial was not completed. Assessment of the 12 patients suggested an effect on pruritus but not on growth. Mautner (1992) reports similar experience with pruritus. He feels there is a need to develop objective measures of neurofibroma growth and has begun to develop a method of tumour volume measurement. In Dr Huson's practice, few patients have suffered severe enough pruritus or pain that they want to take regular medication for it. The initial studies of Riccardi with ketotifen must be regarded as encouraging but preliminary. There is a need for a multicentre double-blind control trial of its use. Objective measures for tumour growth are difficult, but are essential so that assessments of several centres can be pooled to provide sufficient data for adequate statistical analysis. Development of trial methodology will be important as other potential treatments are developed, e.g. using antiangiogenic factors (Chapter 1) or through further understanding of gene action (Chapter 2).

(b) Management of disease complications

The authors of the respective chapters in this book deal with these as appropriate to their specialty. It helps if those involved in providing overall care of NF1 patients liaise with consultants in different specialties who have a particular interest in treatment of the NF1 complications in their discipline, e.g. orthopaedic surgeons with an interest in scoliosis or pseudoarthrosis.

15.3.4 The organization of health care for patients with NF1

Any one patient with NF1 can need to be seen by a number of different specialties at different times in their life. One of the principal complaints from people with NF1 to lay organizations (C. Peperell, personal communication) is that their health care is not coordinated and that they are not given an overview of the disease. Each specialist just treats their particular 'part' of the patient. These problems led to the formation of multidisciplinary neurofibromatosis clinics or programmes in the USA (Riccardi, 1981; Korf, 1990; Listernick and Charrow, 1990). In this setting patients are offered coordinated care and follow-up by a group of health professionals, which may include a paediatrician, geneticist, ophthalmologist, dermatologist, neurologist, neurosurgeon, orthopaedic surgeon, otolaryngologist, plastic surgeon, genetic counsellor, social worker and psychologist. Usually one of the group acts as the overall coordinator of patient care and involves other specialists at specific times in the patient's life (e.g. regular ophthalmic assessment during childhood for optic gliomas) or because of specific symptoms.

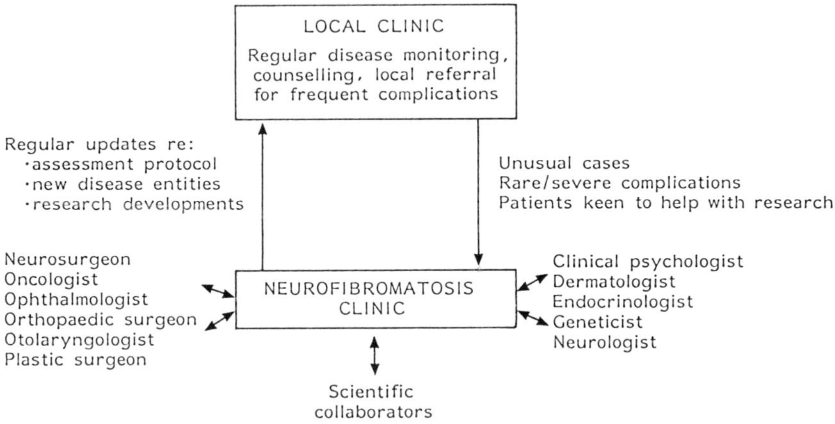

Figure 15.2 Suggested plan for organization of health care of NF1 sufferers. (Reproduced from Huson, 1990, by permission of Elsevier Science Publishers BV.)

In view of the fact that most patients with NF1 will not have a major disease complication during their life, we do not believe that all NF1 patients need to attend a specialist neurofibromatosis clinic on a regular basis. We prefer the model shown in Figure 15.2. Any country needs a number of specialist neurofibromatosis clinics, the number being dependent on the population. The clinics should be developed by individuals with a particular interest in neurofibromatosis, who should collaborate with interested specialists and scientists in appropriate fields. Such centres should be available for diagnostic assessment of unusual cases, to assess cases with particular severe manifestations and to coordinate research programmes. At the neurofibromatosis clinic in Oxford, there is a steady flow of patients and their families who feel they are not getting appropriate follow-up and come for an overall assessment. It usually turns out that having read about the work of neurofibromatosis clinics in the USA, they are worried that they are not being followed up intensively enough. After assessment at the Oxford clinic, and having been given an overview of the pros and cons of the various approaches to neurofibromatosis management, they are usually more than happy to return to local follow-up. We believe that most NF1 patients should be cared for in the 'local setting', either by a hospital consultant or family physician. The question of which specialist should follow up NF1 patients is a difficult one. Because many NF1 complications present in childhood, we usually recommend annual follow-up by a consultant paediatrician during this period. Care at the local level may be improved by one particular paediatrician in a district hospital following all the NF1 children. In adults the family physician or any one of a number of specialists (e.g. clinical geneticist, neurologist or dermatologist) are equally appropriate. Many families appreciate at least one session with a clinical geneticist for an overview of the genetics of NF1 and how it applies to their family.

Many patients with NF1 who do not have a major medical problem at a particular time feel they are wasting their doctor's time just in talking about NF1 in general and their fears about the disease. Through a need to share these experiences, lay organizations have developed in many countries (these are listed on p. xv). The lay organizations provide a vital role in supplying information and in offering help and support to individuals with NF1 and their families. Patients are also helped by having a non-medical health professional with particular skills in counselling who they can contact for support. This may be a specialist genetic nurse or genetic counsellor in patients who have attended a genetics clinic (Bernhardt and Halperin, 1990; Wilson and Yahr, 1990). The British neurofibromatosis patients' association, have recently funded two family support workers to help fulfil this role. One is based in Oxford and helps to coordinate the neurofibromatosis clinic. The family support worker is able to offer ongoing support to families between clinic appointments and offers specific activities such as meetings of groups of NF1 patients with particular disease problems or at particular times in their lives (e.g. groups of adolescents coming to terms with their NF1).

15.4 GENETIC COUNSELLING IN NF1

15.4.1 Introduction

The essential features of the process of genetic counselling are summarized in the following definition (Harper, 1988):

> Genetic counselling is the process by which patients or relatives at risk of a disorder which may be hereditary are advised of the consequences of the disorder, the probability of developing and transmitting it and of the ways this may be prevented or ameliorated.

Prior to giving genetic advice the counsellor must ensure the diagnosis of the condition in question is correct. For NF1, as discussed in Chapter 7, confirming the diagnosis and explaining dominant inheritance is usually straightforward. Informing the patient and their family about the various complications of NF1 is a very difficult counselling task. One has to strike a fine balance between providing adequate information and causing unnecessary alarm. In our experience, NF1 families prefer to have as much information as possible about their condition. The speed at which this information can be absorbed and the best method of delivering it vary from family to family. Some doctors believe that to discuss all the aspects of NF1 with a family is unnecessary as some of the complications are so rare, and knowledge of them may cause unnecessary distress. If this is not done, however, and the patient gets information via a newspaper or television programme, the information about a particular disease aspect may be exaggerated or wrong. The patient is then left with a feeling of mistrust towards their physician for not having informed them in the first place and an exaggerated fear about the particular problem because of wrong information. Research in other chronic neurological diseases (Huntington's disease and multiple sclerosis) has shown that honest communication actually generated constructive behaviours, including family understanding and acceptance of the illness and positive sick role expectations (Power and Sax, 1978).

15.4.2 Explaining the natural history of NF1

As discussed above, this is an extremely difficult task. We usually begin with a description of the major defining features and of the timing of their appearance. With regard to the complications of NF1, very few families are able to cope with a list of all the disease complications, how they may present and what are the available treatment options. In children, learning difficulties are so frequent that they are worth discussing with all parents, particularly as to how mild difficulties may present to avoid the child being labelled as 'just lazy' at school. For the other complications, rather than working through a long list, we have found it useful to group them together as they will affect an individual's lifestyle and discuss them in these terms (Table 15.3). The important balance to achieve is for the patient to accept that most people with NF1 don't have major medical problems, but when they do occur, the earlier they are detected and treated then the better the outcome. Patients therefore must have some awareness of disease complications and in a way be encouraged to act as 'their own physicians' and always to ask if NF1 could be responsible for any unusual symptoms they are experiencing. The importance of being aware of the different complications is illustrated by several children with pseudoarthrosis seen by one of the authors (S.M.H.). On initial assessment in several of these children there has been an unnecessary initial suspicion of child abuse, either because the significance of the family history of NF1 was not appreciated or the children were very young, the café au lait spots not terribly obvious and the association of pseudoarthrosis and NF1 not appreciated by the examining doctor.

15.4.3 Recurrence risks for parents of an isolated case

The reports of cases with limited expression of the NF1 gene having affected children (Riccardi and Lewis, 1988; Chapter 7) mean that detailed cutaneous and slit-lamp examination of the parents of an apparently

Table 15.3 Frequency of NF1 complications for counselling purposes (from Huson, Compston and Harper, 1989, with permission)

	%
Intellectual handicap	
moderate–severe retardation	3.2
minimal retardation or learning difficulties	29.8
total	33.0
Developing in childhood and causing lifelong morbidity	
severe plexiform neurofibromas of head and neck	1.2
scoliosis, requiring surgery	5.2
severe pseudoarthrosis	2.1
total	8.5
'Treatable' complications that can develop at any age	
aqueduct stenosis	2.1
epilepsy	4.2
spinal neurofibromas	2.1
visceral neurofibromas	2.1
endocrine tumours	3.1
renal artery stenosis	2.1
total	15.7
CNS and malignant tumours	
optic gliomas	0.7
other CNS tumours	0.7–1.5
rhabdomyosarcoma	1.5
peripheral nerve malignancy	1.5
total	4.4–5.2

isolated case is essential before counselling is given. In the absence of any abnormalities, in our opinion, there is no significant increased risk of a further affected child. We are aware of only two reported cases of recurrence in a second sibling when the parents were apparently normal (Riccardi and Lewis, 1988), and these might have happened by chance rather than representing gonadal mosaicism.

If limited NF1 features are found in the parent of an apparently isolated case, they usually appear in a segmental distribution and it is presumed that the parent also has gonadal involvement (i.e. they are gonosomal mosaics). At the present time it is impossible to give accurate recurrence risks in this situation, and we usually quote an empirical risk in the region of 5%. It must be emphasized that the area of skin showing NF1 involvement does not necessarily lie in relation to the gonads and so individuals with segmental NF, whatever the distribution, must also be aware of a similar risk of them having children with NF1.

15.4.4 Risk figures for prospective parents

The 50% risk of autosomal dominant inheritance is straightforward. The penetrance of NF1 approaches virtually 100% by the age of 5 years. It is important to stress the extreme variability of NF1 and the fact that the complications do not breed true even within families. This is particularly important if the affected parent has a disease complication, as they often think children will have the same presentation of NF1. We usually discuss the risk of the groups of complications as shown in Table 15.3. The risks to offspring of an affected parent are shown below; the frequencies for complications given in Table 15.3 have been halved and rounded to the nearest 0.5%:

- intellectual handicap, 16.5% (moderate/severe retardation 1.5%, minimal retardation/learning difficulties 15%);
- complications developing in childhood and causing lifelong morbidity, 4.5%;
- treatable complications that can develop at any age, 8%;
- malignant or CNS tumours, 2.3%.

For some couples, this approach is too complex and then it is important to try and identify what complications the couple would find a particular problem if they occurred in the child and talk about the risk of them occurring. If one assumes that these may include moderate to severe mental retardation, the different complications that develop in childhood and cause lifelong morbidity and the risk of developing a brain tumour or malignant tumour elsewhere, then the combined chance to the offspring of an affected parent is 8%. With the advent of molecular genetic diagnosis of NF1 (section 15.4.6), prenatal diagnosis is now an option for some prospective parents. In practice, however, our experience is that many parents decide that the risk of having a child with one of the severe complications is relatively small, and proceed to have children without prenatal diagnosis. Many comment that if a test was available that would detect the different levels of disease severity, then a prenatal diagnostic test would be worthwhile.

15.4.5 Follow-up of children at risk of NF1

Because café au lait spots are present in all gene carriers by the age of 5 years at the very latest, we usually recommend children at risk are checked once a year until that time. If there are no café au lait spots present within the first year of life, it is extremely likely that the child has not inherited NF1. We have, however, seen a few children, particularly those with pale skins, who had only one or two small café au lait spots by the first birthday but developed more during the second and third year of life. If parents find the process of waiting to see if café au lait spots are going to appear or not difficult, or if by the age of 5 years there are equivocal features, then molecular genetic diagnosis can sometimes can be used to clarify the diagnosis (section 15.4.6).

15.4.6 Prenatal and presymptomatic diagnosis for NF1

Before the application of molecular genetic techniques to the prenatal and presymptomatic diagnosis of NF1, there was no 'test' available for the disease either prenatally or presymptomatically. The clinical diagnosis in early childhood relied on the appearance of café au lait spots with or without other disease features. As the severe complications that result in structural abnormalities are rarely obvious at birth, ultrasound scanning during pregnancy would not be expected to pick up abnormalities related to NF1.

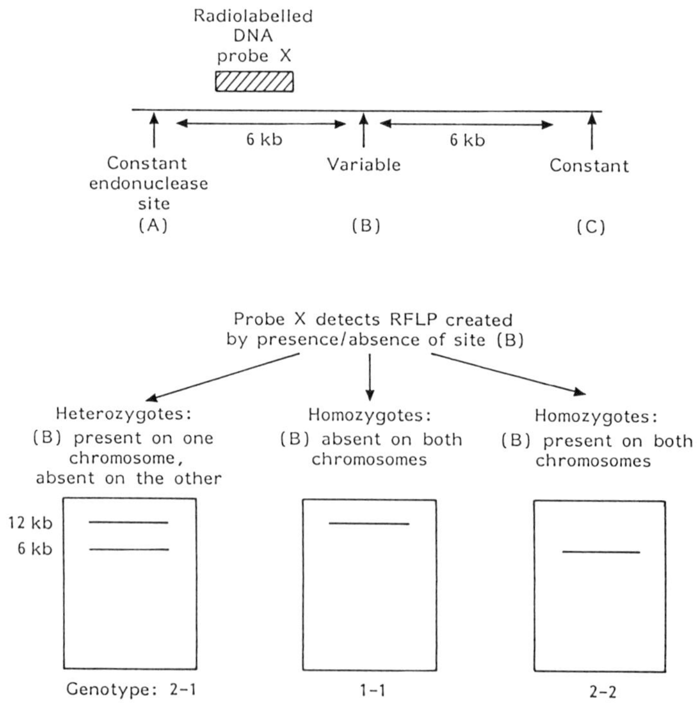

Figure 15.3 Detection of an RFLP by a DNA probe and corresponding genotypes on an autoradiograph. The DNA probe (X) binds to the complementary strand of the subject's DNA; near this are three sites where a given restriction endonuclease can cut the DNA. Sites (A) and (C) are present in the whole population, but the presence of (B) is variable giving rise to an RFLP.

Benjamin *et al.* (1993) assessed the demand for prenatal testing by the NF1 patients on the North Western Region Genetic Family Register. Of 29 individuals considering having children, three (10%) wanted the option of a prenatal test with a view to termination of an affected offspring. A further nine (31%) wanted a test just to know as early as possible the child's disease status. No-one has objectively examined the demand for early presymptomatic DNA testing of NF1. Molecular genetic techniques used to map and isolate genes, described in Chapter 2, have the immediate benefit to the patient of providing genetic markers that 'track' the disease gene through the family (Pembrey, 1987; Weatherall, 1991). In this context the marker gene is used to detect a variation in the DNA called a restriction fragment length polymorphism (RFLP). When DNA is cut with a particular kind of enzyme, called a restriction endonuclease, the number of sites where these enzymes can cut varies within the population. The presence/absence of some of the sites is inherited as a Mendelian trait, which give rise to the RFLPs. In Figure 15.3 the diagram demonstrates how such a polymorphism works to create a two-allele system where people can be homozygote 1–1 or 2–2 or heterozygote 2–1. The method of labelling of the alleles is arbitrary, but is usually numerical or alphabetical and starts with the largest alleles. In Figure 15.4 the marker is tracked through a family. In this family the grandfather (I–1)

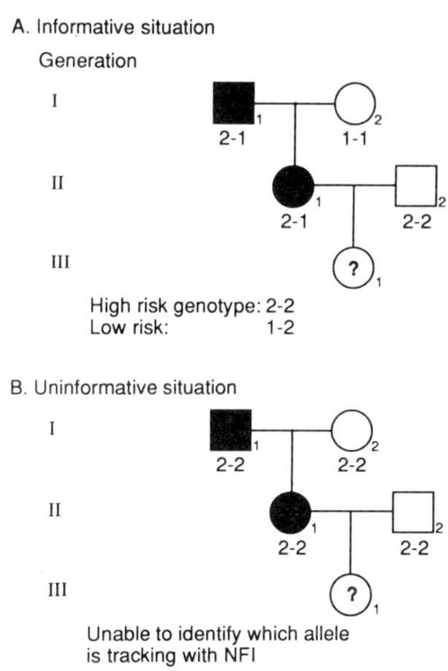

Figure 15.4 Use of genetic markers in presymptomatic diagnosis. (A) Informative situation – NF1 is tracking with the 2 allele. (B) Uninformative situation – all affected family members are homozygous 22, the chromosome 17 carrying the NF1 mutation cannot be identified.

has NF1, which he passed to his daughter (II–I), who would now like to know if her newborn baby (III–I) is affected. In the informative situation the 2 allele is going with NF1 (Figure 15.4a). If the child has a 2–2 genotype she is at high risk of NF1; if she has a 1–2 genotype she is at low risk as the 1 allele is inherited from her unaffected maternal grandmother and the 2 allele from her father. Obviously, if everyone in the family has the same marker typing then the situation is uninformative; this is illustrated in Figure 15.4b. The development of markers with multiple alleles within and around the *NF1* gene has decreased the number of uninformative families, particularly the Alu repeat polymorphism (Xu *et al.*, 1991), the compound nucleotide repeat (Andersen *et al.*, 1993) and the CA/GT repeat polymorphism (in intron 27, Weiss, personal communication).

For NF1, as there are now markers both within and on either side of the gene (Chapter 2), very accurate predictions, virtually 100% certain, can be made. The limitations of the 'gene tracking' approach are that it can usually only be applied in families where two or more people are affected and blood specimens for DNA analysis are usually needed from both of them. Blood samples from the unaffected spouses are also often needed so that it can be seen which markers the children inherited from the affected parent and which from the unaffected parent. The fact that 50% of cases with NF1 are due to new mutation severely limits the use of gene markers for molecular genetic diagnosis of NF1. In half the families there are therefore not enough people in the family to enable prediction to be done. However, once a person with NF1 due to a new mutation has had one or more children and their disease status is known, marker studies can be used for prenatal and presymptomatic diagnosis of subsequent pregnancies (Lazaro *et al.*, 1992). Also, because not all markers are helpful in every family, it can take several weeks to see if a family is 'informative' (Figure 15.4) and therefore this phase of the marker testing is better done before a pregnancy. If the results for a couple are informative for prenatal testing, a specimen of fetal DNA can be obtained from a chorionic villus sample taken at around 10–11 weeks of pregnancy. This technique risks causing a miscarriage in about 2% of cases (Silverman and Wapner, 1992).

Once a gene has been isolated, the most accurate test is to find the specific mutation that has caused the disease in that family, rather than use marker genes. For NF1, this has the advantage that it would be available to people who represent new gene mutations for prenatal and presymptomatic testing in their children. Although the gene was isolated in 1990, it is proving difficult to identify mutations with available techniques. Only approximately 10% of cases tested in one large series had identifiable mutations (Upadhyaya *et al.*, 1992). The techniques used are time-consuming. Mutation testing is unlikely to become routinely available until an easier method with a greater pick-up rate is available. Once a lot of mutations have been identified, it will be possible to undertake genotype/phenotype correlation to see if any particular mutation is associated with a particular disease complication or particularly severe expression of a disease feature such as dermal neurofibromas. From the work of Easton *et al.* discussed in Chapter 7, we anticipate that mutation analysis is probably not going to be helpful with phenotype analysis for NF1.

Even with the linked genetic markers available for NF1, the demand from families has been small. Ward *et al.* (1990) and Hofman and Boehm (1992) have described preliminary experience in the USA and Upadhyaya *et al.* (1992) the experience in the UK. We were providing a service for a large part of England and Wales, and taking referrals from other countries. In 2 years, six prenatal diagnostic tests were performed, 11 couples (and relevant members of their families) were tested for marker informativeness for future prenatal diagnosis and presymptomatic tests were carried out for six at-risk individuals. Of the six prenatal diagnoses, there were four low-risk and two high-risk predictions. One of the high-risk pregnancies was terminated because of a coincidental abnormal karyotype; the other continued to term and a child with multiple café au lait spots was born. Overall this is a relatively low uptake of molecular genetic testing. With regard to prenatal testing, many couples we have counselled would not consider a test unless it could predict disease severity. Other families, where a person has had particularly severe problems, were so anxious about NF1 that prenatal diagnosis with termination of pregnancy was their preferred option. Yet other couples decide to have a prenatal test just to determine the child's disease status. Some couples find the uncertainty and waiting during pregnancy an extremely difficult time and prefer to have the result to help them come to terms with the situation if the child has inherited the gene prior to birth. For some couples, this decision-making process is made particularly difficult if the way that they view the disease is different. Some affected individuals feel that they do not want to take the responsibility of passing NF1 onto their children, but their partners are more objective about the actual risk figures of severely affected children. One couple we counselled had particular difficulties when one of them had attended a lay group meeting and the other had not. At the meeting the affected partner had seen people with NF1 complicated by severe facial plexiform neurofibromas and was extremely distressed. From that time, the risk that she was given of 1 in 100 of this complication arising was unacceptable, yet her husband still saw it as a very acceptable risk to take.

We have no personal experience of parents requesting presymptomatic testing in the Oxford neurofibromatosis clinic, as they have been happy to wait for clinical clarification of the situation. Although our experience and that of other centres involved in DNA testing suggests that some individuals still remain anxious about NF1 despite normal physical examination, in this context or in the presence of equivocal clinical findings, molecular diagnosis is of value.

15.5 CONCLUSIONS

Although the various disease features of NF1 have been recognized since the latter part of the nineteenth century, only in the last two decades has an overall awareness of NF1 begun to develop amongst health professionals. This is beginning to improve patient care, but the best ways to deliver care need to be re-evaluated continually. The recent cloning of the *NF1* gene has contributed significantly to our understanding of the pathogenesis of NF1 (Chapter 2). It is hoped that this understanding will eventually help prevent or treat some of the disease complications. To maximize the benefit to NF1 patients of such developments, it is important that clinical researchers begin to work closely together to address issues such as objective measures of neurofibroma growth and disease severity grading. Although NF1 is 'common' in terms of genetic diseases in general, its complications are sufficiently rare that multicentre international treatment trials will be necessary.

Alongside these medical developments must come an increased awareness of the psychosocial issues surrounding NF1. The medical profession needs to involve other health professionals, such as psychologists and social workers, in supporting NF1 patients and their families. We must remember the particular problems associated with the uncertainty of long-term prognosis and cosmetic burden of the disease. We must also remember the mixed blessings of the association of the Elephant Man and NF1. The next two chapters demonstrate that the true diagnosis of Merrick's condition still causes fascination to the medical profession, but for NF1 families the association with the Elephant Man has often not been helpful. We can, however, learn a lesson in human dignity from the way Merrick coped with his illness (Montague, 1971). There is no doubt that a fundamental change in the lives of individuals with NF1 would occur if society's attitude to appearance changed. On this matter, we can only echo the words of Ellis (1990), who, in summarizing an article on psychosocial aspects of appearance in NF1, wrote:

> The competitiveness in our society and our way of evaluating our qualities by comparison with others rather than by what they do for ourselves reduces pleasure in life for all of us. If we think about appearance less in terms of standards that we ought to meet, the changes in appearance due to illness, like those due to ageing, need not be a cause for shame or inferiority, but simply one aspect of the person. Particularly as we grow older, a heavy emphasis on beauty and health needs to give way to more enduring qualities, such as

courage, humour, and compassion. Thus we affirm our awareness of the value and dignity of human beings and their right to respectful and humane treatment no matter how they look.

REFERENCES

Ablon, J. (1992) The psychological implications of uncertainty, diagnosis, chronicity and prognosis in NF, in *Psychosocial Aspects of the Neurofibromatoses: Impact on the Individual, Impact on the Family*, The National Neurofibromatosis Foundation, New York, pp. 49–66.

Ablon, J. (1993) The 'Elephant Man' as 'Self' and 'Other'. The psychosocial costs of a misdiagnosis. *Soc. Sci. Med.* In press.

Andersen, L.B., Tarle, S.A., Marchuk, D.A. *et al.* (1993) A highly informative compound tetranucleotide repeat in the neurofibromatosis (*NF1*) gene. *Hum. Mol. Genet.*, **2**, 1083.

Benjamin, C.M., Colley, A., Donnai, D. *et al.* (1993) Neurofibromatosis type 1: knowledge, experience and reproductive decisions of affected individuals and families. *J. Med. Genet.*, in press.

Bernhardt, B. and Halperin, J.C. (1990) Genetic counselling for neurofibromatosis, in *Neurofibromatosis: A Handbook for Patients, Families and Healthcare Professionals* (eds A.E. Rubenstein and B.R. Korf), Thieme, New York, pp. 201–8.

Chaglassian, J.H., Riseborough, E.J. and Hall, J.E. (1976) Neurofibromatosis scoliosis: natural history and results of treatment in thirty-seven cases. *J. Bone Joint Surg. [Am.]*, **58A**, 695–702.

Cuckle, H.S. and N.J. (1984) Principles of screening, in *Antenatal and Neonatal Screening* (ed. N.J. Wald), Oxford University Press, Oxford.

Duffner, P.K., Cohen, M.E., Seidel, F.G. and Shucard, D.W. (1989) The significance of MRI abnormalities in children with neurofibromatosis. *Neurology*, **39**, 373–8.

Easton, D.F., Ponder, M.A., Huson, S.M. and Ponder, B.A.J. (1993) An analysis of variation in expression of NF1: evidence for modifying genes. *Am J. Hum. Genet.*, **53**, 305–13.

Ellis, S.A. (1990) Psychosocial aspects of appearance in neurofibromatosis, in *Neurofibromatosis: A Handbook for Patients, Families and Healthcare Professionals* (eds A.E. Rubinstein and B.R. Korf), Thieme, New York, pp. 225–30.

Friedman, J., Birch, P., Greene, C. and the NNFF International Database Participants (1993) National Neurofibromatosis Foundation International Database. *Am. J. Med. Genet.*, **45**, 397–9.

Griffiths, D.F.R., Williams, G.T. and Williams, E.D. (1987) Duodenal carcinoid, phaeochromocytoma and neurofibromatosis: islet cell tumor, phaeochromocytoma and the von Hippel Lindau complex: two distinctive neuroendocrine syndromes. *Q. J. Med.*, **64**, 769–82.

Harper, P.S. (1988) *Practical Genetic Counselling*, 3rd edn, Wright, London.

Hartley, A.L., Birch, J.M., Marsden, H.B. *et al.* (1988) Neurofibromatosis in children with soft tissue sarcoma. *Paediatr. Hemat. Oncol.*, **5**, 7–16.

Hofman, K.J. and Boehm, C.D. (1992) Familial neurofibromatosis type 1: clinical experience with DNA testing. *J. Pediatr.*, **120**, 394–8.

Hope, D.G. and Mulvihill, J.J. (1981) Malignancy in neurofibromatosis. *Adv. Neurol.*, **29**, 33–55.

Horwich, A., Riccardi, V.M. and Francke, U. (1983) Brief clinical report:

Aqueductal stenosis leading to hydrocephalus – an unusual manifestation of neurofibromatosis. *Am. J. Med. Genet.*, **14**, 577–81.

Huson, S.M. (1989) Clinical and genetic studies of von Recklinghausen neurofibromatosis, MD thesis, University of Edinburgh.

Huson, S.M. (1990) Clinical and genetic studies of neurofibromatosis type 1 (NF1), in *Tuberous Sclerosis and Neurofibromatosis: Epidemiology, Pathophysiology, Biology and Management* (eds Y. Ishibashi and Y. Hori), Elsevier, Amsterdam.

Huson, S.M., Harper, P.S. and Compston, D.A.S. (1988) Von Recklinghausen neurofibromatosis: a clinical and population study in South East Wales. *Brain*, **111**, 1355–81.

Huson, S.M., Compston, D.A.S. and Harper, P.S. (1989) A genetic study of von Recklinghausen neurofibromatosis in South East Wales II: Guidelines for genetic counselling. *J. Med. Genet.*, **26**, 712–21.

Ilgren, E.B., Kinnier-Wilson, L.M. and Stiller, C.A. (1985) Gliomas in neurofibromatosis: a series of 89 cases with evidence for enhanced malignancy in associated cerebellar astrocytomas. *Pathol. Ann.*, **20**(1), 331–58.

Korf, B.R. (1990) Diagnosis of neurofibromatosis and clinical overview, in *Neurofibromatosis: A Handbook for Patients, Families and Healthcare Professionals* (eds A.E. Rubenstein and B.R. Korf), Thieme, New York, pp. 15–28.

Lazaro, C., Ravella, A., Casals, T. *et al.* (1992) Prenatal diagnosis of sporadic neurofibromatosis 1. *Lancet*, **339**, 119–20.

Lewis, R.A., Gerson, L.P., Axelson, K.A. *et al.* (1984) Von Recklinghausen neurofibromatosis II. Incidence of optic gliomata. *Ophthalmology*, **91**, 929–35.

Listernick, R. and Charrow, J. (1990) Neurofibromatosis type 1 in childhood. *J. Pediatr.*, **116**, 845–53.

Listernick, R., Charrow, J., Greenwald, M.J. and Esterly, N.A. (1989) Optic gliomas in children with neurofibromatosis type 1. *J. Pediatr.*, **114**, 788–92.

Listernick, R., Charrow, J. and Greenwald, M. (1992) Emergence of optic pathway gliomas in children with neurofibromatosis 1 following normal neuroimaging studies. *J. Pediatr.*, **121**, 584–7.

Mautner, F. (1992) Actual aspects of treatment of NF1 patients with neurofibromatosis. Presentation at the NNFF International Neurofibromatosis Symposium, Vienna.

Messner, R.L. and Smith, M.N. (1986) Neurofibromatosis: relinquishing the masks; a quest for quality life. *J. Adv. Nurs.*, **11**, 459–64.

Messner, R.L., Gardner, S. and Messner, M. (1985) Neurofibromatosis – an international enigma: a framework for nursing. *Cancer Nurs.*, **8**, 314–22.

Messner, R.L., Messner, M. and Lewis, S. (1985) Neurofibromatosis: a familial and family disorder. *J. Neurosurg. Nurs.*, **17**, 221–9.

Modlin, I.M., Farndon, J.R., Shepherd, A. *et al.* (1979) Phaeochromocytoma in 72 patients: clinical and diagnostic features, treatment and long term results. *Br. J. Surg.*, **66**, 456–65.

Montague, A. (1971) *The Elephant Man: A Study of Human Dignity*, Dutton, London.

Morrissy, R.T., Riseborough, E.J. and Hall, J.E. (1981) Congenital pseudoarthrosis of the tibia. *J. Bone Joint Surg.*, **63B**, 367–75.

NIH Consensus Development Conference Statement (1988) Neurofibromatosis. *Arch. Neurol.*, **45**, 575–8.

Pembrey, M. (1987) Impact of molecular biology on clinical genetics. *Br. Med. J.*, **295**, 711–13.

Power, P.W. and Sax, D.S. (1978) The communication of information to the neurological patient: some implications for family coping. *J. Chron. Dis.*, **31**, 57–65.

Riccardi, V.M. (1980) The pathophysiology of neurofibromatosis: IV. Dermatologic insights into heterogeneity and pathogenesis. *J. Am. Acad. Dermatol.*, **3**, 157–66.

Riccardi, V.M. (1981) Von Recklinghausen neurofibromatosis. *N. Engl. J. Med.*, **305**, 1617–27.

Riccardi, V.M. (1987) Mast-cell stabilisation to decrease neurofibroma growth. *Arch. Dermatol.*, **123**, 1011–16.

Riccardi, V.M. (1990) The potential role of trauma and mast cells in the pathogenesis of neurofibromatosis, in *Tuberous Sclerosis and Neurofibromatosis: Epidemiology, Pathophysiology, Biology and Management* (eds Y. Ishibashi and Y. Hori), Elsevier, Amsterdam, pp. 167–90.

Riccardi, V.M. (1992) *Neurofibromatosis: Phenotype, Natural History and Pathogenesis*, 2nd edn, The Johns Hopkins University Press, Baltimore.

Riccardi, V.M. and Eichner, J.E. (1986) *Neurofibromatosis: Phenotype, Natural History and Pathogenesis*, The Johns Hopkins University Press, Baltimore.

Riccardi, V.M. and Lewis, R.A. (1988) Penetrance of von Recklinghausen neurofibromatosis: a distinction between predecessors and descendants. *Am J. Hum. Genet.*, **42**, 284–9.

Silverman, N.S. and Wapner, R.T. (1992) Chorionic villus sampling, in *Prenatal Diagnosis and Screening* (eds D.J.H. Brock, C.H. Rodeck and M.A. Ferguson-Smith), Churchill Livingstone, Edinburgh.

Upadhyaya, M., Fryer, A., MacMillan, J. *et al.* (1992) Prenatal diagnosis and presymptomatic diagnosis of neurofibromatosis type 1. *J. Med. Genet.*, **29**, 180–3.

Upadhyaya, M., Shen, M., Cherryson, A. *et al.* (1992) Analysis of mutations at the neurofibromatosis 1 (NF1) locus. *Hum. Mol. Genet.*, **1**, 735–40.

Ward, K., O'Connell, P., Carey, J.C. *et al.* (1990) Diagnosis of neurofibromatosis 1 by using tightly linked, flanking markers. *Am. J. Hum. Genet.*, **46**, 943–9.

Weatherall, D.J. (1991) *The New Genetics and Clinical Practice*, 3rd edn, Oxford University Press, Oxford.

Wilson, M.A. and Yahr, M.S. (1990) Impact of neurofibromatosis on the family, in *Neurofibromatosis: A Handbook for Patients, Families and Healthcare Professionals* (eds A.E. Rubenstein and B.R. Korf), Thieme, New York, pp. 216–24.

Winter, R.B., Moe, J.H., Bradford, D.S. *et al.* (1979) Spine deformity in neurofibromatosis. *J. Bone Joint Surg.*, **61**, 677–94.

Xu, G., Nelson, L., O'Connell, P. and White, R. (1991) An Alu polymorphism intragenic to the *NF1* gene. *Nucleic Acids Res.*, **19**, 3764.

16

Did the Elephant Man have neurofibromatosis 1?

G.R. Seward

16.1 INTRODUCTION

There is now a body of opinion that supports the Proteus syndrome as a diagnosis for Joseph Merrick, the Elephant Man, rather than neurofibromatosis, but his story played an important part in the development of the perception of von Recklinghausen's disease. The available evidence of his medical history is set out in this chapter. The reasons that led contemporary physicians and early commentators to a diagnosis of neurofibromatosis can be readily discerned. However, many of Joseph Merrick's features are unique to him. Alternative diagnoses, particularly Proteus syndrome (Chapter 17), have only recently been delineated and were not available to nineteenth and early twentieth century clinicians.

16.2 HIS LIFE STORY

16.2.1 Early years

Joseph Carey Merrick was born on 5 August 1862 at 50 Lee Street, Leicester to Mary Jane Merrick, née Potterton, and Joseph Rockley Merrick (Howard and Ford, 1980). His father was aged 24 years at this time and his mother, who was a cripple, was aged 25 years. It is probable that he was normal in appearance as an infant, but a firm swelling of the right cheek became apparent at 21 months and this extended forwards under the upper lip. The other soft-tissue swellings began to be evident at about 5 years of age and the skeletal abnormalities somewhat later.

His brother, William Arthur Merrick, who was normal, was born on 8 January 1866 and his sister Marion Eliza on 28 September 1867. The sister was crippled from birth and lived only 23½ years before dying of 'myoletic convulsions' (Ford, 1989, personal communication).

Joseph fell when he was 4–5 years of age, injuring his left hip. When he was 10 years old his mother died of bronchopneumonia. His father remarried in 1875 and in the same year Joseph, now aged 12 years, left school and took a job rolling cigars. He had to give this up at the age of 15 years because of increasing clumsiness of his deformed right hand. A mass protruded between his teeth and eventually reached 20–23 cm in length and some 85–113 g of it were removed under a general anaesthetic at the Leicester Infirmary, probably in 1882. No histological examination was made of the specimen.

16.2.2 He meets Treves

It was to 123 Whitechapel Road (now 259) that Tom Norman, a showman who exhibited freaks, brought Merrick towards the end of November 1884. There, Frederick Treves' house surgeon, Dr Reginald Tuckett, saw him and then told Treves about the Elephant Man.

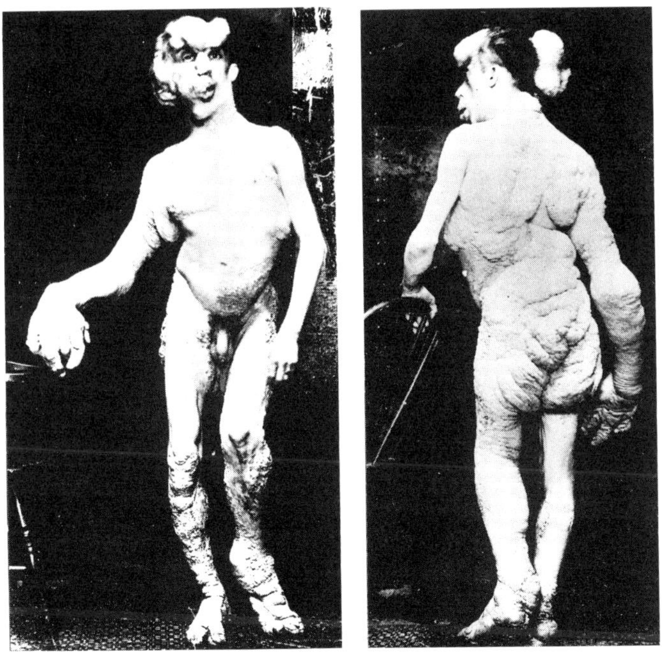

Figure 16.1 Two of the four photographs taken in 1886. Note particularly the line of separate hemispherical tumours on the inner aspect of the right thigh and the front of the left. There is a darker zone of skin over the lower left quadrant of the abdomen which spans the boundary between upward and downward facing planes. The axillary fold is similar to the folds of a plexiform neurofibromatosis.

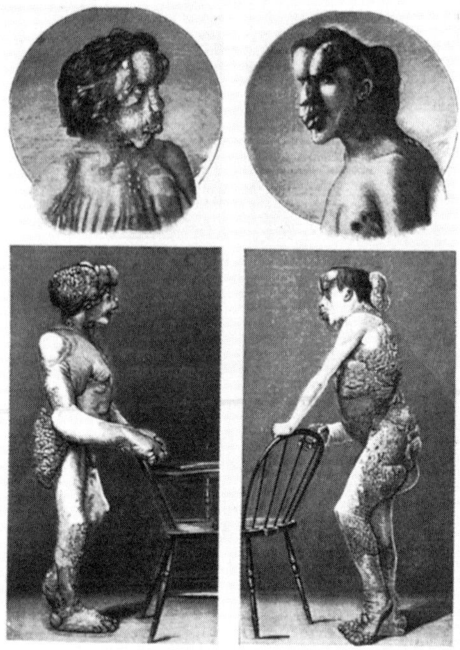

Figure 16.2 Lithographs made from the other two photographs of this series.

Treves saw the Elephant Man and negotiated to take him, now aged 24 years, to his room at the London Hospital Medical College across the road. On this occasion, and on his admission to the London Hospital 2 years later, photographs were taken (Figure 16.1). Lithographs (Figure 16.2) were subsequently prepared from these for the *British Medical Journal* of 11 December 1886 (Unsigned Comment, 1886). Treves demonstrated Merrick at a meeting of the Pathological Society of London on 2 December 1884, on which occasion Sir John Bland Sutton was present (Treves, 1884), and then gave clinical details and showed photographs at a further meeting on 17 March 1885 (Figure 16.3). It was this presentation that the dermatologist Dr Henry Radcliffe Croker attended (Treves, 1885a), an account of which was later published in the Society's Transactions (Treves, 1885b).

Following an unhappy continental tour under an Austrian manager, he returned to England and was accommodated in an attic room at The London Hospital. Subsequently he was housed in two rooms in the semi-basement of the East Wing looking out onto Bedstead Square. A further photograph was taken during this time, which shows him dressed smartly in a three-piece suit with a shirt, collar and tie, which

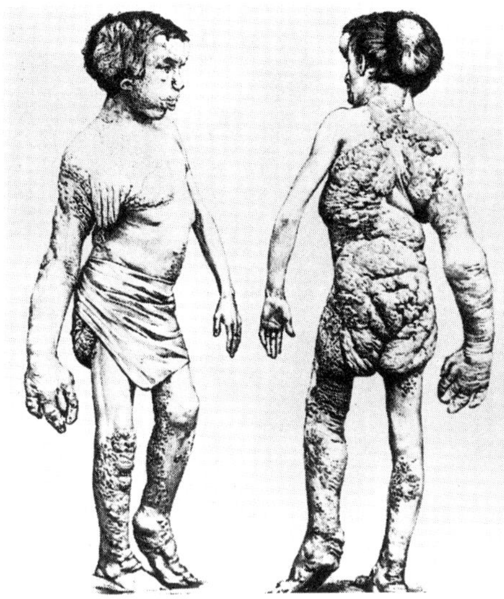

Figure 16.3 The lithographs made from photographs taken in 1884 and used to illustrate Treves' 1885 paper.

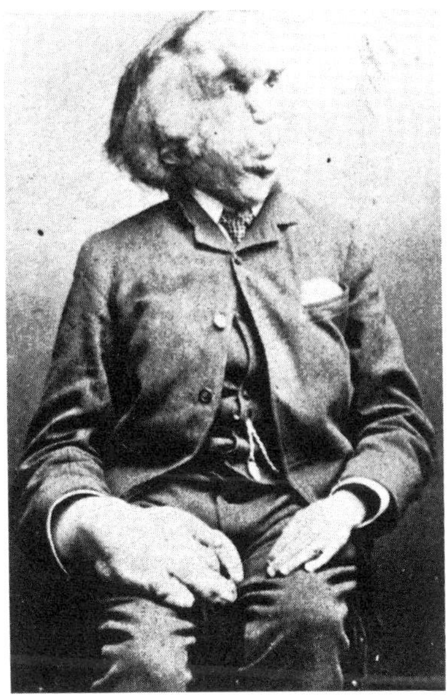

Figure 16.4 A photograph taken around the time that further clinical photographs were taken in 1889, which show Merrick fully dressed.

must have been made specially for him (Figure 16.4). Other full-length clinical photographs were taken in 1889.

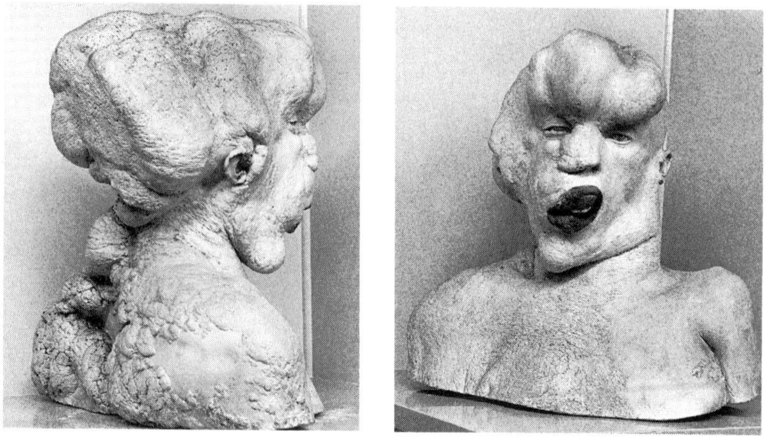

Figure 16.5 The cast of the head and shoulders showing particularly the three supraorbital ridges and the great mass of soft tissue on the back of the head. The upper incisors painted on the cast of the maxillary mass are fanciful. The whole was composed of soft tissue.

16.2.3 His death

Merrick was in the habit of taking a nocturnal stroll in the garden, and did so on the evening of Thursday, 10 April 1890. The account of the following day's events as given at the inquest on 15 April are probably the most reliable (Unsigned Report, 1890).

He normally stayed in bed until noon. Nurse Ireland from Blizard Ward saw him on the Friday morning, when he appeared in his usual health, and she left him sitting up in bed. At 1.30 pm a ward maid arrived with his lunch and left it for him, but he did not touch it. Shortly after 3 pm, Mr Hodges, Treves' house surgeon, paid a routine call. He found Merrick lying across his bed and saw at once that he was dead. He did not touch the body until the arrival of Mr Ashe, a more senior colleague, at 3.30 pm when they examined him together to try to find a cause for his sudden death. At the inquest, Mr Ashe's opinion was that the cause of death was asphyxia. The back of his head was greatly deformed, and while the patient was taking a natural sleep, the weight of his head overcame him, and so suffocated him. The jury accepted this view and returned a verdict that the cause of his death was due to suffocation from the weight of his head pressing upon the windpipe.

In his book *The Elephant Man and Other Reminiscences*, Treves describes him as lying on his back as if asleep and he had evidently died suddenly and without a struggle as the coverlet of the bed was not disturbed. When he assumed the recumbent position the massive skull was inclined to

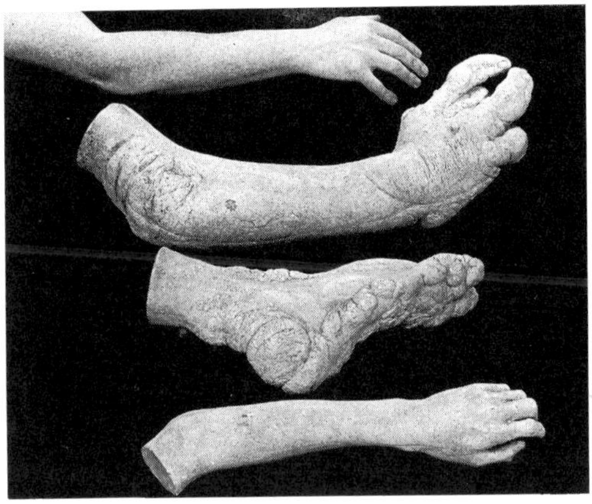

Figure 16.6 The limb casts with the arm of a normal young male at the top.

drop backwards with the result that he experienced no little distress. He normally sat up in bed with his back supported by pillows, his knees drawn up and his arms clasped round his legs while his head rested on the points of his bent knees.

No official necropsy was performed. The body was transferred to the Department of Anatomy where casts were made of his head and limbs (Figures 16.5 and 16.6). Skin samples were taken and preserved and the bones mounted as a skeleton (Figure 16.7). During the early part of the 1939–45 war, the containers in which the skin specimens were kept dried out. Part of the building was damaged and dry rot started in the adjacent woodwork and spread to involve the specimens, so the affected material was burnt when repairs were put in hand.

16.3 HIS PHYSICAL APPEARANCE

Evidence for the appearance of Joseph Carey Merrick comes from several sources: the writings of Sir Frederick Treves; lithographs made from photographs taken in 1884 (Figure 16.3); clinical photographs probably taken at The London Hospital Medical College around 1886 (Figure 16.1); an undated photograph of Merrick fully clothed taken perhaps in 1889 during his time at The London Hospital (Figure 16.4); further full-length photographs taken in 1889; and the post-mortem casts stored at The London Hospital Medical College. The description given by Treves (1923) was published nearly 40 years after the events it describes, so the report of his presentation to the Pathological Society of London on 17 March 1885 is probably more accurate (Treves, 1885b).

He was 1.57 m in height with a kyphoscoliosis that turned his sternum towards the right. The right shoulder was tilted downwards, and this was

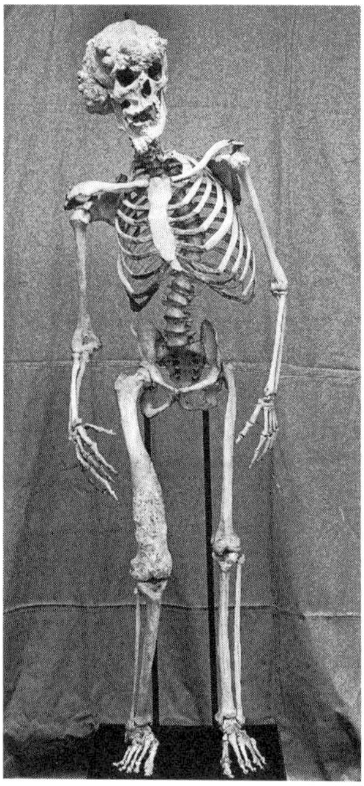

Figure 16.7 An overview of the skeleton from the front showing the fibrous pseudoarthrosis of the trochanters of the left femur, with the pelvis, deformed left ilium, kyphoscoliosis and enlarged right clavicle.

accentuated when the weight of the right arm hung upon it. He bore his weight on the right leg, holding the left flexed and medially rotated at the hip with the left foot in equinus and the pelvis tilted down on the left.

His head, measured in life and on the cast, was 91 cm in circumference. The left cheek, temple and ear were normal, but the forehead was raised up into three smooth surfaced swellings, of which both the largest and the smallest were disposed over the right eye and the other over the left eye (Figures 16.1a and 16.5b). It was largely these swellings that gave him a fanciful resemblance to an Indian elephant. The left nostril was normal, but the right side of the nose was elevated by a swelling that spread out onto the cheek, merged with the upper lip and also protruded from behind the central part of the upper lip. The right side of the head was substantially enlarged by a lobulated mass, which pushed a normal-looking pinna outwards and downwards. This mass was continuous with a trilobed 'bag' of tissue on the back of the head. The left side of the head between the posterior 'bag' and the frontal swelling was normal in shape and covered with black hair. Short, scanty hairs grew on the swellings interspersed with lanky tufts. A swelling over the mandible below the right angle of the mouth gave a false impression that the chin deviated to the right (Figure 16.1a). The cranial nerves functioned normally.

The right arm appeared enormous, partly because it was enlarged, but partly because the right shoulder sagged under its weight. The upper arm and forearm were thickened with the wrist 30 cm in circumference. His right hand was greatly enlarged with the thumb, middle and little finger curled towards the palm and the index and ring finger curved towards one another like a lobster's claw (Figures 16.4 and 16.6). The largest was 13 cm in diameter. Both lower legs were substantially enlarged by lobulated swellings, the left more so than the right, and these extended to deform the feet.

The right anterior and posterior axillary folds formed substantial pendulous masses. A flatter elevation of tissue covered the left side of the chest from the nipple line anteriorly to the midline posteriorly and down to join the buttocks. Both buttocks were enlarged by great drooping, lobulated masses that reached mid-thigh and which on the left became confluent with a thickening of the back of the left thigh. In life they may have been some 15 cm thick.

Treves aptly described the surface of the major swellings as 'like a brown cauliflower'. There was a substantial soft-tissue component to all the swellings, even where they covered bony enlargements. The tissue was soft and could be drawn out into folds or the skin moved freely over the abnormal subcutaneous layer. Some of the swellings were smooth-surfaced, but the majority had a 'papillomatous' surface. The photographs show separate hemispherical elevations on the medial side of the right thigh and groin and lateral aspect of the left thigh, which were perhaps 2 cm in diameter. Where the pebble-like elevations on the surface of the swellings are less closely spaced, they too are hemispherical. Where tightly packed, they take on a polygonal shape or irregular lobules, as seen in the casts, separated by fissures. Elsewhere the skin is coarse, and the surface textured by numerous shallow intersecting cracks.

Treves describes the skin colour as normal. Over prominent masses and dependent parts it was dusky or purplish, but in no part was there any naevoid growth. Merrick himself described the skin colour over the enlargements as the same as that of an elephant's skin (grey or brown?). The clinical photographs support the view that the skin colour was generally normal. The photographs have the appearance of being taken with flash, which casts some marked shadows. Nevertheless, there is a suggestion of pigmentation over the lower left quadrant of the abdomen and left inguinal region (Figure 16.1); this is seen in three different views and hence with different lighting.

16.4 THE SKELETON

The skeleton is mounted with the left leg straight and the longer right one bent (Figure 16.7). In life he stood on the straightened right leg with the left thigh flexed and medially rotated and the foot in equinus. The posture was consistent with his diseased hip. His pelvis is asymmetrical. The right side is close to normal, but the left ilium is thin, vertical and anteroposteriorly aligned (Figure 16.7). There is a marked scoliosis, which appears to be compensatory for the differences in support to the pelvis accorded by the two legs and by the weight of the right arm, which drags the right shoulder down. The curvature in the lumbar region is to the right with rotation of the vertebral bodies to the right. A substantial compensatory curvature to the left goes from L1 to T1 but without rotation of the bodies (Figure 16.7). Only a minimal degree of kyphosis is apparent. Some vertebrae are abnormal in shape secondary to the scoliosis and on the left side the transverse processes are enlarged and rough in the mid and upper thoracic region. The lamina of C4 is thickened and there is a large boss 2.5 cm thick on the left side of the arch of the atlas. The foramina are not enlarged. The shape of the thoracic cage is modified by the scoliosis. The right ribs 1–6 are more slender than average and the right 7th rib is thickened (Figure 16.7).

The right clavicle is 18.5 cm long and obviously thicker than normal (Figure 16.7). The left clavicle is only 15 cm long, slender and with a reduction in anatomical features. The right scapula is of normal size, while the left is smallish, thin and with a shallow suprascapular notch. The right humerus is 30 cm long. The lower end is thicker than normal with a greatly enlarged, rough, medial epicondyle, which is perforated by a 5 mm and × 2 mm diameter foramen towards the top. The left humerus is of normal shape but slender, and 28 cm long. The right ulna is 29 cm long with a greatly enlarged olecranon process, which may have prevented straightening of the arm. The surface of the bone is nodular and roughened so that it is thickened overall. The left ulna is slender, but of normal shape and 23.5 cm long. The bones of the left hand are generally normal in shape, but delicate in form. The right carpal bones are large and their surfaces and those of the metacarpals and phalanges of the index, ring and little finger are porous. The thumb bones are normal. The index finger bones are of normal length. The middle finger is shorter than the index and the ring finger greatly elongated being 3.5 cm longer than the index finger. The little finger is equal in length to the middle finger.

The right femur is 44 cm long. The proximal end is relatively normal in shape, and 3.5 cm in diameter just below the trochanters, but 7 cm wide and 5.5 cm thick in its lower third. Here the surface has a porosity resembling that seen in Paget's disese. The patella is recessed into the lower end (Figure 16.7). In contrast, the left femur is strikingly slender and straight and only 40 cm in length (trochanter to condyles). The upper third of the shaft is 2.0 cm wide and 2.3 cm thick, while the lower third is 2.5 cm wide and 2 cm thick. The entire femoral head has been destroyed, and with it much of the neck, which has been reduced to a beak-shaped spike that articulates with a flattened and markedly irregular acetabulum. Accessory facets for both the greater and lesser trochanters are seen (Figure 16.7). The right tibia is mildly bowed anteroposteriorly and thickened at the upper end to a diameter of 4.3 cm. The surface is roughened, spotted with numerous small foramina, and is 35 cm long. The left tibia is slightly longer (36.5 cm) but slender, of almost uniform thickness along its length and straight. By contrast the right fibula is slender and the left thicker than normal. The bones of the feet are relatively normal.

16.5 THE SKULL

The left temporal and parietal bones with the adjacent part of the occipital bone are largely normal. The rest of the calvarium is thickened by about 1 cm (Figures 16.8 and 16.9). Over the central part of the skull, the elevations are smooth, but covered with low, rounded eminences (Figure 16.8).

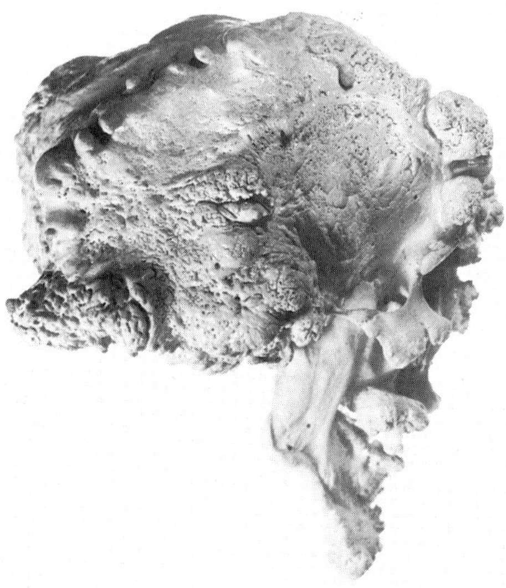

Figure 16.8 The right side of the skull showing the variety of surface characteristics of the bony enlargements, and in particular, the line of pedunculated knobs across the parietal bone.

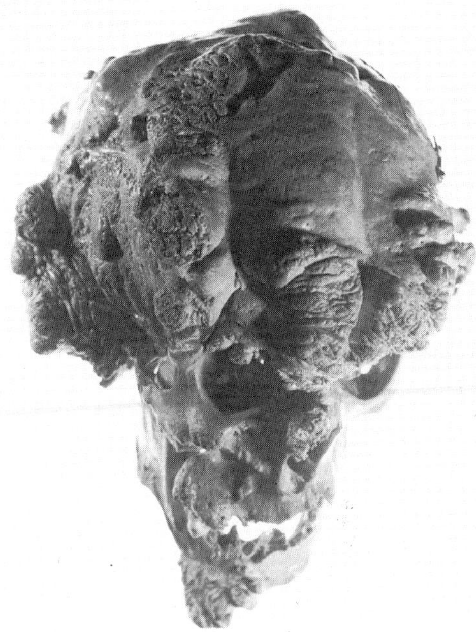

Figure 16.9 The vault of the skull showing the deep groove with lateral tributaries and numerous fine fissures running into it. The groove ends at the enlarged right supraorbital notch.

Three thicker zones of craggy, rough-surfaced bone run backwards from the orbits and nasion. The tallest of these starts over the lateral margin of the right orbit and extends backwards in a curve to the left beyond the vertex. It corresponds to the lowest of the soft-tissue supraorbital swellings. It is separated from the next and shortest ridge by a steep-sided branching groove, which starts at a large, 8 mm wide supraorbital notch (Figures 16.9 and 16.10). The larger, smooth soft-tissue swelling must have surmounted both this groove and the second bony excrescence, suggesting it was related to an enlarged supraorbital nerve. The third mass of rough bone starts over the medial two-thirds of the left orbital margin and extends backwards just to the fronto-parietal suture. The left-hand soft-tissue eminence covered this mass. The left supra-orbital margin is rounded.

The thickening of the skull is maximal over the right temporal region and occipital region with an extension across the posterior part of the base of the skull. The surface here is lobulated and broken up by fissures and foramina. A row of rounded, almost pedunculated swellings extends backwards across the right parietal bone (Figure 16.8). The distance from the nasion to the convexity of the occiput is 22.5 cm.

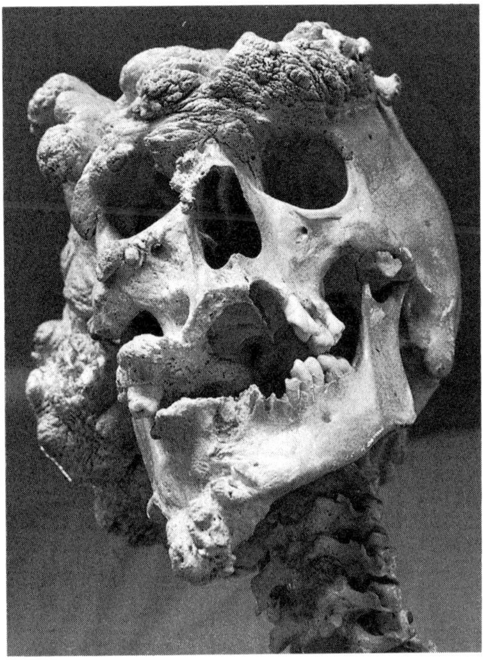

Figure 16.10 The front of the skull. The three bony ridges are seen in silhouette. The valleys on either side of the middle ridge meet in a groove which runs to the enlarged supraorbital notch. The size of the two infraorbital foramina can be compared, the right being the larger. The enormous concavity of the right side of the palate is shown; the contained mass displaced the alveolar process laterally. Above the alveolar process is the equally deep concavity of the front of the maxilla. The two masses were confluent behind the upper lip.

The skull is 57.5 cm in circumference measuring from nasion to occiput, but the distance round on the right side is 35 cm and only 22.5 cm on the left. The circumference of the cast of his head was 91 cm.

The right lateral pterygoid plate and hamulus are one-third larger than those on the left. The right tympanic bone and mastoid process are also enlarged, but are almost buried in the adjacent bony masses. The right foramen lacerum is reduced in size. The right zygomatic bone is thickened and has an irregular surface (Figures 16.8 and 16.10), while the left is delicate.

The orbits and nasal fossae are the same size, but the nasal fossae deviate towards the right. The left maxilla is less deep vertically than the right, but the right alveolar process is displaced entirely lateral to the line of the zygomatic buttress above (Figure 16.10). It forms a bulbous balcony of porous bone between the deep infraorbital depression and a wide palatal depression (Figure 16.10), and contains a single upper molar. These depressions together must have contained the great mass of soft tissue that enlarged the right cheek and pushed out between the lips. The right infraorbital foramen (5 mm in diameter) is noticeably larger than the left (2 mm in diameter) (Figure 16.10). An enormous right pterygoid hamulus overshadows a large, deeply placed greater palatine foramen (3 mm in diameter) grouped with two accessory foramina, while the foramen on the left is a more normal 1 mm × 2 mm in diameter. The anterior alveolar process is flattened and devoid of evidence of sockets.

Inside the skull the right petrous bone is large and lumpy, but the internal auditory meati appear normal and of equal size. The base of the posterior fossa is concave.

16.5.1 The mandible

The right side of the mandible is strikingly thickened. Indeed, the right coronoid process is enlarged both in length and thickness with a posterior border that arises from just anterior to the condyle so that the sigmoid notch is practically non-existent (Figure 16.11). From the lower border of the angle to the coronoid tip, the jaw measures 9.5 cm (5.5 cm on the left). The hyperplasia of the coronoid, together with a hook-like exostosis arising from the medial side of the zygomatic arch anterior to the coronoid, must have severely limited jaw opening. The mandibular foramen on the right is enormous (Figure 16.12), being over 10 mm in diameter, and is at the lower end of a deep groove, which is overhung by a large lingula in front. The groove undermines the upper end of the insertion of the medial pterygoid muscle. Even the groove for the nerve to

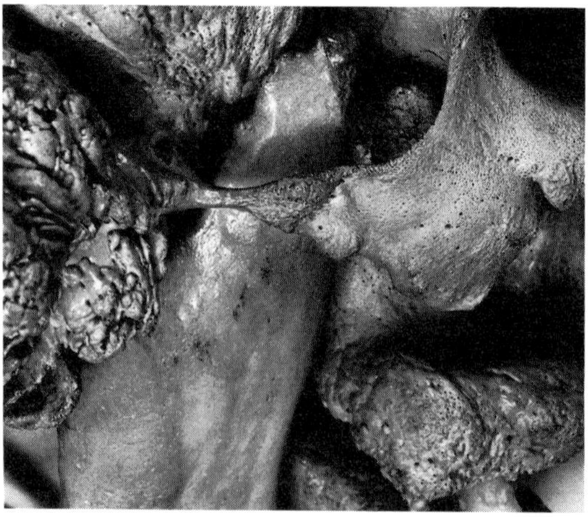

Figure 16.11 The greatly elongated right coronoid process.

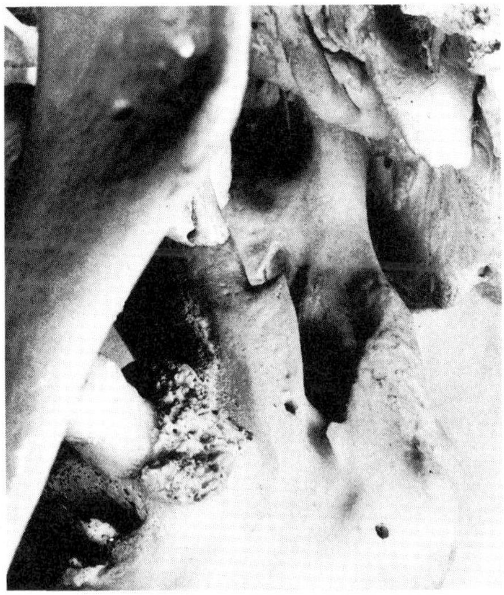

Figure 16.12 A close-up view of the enormous entrance to the right inferior dental canal and the overlapping lingula. The wide groove for the nerve to the mylohyoid is seen complete with a hook of bone; probably part of the insertion of the medial pterygoid muscle.

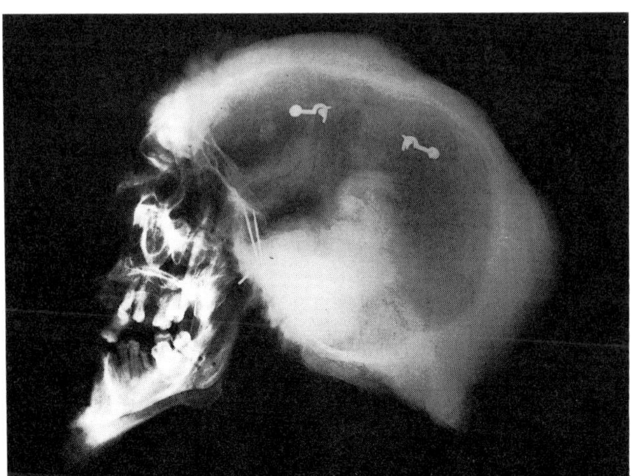

Figure 16.13 A lateral radiograph of the skull showing the shape of the cranial cavity.

the mylohyoid is 3 mm across and with a hook of bone crossing it from behind and below. Interestingly, the right mental foramen is small.

The right molar alveolar process is enlarged by a mass of bone on the

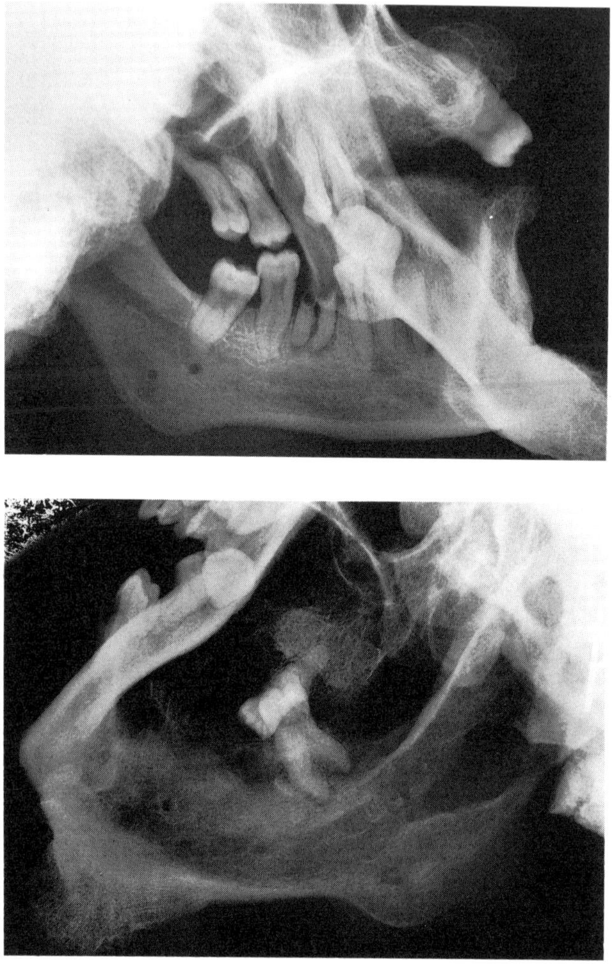

Figure 16.14 (A) Left and (B) right oblique lateral radiographs of the mandible. There is loss of trabeculae in the lower part of the right mandibular body in continuity with the mandibular foramen.

lingual side and is lingually inclined. Laterally, protruding from the lower border below the canine and premolar region, there is a substantial wedge of bone with a rough edge (Figure 16.10).

The left side of the mandible is smallish, with a short coronoid process.

16.5.2 Radiographs of the skull

The exostoses are composed of a close honeycomb of trabeculae, which are of lamella bone density and not like woven bone. In part, the surface

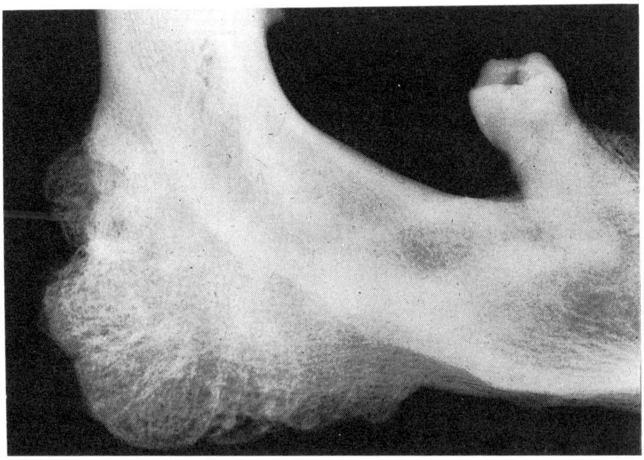

Figure 16.15 Detail of the exostosis, which shows the difference from fibrous dysplasia of bone.

of the enlargements is smooth, but elsewhere is irregular with grooves and canals disposed vertically to the surface.

The general outline of the cranial cavity is normal except for the outward concavity of the floor of the posterior fossa (Figure 16.13). The frontal sinuses are small, but the maxillary sinuses are of normal size and shape.

The left mandible is of normal structure (Figure 16.14A) The right side has a normal cortex, but there is a broad zone of absent medullary trabeculae from the mandibular foramen to the mental foramen region (Figure 16.14B). Where present, the medullary trabeculae are thin and closely aggregated, but not in the characteristic pattern of fibrous dysplasia. The deeper portion of the large exostosis is composed of linear trabeculae arranged parallel to the lower border. Towards the lower edge they become radially disposed with narrow vascular channels at intervals (Figure 16.15).

16.6 THE PROBLEMS

There are three matters concerning Joseph Merrick about which there is uncertainty: the disease that affected his left femoral head; the cause of his death; and of greatest relevance to this book, the cause of his deformity.

16.6.1 What was the disease affecting his left hip?

A pyogenic arthritis of the hip would have caused bony ankylosis, but Merrick's joint was not ankylosed. Perthes' disease would have caused the femoral epiphysis to become crushed and flattened. Tuberculosis of the hip joint secondary to an occult primary focus is the most likely diagnosis. The fibrous ankylosis that usually followed tuberculous disease of a joint would account for the accessory articular facets.

16.6.2 What was the cause of death?

Merrick normally slept with his head resting forwards on the points of his knees. This is just the position adopted by patients if they have potential respiratory obstruction from an enlarged tongue or if there is a bilateral fracture of the body of the mandible such that the tongue drops backwards. He would have reduced space in his mouth for his tongue because of the palatal mass. The combined effect of the coronoid hyperplasia and the hook-shaped exostosis on the inside of the zygomatic arch would have limited mouth opening to about 1 cm anteriorly. With both the inferior dental nerve and the nerve to the mylohyoid greatly enlarged, it is probable that the lingual nerve was also thicker than normal and associated with enlargement of the right side of the tongue. A bulky tongue in the confined space of an oral cavity reduced in size by a palatal swelling would certainly cause respiratory difficulty if the head was tilted backwards.

Merrick was sitting in bed propped up on pillows when the maid took in his lunch, so he had not tried to sleep during the night 'like ordinary men'. He was found lying across the bed, which suggests that he was getting up when he died and subsequently fell backwards. The large mass on the back of his head could have tilted it forwards, compressing his neck, which seems to have been the understanding at the inquest. Other possibilities include intracranial tumour with coning of the medulla and a fit of coughing that precipitated respiratory obstruction.

16.6.3 What did the Elephant Man suffer from?

The first medical syndrome with any resemblance to Joseph Merrick's condition was von Recklinghausen's disease. However, it was not until 1882 that von Recklinghausen's monograph was published, and it was in German. It is therefore unlikely that Bland-Sutton, Treves and Crocker were familiar with his work when they saw Merrick towards the end of 1884. It was probably Crocker who measured his head, right wrist and finger, and thus he examined him closely. Subsequently, in 1905 he was of the opinion that Merrick suffered from neurofibromatosis (Crocker, 1905). Professor Turnbull, Director of the Bernhardt Baron Institute of Pathology at The London Hospital from 1906 until he retired in 1946, was one of the foremost authorities on diseases of the bone. Dr Donald Hunter says in a letter (personal communication, 1968) that Turnbull believed that the Elephant Man suffered from neurofibromatosis. Weber, who saw Merrick while he was at The London Hospital, also subscribed to the same diagnosis (Weber 1909, 1930). It is of course unfortunate, and indeed surprising, that no histological examination was made, at least from the skin specimens that survived until the 1940s. However, histological examination of surgical and postmortem specimens was not routinely made until the turn of the century.

In my current view, the clinical appearances, while undoubtedly extreme, are not entirely inconsistent with neurofibromatosis.

The cutaneous abnormalities have been used to support a diagnosis of neurofibromatosis. The pendulous folds of skin and subcutaneous tissue, soft in texture and with the skin moving easily over the deeper tissues (Unsigned Comment, 1886), fit the diagnosis of plexiform neurofibromas closely and are less characteristic of lipomas or haemangiomas. The discrete, rounded lesions such as are seen on the inner aspect of the right thigh are similar to the peripheral lesions seen in NF1. Closely packed, rounded excrescences are seen on the surface of many of the larger masses, which are larger than the finger-like elements of a veruccous epidermal naevus.

A question that is often posed is why no reference was made to café au lait patches and spots. Treves described his skin as of normal colour, yet says the surface of the 'fungous-looking skin' was comparable to a brown cauliflower. A thickened keratinized layer and accumulated dirt and secretions on the rough skin could make it brown, or did it have a pale brown pigmentation? The photographs show a dark shadow, darker still in and above the groin, on the left side of the abdomen. This could be no more than a shadow on the underside of a convexity, but it is more intense than other shadows and the appearance persists in other views where the lighting was different. Café au lait marks are not always obvious and could have been overlooked by observers unaware of their significance.

The skeleton remains the best enduring evidence as to his disease. Paget's disease, fibrous dysplasia of bone, melorrheostosis and similar conditions produce local thickening and enlargement of bones, but not elongation of specific bones. Until recently, vascular malformations and plexiform neurofibromatosis were the only two conditions known to produce increased length of individual bones as opposed to local gigantism. Indeed, it is probably increased vascularity of the tissues, even in plexiform neurofibromatosis, that is the cause of the increased growth.

Despite the reddish-purple appearance of some of the smaller excrescences on the skin, Treves was certain the lesions were not naevoid. The absence of evidence of enchondromata excludes Maffucci's syndrome, in which there is a similar soft-tissue deformity of the extremities, but with a substantial haemangiomatous element.

The currently proposed diagnosis of Proteus syndrome (Wiedemann *et al.*, 1983; Tibbles and Cohen, 1986; Clark *et al.*, 1987) is attractive. Moccasin feet are a characteristic of this condition. Gigantism of the extremities of very variable extent is a feature but not infrequently with obvious local increased vascularity. The soft-tissue masses are commonly fibrous, fatty or haemangiomatous. Exostoses occur in the skull, but gross enlargement of the head, when present, has been due to hydrocephalus. This suggested diagnosis has gained strong support, but if correct, abnormalities not observed in contemporary patients, but recorded for Merrick, will have to be added to the many features already included.

The bony enlargements of the cranial vault and the appearance of the lower third of the right femur have been compared to fibrous dysplasia of bone. There is indeed a similarity in the sponge-like arrangement of the thin bony trabeculae, but the density of these is similar to lamellar bone not the woven bone of fibrous dysplasia, and the spikey surface seen in many places and the nodular surface seen elsewhere on the vault of the skull is different from the smooth expansion normally seen with fibrous dysplasia. Indeed, the latter condition would not, on its own, account for the substantial soft-tissue masses that overlie the bony knobbles.

While in Merrick the abnormalities are extreme, a number of features can be matched from confirmed cases of plexiform neurofibromatosis, e.g. the enlargement of a limb in both length and width. Where the periosteum under a plexiform mass is involved, the porous bone as seen in Merrick's femur is described. It is also characteristic that some of the other bones are thinner and more delicate than normal, and this is clearly the case in Merrick's skeleton. Whether neurofibromatosis or Proteus syndrome is favoured, the enormous exostoses on the skull are not typical. Smaller exostoses can be found in both conditions. An angular kyphosis results where the body of a vertebra has been affected by a neurofibroma, and this Merrick did not have. Scoliosis may compensate for unequal leg length, and in Merrick this would probably have resulted from the elongation of the right leg, even if the left hip joint had not been diseased.

It is in the skull that the best supporting evidence is found. The right supraorbital groove, infraorbital foramen (Figure 16.10), palatine foramina, mandibular foramen (Figure 16.12) and the groove for the mylohyoid nerve are all greatly enlarged. Each is directly associated with a substantial soft-tissue mass – the supraorbital groove with the considerable lump over the right eye, the infraorbital foramen with the enlarged cheek, and the palatine foramina with the palatal mass. Clearly the latter two were not haemangiomatous as the large lump between the lips was excised without recorded gross haemorrhage. Enlargement of nerves rather than vessels is therefore the likely cause of these enlarged foramina. The funnel-shaped opening of the canal for the mandibular nerve is typical of the appearance in neurofibromatosis. Similar appearances have not so far been described in cases of Proteus syndrome.

REFERENCES

Clark, R.D., Donnai, D., Rogers, J. *et al.* (1987) Proteus syndrome: an expanded phenotype. *Am. J. Med. Genet.*, **27**, 99–117.

Crocker, H.R. (1905) *Diseases of the Skin: A Review of 15 000 Cases of Skin Disorders*, Lewis, London.

Howard, M. and Ford, P. (1980) *The True History of the Elephant Man*, Allison & Busby, London.

Tibbles, J.A.R. and Cohen, M.M. (1986) The Proteus syndrome: the Elephant Man diagnosed. *Br. Med. J.*, **293**, 683–5.

Treves, F. (1884) Congenital deformity, in Reports of Societies: Pathological Society of London, 6 December 1884. *Br. Med. J.*, **ii**, 1140.

Treves, F. (1885a) A case of congenital deformity. *Trans. Pathol. Soc. Lond.*, **36**, 494–8.

Treves, F. (1885b) Congenital deformity, in Reports of Societies: Pathological Society of London, 17 March 1885. *Br. Med. J.*, **i**, 595–6.

Treves, F. (1923) *The Elephant Man and Other Reminiscences*, Cassell, London.

Unsigned Comment (1886) The Elephant Man. A commentary on a letter in *The Times* from Mr Carr Gomm. *Br. Med. J.*, **ii**, 1188–9.

Unsigned Report (1890) Death of the Elephant Man. *Br. Med. J.* **i**, 916–17.

Weber, F.P. (1909) Cutaneous pigmentation as an incomplete form of Recklinghausen's disease, with remarks on the classification of incomplete and anomalous forms of Recklinghausen's disease. *Br. J. Dermatol.*, **21**, 49–55 (Elephant Man comment, p. 53).

Weber, P.F. (1930) Periosteal neurofibromatosis, with a short consideration of the whole subject of neurofibromatosis. *Q. J. Med.*, **23**, 151–65 (Elephant Man comment, p. 159).

Wiedemann, H.R., Burgio, G.R., Aldenhoff, P. *et al.* (1983) The Proteus syndrome. *Eur. J. Pediatr.*, **140**, 5–12.

17

Proteus syndrome

R.D. Clark

17.1 INTRODUCTION

Although Joseph Merrick was the first patient with Proteus syndrome to be mistakenly diagnosed with neurofibromatosis 1 (NF1) (Tibbles and Cohen, 1986), he will certainly not be the last. Several of the over 50 reported cases of Proteus syndrome have been initially diagnosed as NF1. There is ample reason to think this problem will continue. Proteus syndrome is a rare and highly variable hamartomatous disorder. Because Proteus syndrome is unknown to most clinicians except clinical geneticists, it continues to be infrequently diagnosed. NF1, however, is common, widely appreciated and routinely diagnosed in all branches of medicine and surgery. Because clinicians are more familiar with NF1, they tend to consider it more often in the differential diagnosis of patients with neurocutaneous stigmata and hemihypertrophy, scoliosis or other disfiguring skeletal anomalies, whereas Proteus syndrome may not even make the list.

The typical case of NF1, with multiple café au lait spots, Lisch nodules, axillary freckling and neurofibromas, would not be confused with Proteus syndrome, which is characterized by asymmetrical overgrowth, exostoses and bulky soft-tissue and vascular tumours. It is only when the plexiform neurofibromas and skeletal complications are severe that the phenotype of NF1 would begin to approach that of even the milder cases of Proteus syndrome. Nevertheless, these overlapping signs have led to considerable diagnostic confusion among Proteus syndrome, NF1, Klippel–Trenaunay–Weber syndrome, Maffucci syndrome, Bannayan–Zonana syndrome and others.

The purpose of this chapter is to describe the clinical manifestations of Proteus syndrome and highlight those features that distinguish it from NF1 and other hamartomatous disorders. It is my hope that wider recognition of Proteus syndrome will lead to more accurate diagnoses, and will help eliminate the stigma that has long been attached to NF1 as 'the Elephant Man disease'. This pejorative term, which has caused patients with NF1 much unnecessary anxiety and pain, should no longer be used by responsible clinicians to describe this disorder.

17.2 PROTEUS SYNDROME

17.2.1 History

Although first reported in contemporary medical literature by Cohen and Hayden (1979), individual case reports of patients with Proteus syndrome can be found as early as 1907 (Wieland, 1907). This condition was not widely appreciated, however, until Wiedemann (1983) reported four cases in the paediatric literature. He aptly named the disorder after Proteus, the prophetic old man of the sea in Greek mythology. To evade capture, Proteus was given the power to change his shape at will. Ironically, the variable phenotype of Proteus syndrome has contributed to its elusiveness as a recognized clinical entity and continues to complicate its diagnosis.

17.2.2 Genetics

Proteus syndrome differs from NF1 in that it is sporadic. In spite of two reports of parental consanguinity (Aylsworth *et al.*, 1987; Toro-Sola, 1987) and one report of a chromosome anomaly (Say and Carpenter, 1988) in patients with features of Proteus syndrome, there is no convincing evidence of a heritable basis for this disease. The ratio of males to females is not skewed, nor is there any evidence of advanced paternal age. There have been no recurrences in siblings or offspring of patients with Proteus syndrome, and no concordant twins, either monozygotic or dizygotic, have been reported.

Happle (1986) speculated that a somatic mutation in a gene, lethal in a non-mosaic state, could be responsible. Indeed, mosaicism may account for the random and asymmetrical pattern of overgrowth in affected individuals as well as the varied pattern of anomalies in the syndrome as a whole. The aetiology of Proteus syndrome remains unknown. However, the pattern of overgrowth suggests a defect in the local regulation or production of specific tissue growth factors or their receptors.

17.2.3 Clinical manifestations

Over 50 patients with Proteus syndrome have been reported. The interested reader is referred to several major reviews (Burgio and

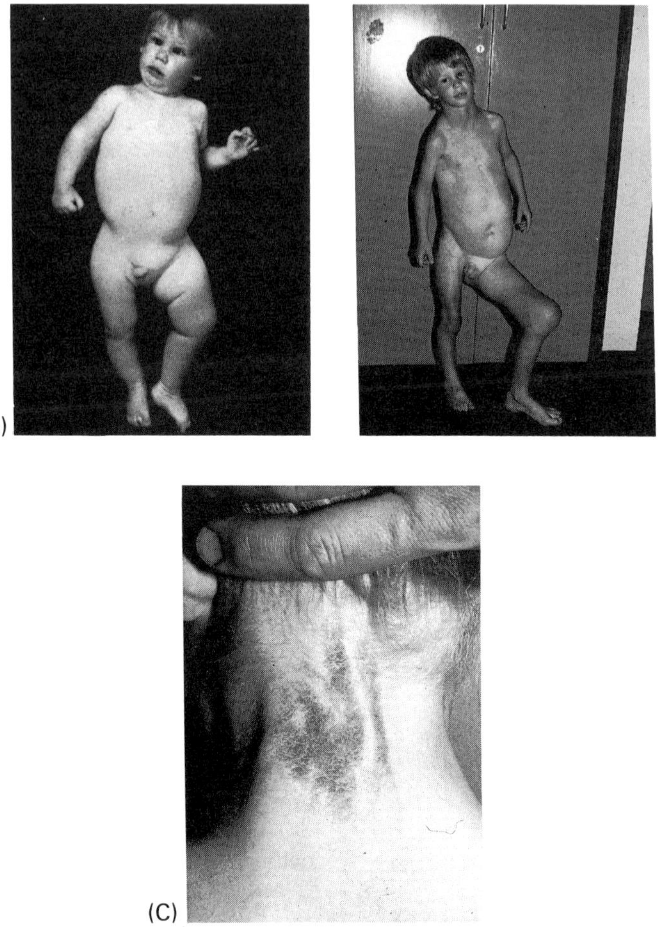

(A) (B) (C)

Figure 17.1 (A and B) The leg length inequality and soft-tissue tumours are present in infancy but become striking by early childhood in this patient. (C) Note the long neck and prominent venous pattern. A pigmented, hyperkeratotic linear naevus is characteristic. (Photographs reproduced with permission from Clark, R.D. *et al.* (1987), published by J. Wiley/A.R. Liss.)

Wiedemann, 1984; Gorlin, 1984; Lezama and Buyse, 1984; Costa *et al.*, 1985; Mucke *et al.*, 1985; Clark *et al.*, 1987; Viljoen *et al.*, 1987). Most publications have dealt with individual case reports or retrospective studies. Data on the clinical manifestations of Proteus syndrome are almost certainly biased in favour of the more severe or unusual cases. Minimal diagnostic criteria have not yet been established and the incidence of Proteus syndrome is unknown.

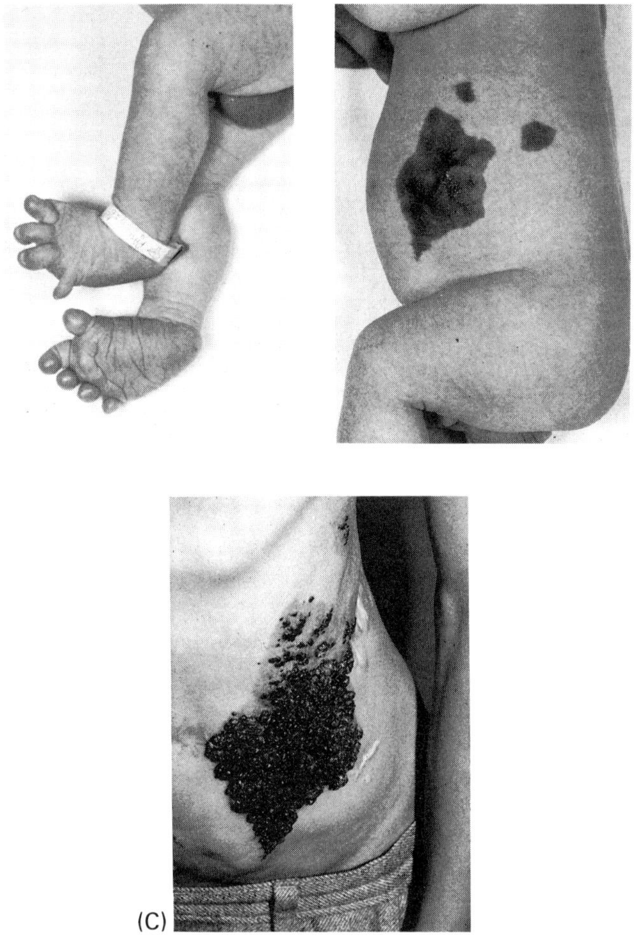

(A) (B) (C)

Figure 17.2 (A) This infant already has deep plantar creases and broad feet with macrodactyly (B). A vascular naevus developed over time to become verrucous with grape-like clusters of highly vascular papules (C). Note also the soft-tissue protruberance in the lower abdomen as an adult.

The typical features of Proteus syndrome are illustrated by several patients in Figures 17.1–17.7. Hallmarks of the disorder are asymmetrical overgrowth of the trunk, extremities or digits; bulky lipomatous or mixed tissue hamartomas (lipo/lymph/haemangiomas); linear epidermal naevi; prominent veins; exostoses of the skull; and partial lipodystrophy. Gyriform hyperplasia of the soles, and occasionally of the palms, is pathognomonic for Proteus syndrome.

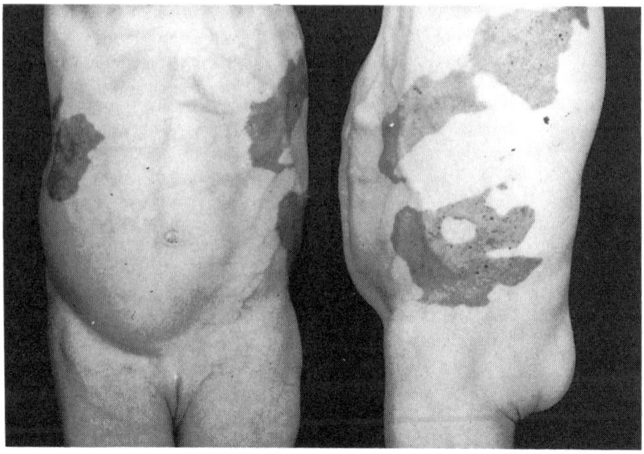

Figure 17.3 This patient exhibits vascular naevi, a soft-tissue mass and prominent veins. The decreased adipose tissue in the 'unaffected' areas, such as the buttocks, is illustrated in this girl. (Photograph on right reproduced from Clark, R.D. *et al*. (1987), published by J. Wiley/A.R. Liss.)

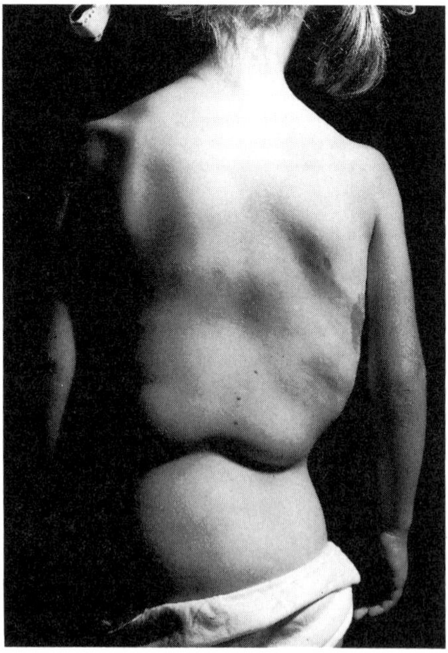

Figure 17.4 In this patient a vascular naevus is seen on the right chest. Here the bulky soft-tissue masses distort the trunk and thorax more than the abdomen.

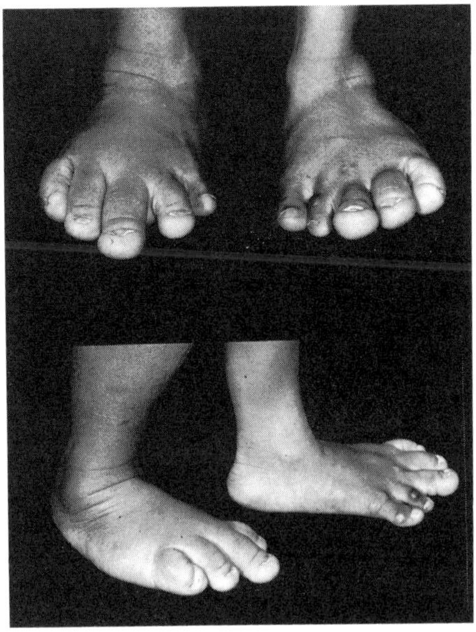

Figure 17.5 The macrodactyly is typically asymmetrical, although in this patient both feet are affected, primarily the lateral toes.

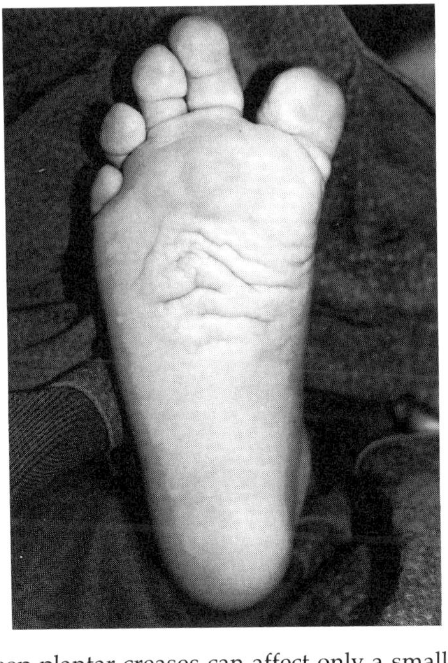

Figure 17.6 The deep plantar creases can affect only a small area of the sole as shown in this patient. (Photograph courtesy of Dr Bruce Blumberg, Kaiser-Permanente Medical Group, San Francisco, CA.)

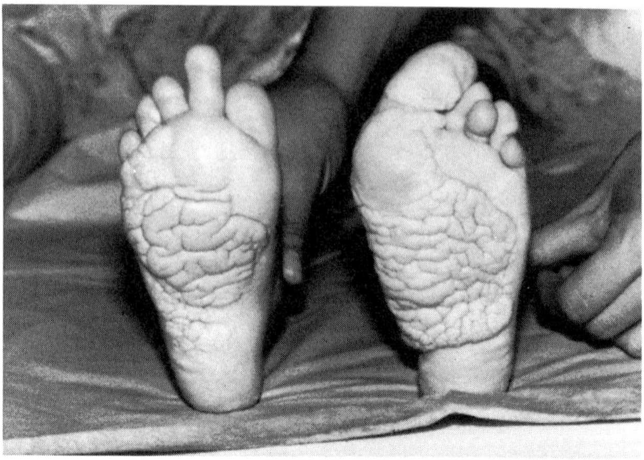

Figure 17.7 This patient illustrates the pathognomonic gyriform pattern of plantar hyperplasia, which has been described as a moccasin lesion. (Photograph courtesy of Dr Sondra Warren-Levin, Walter Reed Army Hospital.)

The major clinical features of Proteus syndrome are summarized in Table 17.1. The number of asterisks increases with the diagnostic significance of the feature. A total of five asterisks or more would make the diagnosis of Proteus syndrome a near certainty. Note the absence of café au lait spots, Lisch nodules, axillary freckling and neurofibromas from this list. Some of the more problematic and distinctive features of Proteus syndrome are discussed below.

17.2.4 Intelligence

Although the intelligence is usually normal in Proteus syndrome, there have been several instances of mental retardation. The cases of Malamitsi-Puchner *et al.* (1987, 1990) and Mayatepek *et al.* (1989) are among the most severely affected. These children had minimal developmental progress, hydrocephaly and seizures.

Macrocephaly is a variable feature and is not necessarily an indicator of poor intellectual function. There have also been well-documented cases of Proteus syndrome with small head circumference, measuring at or below the third percentile.

17.2.5 Patterns of overgrowth

Asymmetry is usually evident at birth or in the first year of life. There is progressive overgrowth of affected areas in childhood, which typically ceases near the time of puberty. The disproportionate growth is usually

Table 17.1 Major features of Proteus syndrome

***	Gyriform hyperplasia of soles
**	Linear epidermal naevi
**	Asymmetrical overgrowth, especially of the trunk, limbs or digits
*	Bulky lipomatous or mixed tissue hamartomas
*	Exostoses, especially of the skull
*	Scoliosis
*	Partial lipodystrophy
	Scoliosis
	Joint limitation or angulation
	Muscle atrophy

The number of asterisks increases with the diagnostic significance of the feature.

manifest as hemihypertrophy, an elongated neck and trunk with scoliosis, enlarged girth or length of one or more limbs and bizarre macrodactyly with angulation and limitation of movement of the affected digits. There is a random pattern of macrodactyly, which may cause gigantism of one digit while sparing its neighbours. The final height has been normal in most affected adults.

Enlargement of the external genitalia is another consequence of the random pattern of overgrowth in Proteus syndrome. Frydman *et al.* (1990) reported a girl with hemihypertrophy, pigmented naevi and subcutaneous tumours with clitoromegaly and scrotal-like hypertrophy of the labia majora. Endocrine evaluation was normal. Patient 1 in the series reported by Viljoen *et al.* (1987) had macro-orchidism and penile hypertrophy.

The presumably unaffected areas, on close inspection, are often abnormal, exhibiting decreased adipose tissue, muscle atrophy and prominent, dilated veins. Atrophy juxtaposed with excess lipomatous tissue creates a clinical picture compatible with partial lipodystrophy in some patients (Lampert *et al.*, 1984). There have been several instances of minimal or no breast development in adult women with Proteus syndrome, in spite of normal endocrine function.

17.2.6 Tumours

The bulky and disfiguring subcutaneous masses, typically on the chest, back and abdomen, are usually histologically benign hamartomas of mixed tissue origin. Often designated as lipomas, they are better described as lipomatous tumours because they usually lack the discrete encapsulated form required for the diagnosis of a true lipoma. Cavernous haemangiomas and lymphangiomas are particularly common. They can reside in the deep structures of the body, as well as superficially. Magnetic resonance imaging is useful in delineating such deep lipomatous tumours (Cremin *et al.*, 1987).

Malignant transformation is rare, although it has been reported. The patient of Malamitsi-Puchner (1990) developed a mesothelioma of the tunica vaginalis of the testis at age 4 years. Hornstein *et al.* (1987) reported two boys with testicular tumours: one with a papillary adenoma of the appendix testis, the other with a yolk sac tumour. Cohen (1993) documents tumours of the central nervous system, parotid gland, ovary and breast. Because the potential for malignant transformation remains unknown, patients with Proteus syndrome should be carefully monitored.

17.2.7 Cutaneous lesions

The cutaneous lesions of Proteus syndrome are varied, distinctive and of diagnostic significance. Unusual hyperplasia of the soles or palms, a pathognomonic sign, is not always present in Proteus syndrome. The lesion can appear as an isolated area of deep rugae or as an extensive fungiform or brain-like distortion of the entire sole. This latter 'moccasin' lesion, demonstrated in the plaster cast of Joseph Merrick's foot, can confirm the diagnosis in many cases.

Linear epidermal naevi, another unusual cutaneous lesion that is common in Proteus syndrome, appear as hyperpigmented warty or hyperkeratotic streaks. Other areas of flat, streaky or whorled hyperpigmentation or hypopigmentation have been reported. Vascular naevi of varying descriptions are common. Engorged or varicose veins have also been noted frequently. Café au lait spots have been reported, but they are infrequently encountered in Proteus syndrome.

17.2.8 Treatment

Therapy is palliative and should be directed at preserving or restoring function. Amputation of overgrown toes or limbs may be necessary to allow ambulation. Debulking subcutaneous tumours is not recommended. Extensive and serious postsurgical complications have been well documented: infection, poor wound healing, keloid formation, regrowth of tissue. Furthermore, when surgical procedures number in the teens, the psychological effect on the young patient may be more profound than learning to cope with a disfiguring affliction.

17.2.9 Differential diagnosis

Although both NF1 and Proteus syndrome may exhibit macrocephaly, hemihypertrophy, scoliosis and cutaneous lesions, there are more differences than similarities between these conditions. The absence of café au lait spots, neurofibromas, Lisch nodules and axillary freckling should discourage the diagnosis of NF1 in patients with Proteus syndrome. Furthermore, the findings of linear epidermal naevi, gyriform plantar hyperplasia and bizarre macrodactyly with angulation and limitation of movement are not part of the clinical spectrum of NF1. Even when plexiform neurofibromas are extensive and disfiguring, they do not resemble the firm, bulky subcutaneous soft-tissue tumours seen in Proteus syndrome.

Klippel–Trenaunay–Weber syndrome of haemangiomas and limb overgrowth presents a more difficult diagnostic problem. It is possible that this disorder exists on a continuum with Proteus syndrome. However, the lack of plantar hyperplasia, linear epidermal naevi, exostoses and bizarre macrodactyly do separate Klippel–Trenaunay–Weber syndrome from Proteus syndrome.

Both Proteus syndrome and osteochondromatosis, which includes Ollier disease and Maffucci syndrome, are non-genetic and asymmetrical disorders affecting bone. One of the main features that distinguishes Proteus syndrome from osteochondromatosis is the nature of the bony lesions. In Proteus syndrome the exostoses are commonly encountered in the skull, while the enchondromata of Ollier disease and Maffucci syndrome are rarely seen in the skull or spine, but characteristically appear in the extremities, especially the digits. However, the digits in Ollier disease and Maffucci syndrome are not overgrown and angulated as seen in Proteus syndrome, rather they are distorted by knob-like protrusions. In Maffucci syndrome, in which enchondromata occur with multiple haemangiomata, bony lesions may progress after puberty and the risk of malignant transformation is 15–18%. In Proteus syndrome, the lesions do not continue to enlarge after puberty and bone malignancy is not seen.

Bannayan–Zonana syndrome, an autosomal dominant trait, consists of macrocephaly and hamartomas, but the typical plantar hyperplasia, hemihypertrophy, macrodactyly and exostoses of Proteus syndrome are not encountered.

Although Proteus syndrome is highly variable and there is considerable overlap with other hamartomatous disorders, the clinical picture is sufficiently distinctive that the diagnosis can usually be made with confidence by the informed physician on clinical grounds.

17.3 CONCLUSION

Proteus syndrome is a rare, sporadic hamartomatous disorder distinct from NF1 and other overlapping conditions. The diagnosis of Proteus syndrome has been established in Joseph Merrick, the so-called 'Elephant Man', beyond a reasonable doubt. This should eliminate the use of this pejorative term that has been unfortunately associated with NF1 for so many years.

The principal features of Proteus syndrome are overgrowth leading to hemihypertrophy, scoliosis and macrodactyly, unusual cutaneous lesions, linear epidermal naevi, gyriform plantar hyperplasia, exostoses of the skull and bulky mixed tissue tumours that often cause disfigurement. The cause of this disorder is unknown, although the random and varied pattern of overgrowth suggests a somatic mutation, perhaps involving the local regulation or control of tissue-specific growth factors or their receptors.

REFERENCES

Aylsworth, A.S. *et al.* (1987) New observations with genetic implications in two syndromes (1) father to son transmission of the Nager acrofacial dysostosis syndrome; and (2) parental consanguinity in the Proteus syndrome. *Am. J. Med. Genet.*, **41** [Suppl.], A43.

Burgio, G.R. and Wiedemann, H.-R. (1984) Further and new details on the Proteus syndrome. *Eur. J. Pediatr.*, **143**, 71–3.

Clark, R.D. *et al.* (1987) Proteus syndrome: an expanded phenotype. *Am. J. Med. Genet.*, **27**, 99–118.

Cohen, M.M., Jr (1993) Proteus syndrome: Clinical evidence for somatic mosaicism and selective review. *Am. J. Med. Genet.*, **47**, 645–52.

Cohen, M.M., Jr and Hayden, P.W. (1979) A new recognized hamartomatous syndrome. *Birth Defects*, **15**, 291–6.

Costa, T. *et al.* (1985) The Proteus syndrome: report of two cases with pelvic lipomatosis. *Pediatrics*, **76**, 984–9.

Cremin, B.J. *et al.* (1987) The Proteus syndrome: the magnetic resonance and radiological features. *Pediatr. Radiol.*, **17**, 486–8.

Frydman, M. *et al.* (1990) Ambiguous genitalia in the Proteus syndrome. *Am. J. Med. Genet.*, **36**, 511–12.

Gorlin, R.J. (1984) Proteus syndrome. *J. Clin. Dysmorphol.*, **2**, 8–9.

Happle, R. (1986) Cutaneous manifestations of lethal genes. *Hum. Genet.*, **72**, 280.

Hornstein, L. *et al.* (1987) Linear nevi, hemihypertrophy, connective tissue hamartomas and unusual neoplasms in children. *J. Pediatr.*, **110**, 404–8.

Lampert, R.P. *et al.* (1984) Partial lipodystrophy in one of twins. *Proc. Greenwood Genet. Center*, **3**, 53–5.

Lezama, D.B. and Buyse, M.L. (1984) The Proteus syndrome. *J. Clin. Dysmorphol.*, **2**, 10–13.

Malamitsi-Puchner, A. *et al.* (1987) Severe Proteus syndrome in an 18-month-old boy. *Am. J. Med. Genet.*, **27**, 119–25.

Malamitsi-Puchner, A. *et al.* (1990) Proteus syndrome: course of a severe case. *Am. J. Med. Genet.*, **35**, 283–5.

Mayatepek, E. *et al.* (1989) Expanding the phenotype of the Proteus syndrome: a severely affected patient with new findings. *Am. J. Med. Genet.*, **32**, 402–6.

Mucke, J. *et al.* (1985) Variability in the Proteus syndrome: report of an affected child with progressive lipomatosis. *Eur. J. Pediatr.*, **143**, 320–3.

Say, B. and Carpenter, N.J. (1988) Report of a case resembling the Proteus syndrome with a chromosome abnormality (letter to the editor). *Am. J. Med. Genet.*, **31**, 987–9.

Tibbles, J.A.R. and Cohen, M.M., Jr (1986) Proteus syndrome: the elephant man diagnosed. *Br. Med. J.*, **293**, 683–5.

Toro-Sola, M.A. (1987) Proteus syndrome and Klippel-Trenaunay-Weber with Sturge Weber sequence in a consanguineous Puerto Rican family. *Am. J. Med. Genet.*, **41** [Suppl.], A108.

Viljoen, D.J. *et al.* (1987) Proteus syndrome in Southern Africa: natural history and clinical manifestations in six individuals. *Am. J. Med. Genet.*, **27**, 87–98.

Wiedemann, H.-R. *et al.* (1983) The Proteus syndrome. *Eur. J. Pediatr.*, **140**, 5–12.

Wieland, E. (1907) Zur Pathologie der dystrophischen Form des angeborenen partiellen Riesenwuchses. *Jahrbuch für Kinderheilkünde*, **65**, 519–84.

18

Neurofibromatosis 2: clinical features, genetic counselling and management issues

P.M. Short, R. L. Martuza and S.M. Huson

18.1 INTRODUCTION

Neurofibromatosis 2 (NF2), with a prevalence of 1 in 210 000 (Evans *et al.*, 1992a), is much less common than neurofibromatosis 1 (NF1). Prevalence only reflects those symptomatic at any one time; the same study gave an estimate of birth incidence of 1 in 33 000–40 562. Until recently, NF1 and NF2 were frequently classified as one disease, which often led to inappropriate investigation and management of families. Wishart (1820) reported the first probable case of NF2. The patient had multiple intracranial tumours with no recorded cutaneous features and was therefore quite different from those reported by von Recklinghausen in 1882. Following von Recklinghausen's report, however, authors described cases of NF1 with intracranial tumours and NF2 with cutaneous features (Henschen, 1915; Cushing, 1917). The two conditions became lumped together and referred to as von Recklinghausen's disease or multiple neurofibromatosis.

Gardner and Frazier reported a large family with NF2 in 1930 and suggested that bilateral acoustic neuromas (now called vestibular Schwannomas) represented a separate, central form of von Recklinghausen's disease. Subsequent reports did not follow this suggested subclassification. In their large study of neurofibromatosis in 1956, Crowe, Schull and Neel did not distinguish between the two forms and reported that 5% of patients with what they called multiple neurofibromatosis had acoustic neuromas. In retrospect it is clear that these patients had NF2.

Young, Eldridge and Gardner reported a follow-up study of the

Gardner and Frazier family in 1970, and again concluded that the disorder was distinct from that described by von Recklinghausen. They suggested it be called central neurofibromatosis. The division of the two types of neurofibromatosis then became widely accepted (Kanter *et al.*, 1980; Riccardi, 1981). Subsequent studies of large NF1 populations have shown no increased incidence of vestibular Schwannoma (Huson, Harper and Compston, 1988; Riccardi, 1992). The quite different natural history of the two conditions has also become more widely appreciated (Huson and Thrush, 1985; Martuza and Eldridge, 1988; Evans *et al.*, 1992b). In NF2 there is significant morbidity and disease-related mortality in the majority of affected individuals. The confusion with NF1 arises because café au lait spots and peripheral nerve tumours can develop in both conditions.

The National Institutes of Health (NIH) Consensus Statement on neurofibromatosis in 1987 gave clear guidelines on nomenclature, recommending neurofibromatosis 2 rather than central or bilateral acoustic neurofibromatosis. In the same year the mapping of the gene for NF1 to chromosome 17 (Chapter 2) and NF2 to chromosome 22 (Chapter 3) confirmed the clinical impression of two distinct diseases. A further nomenclature change with regard to NF2 was made at the recent NIH Consensus Conference on 'acoustic neuroma' (1992). Noting that the tumours are histologically Schwannomas arising on the vestibular branch of the eighth cranial nerve, the Conference recommended replacing the term acoustic neuroma with vestibular Schwannoma.

18.2 CLINICAL FEATURES

The morbidity and mortality caused by NF2 are largely due to the presence of the vestibular Schwannomas and other cranial or spinal tumours. The frequency of these and other disease features in the large series of NF2 patients reported by Evans *et al.* (1992b) are shown in Table 18.1.

18.2.1 Diagnostic criteria

The NIH Consensus Conference on neurofibromatosis agreed the following diagnostic criteria for NF2:

1. bilateral eighth nerve masses seen with appropriate imaging techniques, e.g. computed tomography (CT) or magnetic resonance imaging (MRI); or
2. a first-degree relative with NF2 and either unilateral eighth nerve mass or two of the following: neurofibroma, meningioma, glioma, Schwannoma or juvenile posterior subcapsular lenticular opacity.

The NIH Consensus Conference on Acoustic Neuroma (1992) slightly modified these criteria to take account of updated imaging techniques

Table 18.1 Clinical features of NF2 in 120 patients

Feature	*Frequency (%)*
Bilateral VS	85
Unilateral VS	6
Meningiomas	45
Spinal tumours (meningiomas, Schwannomas)	26
Astrocytomas[a]	4
Ependymoma[a]	3
Skin tumours	
Overall	68
>10 skin tumours (maximum number was 27)	10
Café au lait spots ($n = 100$)	
1–6 spots	43
1 spot	24
2 spots	11
3 spots	4
4 spots	3
6 spots	1
Cataracts and lens opacities ($n = 55$)[b]	60

VS = vestibular Schwannoma.
[a] All located in brain stem and/or upper cervical cord.
[b] Only 55 individuals had slit lamp examination.
Adapted from Evans *et al.* (1992b).

and so that first-degree relatives only required one, rather than two, of the disease features listed in the NIH Criteria. The revised criteria are as follows:

1. bilateral eighth cranial nerve masses seen by MRI with gadolinium; or
2. a parent, sibling or child with NF2 and either unilateral eighth cranial nerve mass or any one of the following: neurofibroma, meningioma, glioma, Schwannoma, posterior capsular cataract or opacity at a young age.

It should be recognized that the 1988 NIH criteria were designed to be very stringent so that false positives would be excluded and not interfere with linkage studies to localize the NF2 gene. Evans *et al.* (1992b) used these criteria in their study of NF2 in the UK and found a number of individuals, with no family history, who clearly had NF2 but did not satisfy the NIH criteria. Four of the cases (aged 26, 27, 52 and 63 years) had meningiomas as the sole neurological manifestation of their condition; each of these had affected first-degree relatives and therefore satisfied the NIH diagnostic criteria. Evans *et al.* point out that provision needs to be

Table 18.2 Diagnostic criteria for NF2

The criteria for NF2 are met by an individual with one of the following combinations of features:

1. Bilateral vestibular Schwannomas
2. A parent, sibling or child with NF2 plus:
   (a) unilateral vestibular Schwannoma, or
   (b) any one of: meningioma, glioma, neurofibroma, Schwannoma, posterior subcapsular lenticular opacities, cerebral calcification
3. Unilateral vestibular Schwannoma plus one or more of the following: meningioma, glioma, neurofibroma, Schwannoma, posterior subcapsular lenticular opacities, cerebral calcification
4. Multiple meningiomas (two or more) plus unilateral vestibular Schwannoma
5. Multiple meningiomas (two or more) plus one or more of the following: glioma, neurofibroma, Schwannoma, posterior subcapsular lenticular opacities, cerebral calcification

Source: Evans *et al.* (1992b).

made for individuals with no family history (50% of cases) as, using theNIH criteria, even with the 1992 modification, the diagnosis can only be made if they have bilateral vestibular Schwannomas. As these lesions often develop some years after the meningiomas and spinal tumours, an expansion of the diagnostic criteria was proposed as shown in Table 18.2; cranial calcification was also added to the list of disease features (section 18.2.7). These criteria are more flexible for use in the clinical setting. The disease features that allowed a diagnosis of NF2 to be made in 120 individuals in the Evans study are shown in Table 18.3. Such criteria are more reasonable when used to make clinical decisions.

18.2.2 Vestibular Schwannomas

Vestibular Schwannomas are the most consistent disease feature of NF2 (Table 18.1) and were the cause of the patients' initial symptoms in the majority of cases in both the large reported series (Kanter *et al.*, 1980; Evans *et al.*, 1992b). Early symptoms include hearing loss with tinnitus or vertigo related to pressure on the cochlear nerve. The hearing loss is characterized as a sensorineural loss in contrast to the conductive hearing loss seen in otosclerosis, a relatively common cause of deafness with onset in the same age group. Other symptoms may include gait instability, facial weakness or facial twitching, a change in facial sensation, headache or a change in vision. Involvement of the facial nerve

Table 18.3 Diagnostic criteria and mean age at onset in 120 cases with NF2

Diagnostic criteria	*Percentage of cases (mean age at onset in years)*
Bilateral VS	41.5 (27)
Bilateral VS + cranial meningiomas	20.0 (20)
Bilateral VS + spinal tumours[a]	7.5 (14)
Bilateral VS + meningioma + spinal tumours	16.0 (19)
FH + unilateral VS	3.0 (17)
FH + cranial meningiomas	2.5 (29)
FH + spinal tumours	1.0 (11)
FH + meningioma + unilateral VS	1.5 (3 and 8)
FH +meningioma + spinal tumour	1.0 (6)
FH + cataract + peripheral nerve tumour	1.0 (19)
FH + cranial Schwannoma	1.0 (42)
FH + cerebral calcification + peripheral nerve tumour	1.0 (8)
Unilateral VS + two meningiomas	1.5 (35)
Meningiomas + spinal + peripheral nerve tumours	1.5 (13)

VS = vestibular Schwannoma; FH = family history.
[a] Includes nerve root and/or intrinsic cord tumours.
Source: Evans *et al.* (1992b).

occurs with compression of the nerve by the enlarging eighth nervetumour. Changing facial sensation may be related to compression of the trigeminal nerve by tumour. Neurofibromas of the trigeminal nerve can be a manifestation of NF2 and produce a spectrum of sensory symptoms that overlap with those secondary to compression from a vestibular Schwannoma. They can also cause symptoms secondary to involvement of the motor root of this nerve (Nager, 1984).

In contrast to isolated unilateral vestibular Schwannomas, the tumours in NF2 tend to cause symptoms at a relatively young age. The mean age of onset of symptoms in the UK study was 27 years (Evans *et al.*, 1992b), whereas unilateral vestibular Schwannomas usually present after the fourth decade. The other difference between the tumours in NF2 and their sporadic counterparts is the difference in the size of the tumours at diagnosis and their appearance at operation. Bess *et al.* (1984) reviewed the audiological findings in a series of 22 patients with bilateral vestibular Schwannomas. Sixty-one per cent of these patients had lesions greater than 1.5 cm in diameter and 26% had tumours with a diameter of 4 cm or more. On pure-tone audiograms, however, 41% of the ears tested had normal hearing (0–25 dB), 29% had mild to moderate degrees of hearing impairment (25–70 dB) and 30% had severe loss (71–95dB). In patients with unilateral vestibular Schwannomas, the pure-tone audiograms are

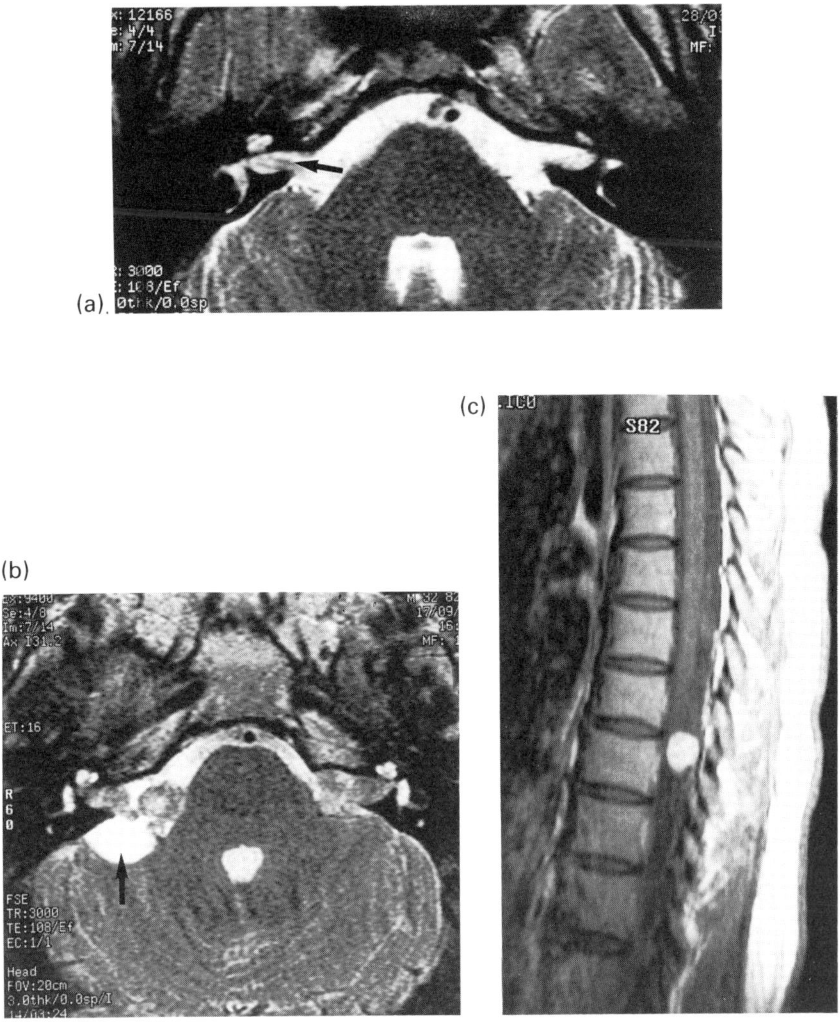

Figure 18.1 (A) Normal appearance of internal auditory meatuses on fast spin echo axial T2 weighted MRI imaging. The seventh and eighth cranial nerves can be seen traversing from the brainstem through the internal auditory canal (arrowed on left of figure). (B) MRI images of enlarged internal auditory meatuses in an affected individual. On both sides there are multiple vestibular Schwannomas along the course of the eighth nerve. There is an arachnoid cyst in association with the lesions on the left of the figure (arrowed). (C) Spinal meningioma detected on routine screening of a 33-year-old patient at risk of the disease. In retrospect, it had been causing local discomfort. Despite the relative lack of symptoms, it was removed because of its size and position.

abnormal in 95% of all cases and in 7% of cases with small tumours < 2 cm in diameter (Hart, Gardner and Howieson, 1983).

Linthicum (1972) and Martuza and Ojemann (1982) have reported differences in tumour growth and behaviour at operation which may explain the relative delay of presentation of bilateral vestibular Schwannomas. Although the tumours in NF2 cannot be distinguished from their unilateral counterparts histologically, at operation using an operating microscope the lesions in NF2 sometimes appear different from the more common unilateral vestibular Schwannoma. The isolated tumour is generally a solitary lesion arising from the vestibular nerve at or near the porus acousticus, where it displaces the facial and often the cochlear nerve so that these nerves lie external to the tumour capsule. Therefore the facial nerve can commonly, and the cochlear nerve occasionally, be spared during a microsurgical total removal of the tumour. In contrast, the tumour in some NF2 patients appears as a multilobulated mass with the facial and cochlear nerves often directly entering the tumour or surrounded by lobules of tumour. Linthicum (1972) originally described the tumours in NF2 as appearing to infiltrate the cochlear nerve. From a pathogenetic viewpoint, it is probably more likely that what is observed are multiple foci of primary tumours. More recently, Sobel (1993) reported histological differences in vestibular Schwannomas from 39 NF2 patients and 293 vestibular Schwannomas from patients with isolated lesions. Varocay bodies, foci of high cellularity and lobular growth patterns were present more frequently in the tumours from NF2 patients. Other characteristics were seen with equal frequency; these were areas of Antoni A and B, nuclear atypia, whorls, scarring, chronic inflammation and sheets of macrophages. Ten of the 39 vestibular Schwannomas from NF2 patients either had meningioma tissue mixed in with them or meningiomas had been removed concurrently at the time of surgery. None of the patients with unilateral vestibular Schwannoma had meningiomas. The rate of growth of the vestibular Schwannomas in NF2 is extremely variable, which has important implications for management (section 18.6.2a).

18.2.3 Other cranial and spinal tumours

(a) Schwannomas

In addition to the eighth nerve, Schwannomas can develop on any of the other cranial nerves (except I and II) and on the dorsal nerve roots of the spinal cord. There may be multiple nerve involvement. The presenting features of the tumours are related to their anatomical localization. With the improved neuroimaging provided by MRI, asymptomatic Schwannomas and meningiomas (Figure 18.1c) are often detected on screening of

NF2 patients. That such lesions would be fairly frequent was predicted from one autopsy series (Huson and Thrush, 1985). In the family reported, five of the six affected members had other tumours of the nervous system apart from vestibular Schwannomas. In three of these, the tumours were only detected at postmortem examination. In the study of Evans *et al.* (1992b), every cranial nerve except the olfactory nerve was involved with either a Schwannoma or meningioma in at least one patient. The trigeminal nerve was the second most frequently involved after the eighth nerve.

Spinal Schwannomas are also relatively common and are often multiple. In a series of 15 patients with NF2, six developed symptomatic spinal root Schwann cell tumours (Martuza and Ojemann, 1982). Their presentation and radiological appearance can be similar to spinal root tumours in NF1, but in NF1 these tumours are neurofibromas and not Schwannomas (Halliday, Sobel and Martuza, 1991).

(b) Meningiomas

Meningiomas are relatively common in NF2, occurring in 45% of patients in the UK study (Evans *et al.*, 1992b). There is no site where they are particularly prone to occur; symptoms are related to location. Intracranial tumours can present with weakness, seizures, sensory changes, visual disturbances, changes in memory or personality and even as transient ischaemic attacks. In terms of misdiagnosis as NF1, the meningiomas can occasionally involve the optic nerve; five of the 120 patients in the study of Evans *et al.* had such a lesion. We have seen the occasional case where these lesions have been misdiagnosed as optic glioma on neuroradiological examination and the patient presumed to have NF1. Spinal meningiomas can present with weakness and numbness, especially of the legs, and changes in bladder function.

The meningiomas in NF2 do not differ pathologically from those occurring sporadically, although multiple tumours are common in NF2. The anatomical location of meningiomas is not different from those occurring in the general population, though the age of onset is earlier. In general, the rate of recurrence of meningiomas is related to whether or not total resection is possible, which is related to anatomical location. The majority of convexity tumours can be entirely resected and have a low recurrence rate. Parasellar meningiomas, which represent the fourth most common location, can be resected in only 50% of cases, but the 5-year recurrence rate is only 19%. By contrast, sphenoid ridge meningiomas can be completely resected in only 28% of cases and have a recurrence rate of 34% (Mirimanoff *et al.*, 1985). These figures are for sporadic meningiomas, actual figures for meningiomas in NF2 are not available.

Meningioangiomatosis is a distinctive lesion with a meningothelial component that can be associated with NF2 (Chapter 6). Although the lesions have been reported adjacent to meningiomas, it is thought that they represent a dysplastic hamartomatous lesion rather than a neoplastic process. In the postmortem series of Rubinstein (1986), four of 11 NF2 cases had meningioangiomatosis; the lesion may not necessarily be symptomatic, but if it is, the symptoms are related to its location. The most frequent site of involvement is the cerebrum.

(c) Glial tumours

Glial tumours are much less common in NF2 than either Schwannomas or meningiomas. They include pilocytic astrocytomas of the brain and spinal cord, and cerebral and spinal ependymomas. Optic nerve gliomas **do not** occur with increased frequency in NF2. In the study of Evans *et al.* (1992b), 4% (5/120) of patients had an astrocytoma and 2.5% (3/120) ependymomas. They were low-grade tumours and affected the lower brain stem or upper cervical cord; one astrocytoma had spread to involve the entire spinal medulla. Syringomyelia can develop in association with intramedullary tumours (Rubinstein, 1986). Other distinctive, but usually asymptomatic, lesions include intramedullary and perivascular Schwannosis, discrete ependymal ectopias and glial microhamartomas (Chapter 6, section 6.2).

18.2.4 Peripheral nerve tumours

These occur less consistently and in much smaller numbers than in NF1. In the recent UK study (Evans *et al.*, 1992b), 68% of patients had peripheral nerve tumours, which varied in number from 1 to 27. There are three types of peripheral nerve tumour in NF2, which, although of different appearance, are usually Schwannomas histologically. The most common, occurring in 48% of patients in the Evans *et al.* (1992b) study, are sometimes referred to as NF2 plaques and have a distinctive appearance (Figure 18.2a). They are discrete, well-circumscribed, slightly raised cutaneous lesions usually less than 2 cm in diameter. Their surface is roughened, may be slightly pigmented and often contains excess hair.

The second type of peripheral nerve tumour appears clinically like the nodular tumours in NF1. They are subcutaneous, often spherical, lesions that develop on the larger peripheral nerves (Figure 18.2b). The nerve is often thickened at either end of the tumour or there may be a number of nodular tumours developing in one particular part of the same nerve. Forty-three per cent of patients in the Evans *et al.* study had these lesions.

The least common type of peripheral tumour is similar to the dermal lesions of NF1 in appearance and has a violaceous colouring. They

(a) (b)

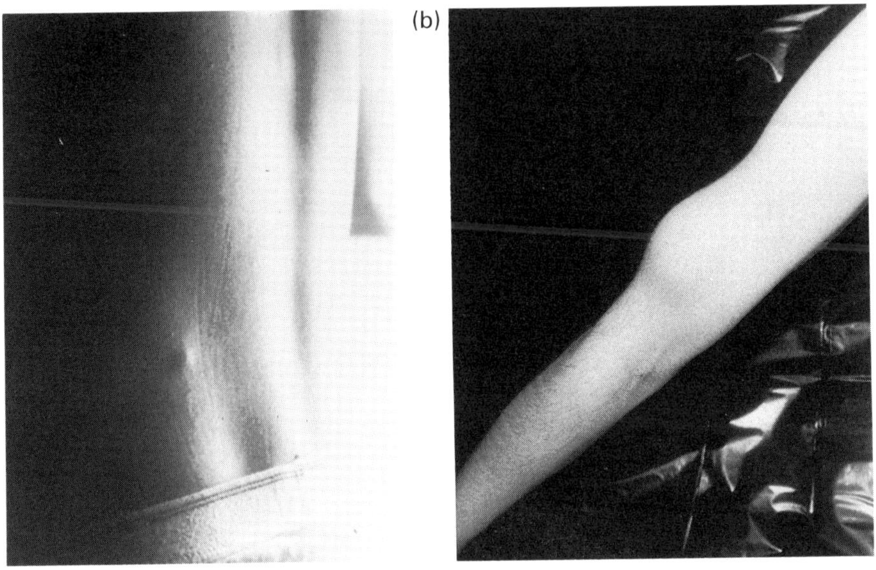

Figure 18.2 Peripheral nerve tumours in NF2. (a) NF2 plaques. These are difficult to illustrate. Clinically, they are slightly raised plaques, the skin appears toughened and there may be hypertrichosis. (b) Nodular Schwannomas of peripheral nerve. (Reproduced with permission from Evans *et al.*, 1992c.)

occurred in 27% of patients in the Evans *et al.* study, but were much fewer in number than would be normally seen in an adult with NF1.

18.2.5 Café au lait spots

Approximately 10% of the general population have one or two café au lait spots (Crowe and Schull, 1953; Kopf *et al.*, 1985). They occur more frequently in patients with NF2; 43% of the patients in the UK study (Evans *et al.*, 1992b) had café au lait spots. Of these, 24 patients had one spot, 11 had two, four had three and three had four spots. Only one patient had six café au lait spots. She also had two skin tumours of the NF2 plaque type, which meant that had she presented prior to her neurological problems and the significance of these plaques not been realized, NF1 would have been suspected rather than NF2. Therefore, although the café au lait spots do occur more frequently than in the general population, they are much less frequent in number than in NF1. By light microscopy, the café au lait spots in NF2 have been shown to contain lower numbers of melanin macroglobules than those in NF1 (Martuza *et al.*, 1985). Axillary and groin freckling are not seen in NF2.

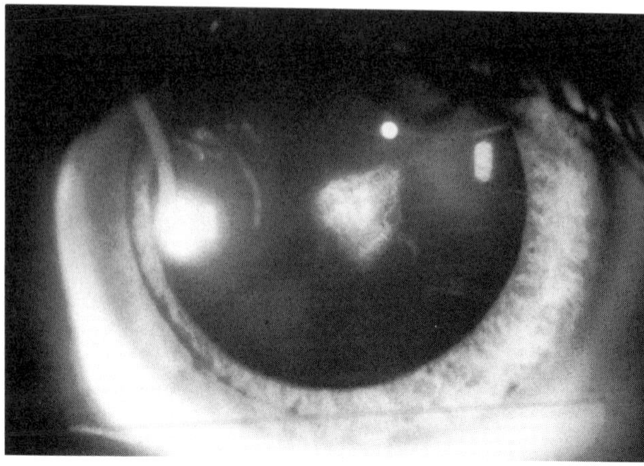

Figure 18.3 A typical 'plaque-like' posterior subcapsular cataract in an affected NF2 patient.

18.2.6 Ophthalmological features

The lens changes associated with NF2, posterior subcapsular lens opacities and sometimes actual cataracts (Figure 18.3), were only recognized relatively recently (Martuza, 1984; Pearson-Webb, Kaiser-Kupfer and Eldridge, 1986). Eighteen of 22 affected individuals (82%) in one study demonstrated these changes (Kaiser-Kupfer *et al.*, 1989). They also drew attention to the fact that the lens opacities appear prior to the vestibular Schwannomas or other tumours, making them a valuable disease marker in individuals at risk. Evans *et al.* (1992b) found opacities in 60% (33/55) of their patients who had slit lamp examination. Fifteen cases had been identified as having cataracts in childhood, of which four cases had minimal vision in the affected eye, probably from birth. In their series, congenital polar cataracts appeared to be at an increased frequency in addition to the posterior subcapsular changes. Lens changes are therefore a valuable marker of NF2 in individuals at risk, and in view of those cases with symptomatic lesions in childhood, individuals at risk should be screened for their presence in infancy.

There have been several single case reports of the presence of combined hamartomas of the retina and retinal pigment epithelium of NF2 (Landau *et al.*, 1990; Good *et al.*, 1991; Sivalingam *et al.*, 1991) suggesting an association with NF2. In the 21 patients examined by Ragge *et al.* (1992), eight had retinal astrocytic hamartomas, of which three were peripapillary, one had a combined retinal and retinal pigment epithelial hamartoma and one had a choroidal hamartoma. The frequency of retinal hamartomas in the series of Ragge *et al.* suggests they are a disease feature in NF2 and that screening tests should include indirect ophthalmoscopy.

Lisch nodules have not been found to be associated with NF2 in the large series of patients who have had slit lamp examination of the iris (Kaiser-Kupfer *et al.*, 1989; Evans *et al.*, 1992b). Charles *et al.* (1989), however, reported a man with six Lisch nodules in one eye, the other eye showing no lesions. This one case does not prove an association with NF2 and Lisch nodules, since another possible explanation is that the patient had very limited segmental NF as well as NF2. Michaels *et al.* (1989) reported a patient who they presumed to have NF1 with bilateral vestibular Schwannomas. The diagnosis of NF1 was made on the basis of six café au lait spots, multiple subcutaneous tumours and one Lisch nodule. Isolated Lisch nodules are occasionally seen in the general population (Huson, Jones and Beck, 1987). It is likely that this patient had NF2 with extreme skin manifestations, rather than NF1.

18.2.7 Other disease features

A mixed peripheral motor and sensorineuropathy can occur in some patients with NF2, although it is an infrequent complication. Evans *et al.* (1992b) found that three out of 100 personally examined cases had a neuropathy, with glove and stocking sensory loss and peripheral weakness. Ohnisshi and Nada (1972) and Thomas *et al.* (1990) have described typical nerve biopsy findings in these cases.

Intracranial calcifications on CT scans not due to tumour and somewhat similar to those in tuberous sclerosis have been reported in a number of patients without signs of tuberous sclerosis but evidence of NF2 (Arts and van Dongen, 1986; van Tassel, Yeakley and Leigh, 1987; Clarke *et al.*, 1990; Mayfrank, Mohadjer and Wullich, 1990). Their frequency in a large series of patients has not been reported, nor is the pathological nature of the lesions known.

18.3 DIFFERENTIAL DIAGNOSIS

The commonest misdiagnosis in our experience is that patients with NF2 and marked cutaneous features are labelled as having NF1. The most helpful distinguishing features are the much lower number of café au lait spots, the absence of axillary freckling and the different appearance of the peripheral tumours in the majority of cases.

Another problem in misdiagnosis is that the possibility of NF2 is not considered when young people present with single vestibular Schwannomas, meningiomas or spinal Schwannomas. We have seen a number of patients diagnosed very late in their disease course because NF2 had not been considered when they presented with an apparently isolated tumour at a young age and other signs of NF2 were not looked for. They were then lost to follow-up until another tumour caused problems.

Riccardi (1982), in his classification of neurofibromatosis, suggests a form of neurofibromatosis where patients have features of both NF1 and NF2 (NF3). A review of the literature in our opinion gives little support to the occurrence of NF3. We are aware of reports of only three individuals who satisfy the NIH criteria for both NF1 and NF2. Two of the patients had no family history and bilateral vestibular Schwannomas, and one had more than six café au lait patches and skin neurofibromas, including a plexiform tumour (Martuza and Ojemann, 1982). The other patient had six café au lait patches, multiple skin tumours and a single Lisch nodule (Michaels *et al.*, 1989). A single Lisch nodule can be a variant within the general population (Huson, Jones and Beck, 1987). A further case in the literature (Sadeh, Martinovits and Goldhammer, 1989) clearly inherited NF1 from one parent and NF2 from the other. It is difficult to know whether the sporadic cases represent new mutations for both NF1 and NF2 or marked expression of the peripheral features of NF2. In the UK study (Evans *et al.*, 1992b) no patient with NF2 had a plexiform neurofibroma. It may be that multifocal Schwannomas in NF2 are sometimes misdiagnosed as plexiform neurofibromas. Further delineation of the NF1/NF2 overlap must await direct mutation analysis in cases with marked cutaneous features. Cawthon *et al.* (1990) reported a patient with a history of bilateral vestibular Schwannomas and multiple paraspinal neurofibromas, diagnosed as NF2, who showed a single strand confirmation polymorphism (SSCP) variant in exon 5 of the *NF1* gene. The authors proposed that if polymorphism could be excluded, this finding would suggest that NF2 is genetically heterogeneous. However, analysis of the patient's parents, to exclude polymorphism, has not been possible nor has a detailed review of the patient's clinical features (D. Viskochil, personal communication). Linkage studies in NF2 families have not shown any evidence of locus heterogeneity (Narod *et al.*, 1992).

As reviewed in Chapter 19, patients with the features of NF1 limited to one segment of the body are well recognized. We are aware of two possible cases of segmental NF2. Riccardi and Ragge (1992) reported a 67-year-old woman who had had a left vestibular Schwannoma removed at 42 years of age. Follow-up studies at age 61 years had shown left-sided cerebral meningiomatosis (on cranial CT) and multiple left-sided paraspinal tumours (on myelography). Cranial MRI at 66 years showed no right-sided lesions. She had no ocular or skin findings. Family history was negative and her three children (aged 44, 42 and 38 years) had no symptoms, two having normal brain stem auditory evoked responses (BAER). In his UK study, Evans (personal communication) had a similar case. This lady was aged 53 years with no family history, and had a unilateral vestibular Schwannoma with three ipsilateral meningiomas and two peripheral Schwannomas. She had one son, in his mid-thirties, who had no symptoms suggestive of NF2. These cases seem very likely to represent somatic mosaicism for the *NF2* gene, akin to cases of segmental NF1.

Bilateral vestibular Schwannomas are unique to NF2. However, multiple meningiomas with no other associated tumours is a recognized autosomal dominant trait (McKusick, 1990). One of us (S.M.H.) has seen one family and is aware of one other (A. Harding, personal communication) where spinal Schwannomas as the only disease feature segregate as an autosomal dominant. As the study of Evans *et al.* (1992b) showed that multiple meningiomas can be the only nervous system tumours in occasional patients with NF2, care has to be taken in managing isolated cases with only multiple meningiomas or Schwannomas; it cannot be assumed that they definitely have NF2. Their children would be at 50% risk, whatever the problem, and they should be screened for NF2 until the natural history of the condition in that family becomes obvious. If a direct genetic test becomes available for NF2 it will be useful to confirm/refute the diagnosis in patients with unusual presentations.

18.4 NATURAL HISTORY

18.4.1 Initial presentation

The first symptoms in the 100 cases studied personally by Evans *et al.* (1992b) are listed in Table 18.4. Presenting symptoms are due to vestibular Schwannomas in most cases. Peripheral tumours or cataract were excluded as they were usually asymptomatic. In the patients who had presented with peripheral tumours prior to onset of central problems, a diagnosis of NF1 had usually been made. The association of the cataracts with NF2 had not been appreciated. Mean age at first symptom ($n = 110$) was 21.6 years (range 2–52 years) and at diagnosis of NF2, 27.6 years (range 5–66 years). An age of onset curve is shown in Figure 18.4. Eleven patients (10%) presented with features before the age of 10 years. In four of these, symptoms were secondary to vestibular Schwannoma (deafness 4 years, facial palsy 3, 7 and 8 years). Another patient presented with deafness at 3 years resulting from a cerebellopontine angle meningioma. Three per cent of patients presented with fits (associated with meningioma aged 5 and 6 years; cerebral calcification 8 years), one with unilateral blindness and amblyopia (optic sheath meningioma, aged 5 years), one with intractable headache (meningioma, aged 2 years) and one with foot drop (aged 6 years). Mean age at onset of deafness was 24.25 years (range 4–50 years) in 87 patients, although two obligate gene carriers with other complications had no evidence of deafness or vestibular Schwannoma on scan at the ages of 52 and 61 years.

Table 18.4 First symptom in 100 cases of NF2

Symptom	*Percentage of cases*
Due to vestibular Schwannoma	
Deafness (unilateral in 35)	44
Tinnitus	10
Vertigo	8
Due to other tumours	
Peripheral weakness	12
Seizures	8
Root pain	4
Numbness and tingling	2
Blindness	1
Asymptomatic at-risk relatives diagnosed on screening	11

Source: Evans *et al.* (1992b).

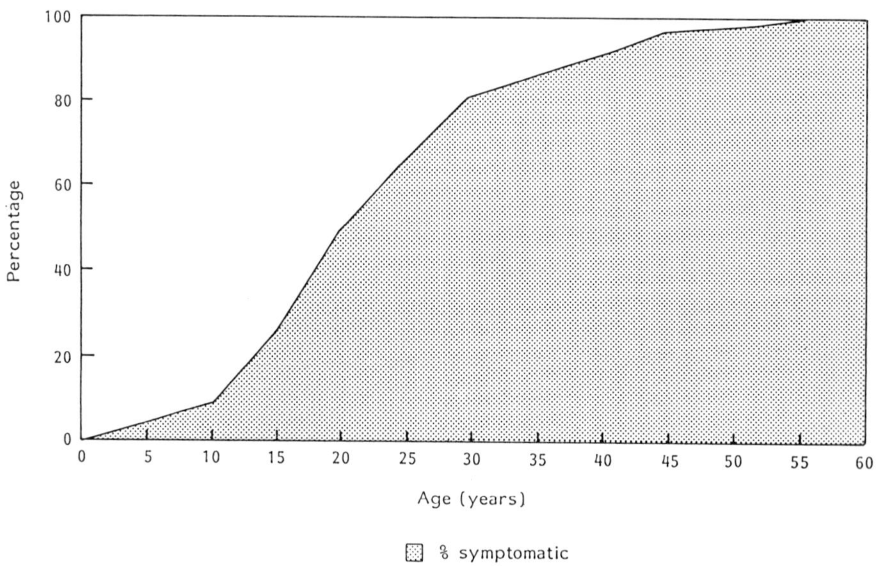

Figure 18.4 Age at onset curve for NF2 based on the 120 patients in the Evans study. (Reproduced with permission from Evans *et al.*, 1992c.)

18.4.2 Morbidity and mortality

The natural history of NF2 in a particular patient is affected by the rate of growth of their vestibular Schwannomas and the number of other tumours they develop. As reviewed in the next section there is inter-family variation, some families having a particularly severe form of NF2 with rapidly growing tumours at multiple sites. The natural history is also affected by the surgical management (section 18.6). Inappropriate operations on large vestibular Schwannomas can hasten the course of the disease. In the large family initially reported by Gardner and Frazier (1930), and then followed up by Young, Eldridge and Gardner (1970), the 20 deceased members who did not undergo surgery had a mean survival (from onset of symptoms) of 18.5 years (range 4–44 years). The nine deceased members who had surgery had a mean survival of 9.2 years (range 3–19 years).

In the recent UK study (Evans *et al.*, 1992b), the mean age at death in 40 cases was 36.25 years. The mean actuarial survival from diagnosis was 15 years, which gave a mean age at death of 42.55 years if mean age at diagnosis was used. Mean actuarial survival in 150 cases was 62 years; however, over 40% would be expected to have died by 50 years and all cases by 70 years.

18.4.3 Effect of gender and pregnancy on natural history

Some studies have suggested a deleterious effect of pregnancy on the natural history of NF2 (Allen, Eldridge and Koerber, 1974). In the study of Kanter *et al.* (1980), eight women developed their first symptoms or experienced exacerbation of their problems during the last trimester of their pregnancies. These findings suggested a hormonal effect on disease course. In addition, in one series of isolated vestibular Schwannomas, these tumours were found to be more common and larger in females than in males (Kasantikul *et al.*, 1980). Schwannomas, meningiomas and neurofibromas had been demonstrated to have specific oestradiol-binding capacity (Martuza, MacLaughlin and Ojemann, 1981). This led to the suggestion that hormonal manipulation may be a therapeutic option worthy of investigation (Martuza and Ojemann, 1982).

The recent UK study (Evans *et al.*, 1992b) did not find evidence of a deleterious effect of pregnancy or gender on the natural history of NF2. There was no instance of death or need for urgent intervention in pregnancy in the study. A few women reported an increase in symptoms during or soon after pregnancy. One patient developed tinnitus, which resolved after pregnancy and only became symptomatic again several years later. Several women who were symptomatic before pregnancy went through up to four pregnancies without recourse to surgery.

With regard to the effect of gender on disease, the mean age at onset of symptoms of 51 women with NF2 was 21.6 years and that for 59 men was 21.1 years. The age at onset of deafness was 24.1 years in women and 24.3

years in men. There was, therefore, no clear difference in disease course between men and women. The UK study therefore suggests that if there is a hormonal effect on the disease process, it is slight.

18.5 GENETICS OF NF2

18.5.1 Inheritance and mutation rate

NF2 is an autosomal dominant condition with almost complete penetrance by the age of 60 years. In the study of Evans *et al.* (1992a), there were no cases of affected sibs born to apparently normal parents and no cases of proven non-penetrance within families. One 67-year-old man was only diagnosed after NF2 developed in his two daughters. Although he had required a hearing aid for some years, he only underwent investigations for vestibular Schwannomas secondary to the diagnosis of NF2 in his daughters. The only obligate carrier where the diagnosis of NF2 was not confirmed was the mother of two affected children who had inherited NF2 from her mother. She died of a myocardial infarction at the age of 36 years with no symptoms. One case of probable non-penetrance was reported by Young, Eldridge and Gardner (1970), although she died in her fifties without specific investigation. Kanter *et al.* (1980) alluded to two possible cases of non-penetrance, but gave no information on age. As these older reports relied on symptoms and the patients had not had full screening, we conclude that if modern diagnostic imaging is used to screen for vestibular Schwannoma, in conjunction with a careful cutaneous and ocular examination, penetrance will be virtually 100% by the age of 60 years.

Approximately half the cases of NF2 are the first in their family and are presumed to be the result of new gene mutation (Martuza and Ojemann, 1982; Glasscock, MacKennan and Levine, 1987; Evans *et al.*, 1992a). The Evans *et al.* study is the only one to calculate the mutation rate, which was 6.5×10^{-6}; this is less than that in NF1 ($3.1 - 10.4 \times 10^{-5}$, Huson *et al.*, 1989), but greater than in von Hippel-Lindau disease (4.4×10^{-6}, Maher *et al.*, 1991).

The mechanism of mutation is unknown, but the UK study (Evans *et al.*, 1992a) showed no evidence that advanced paternal age was a factor. As half the cases are new mutations and the disease prevalence appears steady, then reduced genetic fitness is expected. This was estimated formally in the UK study (Evans *et al.*, 1992a). Overall fitness was reduced by approximately 50%, with relative fitness in males (0.27) being more markedly reduced than in females (0.76). The reduced fitness in males could be partially explained by later expected age at marriage and of birth of their first child.

18.5.2 Maternal effect on disease severity

Although there is no difference in disease course between males and females, there is a difference in natural history depending on whether the gene is inherited from the mother or father. Those individuals with maternal inheritance of NF2 have an earlier age of presentation and more rapid course. This suggests that gene modification by imprinting (Hall, 1990) could be involved in NF2. A maternal gene effect was first suggested by Kanter and Eldridge (1978). They found an age at onset in maternal cases of 18.3 years and in paternal cases of 24.1 years. Evans *et al.* (1992a) confirmed this finding, with a very similar difference in age at onset (maternal cases 18.2 years, paternal cases 24.5 years). In addition there was a general impression of a worse clinical course in maternally inherited cases; the average age of death in six maternally inherited cases was 24.33 years, compared with 39.33 years in three paternally inherited cases.

18.5.3 Genetic heterogeneity

In contrast to NF1, all studies of NF2 have shown strong intrafamilial correlation and disease course but marked interfamilial variation. As early as 1937, it was suggested that NF2 could be divided into a severe and mild form (Worster-Drought, Dixon and McMenemey, 1937). Attention has been recently refocused on this possibility (Mayfrank *et al.*, 1990; Eldridge, Parry and Kaiser-Kupfer, 1991). Eldridge and his colleagues propose a severe form of NF2 with early onset of bilateral vestibular Schwannomas and multiple other tumour types, and a mild form where the vestibular Schwannomas are of later onset and rarely associated with other tumours. As the initial report of NF2 by Wishart (1820) would be classified severe, and the Gardiner family (Gardiner and Frazier, 1930) mild, Eldridge *et al.* suggest the two forms be eponymously titled Gardiner (mild) and Wishart (severe) type. They also suggest that the family reported by Lee and Abbott (1969) with a predominance of meningiomas may represent a third type.

The UK study (Evans *et al.*, 1992a,b) found relatively uniform presentation of the disease within families, but some variation in age of presentation. There were the two broad types of families previously described who had the following features.

- **Mild (Gardiner, type 2A)**. Characterized by relatively late onset (> 15 years and usually > 25 years) of bilateral vestibular Schwannomas, with only minimal skin manifestations and occasional other CNS tumours (no more than one spinal tumour or meningioma). Progression of tumours is often very slow.
- **Severe (Wishart, type 2B)**. With early onset (< 30 years, usually < 25

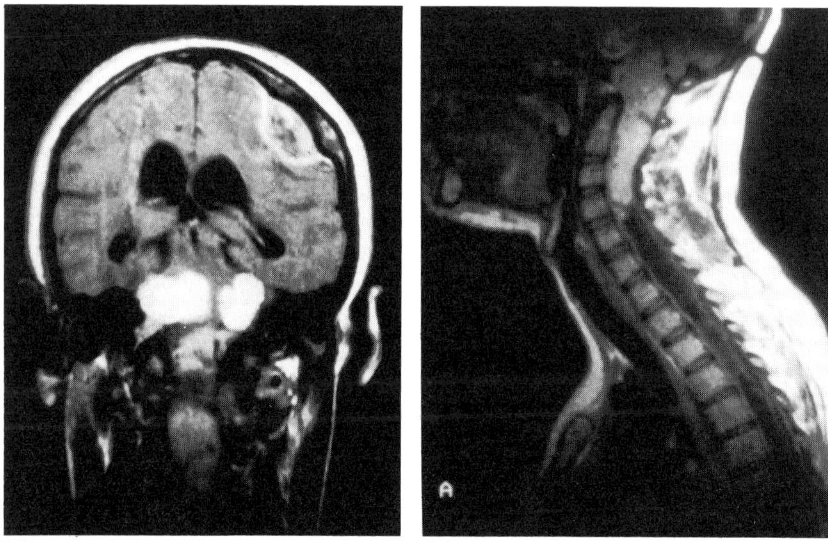

(a) (b)

Figure 18.5 An 18-year-old patient with severe NF2. (A) A Coronal T1 weighted gadolinium-enhanced MR image demonstrating bilateral enhancing vestibular Schwannomas, dramatically compressing the brain stem. The brain stem and upper cervical cord are also expanded by an enhancing mass consistent with a brain stem glioma. There is also a left convexity meningioma. (B) A sagittal T1 weighted gadolinium-enhanced image of the cervical spine demonstrates the inferior extent of the brain stem glioma, terminating at C4/C5, and an associated syrinx involving the cervical and thoracic cord.

years) and meningiomas and spinal tumours in large numbers (at least two of one type and usually multiples) in addition to bilateral vestibular Schwannomas, which are the presenting feature in only 50% of cases (Figure 18.5). Disease course is often rapid causing severe handicap or death before reproductive age.

The peripheral features of NF2 (eye changes, café au lait spots and neurofibromas) were present in both forms but more pronounced in type 2B. No evidence was found to support a third (Lee–Abbott) type of NF2.

In the UK study, however, a significant number of cases (12 out of 120) did not fit exactly into this classification. For example, there were two cases with multiple meningiomas and a unilateral vestibular Schwannoma presenting at 30 and 43 years, respectively. A 28-year-old woman, whose father had typical type 2A disease with onset aged 28 years, presented at 6 years of age with seizures owing to a meningioma and has since developed a spinal tumour. Another woman with a family history of type 2A disease presented aged 8 years with a vestibular

Schwannoma and now has a meningioma at 21 years. In contrast to typical 2B cases, however, these two women remain extremely well and their disease course and tumour growth have been slow. None of the families studied showed a child of a patient with a type 2B classification having a type 2A presentation. Only four out of 60 type 2A cases presented with symptoms not resulting from a vestibular Schwannoma compared with 23 out of 60 type 2B cases who presented with symptoms resulting from a spinal tumour or meningioma.

Subclassifying NF2 purely on the age at presentation is artificial, particularly in view of the maternal age effect on disease course. Although age at presentation is significant in dividing the two types, they are also distinguishable by the rate of growth of the tumours and the number of other lesions apart from bilateral vestibular Schwannomas. In view of the recent identification of a molecular basis for anticipation in myotonic dystrophy (Harley *et al.*, 1992), another mechanism to be considered to explain variable age at onset is anticipation. In the UK study there were not enough multigeneration families identified to address the issue definitively. It is of interest that in the initial report of the largest NF2 family known (Gardiner and Frazier, 1930) the authors drew attention to the decrease in age at death in successive generations (72, 64, 42, and 28 years in generations 1–4, respectively).

At the present time the division of NF2 into two definite clinical types is therefore not clear cut, although at a practical level the very different disease course and manifestations in some families remain constant and can be used to guide management of individual families. As reviewed by Dr Rouleau in Chapter 3, there is no evidence of locus heterogeneity at the present time, with all families studied mapping to the same region of chromosome 22. However, as it is large families that are used for linkage studies, the majority of them will have mild neurofibromatosis by definition, and therefore to address fully the question of heterogeneity at the molecular level we will have to wait for direct mutation analysis. When this is available, we will be able to investigate definitively allelic and non-allelic heterogeneity in NF2.

18.6 MANAGEMENT OF NF2

18.6.1 Overview

The successful management of NF2 patients involves coordination between several different medical specialties, principally neurosurgeons, otolaryngologists, ophthalmologists and geneticists. Patients also need ongoing support from other health professionals such as teachers of communication to the deaf and social workers. Several studies have shown improved surgical outcome when vestibular Schwannoma surgery in NF2 is performed in centres specializing in this kind of surgery (NIH Consensus Statement, 1992; Evans *et al.*, 1993). Other reports have focused on the lack of information given to families, particularly preparation for hearing loss at the time before vestibular Schwannoma surgery (Huson and Thrush, 1985). In the recent UK study (Evans *et al.*, 1992c) very few of the families had any understanding of the natural history or genetic nature of their condition. Only 44 out of 120 patients had received genetic counselling and many people were unaware that NF2 could be inherited.

18.6.2 Management of affected individuals

As discussed above, the coordination of medical care and ongoing psychosocial support to patients is extremely important in the care of patients with NF2. Although it is the vestibular Schwannomas themselves that usually present the most difficult challenge in patient management, it is important that those operating on vestibular Schwannomas in NF2 are aware of the risk of other tumours developing. NF2 patients undergoing vestibular Schwannoma surgery should always have a spinal MRI scan preoperatively to exclude spinal tumours, which could affect the outcome of surgery.

(a) Investigation and management of vestibular Schwannomas

As discussed in section 18.2.2, vestibular Schwannomas cause the initial symptoms in most patients with NF2. Their early diagnosis is important as tumour size is one of the major preoperative factors for postoperative preservation of useful hearing and facial nerve function. Although early diagnosis is achievable in known NF2 families when the children at risk are monitored from birth, in patients with NF2 and no family history there is often delay in diagnosis. As reviewed in section 18.2.2, it has been shown that the vestibular Schwannomas in NF2 tend to cause symptoms at a later stage than their solitary unilateral counterparts (Hart, Gardiner and Howieson, 1983). Once vestibular Schwannomas have been identified, it is important that their effect on vestibular nerve function is discussed with the patient. There have been reports of patients 'getting lost underwater' and even drowning because of this (Kanter *et al.*, 1980).

In the diagnostic assessment of patients suspected of having NF2, detailed cutaneous and ophthalmic assessment for peripheral signs of the disease is important. For example, a young person presenting with bilateral deafness and a history of having had a peripheral nerve tumour removed or a congenital cataract will very likely have NF2. The actual diagnosis of the vestibular Schwannomas depends on audiometric testing and neuroimaging.

Although standard audiometric tests, including vestibular nerve function tests, are important perioperative measures of eighth nerve function, it has been shown that they are not particularly useful detectors of small vestibular Schwannomas, particularly in NF2 (Bess *at al.*, 1984). BAER testing is a much better diagnostic procedure. It is abnormal in 96% of all unilateral tumours and in 91% of small tumours (< 2 cm diameter; Hart, Gardiner and Howieson, 1983). It has also been shown to be extremely sensitive in NF2. All 14 patients in the series of Bess *et al.* (1984) had abnormal BAERs. Glasscock *et al.* (1979) reported the assessment of an individual at risk for NF2 with a normal CT scan but abnormal BAERs. In view of this abnormality, posterior fossa meatography was performed and showed small bilateral tumours, 1.5 and 2 cm in diameter.

Abnormalities seen on BAER in individuals with vestibular Schwannomas include a prolongation in the time difference between wave I and wave V, and in cases with known hearing loss, an absence of wave I. In those cases of absent wave I, information can be obtained from normative values for wave V latency, taking into account results of routine audiograms and by comparison with the patient's other ear. The latency between wave I and wave V is referred to as 'central conduction time'. Eggermont and Don (1986) have concluded that cases with prolonged central conduction time using a whole click response but with a nearly normal I–V delay in the narrow band responses are indicative of small intracanalicular vestibular Schwannomas.

Developments in neuroimaging techniques have made the detection of vestibular Schwannomas in NF2 much easier. Internal auditory canal flaring on skull radiographs is not necessarily associated with the presence of vestibular Schwannoma and is not sensitive enough to be used as a diagnostic test. The use of CT and MRI is indicated for the detection of vestibular Schwannomas. CT scanning is sensitive to 77% of all unilateral vestibular tumours. With air contrast CT cisternography the sensitivity was increased to 95% in one series (Hart, Gardiner and Howieson, 1983). As the resolution of CT scanners has improved, so has the level of detection of small tumours, although as noted above, some cases with abnormal BAERs had normal CT scans at the time of initial assessment. With the advent of MRI the level of sensitivity of neuroimaging has increased to the point that with very small tumours the BAERs can be normal. On MRI studies of patients with NF2, enlargement of the seventh and eighth nerve complex can be detected down to 0.5 cm in diameter. The use of gadolinium-DTPA enhancement improves sensitivity. Cranial neuroimaging may give other clues to the diagnosis of NF2, such as the presence of tumours on other cranial nerves, meningiomas, or the calcified, tuberous sclerosis-like lesions mentioned in section

18.2.7 (on MRI these appear as hypointense lesions on long TR/TE images; Aoki *et al.*, 1989).

The management of vestibular Schwannomas in NF2 must take into account the risk of hearing impairment in both ears and the disabling consequences of acquired deafness. Assessment of the patient must also account for the presence of other tumours and the management of different tumours prioritized. For example, aggressive vestibular Schwannoma surgery may not be appropriate in a patient with an inoperable expanding intramedullary spinal tumour.

Early series (Young, Eldridge and Gardiner, 1970) showed that patients who had surgery had a shorter survival than those who did not. In the recent UK series (Evans *et al.*, 1993), vestibular Schwannoma surgery was assessed in 74 patients who had had operations over a 35-year period. One hundred and eighteen vestibular Schwannomas had been totally/subtotally removed from 74 patients, including removal of three asymptomatic tumours. Useful hearing preservation was only achieved in nine out of 118 operations (7.6%) and good facial nerve function in 32 out of 118 operations (27%). Hearing was lost in all three asymptomatic ears. However, the operations had been performed over a 25-year period during which there has been a marked improvement in neuroimaging and surgical technique; in recent years the operations performed in specialized centres showed better outcomes. In two centres with a particular interest in vestibular Schwannoma surgery, hearing preservation was achieved in 15% and good facial nerve function in 45% of operations compared with 6% and 23%, respectively, for the remaining centres. The difference was not statistically significant for hearing preservation by χ^2 testing ($p = 0.17$) but was for facial nerve function ($p = 0.05$). Improved surgical outcome in specialized centres is recognized both in NF2 and isolated vestibular Schwannoma surgery (NIH Consensus Statement, 1992), although even in these centres it is well recognized that surgery on vestibular Schwannomas in NF2 is extremely difficult and the best form of management is still unclear.

Improvement in surgical techniques for vestibular Schwannoma led the NIH Consensus Statement on Neurofibromatosis (1988) to advocate a relatively aggressive approach to vestibular Schwannoma surgery in NF2 with a view to removing the tumours at the earliest opportunity. The results of surgery on small tumours in NF2 have, however, been less successful than in unilateral cases (Glasscock *et al.*, 1989). This led the NIH Conference on Vestibular Schwannoma in 1992 to recommend more conservative approaches such as subtotal intracapsular resection or simple observation of the patient's progress.

Management of bilateral vestibular Schwannomas in NF2 patients demands careful evaluation of audiological examinations and neuroimaging studies. In patients with no symptoms or mild stable symptoms, where MRI shows no increase in tumour size, conservative observation is indicated. When audiological studies show worsening on one side or neuroimaging studies show rapid increase in tumour size and there is stable and 'useful' hearing in the opposite ear, complete surgical removal should be considered. 'Useful' hearing is defined as speech reception threshold no poorer than 70 dB and a speech discrimination score of at least 15% (Nadol *et al.*, 1987). Complete removal is also recommended for a tumour of any size when no hearing is present on the tumour-bearing side and neurological symptoms are present, or in a similar patient with no hearing on the tumour-bearing side without symptoms who might become symptomatic with minimal enlargement of the tumour. The surgical approach most favoured in cases of small tumours with the possibility of preservation of hearing is the micro-operative suboccipital approach. Return to previous level of activity was achieved in 95% of patients with small and medium tumours using that approach in one series (Ojemann and Martuza, 1990). The use of intraoperative monitoring of seventh and eighth nerve function is recommended to alert the surgeon to compromise of hearing and facial nerve function. For those with one hearing ear, with progressive hearing loss related to enlarging tumour in which complete removal could sacrifice remaining hearing, internal auditory canal decompression and subtotal removal has provided continued useful hearing for a number of years (Martuza, 1990).

An alternative to surgery that has been recently explored is focused stereotactic radiation. The most extensive experience of the technique has used the gamma knife. This technique has provided stabilization of vestibular Schwannoma size, but with variable results in saving hearing and preserving facial nerve function (Noren, Arndt and Hindmarsh, 1983; Khonsary, Rand and Wilson, 1986).

The discussion of possible side-effects of any surgery with the patient and their families is very important. Particular reference should be given to possible deafness and the preparation of the patient for this with an introduction to other forms of communication such as lip reading or sign language as appropriate. Approaches to management of postoperative facial nerve palsy are discussed by Drs Angel, Persing and Edgerton in Chapter 14 (section 14.3.4a).

(b) *Management of other tumours*

The other tumours NF2 do not present such a difficult management challenge as the vestibular Schwannomas. The size, location and related symptoms all need to be considered in tumour management. There is no difference in the surgical approach to the other tumours that occur in NF2 than when they occur in isolation. Neurophysiological monitoring is important during surgery on the nodular peripheral nerve tumours to help avoid peripheral nerve damage if possible.

Gliomas in NF2 are usually low-grade and may not need treatment. Serial neuroimaging should be used to monitor their growth. If there is growth, stereotactic biopsy can be used to determine malignant potential. Intraspinal gliomas and ependymomas can lead to the development of syringomyelia and serial MRI scans will monitor for the development of this; appropriate treatment of the syringomyelia may halt or slow the progression of symptoms.

18.6.3 Genetic counselling and the management of at-risk individuals

Genetic counselling is an important part of the management of people with NF2. Children of individuals at risk have a 50% risk of inheriting the condition. In approximately half the individuals who present, there will be no obvious family history (Evans *et al.*, 1992a). Before concluding they represent new mutations, it is important to ensure a very detailed family tree has been drawn up and, unless they are over 60 years of age, to screen the parents for NF2 with cutaneous and ophthalmological examination (including indirect ophthalmoscopy and slit lamp examination), BAERs and cranial MRI.

A protocol for screening subjects at risk of NF2 is shown in Figure 18.6. As 10% of the cases are symptomatic before 10 years of age (Evans *et al.*, 1992b), screening is warranted from early childhood. The presence of congenital or very early cataracts necessitates detailed early ophthalmological screening and slit lamp evaluation should be used in addition to ophthalmoscopy at least every 5 years. Screening for vestibular Schwannoma should begin in the early teens and BAER should be performed annually. Cranial neuroimaging can be reserved when an abnormality is detected on clinical or audiological examination until the late teens. At that time, a normal cranial MRI scan will approximately halve the risk of having inherited NF2 and will facilitate reproductive decision-making. Gadolinium-enhanced MRI scans are the imaging technique of choice, because they detect smaller tumours than CT and avoid the risk of radiation. A normal cranial scan at 30 years of age will make inheritance very unlikely, except in late-onset families, and will lead to cessation of formal screening in most people. Where onset in the family has been late, screening should be continued as appropriate to that family.

The developments in molecular genetics of NF2 described by Dr Rouleau in Chapter 3 will gradually make the above screening protocol unnecessary for all at-risk individuals. It will be possible to use DNA diagnosis to identify those who are at high or low risk of inheriting the disease gene (if linked markers are used) or to identify directly the gene mutation (when direct mutation analysis becomes available).

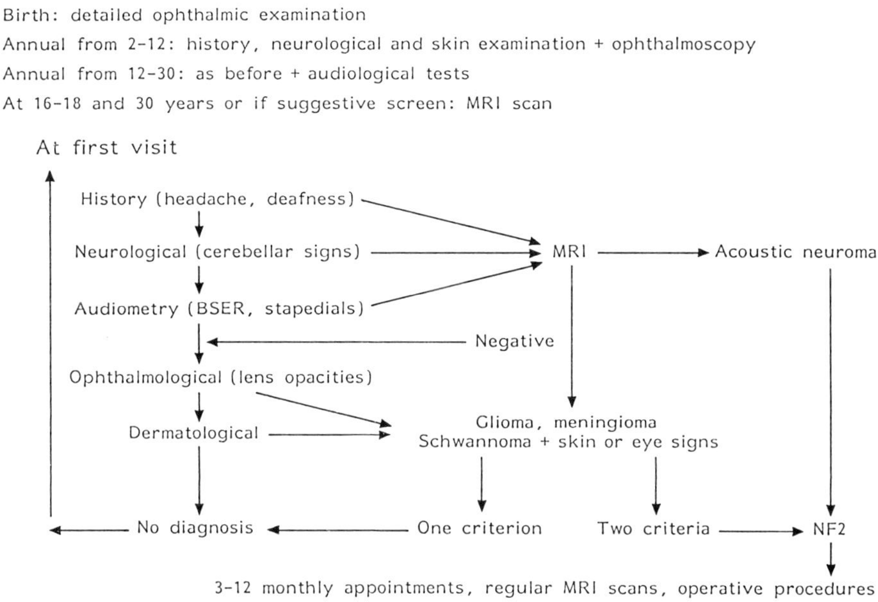

Figure 18.6 Screening protocol for individuals at risk of NF2. (Reproduced with permission from Evans *et al.*, 1992c.)

At the present time, in families with two or more affected individuals, linked genetic markers can be used in presymptomatic and prenatal testing (Narod *et al.*, 1992). The principles of using linked markers in presymptomatic and prenatal diagnosis of genetic disease are the same whatever the condition, and are explained in relation to NF1 in Chapter 15 (section 15.4.6). Linked markers have a small margin of error, which is proportional to their distance from the disease gene, and this error falls significantly if two markers are used that flank the disease gene and are both informative in the family. With close flanking markers the margin of error is usually less than 1%. Individuals shown to have inherited a low-risk marker allele would not need to be followed as frequently as recommended in Figure 18.6 for those where DNA testing is not available. Where there is a margin of error in the DNA test, screening with BAERs and cranial MRI should probably be performed in the late teens as a double check on disease status. The recent cloning of the NF2 gene brings the possibility of direct mutation testing. Providing the mutation in the family can be identified at-risk individuals, regardless of family structure, will be able to be tested with a 100% accuracy and only those shown to carry the disease gene will proceed with the kind of follow-up recommended in Figure 18.6.

18.6.4 Supraregional care for NF2

In contrast to NF1 where all affected individuals do not need specialized care, for NF2 we strongly recommend that affected patients and their families are under the care of specialist centres with a team of health professionals who have a particular interest in vestibular Schwannoma surgery and the management of NF2 families. Experience on both sides of the Atlantic (NIH Consensus Statement, 1992; Evans *et al.*, 1993) suggests that treatment in such centres improves the morbidity associated with surgery in NF2. The patients also benefit from the coordination of their care by one team of doctors and the input of other health professionals with experience of the disease. In a country the size of the UK, only two or three such centres would be needed. The cloning of the *NF2* gene may provide insights into pathogenesis and suggest possible preventive treatment. Specialist centres with experience in NF2 management would ensure clinical application of such developments, with careful appraisal, at the earliest opportunity.

18.7 FUTURE PROSPECTS

NF2 is a serious neurogenetic disorder associated with significant morbidity and mortality in the majority of affected individuals. In this chapter, we have reviewed the difficult problems associated with successful management of patients with the disease. It must be emphasized, however, that the published material is based on retrospective series collected before diagnosis by cranial MRI was available and surgical techniques were less well-developed than they are today. The last few years have seen considerable improvement in both these areas, but even then neurosurgeons and otolaryngologists still find the vestibular Schwannomas in NF2 much more difficult to remove successfully than their unilateral isolated counterparts. In NF2, the importance of coordination of care and long-term follow-up of affected individuals cannot be overstressed, nor that of offering their at-risk relatives genetic counselling and presymptomatic screening.

As reviewed in Chapters 1 and 3, the pathogenesis of NF2 is not understood other than that the clinical features of the disease would suggest that the gene is a tumour suppressor. This is based on the similarity of NF2 to the model of isolated and familial retinoblastoma that Knudson (1971) used to formulate his 'double-hit' hypothesis of tumour formation. Molecular genetics studies (Chapter 3) have shown that the mechanism of tumorigenesis in NF2 is exactly the same. The recent cloning of the *NF2* gene gives the prospect of detailed understanding of pathogenesis of the condition and the possible development of treatment that would prevent or modify tumour development in affected individuals.

ACKNOWLEDGEMENTS

We would like to thank Dr Gareth Evans for helpful discussions about NF2 during the preparation of this chapter, and Drs Nicola Ragge for supplying Figure 18.3, and Drs Phillip Anslow, Andrew Molyneux and Shelley Renowden for supplying the MRI illustrations (Figures 18.1 and 18.5).

REFERENCES

Allen, J., Eldridge, R. and Koerber, T. (1974) Acoustic neuroma in the last months of pregnancy. *Am. J. Obstet. Gynecol.*, **119**, 516–20.

Aoki, S., Barkovich, A.J., Nishimura, K. *et al.* (1989) Neurofibromatosis types 1 and 2: cranial MR findings. *Radiology*, **172**, 527–34.

Arts, W.F.M. and van Dongen, K.J. (1986) Intracranial calcified deposits in neurofibromatosis. *J. Neurol. Neurosurg. Psych.*, **49**, 1317–20.

Bess, F.H., Forrest Josey, A., Glasscock, M.E. and Wilson, L.K. (1984) Audiological manifestations in bilateral acoustic tumours (von Recklinghausen's disease). *J. Speech Hear. Disord.*, **49**, 177–82.

Cawthon, R.M., Weiss, R., Xu, G. *et al.* (1990) A major segment of the neurofibromatosis type 1 gene: CDNA sequence, genomic structure and point mutations. *Cell*, **62**, 193–201.

Charles, S.J., Moore, A.T., Yates, J.R.W. and Ferguson-Smith, M.A. (1989) Lisch nodules in neurofibromatosis type 2. Case report. *Arch. Ophthalmol.*, **107**, 1571–2.

Clarke, A., Church, W., Gardner Medwin, D. and Sengupta, R. (1990) Intracranial calcification and seizures: a case of central neurofibromatosis. *Dev. Med. Child Neurol.*, **32**, 729-32.

Crowe, F.W. and Schull, W.J. (1953) Diagnostic importance of the café au lait spot in neurofibromatosis. *Arch. Intern. Med.*, **91**, 758–66.

Crowe, F.W., Schull, W.J. and Neel, J.V. (1956) *A Clinical, Pathological and Genetic Study of Multiple Neurofibromatosis*, Charles C. Thomas, Springfield, Illinois.

Cushing, H. (1917) *Tumours of the Nervus Acusticus and the Syndrome of the Cerebellopontine Angle*, W.B. Saunders, Philadelphia.

Eggermont, J.J. and Don, M. (1986) Mechanisms of central conduction time prolongation in brain-stem auditory evoked potentials. *Arch. Neurol.*, **43**, 116–20.

Eldridge, R., Parry, D.M. and Kaiser-Kupfer, M.I. (1991) Neurofibromatosis 2: clinical heterogeneity and natural history in 39 individuals in 9 families and 16 sporadic cases. Proceedings of the Eighth International Congress on Human Genetics. *Am. J. Hum. Genet.*, **49**, 133, A676.

Evans, D.G.R., Huson, S.M., Donnai, D. *et al.* (1992a) A genetic study of type 2 neurofibromatosis in the north west of England and the UK. I. Prevalence, mutation rate, fitness and confirmation of maternal transmission effect on severity. *J. Med. Genet.*, **29**, 841–6.

Evans, D.G.R., Huson, S.M., Neary, W. *et al.* (1992b) A clinical study of type 2 neurofibromatosis. *Q. J. Med.*, **304**, 603–18.

Evans, D.G.R., Huson, S.M., Neary, W. *et al.* (1992c) A genetic study of type 2 neurofibromatosis. II. Guidelines for genetic counselling. *J. Med. Genet.*, **29**, 847–52.

Evans, D.G.R., Ramsden, R., Huson, S.M. *et al.* (1993) Type 2 neurofibromatosis: the need for supraregional care? *J. Laryngol. Otol.*, **107**, 401–6.

Gardiner, W.J. and Frazier, C.H. (1930) Bilateral acoustic neurofibromatosis: a clinical study and field survey of a family of five generations with bilateral deafness in thirty-eight members. *Arch. Neurol. Psychol.*, **23**, 266–302.

Glasscock, M.E., Jackson, C.G., Tosey, A.F. *et al.* (1979) Brain stem evoked response audiometry in a clinical practice. *Laryngoscope*, **7**, 1021–39.

Glasscock, M.E., McKennan, K.X. and Levine, S.C. (1987) Acoustic neuroma surgery: the results of hearing conservation surgery. *Laryngoscope*, **97**, 785–9.

Glasscock, M.E., Woods, C.I., Jackson, C.G. and Welling, B. (1989) Management of bilateral acoustic tumours. *Laryngoscope*, **99**, 475–84.

Good, M.V., Brodsky, M.C., Edwards, M.S. and Hoyt, W.F. (1991) Bilateral retinal hamartomas in neurofibromatosis type 2. *Br. J. Ophthalmol.*, **75**, 190.

Hall, J.G. (1990) Genomic imprinting: review and relevance to human disease. *Am. J. Hum. Genet.*, **46**, 857–73.

Halliday, A.L., Sobel, R.A. and Martuza, R.L. (1991) Benign spinal nerve sheath tumours: their occurrence sporadically and in neurofibromatosis types 1 and 2. *J. Neurosurg.*, **74**, 248–53.

Harley, H.G., Brook, D.J., Rundle, S.A. *et al.* (1992) Expansion of an unstable DNA region and phenotypic variation in myotonic dystrophy. *Nature*, **355**, 545–51.

Hart, R.G., Gardiner, D.P. and Howieson, J. (1983) Acoustic tumors; atypical features and recent diagnostic tests. *Neurology*, **33**, 211–21.

Henschen, F. (1915) Zur histologie und pathogenese der kleinhirnbrucken-winkeltumoren. *Arch. f. Psychiatr.*, **56**, 21.

Huson, S.M. and Thrush, D.C. (1985) Central neurofibromatosis. *Q. J. Med.*, **55**, 213–24.

Huson, S.M., Jones, D. and Beck, L. (1987) Ophthalmic manifestations of neurofibromatosis. *Br. J. Ophthalmol.*, **71**, 235–8.

Huson, S.M., Harper, P.S. and Compston, D.A.S. (1988) Von Recklinghausen neurofibromatosis: a clinical and population based study in South East Wales. *Brain*, **111**, 1355–81.

Huson, S.M., Compston, D.A.S., Clark, P. and Harper, P.S. (1989) A genetic study of von Recklinghausen neurofibromatosis in South East Wales. I. Prevalence, fitness, mutation rate, and effect of parental transmission on severity. *J. Med. Genet.*, **26**, 704–11.

Kaiser-Kupfer, M.I., Freidlin, V., Datiles, M.B. *et al.* (1989) The association of posterior capsular lens opacities with bilateral acoustic neuromas in patients with neurofibromatosis type 2. *Arch. Ophthalmol.*, **107**, 541–4.

Kanter, W. and Eldridge, R. (1978) Evidence of a maternal effect in central neurofibromatosis. *Lancet*, **ii**, 903.

Kanter, W.R., Eldridge, R., Fabricant, R. *et al.* (1980) Central neurofibromatosis with bilateral acoustic neuroma: genetic, clinical and biochemical distinctions from peripheral neurofibromatosis. *Neurology*, **30**, 851–9.

Kasantikul, V., Netsky, M.G., Glasscock, M.E. and Hays, J.W. (1980) Acoustic neurilemmoma: clinicoanatomic study of 103 patients. *J. Neurosurg.*, **52**, 28–35.

Khonsary, A., Rand, R.W. and Wilson, G.H. (1986) Stereotactic radiosurgery of acoustic neuromas, in *Surgery In and Around the Brain Stem and Third Ventricle* (ed. M. Samii), Springer-Verlag, Berlin, pp. 559–69.

Knudson, A.G., Jr (1971) Mutation and cancer: statistical study of retinoblastoma. *Proc. Natl. Acad. Sci. USA*, **68**, 820–3.

Kopf, A.W., Levine, L.J., Rigel, D.S. *et al.* (1985) Prevalence of congenital-nevus-like nevi, nevi spilli and café au lait spots. *Arch. Dermatol.*, **121**, 766–9.

Landau, K., Dossetor, F.M., Hoyt, W.F. and Muci-Mendoza, R. (1990) Retinal hamartoma in neurofibromatosis 2. *Arch. Ophthalmol.*, **108**, 328–9.

Lee, D.K. and Abbott, M.L. (1969) Familial central nervous system neoplasia. *Arch. Neurol.*, **20**, 154–60.

Linthicum, J.J.P. (1972) Unusual audiometric and histological findings in bilateral acoustic neuromas. *Ann. Otol. Rhinol. Laryngol.*, **81**, 433–7.

Maher, E.R., Iselius, L., Yates, J.R.W. *et al.* (1991) von Hippel Lindau disease: a genetic study. *J. Med. Genet.*, **28**, 443–7.

Martuza, R.L. (1984) Genetics in neuro-oncology. *Clin. Neurosurg.*, **31**, 417–40.

Martuza, R.L. (1990) Pathogenesis and treatment of nervous system tumors in NF2, in *Tuberous Sclerosis and Neurofibromatosis: Epidemiology, Pathophysiology, Biology and Management* (eds Y. Ishibashi and Y. Hori), Elsevier, Amsterdam, pp. 281–7.

Martuza, R.L. and Eldridge, R. (1988) Neurofibromatosis 2. *N. Engl. J. Med.*, **318**, 684–8.

Martuza, R.L. and Ojemann, R.G. (1982) Bilateral acoustic neuromas: clinical aspects, pathogenesis and treatment. *Neurosurgery*, **10**, 1–12.

Martuza, R.L., MacLaughlin, D.T. and Ojemann, R.G. (1981) Specific estradiol binding in Schwannomas, meningiomas and neurofibromas. *Neurosurgery*, **9**, 665–71.

Martuza, R.L., Philippe, I., Fitzpatrick, T.B. *et al.* (1985) Melanin macroglobules as a cellular marker of neurofibromatosis: a quantitative study. *J. Invest. Dermatol.*, **85**, 347–50.

Mayfrank, L., Mohadjer, M. and Wullich, B. (1990) Intracranial calcified deposits in neurofibromatosis type 2. A CT study of 11 cases. *Neuroradiology*, **32**, 33–7.

Mayfrank, L., Wullich, B., Wolff, G. *et al.* (1990) Neurofibromatosis 2: a clinically and genetically heterogeneous disease? Report on 10 sporadic cases. *Clin. Genet.*, **38**, 362–70.

McKusick, V.A. (1990) *Mendelian Inheritance in Man*, 9th edn, Johns Hopkins University Press, Baltimore.

Michaels, V.V., Whisnant, J.P., Garrity, J.A. and Miller, G.M. (1989) Neurofibromatosis type 1 with bilateral acoustic neuromas. *Neurofibromatosis*, **2**, 213–17.

Mirimanoff, R.O., Dosoretz, D.E., Linggood, R.M. *et al.* (1985) Meningioma: analysis of recurrence and progression following neurosurgical resection. *J. Neurosurg.*, **62**, 1824.

Nadol, J.B., Levine, R., Ojemann, R.G. *et al.* (1987) Preservation of hearing in surgical removal of acoustic neuromas of the internal auditory canal and cerebellopontine angle. *Laryngoscope*, **97**, 1287–94.

Nager, G.T. (1984) Neurinomas of the trigeminal nerve. *Am. J. Otolaryngol.*, **5**, 301–33.

Narod, S.A., Parry, D.M., Parboosingh, J. *et al.* (1992) Neurofibromatosis type 2 appears to be a genetically homogeneous disease. *Am. J. Hum. Genet.*, **51**, 486–96.

National Institutes of Health Consensus Development Conference Statement (1988) Neurofibromatosis. *Arch. Neurol.*, **45**, 575–8.

National Institutes of Health Consensus Development Conference Statement (1992) Acoustic neuroma. *Neurofibromatosis Research Newsletter*, **8**, 1–7.

Noren, G., Arndt, J. and Hindmarsh, T. (1983) Stereotactic radiosurgery in cases of acoustic neurinoma: further experiences. *Neurosurgery*, **13**, 12–22.

Ohnishi, A. and Nada, O. (1972) Ultrastructure of the onion bulb-like structure observed in the sural nerve in a case of von Recklinghausen's disease. *Acta Neuropathol. (Berl.)*, **20**, 258–63.

Ojemann, R.G. and Martuza, R.L. (1990) Acoustic neuroma, in *Neurologic Surgery*, 3rd edn (ed. J. Youmans), W.B. Saunders, Philadelphia, pp. 3316–50.

Pearson-Webb, M.A., Kaiser-Kupfer, M.I. and Eldridge, R. (1986) Eye findings in bilateral acoustic (central) neurofibromatosis: association with presenile lens opacity and cataracts but absence of Lisch nodules. *N. Engl. J. Med.*, **315**, 1553–4.

Ragge, N.K., Baser, M., Falk, R.E. *et al.* (1992) Presymptomatic diagnosis of NF2: ocular expression. *Am. J. Hum. Genet.*, **51** (Suppl.), A31(113).

Riccardi, V.M. (1981) Von Recklinghausen neurofibromatosis. *N. Engl. J. Med.*, **305**, 1617–27.

Riccardi, V.M. (1982) Neurofibromatosis: clinical heterogeneity. *Curr. Probl. Cancer*, **7**, 1–34.

Riccardi, V.M. (1992) *Neurofibromatosis: Phenotype, Natural History and Pathogenesis*, 2nd edn, Johns Hopkins University Press, Baltimore.

Riccardi, V.M. and Ragge, N. (1992) Unilateral NF2. NNFF Annual Clinical Care Symposium, San Francisco.

Rubinstein, L.J. (1986) The malformed central nervous system lesions in the central and peripheral forms of neurofibromatosis. *Ann. N.Y. Acad. Sci.*, **486**, 14–29.

Sadeh, M., Martinovits, G. and Goldhammer, Y. (1989) Occurrence of both neurofibromatosis 1 and 2 in the same individual with a rapidly progressive course. *Neurology*, **39**, 282–3.

Sivalingham, A., Augsburger, J., Perilongo, G. *et al.* (1991) Combined hamartoma of the retina and retinal pigment epithelium in a patient with neurofibromatosis type 2. *J. Ped. Ophthalmol. Strab.*, **28**, 320–2.

Sobel, R.A. and Wang, Y.J. (1993) Vestibular (acoustic) Schwannomas: histological features in neurofibromatosis 2 and unilateral cases. *J. Neuropathol. Exp. Neurol.*, in press.

Thomas, P.K., King, R.H.M., Chiang, T.R. *et al.* (1990) Neurofibromatous neuropathy. *Muscle Nerve*, **13**, 93–101.

van Tassel, P., Yeakley, J.W. and Lee, K.F. (1987) Cerebellar calcification in central neurofibromatosis: CT in two cases. *AJNR*, **8**, 913–15.

von Recklinghausen, F. (1882) *Ueber die multiplen Fibroma der Haut und ihre Beziehung zu den multiplen Neuromen*, A. Hirschwald, Berlin.

Wishart, J.H. (1820) Case of tumours in the skull, dura mater, and brain. *Edinb. Med. Surg. J.*, **18**, 393–7.

Worster-Drought, D., Dickson, W.E.C. and McMenemey, W.H. (1937) Multiple meningeal and perineural tumors with analogous changes in the glia and ependyma (neurofibroblastomatosis). *Brain*, **60**, 88–117.

Young, D.R., Eldridge, R. and Gardiner, W.J. (1970) Bilateral acoustic neuroma in a large kindred. *JAMA*, **214**, 347–53.

19

Alternate and related forms of the neurofibromatoses

D. Viskochil and J.C. Carey

19.1 INTRODUCTION

The neurofibromatoses are a heterogeneous set of conditions having clinical manifestations commonly seen in the classical forms of neurofibromatosis (NF) types 1 (NF1) and 2 (NF2). Both NF1 and NF2 display wide variability in clinical expression making it difficult to classify many conditions that have overlapping NF clinical manifestations. The development and use of objective diagnostic guidelines for NF1 and NF2 appropriately excludes many cases that have clinical features of NF but do not fulfil the established diagnostic criteria. In order to provide more accurate healthcare counselling, medical conditions demonstrating atypical clinical manifestations of NF have been classified separately from the distinctive forms of NF1 and NF2. This chapter will examine the clinical presentations of the variant forms of the neurofibromatoses, including the NF-overlap syndromes, and classify them with respect to the prototypical phenotypes of NF1 and NF2.

NF1 and NF2 have distinct clinical signs that usually make their respective diagnoses relatively straightforward. However, variability in clinical expression, high sporadic mutation rates and age-related penetrance all tend to make diagnosis difficult in some instances. This becomes an issue in genetic counselling because both NF1 and NF2 are inherited in an autosomal dominant fashion, whereas the overlap syndromes associated with NF generally do not have well-defined inheritance patterns. Distinguishing the various forms of NF should enable one to provide more accurate genetic counselling of recurrence risks and prognosis. The difficulties associated with any classification scheme that attempts to distinguish different forms of NF cannot be overstated. Nevertheless, the exercise of exploring the variant forms of

NF and acknowledging the limitations in clinical diagnosis and prognosis may be of future benefit for those afflicted with any of the forms of NF.

19.2 SUBCLASSIFICATION OF THE NEUROFIBROMATOSES

Historically, the classification of the neurofibromatoses has been based on clinical grounds only. Riccardi (1982) initially devised a scheme to account for heterogeneity of NF, which has been revised as a chapter in the two editions of Riccardi's book *Neurofibromatosis: Phenotype, Natural History and Pathogenesis* (Riccardi and Eicher, 1986; Riccardi, 1992). Riccardi presented seven types of NF (Table 19.1) as a tentative classification scheme to serve as a starting place for students of NF. On review, Riccardi's classification scheme shows that NF-1 (von Recklinghausen NF), NF-2 (bilateral acoustic NF) and NF-3 (mixed NF) are discrete clinical conditions belonging to distinct categories. NF-4 (variant NF) is minimally helpful to classification because it serves as a wastebasket category and, as aptly pointed out, such cases may simply represent the extreme clinical manifestations of NF1. The category NF-5 (segmental NF) is restrictive in its diagnostic criteria and excludes many localized presentations of NF1 features. A more encompassing classification scheme devised by Roth, Martines and James (1987) is more appropriate for the variety of segmental NF clinical presentations. NF-6 (multiple, familial café au lait spots) is a rare, autosomal dominant condition presenting with multiple café au lait spots and no other symptoms or signs of NF. This condition does not map to the *NF1* locus (Charrow, Listernick and Ward, 1992). NF-7 (late-onset NF) is not a distinct form of NF aside from the definition that NF features present later in life, after the third decade. This feature does not justify a specific classification, but should alert us to the pathogenesis of NF with respect to ageing (Huson, Compston and Harper, 1989). Many of the segmental cases of NF present after the age of 30 years, which suggests that the late-onset form of NF may be caused by somatic mutations arising in the ageing process. The remaining two headings in Riccardi's classification, NF-NOS (not otherwise specified) and Other NF types, are not helpful because there are no common clinical findings unifying the cases in a medically significant way. Even though there are some inadequacies in this classification scheme, until the pathophysiology of the variant forms of NF is deciphered, any scheme will be fraught with similar inadequacies and reflect the biases of the respective authors. As Riccardi (1984) stated '...we just do not know enough about NF to be too rigid or too exclusive in any current classification system. We need one that will provide order now and still allow for adjustments and subclassifications over time'.

Table 19.1 Classification of the different types of neurofibromatosis proposed by Riccardi (1982, 1992)

Type	*Descriptive title*	*Inheritance*	*Presence/absence of defining features of NF1*			*Major clinical features*
			CAL	*NF*	*LN*	
NF-1	von Recklinghausen	AD	+	+	+	Numerous complications affecting all body systems
NF-2	Acoustic	AD	+	+	0	Major feature is bilateral vestibular Schwannomas, occasionally with meningiomas. The CAL and NF are less numerous than in NF-1
NF-3	Mixed	AD	+	+	?	Major feature is multiple CNS tumours (Schwannomas, gliomas, meningiomas). Defining features may be as marked as in NF-1, more usually as in NF-2
NF-4	Variant	Probably AD	±	?	?	Absence of typical features of NF-1 or NF-2 and/or presence of additional, possibly unique features
NF-5	Segmental	? Somatic mutation	L	L	L	Features of NF-1 but limited to one area/segment of the body
NF-6	CAL only	AD	+	–	–	CAL spots alone segregating as AD. One family cited also have pectus excavatum and dull intelligence.
NF-7	Late onset	Non-familial	–	+	–	Patients develop NF as their only feature, onset after third decade
NF-NOS	Not otherwise specified					To include patients not covered by NF-1 through NF-7
Other neurofibromatosis types						
	Gastrointestinal neurofibromatosis	AD	–	–	–	Neurofibromas limited to gastrointestinal tract
	Multiple Schwannomatosis	Not specified	–	–	–	Multiple Schwannomas which may affect the skin and spinal cord but no cranial involvement
	Familial brain tumours	AD	–	–	–	e.g. Multiple meningiomas with no other NF1 or NF2 features

CAL = café au lait spots; NF = dermal neurofibromas; LN = Lisch nodules; L = limited distribution.
Table compiled by S.M. Huson and D. Viskochil.

19.2.1 A new approach to NF subclassification

As an alternative to the clinically based classification schemes for the neurofibromatoses, identification of the NF1 gene (Cawthon *et al.*, 1990; Viskochil *et al.*, 1990; Wallace *et al.*, 1990) and mapping of the NF2 gene (Rouleau *et al.*, 1987) provide a framework for classification based on a molecular approach. Familial, variant forms of NF can now be examined for genetic linkage at the NF1 and NF2 loci. Linkage of NF-overlap syndromes would suggest that the specific NF entity maps to the locus either as an allele or a contiguous gene. Mutational analysis of the genes might identify single gene mutations or allelic variants in affected individuals. Potentially, this information should enable one to diagnose unusual presentations of NF and better define the spectrum of clinical manifestations found in NF1 and NF2. Furthermore, genomic DNA screening of individuals diagnosed with NF-overlap syndromes, using probes from the *NF1* and *NF2* genes, might identify the presence of hypothesized deletions encompassing contiguous genes at the respective loci. Finally, an understanding of the function of the encoded proteins for NF1 and NF2 may identify shared cellular biochemical pathways whereby alleles of non-NF components of such shared pathways might cause the overlapping clinical features in NF. It is unfortunate that, except for the splitting of NF2 from NF1, our present understanding of the pathophysiology of NF does not allow us to classify the other variant NF forms on a molecular basis (e.g. contiguous genes, allelic forms, somatic mosaicism, or shared biochemical pathways). Until that time, the neurofibromatoses should be classified by clinical presentation.

Based on the clinical and molecular aspects of NF we propose that the so-called variant forms of NF be divided into two broad categories, alternate and related forms of NF, as follows:

1. alternate forms
    - (a) mixed NF
    - (b) localized NF
        - (i) segmental
        - (ii) gastrointestinal
        - (iii) spinal
        - (iv) multiple café au lait spots
    - (c) Schwannomatosis
2. related forms
    - (a) Noonan/NF1
    - (b) Watson syndrome
    - (c) duodenal carcinoid/phaeochromocytoma/NF1
    - (d) juvenile xanthogranuloma/NF1.

Alternate forms of NF1 and NF2 are defined as those conditions having some of the respective clinical features of either NF1 or NF2 yet not demonstrating the 'typical' clinical presentation. The clinical manifestations of the alternate forms of NF generally fit with the spectrum of clinical features observed in NF1 and NF2. Related forms of NF1 and NF2 constitute a set of conditions that have classical clinical features of NF in addition to distinctive clinical features not typically seen in either NF1 or NF2. The related forms of NF may or may not satisfy the clinical criteria for diagnosis, but must have some features that go beyond what can be attributed to the clinical spectrum of NF. The presence of such features thereby excludes either NF1 or NF2 as a diagnosis.

Defining a classification scheme distinguishing alternate forms of NF from related forms of NF is not simply a semantic exercise. In considering a molecular approach to classification, one can venture that alternate forms of NF may be caused by allelic forms of *NF1* and *NF2* (including somatic mosaicism) whereas non-allelic aetiologies of NF variants such as contiguous genes or shared biochemical pathways may account for the more extensive clinical expression of the related forms of NF. Prior to presenting the alternate and related forms of NF, one needs to examine the variability of clinical expression of NF1 and NF2, the two classical forms of NF.

19.3 NEUROFIBROMATOSIS 1

NF1 is the most prevalent form of the neurofibromatoses with a birth incidence of 1 in 2500–3300 (Crowe, Schull and Neel, 1956). The *NF1* gene has been cloned by the mapping approach (Cawthon *et al.*, 1990; Viskochil *et al.*, 1990; Wallace *et al.*, 1990); however, complete DNA diagnosis is not yet available. Therefore, NF1 remains a clinical diagnosis whereby a set of clinical criteria need to be satisfied (NIH Consensus Development Conference Statement, 1988). Clinical manifestations include multiple café au lait macules, neurofibromas, axillary and groin freckling, optic gliomas, Lisch nodules and specific osseous lesions. The frequency of clinical signs making up the diagnostic criteria in individuals diagnosed with NF1 is discussed in Chapter 7. In order to evaluate fully the variant forms of NF, one must appreciate both the frequency and the degree of variation of these signs in the general population.

Café au lait macules were first used as a diagnostic clinical sign of NF1 by Crowe and Schull (1953) and expanded in their epic monograph on NF in Michigan (Crowe, Schull and Neel, 1956). Crowe, Schull and Neel (1956) and Whitehouse (1966) observed that even though individuals in the general population have café au lait spots, rarely do they have more than six in the absence of other more distinctive features of NF1. Riccardi and Eichner (1986) used the finding of six café au lait spots to 'heighten the clinical concern' in the evaluation for NF1 diagnosis rather than as an immutable sign of the condition. Furthermore, exclusion of familial, multiple café au lait spots (NF-6, Riccardi and Eichner, 1986) from mapping to the *NF1* locus (Charrow, Listernick and Ward, 1992) demonstrates genetic heterogeneity for one feature of NF1, café au lait spots. Thus, in evaluating unusual clinical presentations of NF, one must keep in mind that even though multiple café au lait spots are almost invariably seen in NF1, they do not, in and of themselves, identify variant forms of NF.

Neurofibromas are the hallmark of the neurofibromatoses. Nevertheless, there are individuals who manifest discrete cutaneous and subcutaneous neurofibromas without other features of NF1. Even so, unlike familial, multiple café au lait spots, there are no reported instances of inherited cutaneous neurofibromas without other findings of NF1. The frequency of cutaneous neurofibromas in the general population has not been established; however, plexiform neurofibromas are rare and almost exclusively found in individuals with NF1. Gliomas of the optic nerve are benign tumours seen in approximately 15% of NF1 individuals. Although the incidence of optic gliomas in the asymptomatic population has not been established, they are rare enough to serve as a specific marker for NF1.

The other features comprising the diagnostic criteria are quite specific. Axillary and inguinal freckling when present with café au lait spots is diagnostic for NF1. The osseous lesions, sphenoid wing dysplasia and tibial pseudoarthroses, rarely occur except in people with NF1. Lisch nodules as a marker for NF1 have taken on new significance with reports of over 90% of adults with NF1 showing bilateral multiple Lisch nodules (Lewis and Riccardi, 1982; Huson, Jones and Beck, 1987; Mulvihill *et al.*, 1990). Slit lamp examination by a qualified ophthalmologist performs two functions: (1) the identification of Lisch nodules establishes one of the diagnostic criteria; and (2) the absence of Lisch nodules in an adult virtually eliminates the diagnosis in parents of offspring with NF1. The Lisch nodule examination is an objective analysis that takes on some importance in the evaluation of variant forms of NF. For example, the lack of Lisch nodules in the presence of unusual features of NF1 could almost be considered an exclusionary feature, thereby classifying such a clinical presentation as a related form of NF. This example demonstrates that application of all the NF1 diagnostic criteria in the evaluation of variant forms of NF is essential for the establishment of overlap syndromes. In addition to the clinical evaluation of NF variant forms, knowledge of both the molecular biology of the *NF1* gene and the functional biochemistry of neurofibromin may be necessary for a better aetiological understanding of some NF1-overlap syndromes.

The *NF1* gene has been isolated and one domain of the encoded peptide stimulates the intrinsic GTPase of p21*ras* (Ballester *et al.*, 1990; Martin *et al.*, 1990; Xu *et al.*, 1990). The gene is almost entirely contained on a 350 kb NotI genomic DNA fragment and it has approximately 50 exons, some of

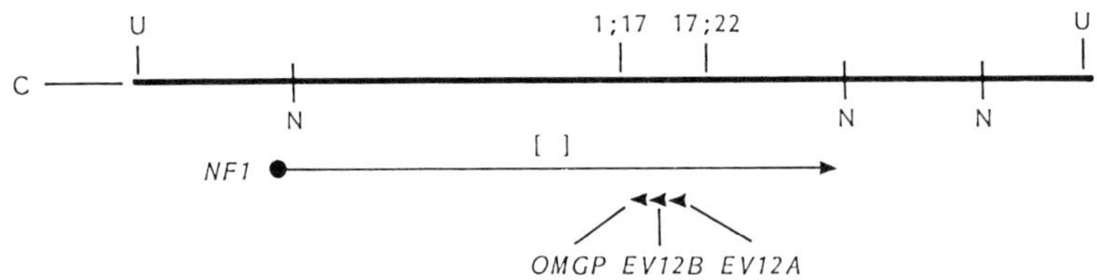

Figure 19.1 Pulsed-field map of the *NF1* locus represented as a 600 kb NruI fragment. *NF1, OMGP, EVI2A,* and *EVI2B* are depicted below the genomic fragment; arrowheads show directions of transcription. The brackets represent the region encompassing the GAP-related domain. The translocation breakpoints that served as markers for physically mapping this locus are shown above the fragment. U = NruI; N = NotI; C = centromere for chromosome 17.

which are alternative splice forms of the transcript (Figure 19.1). The NF1 transcript has been identified in numerous cell types by using RNA-PCR methodology; however, the levels of *NF1* gene expression from different tissues have not been rigorously demonstrated. The NF1 protein has significant amino acid homology to two yeast proteins, IRA1 and IRA2, and mammalian p120GAP (GTPase activating protein) (Xu *et al.*, 1990). The amino acid homology with IRA1 and IRA2 extends much further than with p120GAP, which extends only through the GAP catalytic domain. Furthermore, there is a 98% amino acid homology with the rodent *NF1* sequence (Buchberg *et al.*, 1990; A. Bernards *et al.* 1993). Biochemical functions outside of the shared catalytic domains of IRA1, IRA2 and neurofibromin have not been identified. By virtue of its GAP-related domain, neurofibromin has been shown to interact with p21*ras*, either as an effector or a negative regulator of the p21*ras* signal transduction pathway. However, the role that neurofibromin may play as a tumour suppressor has yet to be established (Skuse, Kosciolek and Rowley, 1989; Menon *et al.*, 1990).

Mutational analysis of the NF1 locus in individuals with NF1 has been carried out by many research groups. Over 300 individuals have been screened by various mutational analysis methods encompassing at least 90% of the structural gene. To date, approximately 10% of individuals have demonstrated a mutation in the *NF1* gene. These mutations include chromosome translocations (Schmidt, Michels and Dewald, 1987; Ledbetter *et al.*, 1989), deletions (Stark, Assum and Krone, 1991; Upadhyaya *et al.*, 1990; Viskochil *et al.*, 1990; Kayes *et al.*, 1992), insertions (Wallace *et al.*, 1990; Thakker and Strachan, personal communication) and exon point mutations (Cawthon *et al.*, 1990; Wallace *et al.*, 1990; Li *et al.*, 1992). An exhaustive search by single strand conformation polymorphism, SSCP-PCR, covering 95% of the coding region of *NF1* in a subset of 40 NF1 patients has thus far identified only one additional SSCP variant that is a probable mutation (Cawthon, personal communication, 1993). This unforeseen difficulty in identifying mutations in the *NF1* gene in individuals with classical presentations for NF1 may also hamper the identification of allelic forms of NF1 in the evaluation of variant forms of NF.

19.4 NEUROFIBROMATOSIS 2

NF2 is also an autosomal dominant condition with an incidence of 1 in 33 000–40 000 individuals (Evans *et al.*, 1992). The clinical features of this condition are distinct from NF1, and McKusick (1992) has listed bilateral acoustic neuroma (NF2) as an autosomal dominant phenotype, #101000. The variability of clinical expression is much less than that of NF1 and there are fewer documented overlap conditions and variant forms of NF2. The diagnostic criteria for NF2 are discussed in Chapter 18, and, except for the age-related penetrance of tumour presentation and the requirement for tumour typing, diagnosis for NF2 is relatively straightforward.

The *NF2* gene has been mapped to the long arm of chromosome 22 (band q11.1–13.1) (Rouleau *et al.*, 1987, 1990; Narod *et al.*, 1992; Wolff *et al.*, 1992) and was recently cloned (see Chapter 3, Note, p. 58). The *NF2* gene product is a tumour suppressor and deletions of this region on chromosome 22 have been associated with a number of intracranial tumours (Seizinger, Martuza and Gusella, 1986). The tumour types seen in NF2 are distinct from those found in NF1. Even the paraspinal 'neurofibromas' in NF2 appear much like Schwannomas rather than the typical neurofibromas, which are comprised of fibroblasts, Schwann cells and mast cells (Halliday, Sobel and Martuza, 1991). Aside from the occasional patient with several café au lait spots and/or multiple peripheral nerve tumours, NF1 and NF2 have very little in common.

The distinction between NF1 and NF2 arose as early as 1930 when Frazier commented in the Abstract of Discussion concluding Gardner and Fraziers' (1930) field survey of an extended family with bilateral acoustic neurofibromas that '. . . the question came up as to whether some specific designation ought not to be given to this syndrome other than von Recklinghausen's disease'. In the mid-1950s Scott (1953) separated the two entities and Rodriguez and Berthrong (1966) discerned the central form of NF in their review of intracranial tumours in von Recklinghausen NF. Young, Eldridge and Gardner (1970) extended the same pedigree that Gardner and Frazier (1930) presented and solidified the proposal that central NF be considered a separate entity; however, they continued to use the reference to NF. It is now quite clear that Lisch nodules and axillary freckling are not seen in NF2; when café au lait spots are observed in NF2 patients they are usually less than six in number. The small cutaneous and subcutaneous neurofibromas occasionally seen in NF2

(Rodriguez and Berthrong, 1966; Martuza and Eldridge, 1988; Evans *et al.*, 1992) are the only clinical features that sometimes cause diagnostic confusion between NF1 and NF2. In view of the different chromosomal locations of these two loci, and the distinct clinical features of NF2, perhaps a more appropriate term for this condition is a purely descriptive one such as familial bilateral vestibular Schwannomatosis. This nomenclature may be an option in the future as other NF-overlap syndromes are better characterized and the term neurofibromatosis takes on a more specific connotation.

Even though the clinical overlap of NF1 and NF2 is limited, the similar manifestations may be due to the sharing of a common biochemical pathway. Tissue specificity and timing of gene expression may play a role in determining the overlap phenotypes, depending on which portion of a shared pathway is affected by *NF1* and *NF2* mutations. Riccardi and Eichner (1986) considered 'NF-2' as an alternate type of NF-1; however, NF2 is distinct from NF1 and in reviewing overlap syndromes of NF it is clear that some variant forms overlap not with NF1 but with NF2. Therefore, NF2 will be considered as a distinct entity and the variant forms of NF2 will be delineated from the variant forms of NF1.

19.5 ALTERNATE FORMS OF NF1 AND NF2

19.5.1 Mixed NF

Riccardi identified a number of individuals with features of both NF1 and NF2, although such patients did not clearly fit either category (1982). He introduced the term NF-3 for the 'mixed type of NF' and noted the following clinical features: (1) presence of café au lait spots, freckling and cutaneous neurofibromas, although not as evident as with NF1; (2) presence of palmar cutaneous neurofibromas; (3) early onset and fulminant expression of bilateral vestibular Schwannomas, meningiomas and spinal/paraspinal neurofibromas; and (4) absence of iris Lisch nodules, posterior capsule cataracts, optic gliomas and other non-specific features of NF1 (Riccardi and Eichner, 1986). In Riccardi's series all affected individuals were sporadic cases.

The central theme in the clinical presentation of 'mixed NF' is the presence of aggressive intracranial tumours, vestibular Schwannomas and typical dermatological signs of NF1. Of historical note, Crowe, Schull and Neel (1956) identified 10 individuals with potential signs of eighth nerve involvement and in nine of these cases, cutaneous signs were also present. However, by excluding their interpretation of nerve deafness as a sign of vestibular Schwannomas, from their study one can retrospectively diagnose five individuals with NF1 and four individuals with

NF2, leaving one possible mixed form of NF. Rodriguez and Berthrong (1966) reviewed 48 reports of multiple primary intracranial tumours in association with 'central NF', of which 30 cases had signs of peripheral neurofibromas. These cases should not be considered 'mixed NF' because they most likely represent NF2 with manifestations of subcutaneous neurofibromas occasionally seen in NF2 (Martuza and Eldridge, 1988). Martuza and Ojemann (1982) identified an individual with bilateral vestibular Schwannomas, more than six café au lait spots, one plexiform neurofibroma and multiple skin nodules consistent with cutaneous neurofibromas. An eye examination was not reported and there was a negative family history. This person has features beyond either NF1 or NF2 and fits the diagnosis of 'mixed NF'. Michels *et al.* (1989) also identified an individual with bilateral vestibular Schwannomas and multiple meningiomas in addition to more than six café au lait spots, multiple subcutaneous neurofibromas and one Lisch nodule. The authors proposed that small acoustic tumours may be more common in NF1 than generally appreciated and they speculated that the clinical category of NF-3 (mixed) may represent an allelic form of NF1. Rubenstein *et al.* (1988) identified two patients with bilateral eighth nerve masses, plus one or more other tumours, more than six café au lait spots and more than 10 dermal neurofibromas. Charles *et al.* (1989) identified an individual with bilateral vestibular Schwannomas, unilateral ganglioneuromas, early lens opacities and multiple unilateral Lisch nodules without cutaneous manifestations of NF1; this individual does not fulfil the diagnostic criteria of NF1 and may represent an atypical NF2 patient with multiple Lisch nodules on one side. One other intriguing case has been reported by Sadeh, Martinovits and Goldhammer (1989), who identified an individual with perhaps a *bona fide* 'mixed' form of NF in that his mother had NF2 and his father had NF1. In his first decade of life he developed bilateral vestibular tumours, multiple meningiomas and manifestations of NF1 including multiple café au lait spots, intertrigenous freckling and subcutaneous neurofibromas. He died at the age of 12 years and the autopsy revealed that every large peripheral nerve root had associated neurofibromas. This case presumably demonstrates the phenotype of a double heterozygote for both the *NF1* and the *NF2* loci, although the identification of mutations at either locus in this family has not been shown. This case identifies a potential synergism of the NF1 and NF2 biochemical pathways; decreased expression of the respective proteins in both conditions may cause a more severe expression of clinical features than typically observed for each condition alone.

There are enough cases of individuals sharing a distinct phenotype with features of NF1 and NF2 to warrant the descriptive term of 'mixed NF' (Nager, 1964; Toyama *et al.*, 1979). The absence of families inheriting 'mixed NF' precludes the use of genetic linkage analysis to ascertain which, if any, locus is affected. This observation also reflects the severity of this condition since no affected individuals have had affected offspring. The underlying aetiology for 'mixed NF' is not known. As with the case report by Sadeh, Martinovits and Goldhammer (1989), 'mixed NF' may simply represent double heterozygotes with mutations affecting both *NF1* and *NF2*. Alternatively, this form of NF could represent an allele of NF1 whereby mutations in a specific domain lead to more aggressive intracranial tumorigenesis (including vestibular Schwannomas) than is usually seen in typical NF1. If this purported domain is integral to a common biochemical pathway, then features of both NF1 and NF2 could be expressed. The identification of genetic mutations in individuals with the mixed form of NF may in fact resolve the pathophysiology of the overlap clinical presentation of NF1 and NF2.

19.5.2 Localized NF

The term 'localized NF', introduced by Takiguchi and Ratz (1984), was coined by Riccardi and Eichner (1986) as a 'generic term referring to the occasional occurrence of one or more neurofibromas, associated café au lait and/or freckling in a restricted area of the body but not distinguishing between an extremely localized manifestation of one of the diffuse forms of NF (NF-1, -2, -3, -4, -7), an isolated (non-NF) neurofibroma, and segmental NF'. 'Localized NF' is defined in this chapter as the presentation of clinical signs of NF1 in a restricted expression pattern. The major forms of 'localized NF' are: (1) the limited cutaneous distribution of NF1, segmental NF; (2) the restricted gastrointestinal expression of neurofibromas; and (3) familial, spinal NF. These forms of NF may represent either somatic mutations in non-terminally differentiated tissue that subsequently affect numerous tissue types of specific geographical distribution, or *NF1* mutations that are tissue-restricted in cellular expression.

(a) Segmental NF

The most common, localized form of NF is that of segmental NF. Succinctly stated, Riccardi's criteria for segmental NF include neurofibromas and café au lait spots (and/or freckling) that are confined to one side of the body. This strict definition for segmental NF has not been adhered to in the clinical literature and it does not encompass the many case reports that may represent altered expression of *NF1* in a restrictive pattern. In an attempt to encompass the many reports of 'localized NF1', Roth, Martines and James (1987) proposed an alternate classification scheme using clinical criteria to separate cases into four categories: true segmental, bilateral segmental, familial, and segmental with deep involvement. Even though this scheme classifies the atypical segmental cases, it fails to address the molecular mechanisms underlying localized expression of NF. We speculate that localized NF is caused by somatic mutations in the *NF1* gene and the clinical pattern of expression is determined by both the timing and the cell type involved in such a mutation. The precedence for such speculation is the observation that identified mutations in the collagen genes are associated with atypical presentations of osteogenesis imperfecta (Sykes, 1990).

Segmental NF, like osteogenesis imperfecta, may be an ideal genetic condition for the evaluation of somatic mutations in man in that (1) the cutaneous manifestations of NF1 lead to easy detection, (2) the condition is dominant so one hit may allow the presentation of skin manifestations, and (3) the mutation rate of this locus is one of the highest. Providing there is no difference in the mutation rate between the germline and somatic tissue, one would expect approximately one somatic mutation per 10 000 cell divisions, which could result in a number of localized manifestations of NF1. To take this argument to the extreme, a solitary neurofibroma in an individual without other NF1 manifestations may represent a single somatic mutation of the *NF1* gene in a clone of terminally differentiated cells within a peripheral nerve sheath. In reviewing 59 reported cases of segmental NF, we emphasize the somatic mutation hypothesis in proposing an alternative classification scheme that is determined by (1) the timing of the mutation (early versus late embryological development) and (2) the source of tissue affected by the mutation.

The reported cases of segmental NF are reviewed in Table 19.2 and are classified in two ways: one according to Roth, Marines and James (1987) and the other according to a scheme based on the somatic mutation hypothesis. Table 19.2 shows the age of diagnosis, age at onset if known, geographical sites affected, features of NF1 that are clinically evident such as café au lait spots, freckling or neurofibromas, and the familial occurrence. The somatic mutation scheme has four categories: single site–single manifestation (i.e. late neural crest mutation leading to a single disease manifestation; single site–multiple manifestations (i.e. early neural crest mutation leading to café au lait spots and neurofibromas in distinct location); multiple site–single manifestation (i.e. bilateral, dermatomal neurofibromas); and multiple site–multiple manifestations (i.e. full NF1 phenotype). A somatic mutation in the zygote could lead to disseminated NF1 whereas a somatic mutation in lateralized migrating neural crest cells from the region of a somite may give the phenotype of segmental NF affecting only one dermatome. Furthermore, a midline mutation early in somite development may lead to a bilateral, dermatomal presentation of NF1 manifestations. The expansion of a mutated primitive cell type from the neural crest into numerous tissue types may

Table 19.2 Segmental NF reports with itemization of age at diagnosis, age at onset, geographical location, tissue involvement, familial occurrence and classification

	Age (years)			Tissue involvement						Classification schemes							
				Neurofibroma		Skin		Eye		Roth				Somatic mutation (tissue/site)			
Author	Diagnosis	Onset	Location	Dermal	Plex.	CLS	Freckling	Lisch nodules	Family history	True	Deep	Hereditary	Bilateral	Sing./ sing.	Sing./ mult.	Mult./ sing.	Mult./ mult.
Gammel (1931)	60		R,L	+	–	+	–	NE	–				+			+?	+?
Streitmann (1955)	46		R	+	–	–	–	NE	–	+				+			
Crowe, Schull and Neel (1956)	37		R	+	–	+	–	NE	–	+						+	
	27	<30	R	+	–	+	–	NE	–	+						+	
	70		B	+	–	–	–	NE	–				+		+		
	39		L	+	–	–	–	NE	–	+				+			
Winkelmann and Johnson (1962)	73		R	+	–	–	–	NE	–	+				+			
	47		R,L	+	–	–	–	NE	–				+		+		
	59		L	+	–	–	–	NE	–	+				+			
	70		R,L	+	–	–	–	NE	–				+		+		
	67		R	+	–	–	–	NE	–	+				+			
Korting and Tupath-Barniske (1966)	41		R	+	–	–	–	NE	–	+				+			
Nicholls (1969)	64		L	+	+	–	–	NE	–		+			+			
	11	<30	R	–	–	+	+	NE	–	+				+			
Miller and Sparkes (1977)	15	<30	R	+	–	+	+	NE	–	+							+
	61		L	+	–	+	+	NE	–	+							+
Sava *et al.* (1975)	9	<30	R	+	–	+	–	NE	–	+						+	
Biemer and Muhbauer (1975)	24	<30	R	+	–	–	–	NE	NE		+			+			
Uhlin (1980)	29	<30	R	+	–	–	–	NE	+	+				+			
Pallara *et al.* (1985)	52		R	+	–	–	–	NE	–	+				+			
	14	<30	L	+	–	–	–	NE	–	+				+			
Dawson (1984)	67		R,L	+	–	+	–	NE	–				+				+
	72		L	+	–	–	–	NE	–	+				+			
Stotts and Steinman (1987)	64		L	+	–	+	–	–	–	+		–				+	

Table 19.2 Continued

Author	Age (years)		Location	Tissue involvement: Neurofibroma		Skin		Eye	Family history	Classification schemes: Roth				Somatic mutation (tissue/site)			
	Diagnosis	Onset		Dermal	Plex.	CLS	Freckling	Lisch nodules		True	Deep	Hereditary	Bilateral	Sing./sing.	Sing./mult.	Mult./sing.	Mult./mult.
Gretzula *et al.* (1988)	16	<30	R	+	–	–	–	–	–	+				+			
Weleber and Zonana (1983)	14	<30	R	–	–	+	–	+	–	+							+
Oranje *et al.* (1985)	10 mths	<30	L	+	–	–	–	NE	–	+				+			
Takiguchi and Ratz (1984)	36	<30	B	+	–	–	–	–	–				+		+		
Rubenstein *et al.* (1983)	59		L	+	–	–	–	–	+			+			+		
	21	<30	L	+	–	–	–	–	+			+		+			
	49		R	+	–	–	–	NE	+			+		+			
	7	<30	B	–	–	+	+	NE	+			+			+		
Koedijk (1987)	32	<30	L,R	+	–	–	–	NE	–				+		+		
Rawlings *et al.* (1987)	66	>30	L	+	+	NE	NE	NE	NE		+					+	
	46	>30	R	+	+	–	–	NE	–		+					+	
	30	<30	R	+	+	–	–	NE	NE		+					+	
	29	<30	R	–	+	–	–	NE	–		+			+			
Roth, Martines and James (1987)	31	<30	L	+	–	–	–	–	–	+				+			
	41	<30	R	+	–	+	–	–	–	+						+	
	52	>30	R	+	–	–	–	–	–	+				+			
	42	>30	B	+	–	+	–	–	–				+				+
Calzavara *et al.* (1988)	68	>30	R	+	–	–	–	–	–	+				+			
Boltshauser, Stocker and Machler (1989)	1	<30	?	–	+	+	–	NE	+			+					+
	40	<30	R	–	–	+	+	+	+			+					+
Sloan, Fretzin and Bovenmyer (1990)	15	<30	R	+	–	–	–	–	–	+				+			
	33	<30	L	+	–	+	–	–	–	+							+

Table 19.2 Continued

				Tissue involvement						Classification schemes							
	Age (years)			Neurofibroma		Skin		Eye		Roth				Somatic mutation (tissue/site)			
Author	*Diagnosis*	*Onset*	*Location*	*Dermal*	*Plex.*	*CLS*	*Freckling*	*Lisch nodules*	*Family history*	*True*	*Deep*	*Hereditary*	*Bilateral*	*Sing./ sing.*	*Sing./ mult.*	*Mult./ sing.*	*Mult./ mult.*
Smith and Heymann (1990)	83	>30	R	+	–	NE	NE	NE	–	+				+			
Trattner *et al*. (1990)	64	>30	B	+	–	–	–	–	–	+				+			
	68		L	+	–	–	–	–	–	+				+			
Jaakkola *et al*. (1990)	69		R	+	–	–	–	NE	–	+				+			
Sanchez Canejo-Mir, Herrera Saval and Camacho Martinez (1989)	28	<30	R	+	–	–	–	–	–	+				+			
Jung (1988)	70	<30	R	+	–	–	–	–	–	+				+			
	41	<30	R	+	–	–	–	–	–	+				+			
	32	<30	L	+	–	+	+	NE	–	+						+	
	66	>30	L	+	–	+	+	NE	–	+						+	
	60	<30	R	+	–	–	–	NE	–	+				+			
	23	<30	L	+	+	–	–	NE	–		+			+			
	41	<30	R	+	–	–	–	NE	–	+				+			
Kaplan and Pestana (1989)	60		L	+	–	+	–	–	–	+							+

Each case is classified by the scheme devised by Roth, Martines and James (1987) and by the scheme suggested by the somatic mutation hypothesis. Sing. = single tissue site involvement or single NF1 feature; mult. = multiple tissue sites or multiple manifestations (tissue site/clinical feature).

R = right; L = left; CLS = café au lait spots; NE = not examined; Plex. = plexiform.

explain the localization of neurofibromas, café au lait macules and freckling to single sites.

The use of classification schemes for segmental NF is important in that it allows one to classify unusual presentations of NF1 and hopefully provide more accurate counselling to affected individuals. For example, individuals diagnosed with bilateral, segmental NF rather than NF1 with incomplete penetrance would carry an extremely low risk of having an affected child. The use of the somatic hit classification scheme serves as a testable hypothesis in that somatic mutations in *NF1* in affected tissue from segmental NF individuals could be sought and, if found, used to screen for germline mosaicism in that individual. Furthermore, somatically generated alleles could serve as cell markers for more fundamental investigations of cell migration in the embryo.

(b) *Gastrointestinal NF*

Gastrointestinal NF is listed in McKusick (1990) as familial intestinal NF with phenotype #162220 (1992); it has been described as a distinct entity by Lipton and Zuckerbrod (1966) and Heimann *et al.* (1988). Heimann *et al.* (1988) proposed the following phenotypic description for this condition: neurofibromas strictly limited to the intestine, adult onset with incomplete penetrance, variable expression, autosomal dominant inheritance pattern and absence of other features of NF1 or NF2. This description fits with localized expression of a phenotype that may be allelic and tissue specific. Since this is familial, one would not expect a somatic hit in a precursor cell. The identification of a chromosomal abnormality in one family with gastrointestinal NF (Verhest *et al.*, 1988), a t(12;14) balanced translocation, may indicate that a modifying gene product or a mutation in a protein of a shared pathway is the reason for this condition. Again, genetic linkage in families and mutations in the *NF1* gene can be sought to clarify the aetiology of this condition.

(c) *Familial, spinal NF*

Familial spinal NF is an autosomal dominant condition, and has been described by Pulst *et al.* (1990) in two families. One family has spinal neurofibromas and café au lait spots and the second family has spinal neurofibromas only. Genetic mapping with close flanking markers for NF1 demonstrated linkage in the first family and excluded linkage in the second. Even though the first family fits the criteria for NF1 (multiple neurofibromas and more than six café au lait spots), no family member has the other typical markers for NF1 such as Lisch nodules, cutaneous neurofibromas or axillary freckling. The distinctiveness of this family presentation, spinal neurofibromas, is the most compelling reason to include it in the localized alternate form of NF1. The second family does not fulfil the criteria for NF1 nor does it map to the *NF1* locus. It simply has inherited paraspinal neurofibromas, although one family member had a neurofibrosarcoma. In the absence of other NF1 symptomatology and exclusion from the *NF1* locus, this family's mutation may involve a separate protein in a shared biochemical pathway.

(d) Autosomal dominant multiple café au lait spots

Riccardi and Eichner (1986) classify families with inherited multiple café au lait spots as their only manifestation of NF1 as NF-6. Exclusion of the NF1 locus in linkage analysis (Charrow, Listernick and Ward, 1992) shows this form of NF to be distinct and non-allelic to NF1, at least in some alleles.

19.5.3 Schwannomatosis

A condition originally described in Japanese patients consisting of multiple cutaneous Schwannomas, CNS tumours and various neurological deficits without other signs of NF has been identified as neurilemmomatosis (Izumi, Rosato and Wood, 1971; Shishiba *et al.*, 1984; Takano *et al.*, 1989). This most likely represents a distinct clinical entity, which Purcell and Dixon (1989) have labelled as Schwannomatosis. In addition to the cutaneous and subcutaneous Schwannomas, the overlapping features of Schwannomatosis and NF consist of CNS tumours commonly found in NF2. Schwannomatosis is generally a sporadic occurrence and these cases may represent a somatic mutation in *NF2*. Alternatively, all cases could be caused by mutation of a distinct gene that shares a common biochemical pathway with the *NF2*-encoded protein. Because large families have not been identified it will be difficult to map this condition with certainty; however, exclusion mapping and mutational analysis of *NF1* and *NF2* in these patients may allow exclusion of the two loci. The delineation of this condition from NF1 can easily be accomplished by examination of tumour histology, thus establishing it as a Schwannoma rather than as a neurofibroma. On the other hand, delineation of Schwannomatosis from NF2 is more difficult.

There are a number of features of Schwannomatosis that are consistent with the diagnosis of NF2. As presented in section 19.4, the histological inspection of cutaneous and subcutaneous nodules in NF2 (once thought to be neurofibromas) usually reveals a pathological diagnosis consistent with a Schwannoma. One individual presenting with neurilemmomatosis in the report by Shishiba *et al.* (1984) has subsequently developed other signs of NF2 (Shishiba, personal communication). Finally, there are now reports of autosomal dominant Schwannomatosis (Riccardi, 1992;

Shishiba, personal communication). Thus, in cases of cutaneous and subcutaneous Schwannomas, efforts should be made thoroughly to evaluate patients for NF2, and if diagnostic criteria are not satisfied, genetic counselling should still be tempered by the possibility of NF2.

19.6 RELATED FORMS OF NF1 AND NF2

19.6.1 Noonan/NF1 syndrome

There have been a number of reports linking NF with the Noonan syndrome. However, both disorders exhibit remarkable variability of clinical expression, and both are diagnosed by physical examination and clinical pattern recognition. Use of the clinical criteria provides a fairly objective diagnosis of NF1 in contrast to the clinical diagnosis of Noonan syndrome, which remains quite subjective. This subjectivity allows the clinician much leeway in interpretation, and a final diagnosis of Noonan/NF may ultimately reflect biases of the diagnostician. There are enough case reports and familial reports linking NF with Noonan to make chance occurrence of the two separate and distinct conditions unlikely, although an examination of the expected incidence of Noonan syndrome (1/1000) and NF1 (1/3500) shows that 1 in 3.5 million individuals could have the Noonan/NF phenotype by chance alone.

Noonan syndrome as a distinct entity was proposed by Opitz *et al.* (1965) and more recently reviewed by Mendez and Opitz (1985). The clinical presentation is highly variable and a set of diagnostic criteria has not been established, although a 'scoring checklist' of common findings has been compiled for Noonan syndrome (Duncan *et al.*, 1981). The clinical features helpful in making this diagnosis are short and webbed neck (pterygium colli), ptosis, short stature, pectus excavatum, posteriorly rotated and cup-shaped ears and congenital heart disease (valvular pulmonic stenosis) (Mendez, 1985). The subjective interpretation of the relative significance of each of these rather 'objective' findings in the overall diagnosis of Noonan syndrome leaves the diagnosis of milder cases somewhat arbitrary. The threshold one crosses to make the diagnosis of Noonan syndrome in an NF individual is often quite subjective, especially when only a few 'Noonan-like' features are identified. The incidence of Noonan syndrome has been reported as high as 1 per 1000 with an obvious familial occurrence in approximately 20% of the reported cases. In the familial cases the Noonan phenotype is inherited as an autosomal dominant condition. The clinical expression is highly variable and the penetrance of Noonan syndrome has not been established.

The commentary provided by Opitz and Weaver (1985) in their editorial comment on the NF1/Noonan syndrome is as applicable as it was in 1985.

They aptly state that no-one should be 'too apodictic about the causal classification and relationship of these two entities', and they then present four possible nosology schemes underlying the Noonan/NF phenotype: (1) a chance concurrence, (2) an unusual variant of the Noonan syndrome, (3) an unusual type of NF1, and (4) a 'new' entity. The cases of Kaplan, Opitz and Gosset (1968), Allanson, Hall and Van Allen (1985), Mendez (1985), Opitz and Weaver (1985) and Saul (1985), which prompted Opitz and Weaver's commentary (1985), were sporadic cases that demonstrated clinical features of both conditions. However, in order for the Noonan/NF syndrome to be considered a distinct genetic condition, one must show that the phenotype segregates in family studies. Therefore, further investigations on the aetiology of the phenotype should concentrate on the familial cases of Noonan/NF syndrome.

The following cases represent a review of the current literature stressing cases presented since the series on Noonan/NF in the *American Journal of Medical Genetics* (Opitz and Weaver, 1985). Shuper *et al.* (1987) identified a 12-year-old boy with learning disabilities, multiple café au lait spots at birth, short stature, bilateral ptosis, downward palpebral slant, low-set ears, prominent pterygium colli, pectus excavatum, cubitus valgus and normal heart as a case of non-familial Noonan/NF. An eye examination was not performed. However, this case does not fulfil the diagnostic criteria for NF1 and should be considered Noonan syndrome with multiple café au lait spots.

Abuelo and Meryash (1988) identified an 18-year-old patient with left ptosis, early failure to thrive, atrial septal defect and valvular and supravalvular pulmonic stenosis, mild to moderate mental retardation, short stature, 'multiple' café au lait spots, axillary freckling, 'several' cutaneous and subcutaneous nodules on the trunk, a short webbed neck, low-set posteriorly rotated ears and unilateral high frequency hearing loss. An eye examination was not performed. The father had multiple café au lait spots, axillary freckling, many cutaneous and subcutaneous nodules, low-set ears and no heart murmur. The father of the proband does not have classical features of Noonan syndrome, even though the proband has Noonan syndrome plus NF1. Assuming the father and his son have the same *NF1* mutation, the absence of typical Noonan syndrome features in one family member suggests that NF1 and classical Noonan syndrome segregate independently in this family. This report does not support the hypothesis that Noonan/NF is a discrete clinical syndrome.

Meinecke (1987) identified a 5-year-old child with short stature, a wide and depressed nasal root with an inner canthal distance of 3.1 cm (75%), bilateral epicanthus, down-slanting palpebral fissures, multiple Lisch nodules, low-set posteriorly rotated ears, short and wide neck, 'multiple café au lait' spots, axillary freckling, no neurofibroma, no heart murmur and 'slight' retardation. The father had 'typical NF1' without stigmata of Noonan, and there was a positive family history of NF1. In this case the proband has minimal objective features of Noonan syndrome and the father certainly does not have Noonan syndrome. This case likely represents the variability of clinical expression in NF1.

Quattrin, McPherson and Putnam (1987) identified a 3-year-old child with developmental delay, hypospadias, 5th percentile for height, ptosis, large ears, an inner canthal distance > 75%, a broad neck in relation to a small body habitus, cryptorchidism, > 13 café au lait spots, tumour of left eyelid of unknown aetiology and a left optic glioma, pectus excavatum, no heart murmur and no Lisch nodules. The proband's mother was 153 cm tall with a triangular-shaped face, an inner canthal distance in the 75th percentile, ptosis, short neck, more than six café au lait spots, axillary freckling, multiple neurofibromas, severe myopia, scoliosis, no Lisch nodules and a normal heart evaluation. This family does not have a classical Noonan phenotype, although it is certainly positive for NF1. Similar to the other cases, this family does not have the most objective findings for Noonan syndrome (pulmonary stenosis and pterygium colli) and likely represents an NF1 family that has some Noonan-like features.

In preliminary studies, Peter Colley (personal communication) has identified a family with a co-segregating Noonan/NF phenotype that also has a genomic DNA rearrangement at the *NF1* locus. The endpoints of this rearrangement have not been characterized, but this family may represent the best case of Noonan/NF for exhaustive investigation of the underlying molecular defect.

In order seriously to consider the Noonan/NF syndrome as a distinct genetic entity, one needs to identify a family with objective features of Noonan syndrome that also satisfy the diagnostic criteria of NF1. Subsequent molecular studies identifying a distinct class of *NF1* mutations would be supportive of an allelic expression aetiology as a cause for Noonan-like features in NF1 (hypothesis number 3 in Opitz and Weaver, 1985). Supportive evidence linking the two as contiguous genes would be the identification of a large submicroscopic deletion at the NF1 locus and subsequent identification of the Noonan gene within the deletion or, at least, demonstration of genetic linkage of autosomal dominant Noonan syndrome to chromosome 17. The Noonan syndrome in autosomal dominant pedigrees has not been mapped to a specific chromosome, although in a set of British families, familial Noonan syndrome was excluded from chromosome 17 (Sharland *et al.*, 1992). This is a crucial observation in the assessment of Noonan/NF as a distinct clinical entity.

Given that classical Noonan syndrome is unlinked to NF1, one could postulate that the Noonan-like features often seen in NF1 likely represent either genetic heterogeneity of Noonan syndrome (in distinction to variability of clinical expression) or a shared biochemical pathway for the products of these two loci. Molecular studies geared to mapping, isolating and characterizing the classical Noonan gene combined with ongoing studies to identify neurofibromin-associated proteins could address the latter possibility. On the other hand, if Noonan syndrome is genetically heterogeneous, then non-classical Noonan families (pedigrees demonstrating similar Noonan-like features as seen in association with NF1, i.e. absence of pulmonic stenosis) would need to be identified and tested for exclusion of linkage to the *NF1* locus. The studies carried out by Sharland *et al.* (1992) were on selected families diagnosed with Noonan syndrome based on strict clinical criteria. This may not be applicable to the milder phenotype usually seen in Noonan/NF individuals; thus, a heterogenetic Noonan-like locus near *NF1* has not been excluded by linkage analysis. Thus, the identification and evaluation of well-defined Noonan/NF families is essential in establishing the aetiology of the shared phenotypes. By pedigree inspection, good documentation of clinical features and molecular studies both to identify mutations and evaluate linkage to candidate loci, one may actually prove that Noonan/NF is simply a chance concurrence.

19.6.2 Watson syndrome

Watson syndrome was first reported by Watson (1967), who described familial cases having pulmonary stenosis, multiple café au lait macules and low normal intelligence. Partington *et al.* (1985) also identified a family with similar features and, excepting the café au lait spots, no other features of NF1. At a D.W. Smith Symposium in 1986, Allanson reviewed Watson's original cases and compared them with four new cases, concluding that Watson syndrome is a discrete entity inherited in an autosomal dominant manner (Allanson and Watson, 1987). McKusick (1990) lists Watson syndrome as phenotype #193520, an autosomal dominant condition with café au lait spots and pulmonic stenosis.

In a recent genetic linkage study, Allanson *et al.* (1991) mapped the Watson syndrome to the NF1 region of chromosome 17 in two families, one from Watson's original report (Watson, 1967) and Partington's family (Partington *et al.*, 1985). All members of the first family had café au lait spots, axillary freckling and reduced intellectual functioning, while five members had pulmonary stenosis, seven had Lisch nodules and three had neurofibromas (but in smaller numbers than is usual in adults). Partington's family had axillary freckling with café au lait spots, and in addition to pulmonic stenosis, low IQ and short stature, one of three had Lisch nodules and one had multiple neurofibromas. Short stature, café au lait spots, axillary freckling, neurofibromas and Lisch nodules are all associated with the NF1 phenotype. The only distinctive features of the

Watson families are pulmonary stenosis and low normal intellect (in all affected individuals); both features are atypical in NF1. Pulmonary stenosis in NF1 is rare and the type of pulmonary stenosis in the Watson syndrome families is distinct from dysplastic pulmonary valvular stenosis seen in Noonan syndrome (Allanson *et al.*, 1991). Thus, the Watson syndrome phenotype is distinctive enough to be considered separate from NF1, and linkage to the NF1 region invites further speculation of the aetiology of this condition with respect to the *NF1* gene.

Two potential explanations for linkage of Watson syndrome to the NF1 locus are *NF1* allelism and disruption of both *NF1* and a contiguous gene. As an example of the former hypothesis, one could speculate that *NF1* alleles that interrupt a specific function of neurofibromin could lead to pulmonary stenosis and low intellectual functioning. Tassabehji *et al.* (1993) identified a 42 bp duplication in exon 28 leading to an in-frame insertion of 14 amino acids in a three-generation pedigree purported to have Watson syndrome: multiple café au lait spots, learning disabilities, absence of neurofibromas and Lisch nodules, variable expression of posteriorly rotated ears, mild pectus excavatum and one individual with axillary freckling and one individual with pulmonary valve stenosis. However, this family does not present with the typical features of Watson syndrome and may represent the variability of expression in NF1. With respect to a contiguous gene syndrome, one could speculate that a separate but physically linked gene could be disrupted in a large chromosomal rearrangement at the *NF1* locus that could affect both *NF1* and the adjacent gene expression, thereby leading to the Watson phenotype. For example, the presence of a pulmonic valve development gene at the *NF1* locus could serve as an explanation for Watson syndrome in that a simple rearrangement could affect both genes; however, familial pulmonary stenosis is uncommon with only one report in the medical literature (Klinge and Laursen, 1975). Regardless of the proposed aetiologies for Watson syndrome, it is clear that the features of NF1 in this condition suggest that a mutation in the *NF1* gene exists and its identification in each of the typical Watson syndrome families may suggest a pathophysiological aetiology of this distinct NF1-related condition.

19.6.3 NF1, phaeochromocytoma and duodenal carcinoid

There have been isolated reports of individuals with NF1 developing carcinoid tumour in the duodenum as a manifestation of the condition (Arnesjo *et al.*, 1973; Hough, Chan and Davidson, 1983; Dayal *et al.*, 1986; Fernandez *et al.*, 1988). In and of itself the association of carcinoid in NF1 does not constitute an overlap syndrome of NF1 but rather another of the many clinical manifestations of the condition. However, some authors suggest that there is a distinctive neuroendocrine syndrome comprised of duodenal carcinoid tumours, phaeochromocytoma and NF1 features. This syndrome, which will be abbreviated CPNF1 (carcinoid of the duodenum, phaeochromocytoma and NF1), was reviewed by Griffiths, Williams and Williams (1987), who proposed it as a clinical entity distinct from other multiple endocrine neoplasia syndromes.

Griffiths, Williams and Williams (1987) reviewed 27 cases of duodenal carcinoid tumour in patients either known or suspected of having NF1. Clinical signs and symptoms of duodenal carcinoid were present in 21 cases and most individuals presented with symptoms in the fourth and fifth decades. They concluded that somatostatin-rich carcinoid of the ampulla of Vater has a strong association with NF1. In contrast to non-NF duodenal carcinoid, the NF-associated duodenal carcinoid was anatomically close to the ampulla of Vater. Phaeochromocytoma was found in six cases, of which half were symptomatic. The association of carcinoid tumour and phaeochromocytoma without NF1 is rare, with only three reported cases as of 1987. The presence of six phaeochromocytomas in this group of 27 cases is certainly higher than the incidence estimate of 1% or lower in individuals with NF1, and it may represent the numerator in the calculation of the incidence of phaeochromocytoma in NF1. Perhaps most of the phaeochromocytomas associated with NF1 in the literature represent a subset of carcinoid/NF. Nevertheless, the interaction of neurofibromin with p21*ras* suggests that CPNF1 could be allelic for classical NF1; mutations in specific domains of neurofibromin could lead to the development of duodenal carcinoid.

19.6.4 NF1/juvenile xanthogranuloma

There are confirmed case reports associating NF with xanthogranulomas (Jensen *et al.*, 1971; Newell *et al.*, 1973). Xanthogranulomas are usually dome-shaped yellowish nodules composed of foamy histiocytes and multinucleated giant cells. Even though the presence of xanthogranulomas in individuals with NF1 may represent the clinical variability of NF1, the association of xanthogranulomas in juvenile chronic myeloid leukaemia (jCML) (Cooper *et al.*, 1984) should alert the clinician to the possibility of leukaemia in an NF1 patient showing xanthogranulomas. Morier *et al.* (1990) has identified 24 cases showing the triple association of jCML, juvenile xanthogranulomas and NF1. The age at diagnosis ranged from infancy through early childhood and the most common sign leading to the diagnosis of NF1 was multiple café au lait spots. This is not surprising since Lisch nodules and neurofibromas generally do not arise in this age group. Fourteen of 24 patients had a positive family history of NF1; however, none of the first-degree relatives were reported to have had either xanthogranulomas or a past history of jCML. Further review of the

Table 19.3 Differential diagnosis for variant forms of NF

Condition	*Inheritance*	*Clinical features*
Cutaneous melanosis	SP	Pigmented or giant hairy naevi
Proteus syndrome	SP	Bony overgrowth, subcutaneous hamartomas, gyriform hyperplasia of hands and feet (Chapter 17)
Klippel–Trenaunay–Weber syndrome	SP	Haemangiomata, hemihypertrophy
Carney syndrome (NAME syndrome)	SP/AD	The acronym NAME stands for Naevi, Atrial myxoma, Myxoid neurofibromata and Ephiledes
MEN 2B	AD	Mucosal neuromas, phaeochromocytoma, thyroid carcinoma
von Hippel–Lindau	AD	Angiomata of the retina, haemangioblastoma of the cerebellum and phaeochromocytoma
Multiple meningioma	SP/AD	Meningiomas without vestibular Schwannomas
Multiple lipomatosis	AD	Multiple benign lipomas (Chapter 7)
Bannayan–Riley–Ruvalcaba syndrome	AD	Multiple lipomas, haemangiomas (Chapter 7)
McCune-Albright syndrome	SP	Polyosteotic fibrous dysplasia, endocrine dysfunction, areas of pigmentation (Chapter 7)
Leopard syndrome	AD	Lentigines, cardiac abnormalities, short stature, deafness (Chapter 7)
Sotos syndrome	SP/AD	Cerebral gigantism, poor coordination
Jaffe-Campanacci syndrome	SP	Multiple non-ossifying fibromas
Aarskog syndrome	X-linked semidominant	Overlap with Noonan/NF

SP = sporadic; AD = autosomal dominant.

literature has failed to identify a familial case of NF1 with a diagnosis of either multiple xanthogranulomatosis or jCML in more than one family member. The absence of a heritable specific phenotype argues against this triple association as a discrete syndrome. One can speculate that a somatic mutation of a separate gene in an individual with NF1 may lead to the expression of xanthogranulomas and/or jCML. The finding of xanthogranulomas in jCML and the identification of families with inherited xanthogranulomatosis suggest that a distinct locus exists and that the rare occurrence of two hits involving both loci may lead to the triple association. It is also possible that the gene products could be involved in the same biochemical pathway in certain cell types.

19.7 DIFFERENTIAL DIAGNOSIS

There are a number of clinical syndromes that must be considered in the clinical evaluation of unusual forms of the neurofibromatoses. For the most part, these conditions are fairly distinct and the differences between the variant forms of NF and the other conditions are relatively obvious. A number of clinical conditions sharing features of NF are listed in Table 19.3. Further consideration of each entity listed with respect to the overlapping NF clinical signs is beyond the scope of this chapter.

19.8 SUMMARY

We are on the threshold of evaluating the *NF1* and *NF2* loci with respect to overlap syndromes of the neurofibromatoses. Genetic mapping of the *NF1* and *NF2* loci, isolation of the genes and characterization of their encoded products provides a framework for the evaluation of the variant forms of NF. The mapping approach in evaluating variant forms of NF should begin with the rigorous clinical assessment of familial cases. The establishment of genetic linkage in families with overlap syndromes might determine if either *NF1*, *NF2* or a separate locus is involved in the phenotype. Conditions mapping to the *NF1* or *NF2* loci could then be screened for mutations in hopes of identifying the aetiologies of the variant forms of NF. The identification of distinctive mutations may provide a molecular-based classification scheme for the variant forms of NF, tentatively divided into alternate and related forms. The application of molecular information toward rigorous clinical classification schemes may provide more appropriate counselling to affected families. It is our intention that this chapter contributes to that end.

REFERENCES

Abuelo, D. and Meryash, D. (1988) Neurofibromatosis with fully expressed Noonan syndrome. *Am. J. Med. Genet.*, **29**, 937–41.

Allanson, J.E. and Watson, G.H. (1987) Watson syndrome: nineteen years on. Presentation at *Proceedings of David Smith Meeting*.

Allanson, J.E., Hall, J.G. and Van Allen, M.I. (1985) Noonan phenotype associated with neurofibromatosis. *Am. J. Med. Genet.*, **21**, 457–62.

Allanson, J.E. *et al.* (1991) Watson syndrome: is it a sub-type of type 1 neurofibromatosis. *J. Med. Genet.*, **28**, 752–6.

Arnesjo, B. *et al.* (1973) Concomitant occurrence of neurofibromatosis and carcinoid of the intestine. *Scand. J. Gastroenterol.*, **8**, 637–43.

Ballester, R. *et al.* (1990) The NF1 locus encodes a protein functionally related to mammalian GAP and yeast IRA proteins. *Cell*, **63**, 851–9.

Bernards, A. *et al.* (1993) Mouse neurofibromatosis type 1 cDNA sequence reveals high degree of conservation of both coding and non-coding MRMA segments. *Human Molecular Genetics*, **2**, 645–50.

Biemer, E. and Muhlbauer, W. (1975) Ein Fall einer lokalisierten neurofibromatosis der rechten gesichtshalfte, in *Plastische und Wienderherstellungs-Chirurie* (ed. H. Hohler), pp. 357–61.

Boltshauser, E., Stocker, H. and Machler, M. (1989) Neurofibromatosis type 1 in a child of a parent with segmental neurofibromatosis (NF-5). *Neurofibromatosis*, **2**, 244–5.

Buchberg, A. *et al.* (1990) Sequence homology shared by neurofibromatosis type-1 gene and IRA-1 and IRA-2 negative regulators of the RAS cyclic AMP pathway. *Nature*, **347**, 291–4.

Calzavara, P. *et al.* (1988) Segmental neurofibromatosis. Case report and review of the literature. *Neurofibromatosis*, **1**, 318–22.

Cawthon, R.M. *et al.* (1990) A major segment of the neurofibromatosis type 1 gene: cDNA sequence, genomic structure, and point mutations. *Cell*, **62**, 193–201.

Charles, S. *et al.* (1989) Lisch nodules in neurofibromatosis type 2. *Arch. Ophthalmol.*, **107**, 1571–2.

Charrow, J., Listernick, R. and Ward, K. (1993) Autosomal dominant multiple café-au-lait spots and neurofibromatosis. *Am. J. Med. Genet.* **45**, 606–8.

Cooper, P.H. *et al.* (1984) Association of juvenile xanthogranuloma with juvenile myeloid leukemia. *Arch. Dermatol.*, **120**, 371–5.

Crowe, F.W. and Schull, W.J. (1953) Diagnostic importance of cafe-au-lait spot in neurofibromatosis. *Arch. Intern. Med.*, **91**, 758–66.

Crowe, F.W., Schull, W.J. and Neel, J.V. (1956) *A Clinical, Pathological, and Genetic Study of Multiple Neurofibromatosis*, Charles C. Thomas, Springfield, IL.

Dawson, T. (1984) Regional eruptive neurofibromatosis. *Br. J. Dermatol.*, **111**(Suppl. 26), 65.

Dayal, Y. *et al.* (1986) Duodenal carcinoids in patients with and without neurofibromatosis. *Am. J. Surg. Pathol.*, **10**, 348–57.

Duncan, W.J. *et al.* (1981) A comprehensive scoring system for evaluating Noonan syndrome. *Am. J. Med. Genet.*, **10**, 37–50.

Evans, D.G.R. *et al.* (1992) A clinical study of type 2 neurofibromatosis. *Q. J. Med.*, **84**, 603–18.

Fernandez, M.T. *et al.* (1988) Von Recklinghausen neurofibromatosis with carcinoid tumor and submucous leiomyomas of the duodenum. *Neurofibromatosis*, **1**, 294–8.

Gammel, J. (1931) Localized neurofibromatosis. *Arch. Dermatol.*, **24**, 712–15.

Gardner, W.J. and Frazier, G.H. (1930) Bilateral acoustic neurofibromas: a clinical study and field survey of a family of five generations with bilateral deafness in 28 members. *Arch. Neurol. Psychiatr.*, **23**, 266–300.

Gretzula, J. *et al.* (1988) Multiple papules in a localized area: segmental neurofibromatosis. *Arch. Dermatol.*, **124**, 1101–2, 1104–5.

Griffiths, D., Williams, G. and Williams, E. (1987) Duodenal carcinoid tumours, phaeochromocytoma and neurofibromatosis: islet cell tumour, phaeochromocytoma and the von Hippel-Lindau complex: two distinctive neuroendocrine syndromes. *Q. J. Med., New Series 64*, **245**, 769–82.

Halliday, A.L., Sobel, R. and Martuza, R. (1991) Benign spinal nerve sheath tumours: their occurrence sporadically and in neurofibromatosis type 1 and 2. *J. Neurosurg.*, **74**, 248–53.

Heimann, R. *et al.* (1988) Hereditary intestinal neurofibromatosis. I. A distinctive genetic disease. *Neurofibromatosis*, **1**, 26–32.

Hough, D.R., Chan, A. and Davidson, H. (1983) Von Recklinghausen's disease associated with gastrointestinal carcinoid tumors. *Cancer*, **51**, 2206–8.

Huson, S.M., Jones, D. and Beck, L. (1987) Ophthalmic manifestations of neurofibromatosis. *Br. J. Ophthalmol.*, **71**, 235–8.

Huson, S.M., Compston, D.A.S. and Harper, P.S. (1989) A genetic study of von Recklinghausen neurofibromatosis in southeast Wales. II. Guidelines for genetic counselling. *J. Med. Genet.*, **26**, 712–21.

Izumi, A.K., Rosato, F.E. and Wood, M.G. (1971) Von Recklinghausen's disease associated with multiple neurilemomas. *Arch. Dermatol.*, **104**, 172–6.

Jaakkola, S. *et al.* (1990) Segmental neurofibromatosis: immunocytochemical analysis of cutaneous lesions. *J. Am. Acad. Dermatol.*, **22**, 617–21.

Jensen, N.E. *et al.* (1971) Naevoxanthoendothelioma and neurofibromatosis. *Br. J. Dermatol.*, **85**, 326–30.

Jung, E. (1988) Segmental neurofibromatosis (NF-5). *Neurofibromatosis*, **1**, 306–11.

Kaplan, D. and Pestana, A. (1989) Cutaneous segmental neurofibromatosis. *South. Med. J.*, **82**, 516–17.

Kaplan, M.S., Opitz, J.M. and Gosset, F.R. (1968) Noonan's syndrome: a case with elevated alkaline phosphatase levels and malignant Schwannoma of the left forearm. *Am. J. Dis. Child.*, **116**, 359–66.

Kayes, L., Riccardi, V., Burke, W. *et al.* (1992) Large de novo DNA deletion in a patient with sporadic neurofibromatosis 1, mental retardation and dysmorphism. *J. Med. Genet.*, **29**, 686–90.

Klinge, T. and Laursen, B. (1975) Familial pulmonary stenosis with underdeveloped or normal right ventricle. *Br. Heart J.*, **37**, 60–4.

Koedijk, J. (1987) Segmental neurofibromatosis. *Br. J. Dermatol.*, **117**, 790–1.

Korting, G. and Tupath-Barniske, R. (1966) Neurofibromatosis disseminata und Herpes zoster im selben segmentmereich. *Dermatol. Wschr.*, **151**, 33–7.

Ledbetter, D.H. *et al.* (1989) Precise localization of NF1 to 17q11.2 by balanced translocation. *Am. J. Hum. Genet.*, **44**, 20–5.

Lewis, R.A. and Riccardi, V.M. (1982) Von Recklinghausen neurofibromatosis: incidence of iris hamartomata. *Ophthalmology*, **88**, 348–54.

Li, Y. *et al.* (1992) Somatic mutations in the neurofibromatosis 1 gene in human tumours. *Cell*, **69**, 275–81.

Lipton, S. and Zuckerbrod, M. (1966) Familial enteric neurofibromatosis. *Med. Times*, **94**, 544–8.

Martin, G.A. *et al.* (1990) The GAP-related domain of the NF1 gene product interacts with *ras* p21. *Cell*, **63**, 843–9.

Martuza, R. and Eldridge, R. (1988) Neurofibromatosis 2 (bilateral acoustic neurofibromatosis). *N. Engl. J. Med.*, **318**, 684–8.

Martuza, R. and Ojemann, R. (1982) Bilateral acoustic neuromas: clinical aspects, pathogenesis, and treatment. *Neurosurgery*, **10**, 1–12.

McKusick, V. (1992) *Mendelian Inheritance in Man. Catalogs of Autosomal Dominant, Autosomal Recessive and X-linked Phenotypes*, 10th edn, Johns Hopkins University Press, Baltimore.

Meinecke, P. (1987) Letter to the editor: Evidence that the 'neurofibromatosis-Noonan syndrome' is a variant of von Recklinghausen neurofibromatosis. *Am. J. Med. Genet.*, **26**, 741–5.

Mendez, H.M.M. (1985) The neurofibromatosis-Noonan syndrome. *Am. J. Med. Genet.*, **21**, 471–6.

Mendez, H.M. and Opitz, J.M. (1985) Noonan syndrome: a review. *Am. J. Med. Genet.*, **21**, 493–506.

Menon, A.G. *et al.* (1990) Chromosome 17p deletions and p53 gene mutations associated with the formation of malignant neurofibrosarcomas in von Recklinghausen neurofibromatosis. *Proc. Natl. Acad. Sci. USA*, **87**, 5435–9.

Michels, V. *et al.* (1989) Neurofibromatosis type 1 with bilateral acoustic neuromas. *Neurofibromatosis*, **2**, 213–17.

Miller, R. and Sparkes, R. (1977) Segmental neurofibromatosis. *Arch. Dermatol.*, **113**, 837–8.

Morier, P. *et al.* (1990) Juvenile chronic granulocytic leukemia, juvenile xanthogranulomas, and neurofibromatosis. Case report and review of the literature. *J. Am. Acad. Dermatol.*, **22**, 962–5.

Mulvihill, J.J. *et al.* (1990) Neurofibromatosis 1 (Recklinghausen disease) and neurofibromatosis 2 (bilateral acoustic neurofibromatosis). *Ann. Intern. Med.*, **113**, 39–52.

Nager, G.T. (1964) Association of bilateral eighth nerve tumors with meningiomas in von Recklinghausen's disease. *Laryngoscope*, **74**, 1220–61.

Narod, S. *et al.* (1992) Neurofibromatosis type 2 appears to be a genetically homogeneous disease. *Am. J. Hum. Genet.*, **51**, 486–96.

Newell, G.B. *et al.* (1973) Juvenile xanthogranuloma and neurofibromatosis. *Arch. Dermatol.*, **107**, 262.

Nicholls, E. (1969) Somatic variation and multiple neurofibromatosis. *Hum. Hered.*, **19**, 473–9.

NIH Consensus Development Conference Statement (1988) Neurofibromatosis. *Arch. Neurol.*, **45**, 575–8.

Opitz, J.M. and Weaver, D.D. (1985) Editorial comment: The neurofibromatosis-Noonan syndrome. *Am. J. Med. Genet.*, **21**, 477–90.

Opitz, J.M. *et al.* (1965) Noonan's syndrome in girls: a genocopy of the Ullrich-Turner syndrome. *J. Pediatr.*, **67**, 968.

Oranje, A. *et al.* (1985) Segmental neurofibromatosis. *Br. J. Dermatol.*, **112**, 107–12.

Partington, M.W. *et al.* (1985) Pulmonary stenosis, café-au-lait spots and dull intelligence: the Watson syndrome revisited (abstract). *Proc. Greenwood Genet. Center*, **4**, 105.

Pullara, M. *et al.* (1985) Cutaneous segmental neurofibromatosis. *J. Am. Acad. Dermatol.*, **13**, 999–1003.

Pulst, S. *et al.* (1991) Familial spinal neurofibromatosis: clinical and DNA linkage analysis. *Neurology*, **41**, 1923–7.

Purcell, S. and Dixon, S.L. (1989) Schwannomatosis. An unusual variant of neurofibromatosis or a distinct clinical entity. *Arch. Dermatol.*, **125**, 390–3.

Quattrin, T., McPherson, E. and Putnam, T. (1987) Vertical transmission of the neurofibromatosis/Noonan syndrome. *Am. J. Med. Genet.*, **26**, 645–9.

Rawlings, C. *et al.* (1987) Segmental neurofibromatosis. *Neurosurgery*, **20**, 946–9.

Riccardi, V.M. (1982) Neurofibromatosis: clinical heterogeneity. *Curr. Probl. Cancer*, **7**, 1–34.

Riccardi, V.M. (1992) *Neurofibromatosis: Phenotype, Natural History, and Pathogenesis*, 2nd edn, Johns Hopkins University Press, Baltimore.

Riccardi, V.M. and Eichner, J.E. (1986) *Neurofibromatosis Phenotype, Natural History, and Pathogenesis*, 1st edn, Johns Hopkins University Press, Baltimore.

Rodriguez, H.A. and Berthrong, M. (1966) Multiple primary intracranial tumors in von Recklinghausen's neurofibromatosis. *Arch. Neurol.*, **14**, 467–75.

Roth, R., Martines, M. and James, W. (1987) Segmental neurofibromatosis. *Arch. Dermatol.*, **123**, 917–20.

Rouleau, G.A. *et al.* (1987) Genetic linkage of bilateral acoustic neurofibromatosis to a DNA marker on chromosome 22. *Nature*, **329**, 5419–23.

Rouleau, G.A. *et al.* (1990) Flanking markers bracket the neurofibromatosis type 2 (NF2) gene on chromosome 22. *Am. J. Hum. Genet.*, **46**, 323–8.

Rubenstein, A. *et al.* (1983) Familial transmission of segmental neurofibromatosis. *Neurology*, **33**(Suppl. 2), 76.

Rubenstein, A. *et al.* (1988) NF1 and 2: distinct genotypes with overlapping phenotypes (abstract). *Am. J. Hum. Genet.*, **43**, A67.

Sadeh, M., Martinovits, G. and Goldhammer, Y. (1989) Occurrence of both neurofibromatoses 1 and 2 in the same individual with a rapidly progressive course. *Neurology*, **39**, 282–3.

Sanchez Canejo-Mir, J., Herrera Saval, A. and Camacho Martinez, F. (1989) Segmental neurofibromatosis. *J. Am. Acad. Dermatol.*, **20**, 681–2.

Saul, R. (1985) Letter to the editor: Noonan syndrome in a patient with hyperplasia of the myenteric plexuses and neurofibromatosis. *Am. J. Med. Genet.*, **21**, 491.

Sava, P. *et al.* (1975) A propos d'un cas de neurofibromatose avec hypertropic segmentaire d'un membro. *Sem. Hop. Paris*, **51**, 1121–7.

Schmidt, M.A., Michels, V.V. and Dewald, G.W. (1987) Cases of neurofibromatosis with rearrangements of chromosome 17 involving band 17q11.2. *Am. J. Med. Genet.*, **28**, 771–5.

Scott, O.L. (1953) Diseases of the skin, in *Clinical Genetics* (ed. A. Sorsby), Butterworths, London.

Seizinger, B., Martuza, R. and Gusella, J. (1986) Loss of genes on chromosome 22 in tumorigenesis of human acoustic neuroma. *Nature*, **322**, 664–7.

Sharland, M., Taylor, R., Patton, M.A. and Jeffery, S. (1992) Absence of linkage of Noonan syndrome to the neurofibromatosis type 1 locus. *J. Med. Genet.*, **29**, 188–90.

Shishiba, T. *et al.* (1984) Multiple cutaneous neurilemmomas as a skin manifestation neurilemmomatosis. *J. Am. Acad. Dermatol.*, **10**, 744–54.

Shuper, A. *et al.* (1987) Noonan's syndrome and neurofibromatosis. *Arch. Dis. Child.*, **62**, 196–8.

Skuse, G., Kosciolek, B.A. and Rowley, P.T. (1989) Molecular genetic analysis of tumors in von Recklinghausen neurofibromatosis: loss of heterozygosity for chromosome 17. *Genes Chromosom. Cancer*, **1**, 36–41.

Sloan, J., Fretzin, D. and Bovenmyer, D. (1990) Genetic counseling in segmental neurofibromatosis. *J. Am. Acad. Dermatol.*, **22**, 461–7.

Smith, S. and Heymann, W. (1990) Segmental neurofibromatosis in an octogenarian. *J. Am. Geriatr. Soc.*, **38**, 807–8.

Stark, M., Assum, G. and Krone, W. (1991) A small deletion and an adjacent base exchange in a potential stem-loop region of the neurofibromatosis 1 gene. *Hum. Genet.*, **87**, 685–7.

Stotts, J. and Steinman, H. (1987) Congenital, segmental pigmented lesions: segmental neurofibromatosis. *Arch. Dermatol.*, **123**, 252, 255.

Streitmann, B. (1955) Neurofibromatosis loclisata. *Z. Haut. Geschlkr.*, **19**, 324–9.

Sykes, B. (1990) Bone disease cracks genetics. *Nature*, **348**, 18–20.

Takano, Y., Hayashi, N., Toshitani, S. and Soji, T. (1989) A case of neurilemmomatosis. *Jpn. J. Dermatol.*, **99**, 67–71.

Takiguchi, P. and Ratz, J. (1984) Bilateral dermatomal neurofibromatosis. *J. Am. Acad. Dermatol.*, **10**, 451–3.

Tassabehji, M., Strachan, T., Sharland, M. *et al.* (1993) Tandem duplication within a neurofibromatosis type 1 (NF1) gene exon in a family with features of Watson syndrome and Noonan syndrome. *Am. J. Hum. Genet.*, **53**, 90–95.

Toyama, M. *et al.* (1979) A family of von Recklinghausen's disease combined with bilateral acoustic neuroma. *No Shinkei Geka.*, **7**, 85–9.

Trattner, A. *et al.* (1990) Segmental neurofibromatosis, *J. Am. Acad. Dermatol.*, **23**, 866–9.

Uhlin, S. (1980) Segmental neurofibromatosis. *South. Med. J.*, **73**, 526–7.

Upadhyaya, M. *et al.* (1990) A 90kb DNA deletion associated with neurofibromatosis type 1. *J. Med. Genet.*, **27**, 738–41.

Verhest, A. *et al.* (1988) Hereditary intestinal neurofibromatosis. II. Translocation between chromosomes 12 and 14. *Neurofibromatosis*, **1**, 33–6.

Viskochil, D.H. *et al.* (1990) Deletions and a translocation interrupt a cloned gene at the neurofibromatosis type 1 locus. *Cell*, **62**, 187–92.

Wallace, M.R. *et al.* (1990) Type 1 neurofibromatosis gene: identification of a large transcript disrupted in three patients. *Science*, **249**, 182–6.

Watson, G.H. (1967) Pulmonary stenosis, café-au-lait spots, and dull intelligence. *Arch. Dis. Child.*, **42**, 303–7.

Weleber, R. and Zonana, J. (1983) Iris hamartomas (Lisch nodules) in a case of segmental neurofibromatosis. *Am J. Ophthalmol.*, **96**, 740–3.

Whitehouse, D. (1966) Diagnostic value of the café-au-lait spot in children. *Arch. Dis. Child.*, **41**, 316–19.

Winkelmann, R. and Johnson, L. (1962) Cholinesterases in neurofibromas. *Arch. Dermatol.*, **85**, 106–14.

Wolff, R. *et al.* (1992) Analysis of chromosome 22 deletions in neurofibromatosis type 2-related tumors. *Am. J. Hum. Genet.*, **51**, 478–85.

Xu, G.F. *et al.* (1990) The catalytic domain of the NF1 gene product stimulates *ras* GTPase and complements IRA mutants of *S. cerevisiae*. *Cell*, **63**, 835–41.

Young, D.F., Eldridge, R. and Gardner, W.J. (1970) Bilateral acoustic neuroma in a large kindred. *JAMA*, **214**, 347–53.

Index

Page numbers appearing in **bold** refer to figures and page numbers appearing in *italic* refer to tables.